Cardiovascular System: Physiology and Disease Mechanisms

Cardiovascular System: Physiology and Disease Mechanisms

Edited by Greyson Taylor

STATES
ACADEMIC PRESS
www.statesacademicpress.com

States Academic Press,
109 South 5th Street,
Brooklyn, NY 11249, USA

Visit us on the World Wide Web at:
www.statesacademicpress.com

ISBN: 978-1-63989-096-5

Cataloging-in-Publication Data

Cardiovascular system : physiology and disease mechanisms / edited by Greyson Taylor.
p. cm.
Includes bibliographical references and index.
ISBN 978-1-63989-096-5
1. Cardiovascular system. 2. Cardiovascular system--Physiology.
3. Cardiovascular system--Diseases. I. Taylor, Greyson.
QP101 .C37 2022
612.1--dc23

Table of Contents

Preface

Cardiovascular system is a system that allows the circulation of blood and transports nutrients and oxygen within the body. Its main components are the heart, blood and blood vessels. It performs pulmonary and systemic circulation. Pulmonary circulation refers to a loop through the lungs where oxygenated blood is present and systemic circulation is a loop through the whole body to provide oxygenated blood. The systemic circulation functions in two parts, namely, macrocirculation and microcirculation. In humans, blood never leaves the network of blood vessels. This type of cardiovascular system is known as closed cardiovascular system. Some of the major diseases which affect the cardiovascular system are arrythmias, congenital heart disease, heart failure and heart attack. This book provides significant information of this discipline to help develop a good understanding of the cardiovascular system. It elucidates the concepts and innovative models around prospective developments with respect to the physiology and disease mechanisms related to the cardiovascular system. This book is meant for students who are looking for an elaborate reference text on this area of study.

The information contained in this book is the result of intensive hard work done by researchers in this field. All due efforts have been made to make this book serve as a complete guiding source for students and researchers. The topics in this book have been comprehensively explained to help readers understand the growing trends in the field.

I would like to thank the entire group of writers who made sincere efforts in this book and my family who supported me in my efforts of working on this book. I take this opportunity to thank all those who have been a guiding force throughout my life.

Editor

Empagliflozin Limits Myocardial Infarction *In Vivo* and Cell Death *In Vitro*: Role of STAT3, Mitochondria and Redox Aspects

Ioanna Andreadou[1†], Panagiotis Efentakis[1†], Evangelos Balafas[2], Gabriele Togliatto[3], Constantinos H. Davos[4], Aimilia Varela[4], Constantinos A. Dimitriou[4], Panagiota-Efstathia Nikolaou[1], Eirini Maratou[5], Vaia Lambadiari[6], Ignatios Ikonomidis[7], Nikolaos Kostomitsopoulos[2], Maria F. Brizzi[3], George Dimitriadis[6] and Efstathios K. Iliodromitis[7]*

[1] Laboratory of Pharmacology, Faculty of Pharmacy, School of Health Sciences, National and Kapodistrian University of Athens, Athens, Greece, [2] Academy of Athens Biomedical Research Foundation, Centre of Clinical Experimental Surgery and Translational Research, Athens, Greece, [3] Department of Medical Sciences, University of Turin, Turin, Italy, [4] Cardiovascular Research Laboratory, Biomedical Research Foundation, Academy of Athens, Athens, Greece, [5] Hellenic National Center for Research, Prevention and Treatment of Diabetes Mellitus and Its Complications, Athens, Greece, [6] 2nd Department of Internal Medicine, Research Institute and Diabetes Center, National and Kapodistrian University of Athens, "Attikon" University Hospital, Athens, Greece, [7] 2nd University Department of Cardiology, Medical School, National and Kapodistrian University of Athens, Athens, Greece

Edited by:
Mariarosaria Santillo, University of Naples Federico II, Italy

Reviewed by:
Derek John Hausenloy, University College London, United Kingdom
Petra Kleinbongard, Universitätsklinikum Essen, Germany

***Correspondence:**
Ioanna Andreadou
jandread@pharm.uoa.gr

[†] These authors have contributed equally to this work.

Empagliflozin (EMPA), a drug approved for type 2 diabetes management, reduced cardiovascular death but is unknown if it reduces myocardial infarction. We sought to investigate: (i) the effect of EMPA on myocardial function and infarct size after ischemia/reperfusion in mice fed with western diet (WD), (ii) the underlying signaling pathways, (iii) its effects on cell survival in rat embryonic-heart-derived cardiomyoblasts (H9C2) and endothelial cells (ECs). To facilitate the aforementioned aims, mice were initially randomized in Control and EMPA groups and were subjected to 30 min ischemia and 2 h reperfusion. EMPA reduced body weight, blood glucose levels, and mean arterial pressure. Cholesterol, triglyceride, and AGEs remained unchanged. Left ventricular fractional shortening was improved (43.97 ± 0.92 vs. $40.75 \pm 0.61\%$) and infarct size reduced (33.2 ± 0.01 vs. $17.6 \pm 0.02\%$). In a second series of experiments, mice were subjected to the above interventions up to the 10th min of reperfusion and myocardial biopsies were obtained for assessment of the signaling cascade. STAT3 was increased in parallel with reduced levels of malondialdehyde (MDA) and reduced expression of myocardial iNOS and interleukin-6. Cell viability and ATP content were increased in H9C2 and in ECs. While, STAT3 phosphorylation is known to bestow infarct sparing properties through interaction with mitochondria, we observed that EMPA did not directly alter the mitochondrial calcium retention capacity (CRC); therefore, its effect in reducing myocardial infarction is STAT3 dependent. In conclusion, EMPA improves myocardial function and reduces infarct size as well as improves redox regulation by decreasing iNOS expression and subsequently lipid peroxidation as shown by its surrogate marker MDA. The mechanisms of action implicate the activation of STAT3 anti-oxidant and anti-inflammatory properties.

Keywords: empagliflozin, cardioprotection, infarct size, cardiac function, molecular signaling, STAT3 pathway

INTRODUCTION

In the EMPA-REG OUTCOME trial, empagliflozin (EMPA), a selective inhibitor of the sodium glucose co-transporter 2 (SGLT2), reduced the risk of the combined endpoint of hospitalization for heart failure or cardiovascular death, in type 2 diabetic patients (T2D) (Fitchett et al., 2016). The mechanism by which EMPA induces cardiovascular benefits is obscure. However, the discrepancy in the Hazards ratios (HRs) for non-fatal myocardial infarctions (HR 0.87 [95% CI 0.70, 1.09]) and non-fatal strokes (HR 1.24 [0.92, 1.67]) indicates that benefits of EMPA may do not involve classical effects on atherosclerosis (Vettor et al., 2017). Although the results of the EMPA-REG trial were impressive, the cardioprotective mechanisms of the drug are still speculative. There is no *in vitro*, or *in vivo* study investigating if EMPA exerts its cardioprotection through the reduction of myocardial infarction after ischemia/reperfusion (I/R) injury. In the present study we investigated the effect of EMPA on myocardial function and infarction after I/R, in a mouse model with diet-induced T2D. In order to achieve this goal we recruited a murine model of diet induced metabolic syndrome, known to manifest T2D. The C57BL/6 mouse strain has been indicated to be prone in T2D and atherosclerosis following a high-fat, WD for prolonged time (Surwit et al., 1988; Phillips et al., 2003). We selected a dose of 10 mg/kg/day of EMPA which has been calculated based on the inter-species pharmacokinetic and metabolic parameters between rodents and humans (e.g., half-life ~1–2 h in rodent and 10–12 h in man). This dose has been previously shown to correspond to the equivalent active dose in humans (Cheng et al., 2016). Additionally, since we know that SGLT2 is highly specifically expressed in the kidney and very minimally in the heart (Chen et al., 2017) we sought to investigate the mechanism by which EMPA may exert cardioprotective effects based on intracellular signaling cascades independent of SGLT2, as it has been shown that EMPA exerts pleiotropic effects in aorta and in adipose tissue (Steven et al., 2017).

To further investigate a direct cardioprotective effect of EMPA, we evaluated its effect on an *in-vitro* model of injury: we exposed rat embryonic-heart-derived cardiomyoblasts (H9C2) and endothelial cells (ECs) to hypoxia/reoxygenation. Moreover, taking under consideration that mitochondria and redox aspects play very important role in cardioprotection (Penna et al., 2013; Pagliaro and Penna, 2015) we also focused on redox signaling and mitochondrial susceptibility to transition.

MATERIALS AND METHODS

For Complete Methods please see Supplementary Material.

In Vivo Experiments

Animals

A total of thirty five male 8-week old C57BL/6J animals were treated according to the Directive 2010/63/UE European Convention for the Protection of Vertebrate Animals used for Experimental and other Scientific Purposes, and conformed to the Guide for the Care and Use of Laboratory Animals published by the US National Institutes of Health (NIH Publication No. 85-23, revised 1985). The experimental protocol used in this study was approved by Ethical Committee of University of Athens and the Veterinary Authorities of Region of Athens Greece (License Number: 1758/24/3/2017).

Experimental Protocol

Mice were fed a Western diet (WD) (TD 88137, Harlan-Teklad; containing 21% fat by weight, 0.15% by weight cholesterol, and 19.5% by weight casein without sodium cholate), for 14 weeks (Surwit et al., 1988; Phillips et al., 2003). At the 8th week of feeding mice were randomized into two groups: (i) Control group ($n = 15$) in which DMSO 5% in Water For Injection (WFI) solution was given through gavage for additional 6 weeks and (ii) EMPA group ($n = 15$), in which EMPA was administered (10 mg/kg/day) in 5% DMSO/WFI through gavage for additional 6 weeks.

The EMPA dose was selected according to previous reports (Oelze et al., 2014; Habibi et al., 2017). At the end of treatment eighteen mice ($n = 9$ per group) subjected to 30 min myocardial ischemia followed by 2h reperfusion to determine the infarct size. Twelve mice ($n = 6$ per group) were subjected to the above interventions up to the 10th min of reperfusion, to obtain myocardial biopsies from the ischemic area for Western Blot analysis.

The following parameters were determined at baseline (Day 0), at the end of 8th week and at the end of the 14th week (end of treatment): body weight (BW), glucose levels. The following parameters were determined at baseline (Day 0), and at the end of the 14th week (end of treatment): cholesterol and triglycerides, arterial pressure, and myocardial function by echocardiography. Malondialdehyde (MDA) as a marker of lipid peroxidation was determined at the end of 8th week and at the end of 14th week, while advanced glycation end products (AGE) were determined at the end of 14th week.

Murine Model of Ischemia-Reperfusion Injury

Anesthesia/surgical preparation

General anesthesia was induced *via* intraperitoneal injection of a mixture containing ketamine, xylazine, and atropine (100, 20, and 0.6 mg/kg respectively). A cuffed tracheal tube was placed via a tracheotomy (ventral midline incision) for mechanical ventilation of the lungs with a 95% O_2 via a volume-cycled animal ventilator (150 strokes/min, tidal volume 200 μl). Consequently, the animals were placed in left-lateral recumbence and the chest was surgically opened with a left thoracotomy. The chest was opened through the left fourth intercostal space. The beating heart was exposed and the pericardium was incised. The left anterior descending coronary artery was ligated with a 6-0 silk suture. The occlusion of coronary artery in this region leads to ischemia of a large area of the anterolateral and apical left ventricular wall. Ischemia was induced by tightening of the suture against a small piece of polyethylene tubing. Ischemia resulted in a change in the color (i.e., cyanotic) of the myocardium and was maintained for 30 min. At the end of the ischemic period, the suture was released in order to induce reperfusion of the myocardium for up to 2 h. In order to determine/quantify the degree of irreversible myocardial injury (i.e., infarction) resulting from the ischemia and reperfusion insult with and without indicated treatment, infarct areas were evaluated. For this reason, myocardium was excised and aorta was catheterized. After the tightening of the suture, Evan's Blue solution (2.5% in Water for Injection-WFI) was infused through the catheter for the identification of the normally perfused part of the myocardium. Afterwards, hearts were frozen for 24 h and then sliced in 1–2 mm sections, which were incubated for 20 min in Triphenyl-Tetrazolium Chloride Solution (TTC, 1% in PBS pH = 7.4) for the identification of the area-at-risk and the infarct area (Bibli et al., 2015).

Histopathology/Histomorphometery

For each heart, the overall size of the myocardial slice (All/A), the area-at-risk (Risk/R) and the infarct (Infarct/I) were determined. R was expressed as a percentage of the A area (R/A %), and I was expressed as a percentage of the R (I/R %) (Bibli et al., 2015).

Blood Biochemistry

Mice were fasted overnight prior to blood sampling. Blood was collected from the tail vein by puncturing the vessel vertically with a 23-gauge needle at baseline, at the 8th week and at the end of the treatment periods. Blood glucose levels were measured by using a hand-held glucometer (Onetouch Verio IQ Lifescan, Johnson & Johnson Company).

For the assessment of lipid levels and MDA measurement, blood samples were collected at the beginning of the treatment period and at the end of the study. Blood was centrifuged and plasma was stored at −80°C. Plasma cholesterol and triglyceride concentrations were measured spectrophotometrically using commercial kits (DiaSys Diagnostic Systems GmbH, Cholesterol FS 10130021, and Triglycerides FS 10571 021). The MDA concentration was determined spectrophotometrically at 586 nm and expressed as μM (Oxford Biomedical Research Colorimetric Assay for lipid peroxidation) as we have previously described (Andreadou et al., 2004).

Arterial Pressure (AP) Monitoring

At baseline and at the end of treatment, non-invasive arterial pressure was measured on awake mice using CODA Monitor tail-cuff system (Kent Scientific Co, Torrington, CT USA). The mice were placed for 10 min inside a heated chamber (34°C) and then positioned in a restrainer over a heating pad. They were allowed a 5 min acclimation period following cuff positioning and 20 consecutive AP determination cycles we conducted. All measurements were recorded on the CODA software and presented in **Table 1**. In case signs of discomfort were present, the animal was returned to the heated chamber and re-examined 1 h later.

Echocardiography

At baseline and at the end of the treatment, M-mode echocardiography was performed as previously described (Papathanasiou et al., 2015) to measure left ventricular (LV) end-diastolic diameter (EDD), LV end-systolic diameter (ESD), and LV posterior wall thickness at diastole (PWT) and to calculate the ratio of LV radius to PWT (r/h) and the percentage of LV fractional shortening FS (%).

TABLE 1 | Cholesterol and triglyceride levels, mean arterial pressure values and echocardiography data at baseline and after 14 weeks of treatment in Control (n = 10) and EMPA (n = 10) groups.

	Control	EMPA
Triglycerides Baseline (mg/dl)	37.91 ± 3.28	54.36 ± 10.12
Triglycerides 14 weeks (mg/dl)	36.93 ± 9.05*	55.41 ± 8.59*
Cholesterol Baseline (mg/dl)	145.5 ± 16	139.2 ± 12
Cholesterol 14 weeks (mg/dl)	233.6 ± 43*	191.9 ± 20.92*
Diastolic AP Baseline (mmHg)	80.51 ± 2.0	79.17 ± 2.2
Diastolic AP 14 weeks (mmHg)	73.18 ± 2.1	70.87 ± 2.1*
Systolic AP Baseline (mmHg)	106.70 ± 2.3	105.35 ± 2.4
Systolic AP 14 weeks (mmHg)	102.55 ± 2.0	96.91 ± 2.2*
Mean Arterial Pressure Baseline (mmHg)	88.9 ± 2.32	87.56 ± 2.4
Mean Arterial Pressure 14 weeks (mmHg)	82.58 ± 2.6	79.22 ± 2.1*
HR Baseline	592.20 ± 5.27	627.90 ± 11.29#
HR 14 weeks	702.37 ± 10.31*	687.20 ± 5.46*
ECHOCARDIOGRAPHY		
LVEDD, mm Baseline	2.90 ± 0.07	2.96 ± 0.06
LVEDD, mm 14 weeks	3.20 ± 0.07*	3.04 ± 0.07
LVESD, mm Baseline	1.54 ± 0.05	1.59 ± 0.03
LVESD, mm 14 weeks	1.90 ± 0.05*	1.71 ± 0.06#
PWd, mm Baseline	0.79 ± 0.01	0.77 ± 0.01
PWd, mm 14 weeks	0.74 ± 0.01*	0.76 ± 0.01#
PWs, mm Baseline	1.27 ± 0.01	1.27 ± 0.01
PWs, mm 14 weeks	1.23 ± 0.01*	1.24 ± 0.01*
FS% Baseline	47.07 ± 0.65	46.14 ± 0.31
FS% 14 weeks	40.75 ± 0.61*	43.97 ± 0.92#
r/h Baseline	1.84 ± 0.06	1.91 ± 0.05
r/h 14 weeks	2.15 ± 0.07*	1.98 ± 0.05

$p < 0.05$ vs. Baseline, #$p < 0.05$ vs. Control group. Left ventricular (LV) end-diastolic (EDD) and end-systolic dimension (ESD); posterior wall thickness (PW) in diastole (d) and systole (s); percentage fractional shortening (FS%); ratio of LV radius to PWT (r/h).

Western Blot Analysis in Myocardial Tissue

Myocardial tissues were pulverized and the powder was homogenized in lysis buffer (1% Triton X-100, 20 mM Tris pH 7.4–7.6, 150 mM NaCl, 50 mM NaF, 1 mM EDTA, 1 mM EGTA, 1 mM Glycerolphosphatase, 1% SDS, 100 mM PMSF, and 0.1% protease phosphatase inhibitor cocktail). After centrifugation at 11,000 g for 15 min at 4°C, supernatants were collected and protein content was assessed using the Lowry method. The supernatant was mixed with Dave's buffer (4% SDS, 10% 2-mercaptoethanol, 20% glycerol, 0.004% bromophenyl blue, and 0.125 M Tris·HCl). The samples were boiled at 100°C for 10 min and stored at −80°C. An equal amount of protein was loaded in each well and then separated by sodium dodecylsulfate-polyacrylamide gel electrophoresis 7.5–11% and transferred onto a polyvinylidene difluoride membrane (PVDF). After blocking with 5% non-fat dry milk, membranes were incubated overnight at 4°C with the following primary antibodies:

p-eNOS (Ser1177), eNOS, p-Akt (Ser473), Akt, p-ERK 1/2 (Thr202/Tyr204), p-GSK3β (Ser9), t-GSK3β, pAMPKα(Ser172), tAMPKα, p-STAT3 (Tyr705), t-STAT3, iNOS, p-NF-κB (p65) (Ser536), t- NF-κB (p65), GAPDH, β-tubulin, β-actin (Cell

Signaling Technology, Beverly, MA, USA) and IL-6 (Santa-Cruz Biotechnology Inc., USA). PVDF membranes were then incubated with secondary antibodies for 2 h at room temperature (goat anti-mouse and goat anti-rabbit HRP; Cell Signaling Technology, Beverly, MA, USA) and developed using the GE Healthcare ECL Western Blotting Detection Reagents (Thermo Scientific Technologies, Bioanalytica, Athens, Greece). Relative densitometry was determined using a computerized software package (NIH, USA), and relative ratios were used for statistical analysis (Bibli et al., 2015, 2016).

Advanced Glycation End-Products (AGE) Fluorescence Measurement

The fluorescence intensity of plasma samples was measured at 440 nm after excitation at 370 nm, using a fluorescence spectrophotometer (Infinite® 200 PRO NanoQuant Plate Reader) operating at room temperature. Emission and excitation slit widths were set at 5 nm. Fluorescence was expressed as the Intergrated Fluorescence intensity in arbitrary units (AU), as previously described (Yanagisawa et al., 1998).

In Vitro Experiments

Effects on Cellular Level

Cell culture and in vitro hypoxia/reoxygenation assay

Endothelial cells (ECs) were purchased from Lonza (Basel, Switzerland) and cultured as described by the manufacturer's instructions. The embryonic rat heart-derived cell line H9C2 was obtained from American Type Culture Collection (Manassas, VA, USA). Cells were maintained in DMEM high glucose (HG) with 10% FBS, 4 mM glutamine and grown to subconfluence prior to experiments. In parallel experiments H9C2 cells were cultured for 24 h either alone or in combination with 1 mg/ml AGE and untreated or treated with EMPA (100 or 500 nM) (Panchapakesan et al., 2013). ECs, maintained for 24 h in 5% FBS, were cultured either alone or in combination with AGE and untreated or treated with EMPA (100 or 500 nM). At day 2, cells were subjected to *in vitro* hypoxia for 24 h (5% CO_2/95% N_2 humidified atmosphere, yielding 1% O_2 concentrations) and subsequently reoxygenated for 3 h (75% N_2, 20% O_2, and 5% CO_2).

ATP content assay

To determine the level of cellular ATP content as an indirect measurement of viable cells, ATP content was performed using ATP assay kit according to manufacturer's instructions (Sigma Aldrich). Briefly, ECs and H9C2, treated as indicated, were subjected to *in vitro* ischemia for 24 h. After reoxygenation, ATP was quantitatively determined by measuring luminescence generated in an ATP-dependent luciferin-luciferase bioluminescence assay. A standard curve was used in each experiment, and the samples were diluted to be in the linear range of the standard curve. All experiments were performed in triplicate.

Cell viability assay

Cell viability was assessed by MTT as described previously (Baldanzi et al., 2002). Cells were seeded on 96-well plates at 5 × 10^3 cells/well. ECs and H9C2 which had either been treated with the indicated stimuli or had been left untreated were subjected to *in vitro* ischemia and reoxygenation. After treatments, cells were incubated with 1 mg/ml MTT for 2 h. Subsequently, the medium was removed and 100 μl of dimethylsulfoxide (DMSO) was added to each well. After 1 h, the 96-well plate was read by an enzyme-linked immunosorbent assay (ELISA) reader at 570 nm for absorbance density values to determine cell viability. All experiments were performed in triplicate.

Western blot analysis in cells

Cells were lysed (50 mM Tris HCl [pH 8.3], 1% Triton X-100, 10 mM PMSF, 100 U/mL aprotinin, 10 μM/mL leupeptin) and protein concentrations were obtained as previously described (Togliatto et al., 2011). Proteins (50 μg) were subjected to SDS-PAGE, transferred into nitrocellulose membrane, blotted with the indicated antibodies (anti-RAGE antibody cat. No. sc-8230, and anti-b-actin antibody cat. No. sc-47778, purchased from Santa Cruz, Biotechnology, Germany) and processed as previously described (Togliatto et al., 2011). Densitometric analysis was used to calculate the differences in the fold induction of protein level normalized to β-actin. Values are reported as relative amounts.

Effects on Subcellular Level

Mitochondrial isolation

Five additional C57BL/6 mice weighting 25–30 g were euthanized by cervical dislocation, and their hearts were quickly excised, rinsed, and cut in the isolation buffer (225 mM mannitol, 75 mM sucrose, 10 mM HEPES-Tris, 1 mM EGTA-Tris, pH 7.4). Then, the tissue was homogenized in the isolation buffer supplemented with 0.1 mg/ml Nagarse by using a glass-Teflon homogenizer. The homogenate was diluted in isolation buffer supplemented with 0.2% w/v bovine serum albumin, centrifuged at 500 g at 4°C, and filtered through a 150-mm mesh for the removal of cellular debris. The supernatant was further centrifuged at 8,000 g to separate the mitochondrial from the cytosolic fraction. The pellet, consisting of mitochondria was washed with isolation buffer without bovine serum albumin and centrifuged at 8,000 g. The final pellet was used for protein determination and further assays.

Calcium retention capacity assay

The calcium retention capacity (CRC) assay was performed as previously described (Chatzianastasiou et al., 2016) in order to determine the susceptibility of mitochondria to undergo permeability transition. Isolated mitochondria were diluted in mitochondrial assay buffer (KCl 137 mM, KH2PO4 2 mM, HEPES 20 mM, EGTA 20 mM, glutamate/malate 5 mM, pH 7.2) at a concentration of 0.25 mg/ml. Extramitochondrial Ca^{2+} was measured by Calcium Green-5N (1 mM) fluorescence using a Fluoroskan Ascent FL plate reader (Thermo Electron, Waltham, MA). Each minute, pulses of 10 mM Ca^{2+} were added to each well, up to a point when the accumulated Ca^{2+} was released due to mitochondrial transition through the opening of the mitochondrial permeability transition pore (PTP). Cyclosporine A (CsA) (1 mg/ml), was used as a positive control. Mitochondria were exposed to different concentrations of EMPA, and their CRC was determined: All experiments performed in five repetitions.

Statistical analysis

All values were denoted as means ± S.E.M. For animal studies and tissue experiments comparisons of numeric variables among the groups were analyzed using unpaired two-tailed Student's *t*-test, while those originating by different time points belonging to the same group were analyzed using paired two-tailed Student's *t*-test. A calculated $p < 0.05$ was considered to be statistically significant.

For mitochondria and cell culture experiments, the D'Agostino-Pearson test was used to test normality. Data on cell viability assay, ATP content assay and on densitometric analysis for Western blots were analyzed using 1-way ANOVA, followed by Tukey's multiple comparison test. The cut-off for statistical significance was set at $p < 0.05$ ($^{*}p < 0.05$, $^{**}p < 0.01$, $^{***}p < 0.001$). All statistical analyses were carried out using GraphPad Prism version 5.04 (Graph Pad Software, Inc.).

RESULTS

EMPA Reduces Body Weight, Mean Arterial Pressure, Glucose, and Lipid Peroxidation Levels without Altering Lipid Levels and Age Products

The experimental protocol of the study is illustrated in **Figure 1A**. In both groups, BW increased after 14 weeks of WD feeding. At the end of treatment, EMPA reduced significantly the BW (**Figure 1B**) and fast blood glucose levels (250 ± 18 mg/dL vs. 172 ± 8 mg/dL, $^{*}p < 0.05$, **Figure 1C**) in comparison to Control. Mean arterial pressure (MAP) was significantly reduced from baseline after 6 weeks treatment in the EMPA group (**Table 1**). Cholesterol and triglyceride levels did not differ between study groups at the end of treatment; however, they were significantly elevated compared to baseline values (**Table 1**). AGE levels were similar between the study groups at the end of treatment period (**Figure 1D**). Reduced levels of the biomarker of lipid peroxidation, malondialdehyde (MDA) in circulation was observed in the EMPA group compared to the Control group (**Figure 1E**, $p < 0.05$).

Cardiac Function Is Improved with EMPA Pretreatment in Mice Treated with WD

Echocardiography revealed a reduction in the myocardial function after 14 weeks WD feeding as shown by the left ventricular fractional shortening (LVFS%; 43.97 ± 0.92 vs. 40.75 ± 0.61%, $p = 0.001$), due to deterioration of both LV end-systolic and end-diastolic dimensions (**Table 1**). These changes were not evident after EMPA treatment (**Table 1**, Figure S2).

EMPA Pretreatment Reduces Myocardial Infarct Size in Mice Treated with WD

Three animals from the Control group and one animal from the EMPA group were excluded for different technical and/or hemodynamic reasons (severe bleeding and infarction detected outside the area at risk). As a result, 14 animals completed the study, Control ($n = 6$) EMPA ($n = 8$). Myocardial infarct size was reduced in EMPA group (33.2 ± 0.01 vs. 17.6 ± 0.02%, $p < 0.05$) (**Figure 2A**), with no difference in the area at risk (**Figure 2B**).

EMPA Pretreatment Induces Cardioprotection through STAT3 Activation, Independently of the Reperfusion Injury Salvage Kinase (RISK) Pathway and AMPKα Activation

EMPA pretreatment did not activate Akt (**Figure 3A**), eNOS (**Figure 3B**), did not phosphorylate GSK3β on its inhibitory site (**Figure 3C**), did not activate p-44/p-42(ERK 1/2) (**Figure 3D**), and had no effect on AMPKα phosphorylation (**Figure 3E**). EMPA increased both STAT3 expression and phosphorylation (**Figure 3F**, $p < 0.05$) compared to the untreated group. Additionally, EMPA did change neither the phosphorylation nor the expression of nuclear factor kappa-light-chain-enhancer of activated B cells (NF-κB) (**Figure 4A**). Pretreatment with EMPA resulted in reduced levels of myocardial inteleukin-6 (IL-6) (**Figure 4B**, $p < 0.05$) and of inducible nitric oxide synthase (iNOS) expression (**Figure 4C**, $p < 0.05$).

Evaluation of the Effects of EMPA on Isolated Heart Mitochondria

In order to determine the direct effects of EMPA on mitochondrial transition, we recruited an *in vitro* experiment on isolated murine heart mitochondria. EMPA tested in concentrations of 50μM −50 nM had no effect on mitochondrial CRC. Cyclosporine was used as a positive control and increased mitochondrial CRC at a dose of 1 μg/ml (**Figures 5A,B**; $^{***}p < 0.001$ vs. all other study groups).

EMPA Protects H9C2 and EC Cells against Hypoxia/Reoxygenation Injury in a Diabetic Milieu

In order investigate a direct cardioprotective effect of EMPA we exposed H9C2 and ECs to hypoxia/reoxygenation. EMPA at 500 nM increased H9C2 cell viability and ATP content (**Figures 6A,C**). More importantly, it was able to protect cells even when AGE was used to mimic the diabetic milieu. Similar results were obtained in ECs (**Figures 6B,D**). Consistent with AGE expression *in vivo*, no changes in receptor for advanced glycation endproducts (RAGE) expression was detected *in vitro* (**Figure 6E**).

DISCUSSION

EMPA treatment in a Type 2 Diabetes animal model, reduced myocardial infarct size, preserved myocardial function after I/R injury, increased cell viability and ATP content in H9C2 and in ECs even when AGE was used to mimic the diabetic milieu. The present study also highlights that EMPA increased STAT3 phosphorylation and expression and reduced myocardial IL-6 and iNOS expressions regulating inflammatory responses and redox signaling in the ischemic myocardium.

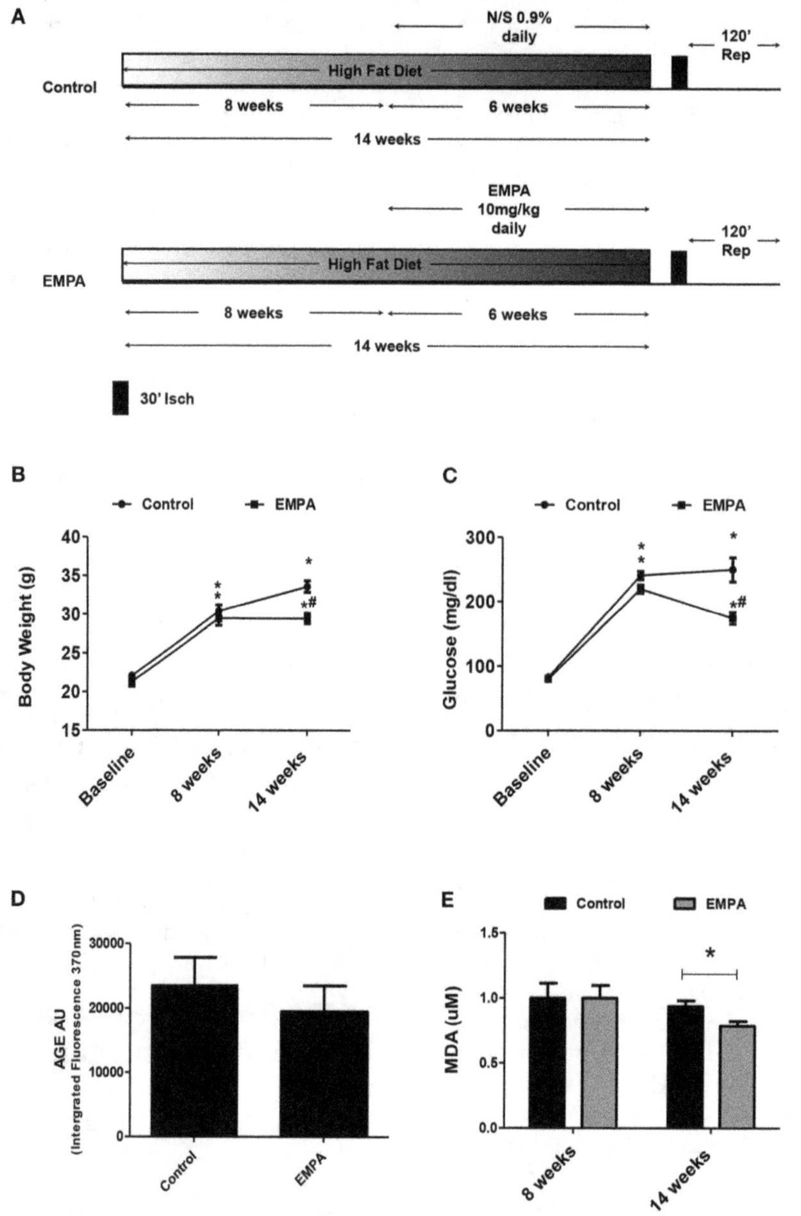

FIGURE 1 | Empagliflozin reduces body weight, glucose levels, and lipid peroxidation levels without altering AGE products. **(A)** Experimental work flow. **(B)** Effects of diet manipulation and empagliflozin treatment on mice BW ($^{*}p < 0.05$ vs. Baseline, $^{\#}p < 0.05$ vs. Control). **(C)** Effects of diet manipulation and empagliflozin treatment on fasting glucose levels ($^{*}p < 0.05$ vs. Baseline, $^{\#}p < 0.05$ vs. Control). **(D)** AGE (AU) measured as Intergrated Fluorescence at emission 370 nm and **(E)** effects of diet manipulation and empagliflozin treatment on circulating MDA (uM) levels ($^{*}p < 0.05$ vs. Control).

Diabetes mellitus increases myocardial susceptibility to I/R injury (Miki et al., 2012). Glycotoxicity plays a major role in this defect by increasing formation of AGE products and the RAGE-induced signaling cascade, leading to vascular dysfunction. RAGE blockade has been demonstrated to be a potential therapeutic approach for treatment of I/R-injury (Park et al., 2015). SGLT2 inhibitors are highly efficient in preventing glucotoxicity, by reducing formation of AGE and induction of RAGE as it is shown in experimental studies (Oelze et al., 2014). In our *in vivo* model EMPA did not alter AGE; additionally, did not alter RAGE expression in H9C2 cells. These findings are consistent with data showing that EMPA, independently of AGE accumulation, exerts pleiotropic protective effects on myocardial function and structure in diabetic db/db mouse (Habibi et al., 2017). In compliance with our findings the administration of EMPA at a similar dose used in our study improved aortic remodeling independently of AGE and RAGE formation in aortic tissue declaring that EMPA activity can be AGE-independent (Oelze et al., 2014).

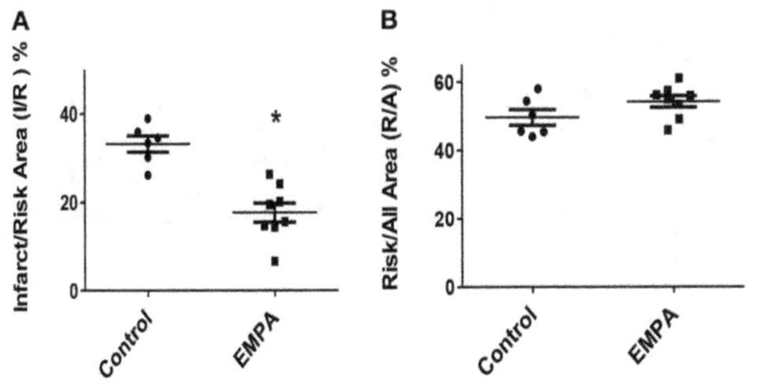

FIGURE 2 | Empagliflozin pretreatment reduces myocardial infarct size in mice treated with WD. **(A)** Representative Graphs of Infarct/Risk Area (I/R) %. Individual animals represented as a scatter plot with dots in the Control group and squares in the EMPA group. Results plotted as Mean ± SEM (*$p < 0.05$ vs. Control). **(B)** Risk/All Area (R/A) %.

Reperfusion Injury Salvage Kinase (RISK) and Survivor Activating Factor Enhancement (SAFE) pathways are the main mediators of cardioprotection leading to reduction of infarct size (Heusch, 2015). We did not find any differences between the EMPA and Control groups in the phosphorylation and expression of Akt, eNOS, ERK1/2, and GSK3β in the ischemic myocardium, indicating a RISK independent pathway in EMPA-mediated cardioprotection. This is in agreement with a recent study demonstrating that EMPA did not phosphorylate Akt or ERK1/2 in cardiomyocytes (Habibi et al., 2017). AMPK is a kinase that serves as a key modulator of cellular bioenergetics, and agents acting on AMPK activation, such as metformin, induce cardioprotective effects (Calvert et al., 2008). Canagliflozin, an SGLT2 inhibitor causes a substantial AMPK activation *in vitro*. In contrast, EMPA caused only a modest AMPK activation at high concentrations, indicating that this effect is unlikely to be relevant *in vivo* (Hawley et al., 2016). We confirmed the above findings *in vivo* showing that EMPA did not phosphorylate AMPK, specifying that its cardioprotective effects are independent of AMPK activation. We must mention that all the above signaling events were tested at the time point of the 10th min of reperfusion. This time point was chosen since many of the cardioprotective mechanisms are activated during the first minutes of reperfusion as previously shown (Andreadou et al., 2012, 2015; Kleinbongard et al., 2017). However, components of the RISK pathway such as Akt may be activated after the 10th min of reperfusion (Kleinbongard et al., 2017); therefore we should clarify that in our protocol there is no activation of RISK pathway and AMPK at this specific time point. In addition to the RISK pathway, SAFE and in particular STAT3 activation, is one of the main mediators of triggering cardioprotection (Andreadou et al., 2015; Kleinbongard et al., 2017). Chronic treatment with the SGLT2 inhibitor, dapagliflozin *in vivo*, activated the STAT3 signaling pathway, which on turn enhanced M2 macrophage activation, resulting in the attenuation of cardiac fibrosis molecularly by myocardial iNOS and IL-6 reduced levels (Lee et al., 2017). This effect was more evident with the use of the specific SGLT2 inhibitor dapagliflozin than with the SGLT1/SGLT2 inhibitor phlorizin, implying that compensatory SGLT1 activation after administration of specific SGLT2 inhibitors may play a role in ventricular remodeling (Lee et al., 2017). We found that 6 weeks administration of EMPA resulted in a significant activation of STAT3 at tyrosine 705. We investigated the phosphorylation on Tyr705, since Tyr705 is the primary phosphorylation site of STAT3 (Andreadou et al., 2015). Moreover, the latter study has deduced that STAT3 activation is mediated through decrease of reactive oxygen species (ROS) accumulation in the myocardium. In compliance with the abovementioned findings we have found that in EMPA treated mice circulating levels of MDA are reduced compared to Control. The decrease in lipid peroxidation biomarker MDA seems to be a key element in redox regulating effects of EMPA.

STAT3 phosphorylation has a direct effect on maintaining mitochondrial integrity and attenuating mitochondrial permeability transition pore (MPTP) opening (Heusch, 2015), a key process that is pivotal for the cardiomyocyte survival after ischemia-reperfusion (Bernardi and Di Lisa, 2015; Hausenloy et al., 2016). Additionally, this pore is important in the induction of ROS induced ROS release (RIRR) and can furtherly lead to increased oxidative decay in the cardiomyocytes (Penna et al., 2013). To elucidate whether EMPA exerts its cardioprotective effects through inhibition of MPTP directly, or if the infarct sparing properties are mediated through STAT3 activation, we evaluated the Ca^{2+} retention capacity of isolated heart mitochondria after a series of Ca^{2+} pulses and increasing EMPA concentrations. Since we observed that EMPA did not alter the mitochondrial susceptibility to permeability transition, we concluded that the effect of EMPA in reducing myocardial infarction is STAT3 dependent. However, we must mention that we tested the efficacy of EMPA on mitochondrial transition under normoxic conditions, addressing the direct link between EMPA's cardioprotective potential and mitochondrial retention capacity. Whether the chronic administration of EMPA may alter mitochondrial susceptibility to transition *in vivo*, when subjected to I/R, as well as the underlying induced signaling cascades is a topic of further investigations. Therefore, our next step focused on the signaling cascade complementary to STAT3 activation.

Activation of STAT3, leads to its translocation to the nucleus to function as a transcriptional factor. STAT3 might exhibit a differential role when translocated to the nucleus as it can bind to the promoter of iNOS directly, inhibiting its expression and mitigating cardiomyocyte apoptosis (Su et al., 2016). This is an important finding, as far as the cardioprotective properties of EMPA are concerned, knowing that iNOS is a key contributing molecule in nitrosative stress as well as it possesses deleterious role in inflammatory processes and that diabetes is *per se* a redox-mediated disease. NO derived from iNOS may react with anion superoxide to form peroxynitrite, which may sustain lipid peroxidation (Sag et al., 2013). Therefore, the decreased MDA levels can be directly correlated with the decreased iNOS expression in the EMPA group.

Furthermore, STAT3 can interfere with key molecules implicated in inflammation. NF-κB is a key mediator of inflammatory response, as it leads to the transcription of

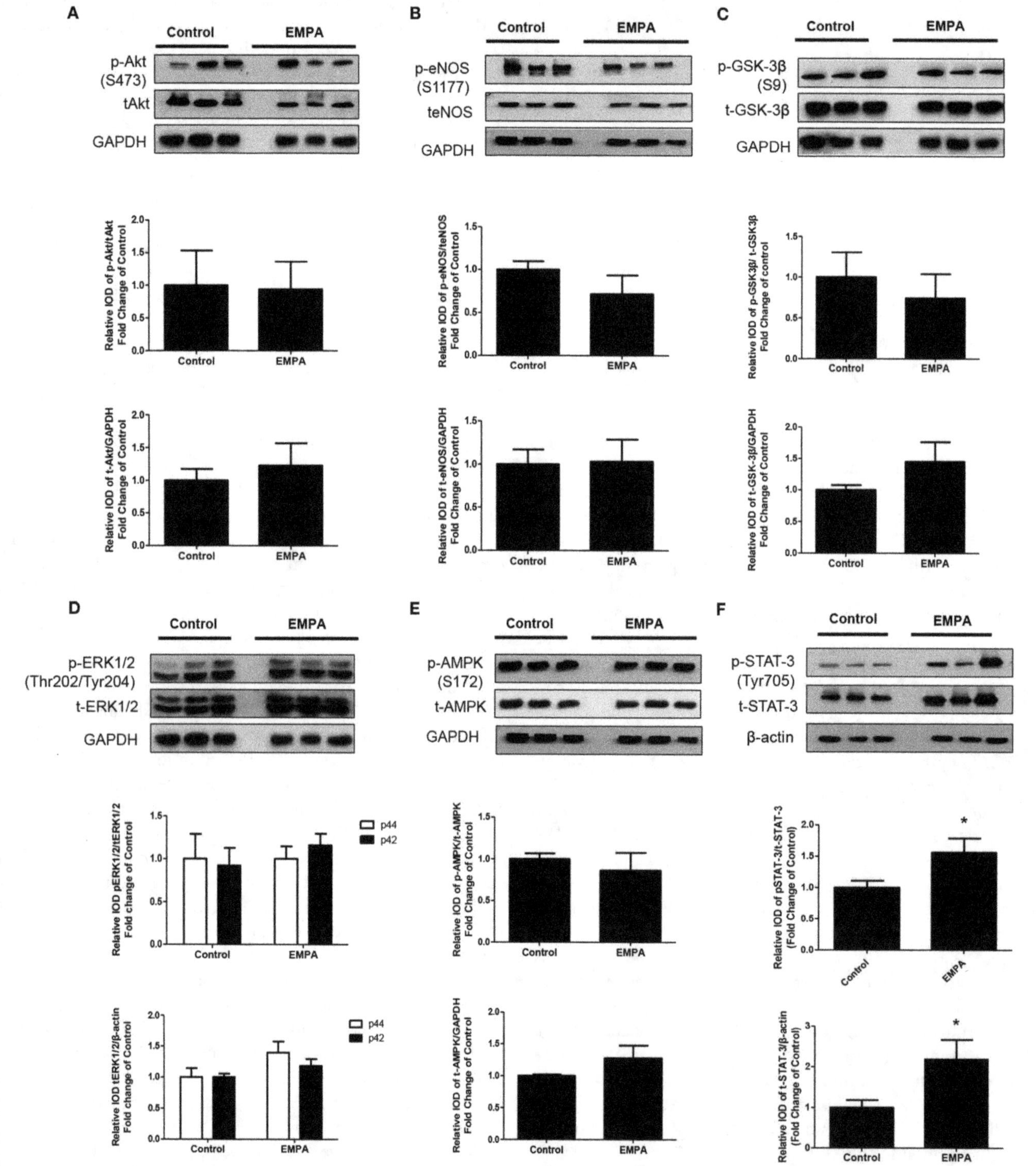

FIGURE 3 | Empagliflozin induces cardioprotection through activation of STAT-3 and independently of RISK pathway and of AMPK activation. Representative western blots and relative densitometry graphs of **(A)** p-Akt (S473)/t-Akt and t-Akt/GAPDH **(B)** p-eNOS(S1177)/t-eNOS and t-eNOS/GAPDH **(C)** p-GSK-3β(S9)/t-GSK-3β and t-GSK-3β/GAPDH **(D)** p-ERK1/2 (Thr202/Tyr204)/t-ERK1/2 and t-ERK1/2/GAPDH **(E)** p-AMPKα(S172)/t-AMPKα and t-AMPKα/GAPDH **(F)** p-STAT3(Tyr705)/t-STAT3 and t-STAT3/β-actin (*$p < 0.05$ vs. Control). p-Akt, t-Akt **(A)** and p-ERK1/2, t-ERK1/2 **(D)** proteins were detected on the same gel and share the same image of GAPDH, serving as loading Control. This was also the case for p-eNOS, t-eNOS **(B)**, p-AMPKα, and t-AMPKα **(E)**.

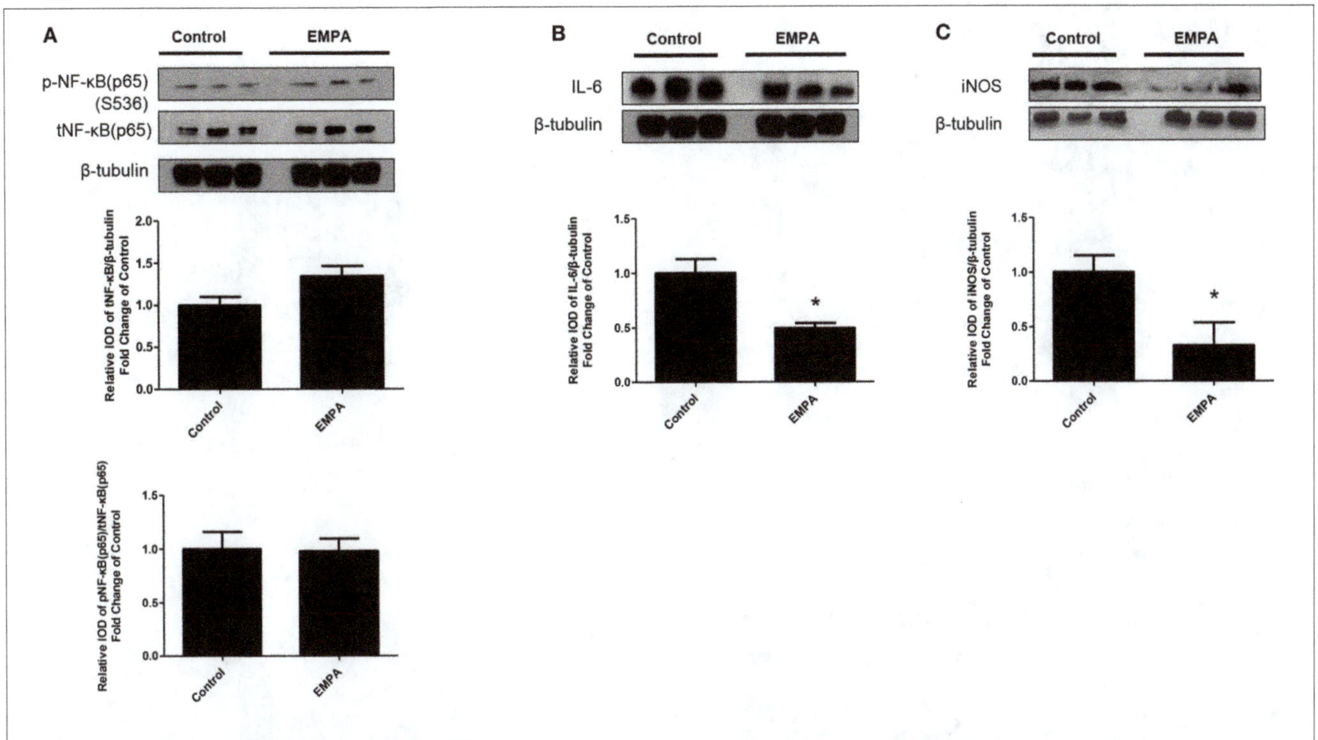

FIGURE 4 | Empagliflozin reduces myocardial iNOS and IL-6 expression. Representative western blots and relative densitometry graphs of **(A)** p-NF-κB (p65) (S536)/ t-NF-κB (p65) and t-NF-κB (p65)/β-tubulin **(B)** IL-6/ β-tubulin ($^{*}p < 0.05$ vs. Control) and **(C)** iNOS/ β-tubulin ($^{*}p < 0.05$ vs. Control). p-NFκB(p65), t-NFkB(p65) **(A)** and IL-6 **(B)** were detected on the same gel and share the same image of β tubulin, serving as loading Control.

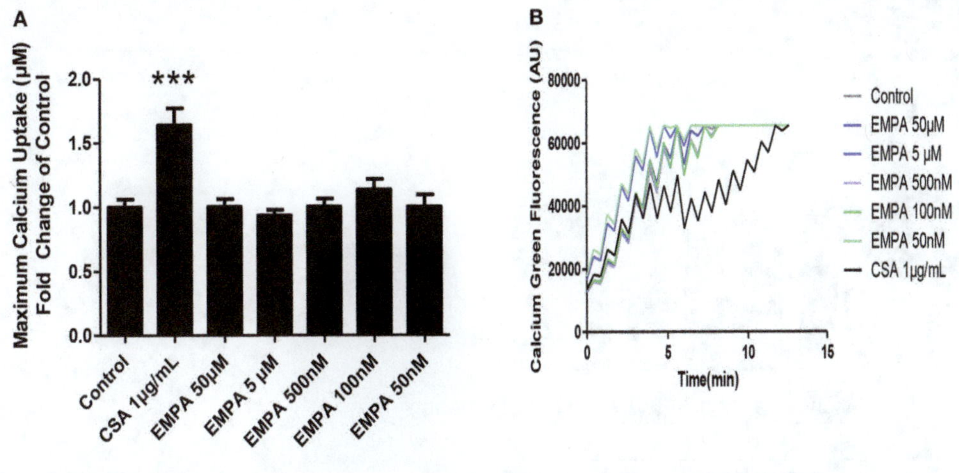

FIGURE 5 | Evaluation of the effects of EMPA on isolated heart mitochondria. Direct effects of empagliflozin on mitochondria. **(A)** Calcium retention capacity of mouse heart mitochondria ($^{***}p < 0.001$ vs. all other study groups) and **(B)** representative Calcium tracing ($n = 5$).

cytokines and apoptosis-related proteins including IL-6 and iNOS in the myocardium (Gordon et al., 2011). Although we observed reduced levels of expression of both IL-6 and iNOS in the myocardium, we did not find any changes in phosphorylation and/or expression of NF-κB in the EMPA group compared to the Control. Among targets that finely tune NF-κB activity, it is proven that STAT3 acts as a suppressor of NF-κB (Gordon et al., 2011). More specifically, STAT3 can directly interact with NF-κB p65 subunit, leading to a dominant inhibition of NF-κB activity and thus indirectly suppressing cytokine induction of the iNOS promoter independently of NF-κB phosphorylation or expression *in vitro* (Yu et al., 2002). This might be the explanation of our aforementioned findings.

It has been assumed that some of the direct effects of EMPA acting independently of SGLT2 inhibition may be in

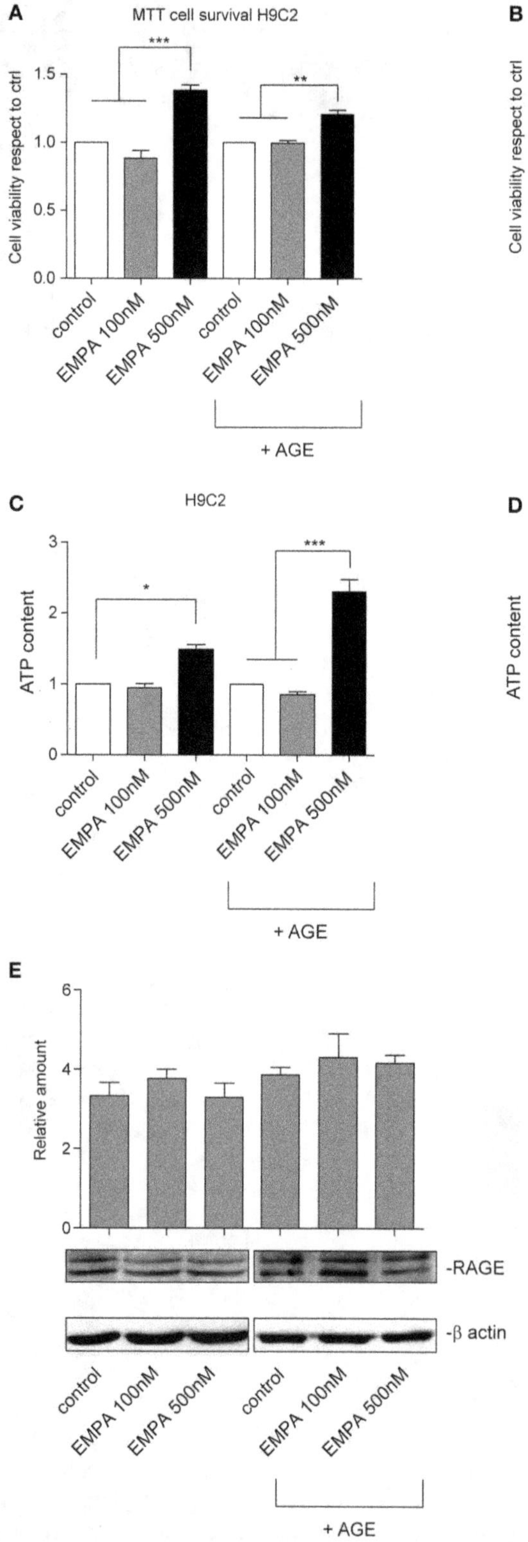

FIGURE 6 | Empagliflozin rescues ECs and H9C2 cells from hypoxia/reoxygenation injury. **(A,B)** MTT assay was used to assess the effect of EMPA in hypoxia/reoxygenation setting. The indicated concentrations were used to treat H9C2 cells **(A)** and ECs **(B)**. Both H9C2 and ECs, either untreated or treated with AGE (1 mg/mL), were subjected to hypoxia/reoxygenation. Data normalized to control are reported as mean ± *SD* and representative of four different experiments performed in triplicate ($n = 12$) (For H9C2, $^{***}p < 0.001$ EMPA 500 nM vs. control and EMPA 100 nM; $^{**}p < 0.01$ EMPA 500 nM + AGE vs. control + AGE and EMPA

(Continued)

FIGURE 6 | 100 nM + AGE; for ECs, $^{**}p < 0.01$ EMPA 500 nM vs. control and EMPA 100 nM; $^{*}p < 0.05$ EMPA 500 nM + AGE vs. control + AGE. **(C,D)** Histogram representation of the relative cellular ATP content. Data are obtained from H9C2 cells and ECs treated as indicated (for H9C2, $^{*}p < 0.05$ EMPA 500 nM vs. control; $^{***}p < 0.001$ EMPA 500 nM + AGE vs. control + AGE and EMPA 100 nM + AGE; for ECs, $^{***}p < 0.001$ EMPA 500 nM vs. control and EMPA 100 nM; $^{**}p < 0.01$ control + AGE vs. EMPA 100 nM + AGE, EMPA 500 nM + AGE vs. control + AGE, $^{***}p < 0.001$ EMPA 500 nM + AGE vs. EMPA 100 nM + AGE). Data are reported as mean ± *SD* and representative of four different experiments performed in triplicate ($n = 12$). **(E)** Cell extracts from H9C2 cells treated, with or without AGE (1 mg/mL), and with Empagliflozin at the indicated concentrations, were subjected to hypoxia/reoxygenation and analyzed for RAGE content, and normalized to β-actin Data are representative of four different experiments performed in triplicate ($n = 12$).

part responsible for the established cardioprotective effects of the drug. In this aspect a recent study showed that EMPA has direct effects on cardiomyocytes through lowering cytoplasmic sodium $[Na^+]c$ and calcium $[Ca^{2+}]c$. These effects are mainly mediated via Na^+/H^+ exchanger (NHE) activity, independently of SGLT2 (Baartscheer et al., 2017). Therefore, we investigated if EMPA has direct effect in H9C2 cells and in ECs under hypoxia/reoxygenation. EMPA is a very potent and selective SGLT2 inhibitor with an IC50 ~3 nM and Cmax from clinical dosing ~500 nM; concentrations between 100 and 500 nM block effectively and selectively SGLT2 without significant inhibition of SGLT1 (Panchapakesan et al., 2013). Based on the above statements we use 100 and 500 nM and interestingly, we observed that treatment with 500 nM EMPA increased cell viability in comparison to the control in absence or in presence of AGE, and increased ATP content in both cell types. The increased ATP is probably the result of improved mitochondrial function since it has been demonstrated that SGLT2 inhibitors may shift whole-body metabolism from glucose to fat oxidation (Vettor et al., 2017), therefore improving oxidative phosphorylation and mitochondrial respiration.

In a very recent study EMPA reduced pro-inflammatory signaling through amelioration of increased interferon-γ (IFN-γ) in an *in vivo* model of T2D (Steven et al., 2017). From a mechanistic sight of view, EMPA reduced epigenetic changes induced by T2D, as it downregulated the activating epigenetic mark histone3 lysine4 trimethylation (H3K4me3) of the promoters of IFN-γ and iNOS. Moreover, EMPA decreased serum oxidative stress biomarkers namely 3-nitrotyrosine and 4-hydroxynonenal and dose-dependently increased aldehyde dehydrogenase (ALDH-2) activity (Steven et al., 2017), a mitochondrial antioxidant enzyme responsible for the detoxification of tissues from MDA (Wenzel et al., 2007). In compliance with the above-mentioned findings we have shown that EMPA reduced circulating MDA levels and improved mitochondrial function as shown in cells by increased ATP cellular content. Thus, we can speculate that these effects along with the observed reduction of iNOS can be attributed to epigenomic changes present in T2D. Moreover, macrophage infiltration present in the context of AMI and T2D (Lee et al., 2017; Steven et al., 2017) can contribute to the induction of a proinflammatory phenotype and oxidative stress in the myocardium, while SGLT2 inhibition is shown to diminish this process. EMPA's redox regulating effects seem to be pleiotropic as it acts both by upregulating endogenous antioxidant mechanisms and interfering with epigenomic changes associated with T2D.

Conclusively, EMPA reduces myocardial infarct size in animals fed with WD through STAT3 activation and regulation of inflammatory responses in the myocardium. Moreover, the decrease in iNOS expression and the concomitant decrease in lipid peroxidation is of great importance. While diabetes is a redox disease, the redox regulation by EMPA in parallel with its glucose-lowering effects can be pivotal in managing diabetes and limiting myocardial infarction. Therefore, the assessment of EMPA effects on myocardial necrosis and the elucidation of the molecular mechanisms responsible for its cardioprotection are of paramount importance. It would allow predicting whether EMPA has such beneficial effects also in diabetic patients without prior cardiovascular disease, or in non-diabetic patients with cardiovascular disease.

STUDY LIMITATIONS

We know that SGLT2 is highly specifically expressed in the kidney and very minimally in the heart (Chen et al., 2017). Therefore, additional studies are essential in order to investigate how EMPA would exert its effects on cardiomyocytes. One of the main limitations of the present study is the mechanistic insight of the role of STAT3 mediating cardioprotection. Additional studies to elucidate the exact cardioprotective mechanism of EMPA by the use of established inhibitors *in vivo* are necessary to answer this question. However, our study is able to stimulate research in investigating the cardioprotective mechanisms of this drug in the setting of I/R injury.

AUTHOR CONTRIBUTIONS

IA, MB, GD, and EI: contributed to conception and design, contributed to acquisition, analysis, and interpretation, drafted the article, critically revised the article and gave final approval; PE, EB, GT, CHD, AV, P-EN, CAD, EM, VL, II, and NK: contributed to acquisition, analysis, and interpretation, critically revised the article, and gave final approval.

REFERENCES

Andreadou, I., Bibli, S. I., Mastromanolis, E., Zoga, A., Efentakis, P., Papaioannou, N., et al. (2015). Transient carotid ischemia as a remote conditioning stimulus for myocardial protection in anesthetized rabbits: insights into intracellular signaling. *Int. J. Cardiol.* 184, 140–151. doi: 10.1016/j.ijcard.2015.01.079

Andreadou, I., Farmakis, D., Prokovas, E., Sigala, F., Zoga, A., Spyridaki, K., et al. (2012). Short-term statin administration in hypercholesterolemic rabbits resistant to postconditioning: effects on infarct size, endothelial nitric oxide synthase and nitro-oxidative stress. *Cardiovasc. Res.* 94, 501–509. doi: 10.1093/cvr/cvs121

Andreadou, I., Iliodromitis, E. K., Mikros, E., Bofilis, E., Zoga, A., Constantinou, M., et al. (2004). Melatonin does not prevent the protection of ischemic preconditioning *in vivo* despite its antioxidant effect against oxidative stress. *Free Radic. Biol. Med.* 37, 500–510. doi: 10.1016/j.freeradbiomed.2004.05.005

Baartscheer, A., Schumacher, C. A., Wust, R. C., Fiolet, J. W., Stienen, G. J., Coronel, R., et al. (2017). Empagliflozin decreases myocardial cytoplasmic Na+ through inhibition of the cardiac Na+/H+ exchanger in rats and rabbits. *Diabetologia* 60, 568–573. doi: 10.1007/s00125-016-4134-x

Baldanzi, G., Filigheddu, N., Cutrupi, S., Catapano, F., Bonissoni, S., Fubini, A., et al. (2002). Ghrelin and des-acyl ghrelin inhibit cell death in cardiomyocytes and endothelial cells through ERK1/2 and PI 3-kinase/AKT. *J. Cell Biol.* 159, 1029–1037. doi: 10.1083/jcb.200207165

Bernardi, P., and Di Lisa, F. (2015). The mitochondrial permeability transition pore: molecular nature and role as a target in cardioprotection. *J. Mol. Cell. Cardiol.* 78, 100–106. doi: 10.1016/j.yjmcc.2014.09.023

Bibli, S. I., Andreadou, I., Chatzianastasiou, A., Tzimas, C., Sanoudou, D., Kranias, E., et al. (2015). Cardioprotection by H_2S engages a cGMP-dependent protein kinase G/phospholamban pathway. *Cardiovasc. Res.* 106, 432–442. doi: 10.1093/cvr/cvv129

Bibli, S. I., Andreadou, I., Glynos, C., Chatzianastasiou, A., Toumpanakis, D., Zakynthinos, S. G., et al. (2016). Exposure to cigarette smoke abrogates the beneficial effect of ischemic postconditioning. *Am. J. Physiol. Heart Circ. Physiol.* 311, H1321–H1332. doi: 10.1152/ajpheart.00925.2015

Calvert, J. W., Gundewar, S., Jha, S., Greer, J. J., Bestermann, W. H., Tian, R., et al. (2008). Acute metformin therapy confers cardioprotection against myocardial infarction via AMPK-eNOS-mediated signaling. *Diabetes* 57, 696–705. doi: 10.2337/db07-1098

Chatzianastasiou, A., Bibli, S. I., Andreadou, I., Efentakis, P., Kaludercic, N., Wood, M. E., et al. (2016). Cardioprotection by H2S donors: nitric oxide-dependent and independent mechanisms. *J. Pharmacol. Exp. Ther.* 358, 431–440. doi: 10.1124/jpet.116.235119

Chen, J., Fan, F., Wang, J. Y., Long, Y., Gao, C. L., Stanton, R. C., et al. (2017). The efficacy and safety of SGLT2 inhibitors for adjunctive treatment of type 1 diabetes: a systematic review and meta-analysis. *Sci. Rep.* 7:44128. doi: 10.1038/srep44128

Cheng, S. T., Chen, L., Li, S. Y., Mayoux, E., and Leung, P. S. (2016). The effects of empagliflozin, an SGLT2 inhibitor, on pancreatic beta-cell mass and glucose homeostasis in type 1 diabetes. *PLoS ONE* 11:e0147391. doi: 10.1371/journal.pone.0147391

Fitchett, D., Zinman, B., Wanner, C., Lachin, J. M., Hantel, S., Salsali, A., et al. (2016). Heart failure outcomes with empagliflozin in patients with type 2 diabetes at high cardiovascular risk: results of the EMPA-REG OUTCOME(R) trial. *Eur. Heart J.* 37, 1526–1534. doi: 10.1093/eurheartj/ehv728

Gordon, J. W., Shaw, J. A., and Kirshenbaum, L. A. (2011). Multiple facets of NF-κB in the heart: to be or not to NF-κB. *Circ. Res.* 108, 1122–1132. doi: 10.1161/CIRCRESAHA.110.226928

Habibi, J., Aroor, A. R., Sowers, J. R., Jia, G., Hayden, M. R., Garro, M., et al. (2017). Sodium glucose transporter 2 (SGLT2) inhibition with empagliflozin improves cardiac diastolic function in a female rodent model of diabetes. *Cardiovasc. Diabetol.* 16:9. doi: 10.1186/s12933-016-0489-z

Hausenloy, D. J., Barrabes, J. A., Bøtker, H. E., Davidson, S. M., Di Lisa, F., Downey, J., et al. (2016). Ischaemic conditioning and targeting reperfusion injury: a 30 year voyage of discovery. *Basic Res. Cardiol.* 111:70. doi: 10.1007/s00395-016-0588-8

Hawley, S. A., Ford, R. J., Smith, B. K., Gowans, G. J., Mancini, S. J., Pitt, R. D., et al. (2016). The Na+/glucose cotransporter inhibitor canagliflozin activates AMPK by inhibiting mitochondrial function and increasing cellular AMP levels. *Diabetes* 65, 2784–2794. doi: 10.2337/db16-0058

Heusch, G. (2015). Molecular basis of cardioprotection: signal transduction in ischemic pre-, post-, and remote conditioning. *Circ. Res.* 116, 674–699. doi: 10.1161/CIRCRESAHA.116.305348

Kleinbongard, P., Skyschally, A., Gent, S., Pesch, M., and Heusch, G. (2017). STAT3 as a common signal of ischemic conditioning: a lesson on "rigor and reproducibility" in preclinical studies on cardioprotection. *Basic Res. Cardiol.* 113, 3. doi: 10.1007/s00395-017-0660-z

Lee, T. M., Chang, N. C., and Lin, S. Z. (2017). Dapagliflozin, a selective SGLT2 inhibitor, attenuated cardiac fibrosis by regulating the macrophage polarization via STAT3 signaling in infarcted rat hearts. *Free Radic. Biol. Med.* 104, 298–310. doi: 10.1016/j.freeradbiomed.2017.01.035

Miki, T., Itoh, T., Sunaga, D., and Miura, T. (2012). Effects of diabetes on myocardial infarct size and cardioprotection by preconditioning and postconditioning. *Cardiovasc. Diabetol.* 11:67. doi: 10.1186/1475-2840-11-67

Oelze, M., Kroller-Schon, S., Welschof, P., Jansen, T., Hausding, M., Mikhed, Y., et al. (2014). The sodium-glucose co-transporter 2 inhibitor empagliflozin improves diabetes-induced vascular dysfunction in the streptozotocin diabetes rat model by interfering with oxidative stress and glucotoxicity. *PLoS ONE* 9:e112394. doi: 10.1371/journal.pone.0112394

Pagliaro, P., and Penna, C. (2015). Redox signalling and cardioprotection: translatability and mechanism. *Br. J. Pharmacol.* 172, 1974–1995. doi: 10.1111/bph.12975

Panchapakesan, U., Pegg, K., Gross, S., Komala, M. G., Mudaliar, H., Forbes, J., et al. (2013). Effects of SGLT2 inhibition in human kidney proximal tubular cells–renoprotection in diabetic nephropathy? *PLoS ONE* 8:e54442. doi: 10.1371/journal.pone.0054442

Papathanasiou, S., Rickelt, S., Soriano, M. E., Schips, T. G., Maier, H. J., Davos, C. H., et al. (2015). Tumor necrosis factor-alpha confers cardioprotection through ectopic expression of keratins K8 and K18. *Nat. Med.* 21, 1076–1084. doi: 10.1038/nm.3925

Park, H., Ku, S. H., Park, H., Hong, J., Kim, D., Choi, B. R., et al. (2015). RAGE siRNA-mediated gene silencing provides cardioprotection against ventricular arrhythmias in acute ischemia and reperfusion. *J. Control. Release* 217, 315–326. doi: 10.1016/j.jconrel.2015.09.006

Penna, C., Perrelli, M. G., and Pagliaro, P. (2013). Mitochondrial pathways, permeability transition pore, and redox signaling in cardioprotection: therapeutic implications. *Antioxid. Redox Signal.* 18, 556–599. doi: 10.1111/bph.12975

Phillips, J. W., Barringhaus, K. G., Sanders, J. M., Yang, Z., Chen, M., Hesselbacher, S., et al. (2003). Rosiglitazone reduces the accelerated neointima formation after arterial injury in a mouse injury model of type 2 diabetes. *Circulation* 108, 1994–1999. doi: 10.1161/01.CIR.0000092886.52404.50

Sag, C. M., Wagner, S., and Maier, L. S. (2013). Role of oxidants on calcium and sodium movement in healthy and diseased cardiac myocytes. *Free Radic. Biol. Med.* 63, 338–349. doi: 10.1016/j.freeradbiomed.2013.05.035

Steven, S., Oelze, M., Hanf, A., Kröller-Schön, S., Kashani, F., Roohani, S., et al. (2017). The SGLT2 inhibitor empagliflozin improves the primary diabetic complications in ZDF rats. *Redox Biol.* 13, 370–385. doi: 10.1016/j.redox.2017.06.009

Su, S. A., Yang, D., Zhu, W., Cai, Z., Zhang, N., Zhao, L., et al. (2016). Interleukin-17A mediates cardiomyocyte apoptosis through Stat3-iNOS pathway. *Biochim. Biophys. Acta* 1863, 2784–2794. doi: 10.1016/j.bbamcr.2016.08.013

Surwit, R. S., Kuhn, C. M., Cochrane, C., McCubbin, J. A., and Feinglos, M. N. (1988). Diet-induced type II diabetes in C57BL/6J mice. *Diabetes* 37, 1163–1167. doi: 10.2337/diab.37.9.1163

Togliatto, G., Trombetta, A., Dentelli, P., Rosso, A., and Brizzi, M. F. (2011). MIR221/MIR222-driven post-transcriptional regulation of P27KIP1 and P57KIP2 is crucial for high-glucose- and AGE-mediated vascular cell damage. *Diabetologia* 54, 1930–1940. doi: 10.1007/s00125-011-2125-5

Vettor, R., Inzucchi, S. E., and Fioretto, P. (2017). The cardiovascular benefits of empagliflozin: SGLT2-dependent and -independent effects. *Diabetologia* 60, 395–398. doi: 10.1007/s00125-016-4194-y

Wenzel, P., Hink, U., Oelze, M., Schuppan, S., Schaeuble, K., Schildknecht, S., et al. (2007). Role of reduced lipoic acid in the redox regulation of mitochondrial aldehyde dehydrogenase (ALDH-2) activity. Implications for mitochondrial oxidative stress and nitrate tolerance. *J Biol Chem.* 282, 792–799. doi: 10.1074/jbc.M606477200

Yanagisawa, K., Makita, Z., Shiroshita, K., Ueda, T., Fusegawa, T., Kuwajima, S., et al. (1998). Specific fluorescence assay for advanced glycation end products in blood and urine of diabetic patients. *Metab. Clin. Exp.* 47, 1348–1353. doi: 10.1016/S0026-0495(98)90303-1

Yu, Z., Zhang, W., and Kone, B. C. (2002). Signal transducers and activators of transcription 3 (STAT3) inhibits transcription of the inducible nitric oxide synthase gene by interacting with nuclear factor kappaB. *Biochem. J.* 367, 97–105. doi: 10.1042/bj20020588

2

Cardioprotective Properties of Human Platelets are Lost in Uncontrolled Diabetes Mellitus: A Study in Isolated Rat Hearts

Isabella Russo[1†], Saveria Femminò[1,2†], Cristina Barale[1], Francesca Tullio[1,2], Stefano Geuna[1], Franco Cavalot[3,4], Pasquale Pagliaro[1,2] and Claudia Penna[1,2*]*

[1] *Department of Clinical and Biological Sciences, AOU San Luigi, University of Turin, Turin, Italy,* [2] *Istituto Nazionale Ricerche Cardiovascolari (INRC), Bologna, Italy,* [3] *Internal Medicine and Metabolic Disease Unit, AOU San Luigi, University of Turin, Turin, Italy,* [4] *Ospedale San Luigi Gonzaga, Orbassano, Italy*

Edited by:
Vincenzo Lionetti,
Scuola Sant'Anna di Studi Avanzati, Italy

Reviewed by:
Lucio Barile,
Cardiocentro Ticino, Switzerland
Domenico Cerullo,
Istituto Di Ricerche Farmacologiche Mario Negri, Italy
Giulio Agnetti,
Johns Hopkins University, United States

***Correspondence:**
Pasquale Pagliaro
pasquale.pagliaro@unito.it
Claudia Penna
claudia.penna@unito.it

† These authors have contributed equally to this work.

Platelets affect myocardial damage from ischemia/reperfusion. Redox-dependent sphingosine-1-phosphate production and release are altered in diabetic platelets. Sphingosine-1-phosphate is a double-edged sword for ischemia/reperfusion injury. Therefore, we aimed to verify whether: (1) human healthy- or diabetic-platelets are cardioprotective, (2) sphingosine-1-phosphate receptors and downstream kinases play a role in platelet-induced cardioprotection, and (3) a correlation between platelet redox status and myocardial ischemia/reperfusion injury exists. Isolated rat hearts were subjected to 30-min ischemia and 1-h reperfusion. Infarct size was studied in hearts pretreated with healthy- or diabetic-platelets. Healthy-platelets were co-infused with sphingosine-1-phosphate receptor blocker, ERK-1/2 inhibitor, PI3K antagonist or PKC inhibitor to ascertain the cardioprotective mechanisms. In platelets we assessed (i) aggregation response to ADP, collagen, and arachidonic-acid, (ii) cyclooxygenase-1 levels, and (iii) AKT and ERK-phosphorylation. Platelet sphingosine-1-phosphate production and platelet levels of reactive oxygen species (ROS) were quantified and correlated to infarct size. Infarct size was reduced by about 22% in healthy-platelets pretreated hearts only. This cardioprotective effect was abrogated by either sphingosine-1-phosphate receptors or ERK/PI3K/PKC pathway blockade. Cyclooxygenase-1 levels and aggregation indices were higher in diabetic-platelets than healthy-platelets. Diabetic-platelets released less sphingosine-1-phosphate than healthy-platelets when mechanical or chemically stimulated *in vitro*. Yet, ROS levels were higher in diabetic-platelets and correlated with infarct size. Cardioprotective effects of healthy-platelet depend on the platelet's capacity to activate cardiac sphingosine-1-phosphate receptors and ERK/PI3K/PKC pathways. However, diabetic-platelets release less S1P and lose cardioprotective effects. Platelet ROS levels correlate with infarct size. Whether these redox alterations are responsible for sphingosine-1-phosphate dysfunction in diabetic-platelets remains to be ascertained.

Keywords: cardioprotection, infarct size, ischemia/reperfusion, platelets, sphingosine-1-phosphate, type 2 diabetes mellitus

INTRODUCTION

The role played by platelets in determining cardiac ischemia/reperfusion (I/R) injury is not clear. Studies, conducted in the nineties, suggested that healthy platelets have cardioprotective properties. Indeed, healthy rat platelets resulted protective against myocardial injury induced by I/R in isolated rat hearts and by hypoxia/reoxygenation in cultured adult rat cardiomyocytes (Yang et al., 1993, 1994, 1998, 1999; Yang and Mehta, 1994; Mehta et al., 1999). Subsequently, in a 2002 study, Mirabet et al. (2002) infused pig platelets - collected before or after coronary occlusion - into Langendorff rat hearts, which were subsequently submitted to I/R. Only the pig platelets collected after reperfusion enhanced I/R injury in rat hearts. The authors concluded that the deleterious effect of platelets on reperfused myocardium depends on their activation status.

Recent studies by Cohen and Downey group have shown that $P2Y_{12}$ receptor antagonists (e.g., Cangrelor, Ticagrelor) targeting platelets may exert a cardioprotective effect. Since the cardioprotective mechanism seems not attributable to inhibition of platelet aggregation (Yang et al., 2013a,b; Cohen and Downey, 2014, 2015), the authors suggest that patients treated with these antagonists are benefiting from protective "conditioning pathways" triggered by factors released by platelets. Indeed, these conditioning pathways are very similar to those activated by brief periods of intermittent non-lethal ischemia, before or after a prolonged ischemia, that are the well-known phenomena of pre- and post-conditioning (Cohen and Downey, 2015; Pagliaro and Penna, 2015; Penna et al., 2015). These conditioning phenomena induce the activation of protective pathways and a consequent reduction of I/R injury.

Many endogenous *molecules* could induce conditioning cardioprotection, eliciting specific pathways (Cohen and Downey, 2015; Pagliaro and Penna, 2015; Penna et al., 2015). Platelets are known to release a plethora of molecules, which mediate platelet effects in a variety of conditions, including cardioprotection against I/R injury (Yang et al., 1993; Penna et al., 2005, 2015). A platelet-derived cardioprotective molecule is *Sphingosine 1-phosphate* (S1P), a bioactive lipid mediator abundantly carried and stored by platelets, whose production and release seem *redox-dependent* and related to thromboxane formation, but mechanisms are poorly understood (Yatomi et al., 1995; Tani et al., 2005; Ulrych et al., 2011; Ono et al., 2013; Russo et al., 2017).

S1P exerts its function through five specific cell surface receptors (S1PRs) on target organs (Tani et al., 2005; Vito et al., 2016) and is a double-edged sword: S1P is a potent proinflammatory and mediator of allergic diseases (Maceyka and Spiegel, 2014; Kulinski et al., 2016; Vito et al., 2016), but it is also a potent protectant against I/R injury (Vessey et al., 2009). The S1P cardioprotection seems mediated by interaction with types 1–3 S1PRs, with subsequent activation of the so-called RISK/SAFE pathways (Vessey et al., 2009; Cohen et al., 2016). However, $S1PR_1$ does not appear cardioprotective *in vivo*, whereas a combination of $S1PR_2$ and $S1PR_3$ activation mediates cardioprotection (Means et al., 2007). Nevertheless, these studies revealed that S1P is an important mediator of cardioprotection and could induce either pre- or post-conditioning.

Several pathological conditions, including type 2 diabetes mellitus (T2DM), reduce the efficacy of ischemic conditioning strategies (Ferdinandy et al., 2014). However, unlike cardioprotection induced by ischemic conditioning, $P2Y_{12}$ antagonist-induced conditioning can result in significant attenuation of I/R injury also in diabetic animals (Bell et al., 2015). These last results open an interesting scenario on the role of platelets in cardioprotection. Therefore, in-depth studies on platelet characteristics and their role in cardioprotection are necessary.

Of note, the S1P dynamic is profoundly altered in diabetic conditions (Fox et al., 2011) and diabetes is indicated as a "pro-thrombotic state" in which, among other alterations, *oxidative stress* and *platelet hyperactivity* play crucial roles in the cardiovascular complications (Jung et al., 2015). Therefore, one can wonder: are diabetic platelets cardioprotective and can reduce I/R damage? Although it is well known that diabetic platelets display a certain degree of activation (Watala et al., 2005; Jung et al., 2015), to the best of our knowledge, no studies ascertained whether the platelet-dependent cardioprotective properties are altered in the platelets of T2DM subjects.

Therefore, after a thorough study of platelet characteristics derived from healthy and T2DM subjects, we aimed to verify whether:

(1) *Human* healthy and diabetic platelets are cardioprotective in an isolated rat heart model;
(2) S1P and RISK-pathways play a role in platelet-induced cardioprotection;
(3) a correlation between platelet redox status (an index of platelet dysfunction) and myocardial I/R injury exists.

To these aims, blood samples were collected from voluntary healthy subjects and from T2DM patients. Platelet samples were analyzed for aggregatory aspects, ROS production and S1P release *in vitro* or were used to be infused in isolated hearts before being subjected to I/R protocols either in the absence or in the presence of S1P receptor blocker and RISK-pathway antagonists.

MATERIALS AND METHODS

Subjects and Platelet Preparation

The study was performed on platelets obtained from 35 healthy volunteers and 16 type 2 diabetes mellitus (T2DM) patients. Healthy subjects were not on any antiplatelet therapy nor did they have any history of cardiovascular disease, metabolic syndrome or diabetes. Patients affected by T2DM were recruited among those attending the Metabolic Disease and Diabetes Unit of the San Luigi Gonzaga Hospital in Orbassano (Turin); six of them were at first diagnosis, the others were poorly controlled with glycated hemoglobin A1c (HbA1c) $> 7.5\%$ even though on antidiabetic drugs. All subjects were without previous cardiovascular events and antiplatelet drugs in the previous 2 weeks. The totality of subjects gave informed consent before the investigation and the Ethics Committee of San Luigi

Hospital approved the study, in accordance with the Declaration of Helsinki. The present study is a "case-control study" that raises potential issues of bias due to patient- and voluntary-donor selection. However, data collection was performed by blinded operators on the origin of platelets. Therefore, there is no subjectivity implied in the assessment or bias under these conditions.

Blood samples were collected from the antecubital vein and laboratory measurements were performed after a 12-h overnight fast. Biochemical parameters, including assessment of fasting glucose, total cholesterol, triglycerides, low-density lipoprotein (LDL) cholesterol, high-density lipoprotein (HDL) cholesterol and HbA1c as well as platelet number were measured using routine laboratory methods, performed by the central laboratory of our Hospital.

For studies concerning platelet function, a venous blood sample was withdrawn without stasis after an overnight fast, and anticoagulated with 3.8% sodium citrate, pH 7.4 (vol/vol: 1/9) for aggregation studies in platelet-rich plasma or with a citrate-dextrose solution (ACD; v/v, 1/6) for experiments on washed platelets. Platelet-rich plasma was obtained by using Platelet Function Centrifuge (BioData Corporation, Horsham, PA, United States) designed to provide a rapid separation of platelet-rich plasma by a centrifugation for 30 s and of platelet-poor plasma by a further centrifugation for 120 s. To prepare washed platelets, ACD-anticoagulated platelet-rich plasma, obtained by centrifugation at 100 × *g* for 20 min, underwent further centrifugation at 2000 × *g* for 10 min and pellet was washed two times at 37°C in HEPES-Na buffer (in mmol/L) (10 HEPES Na, 140 NaCl, 2.1 $MgSO_4$, 10 D-glucose, pH 7.4).

Platelet Aggregation Studies

Platelet aggregation studies were carried out in both platelet-rich plasma and whole blood. Aggregation tests in platelet-rich plasma followed light-scattering changes as described by Born (1962) using an eight-channel aggregation system (Platelet Aggregation Profiler, Model PAP-8, BioData Corporation) and were induced by ADP (10 μmol/L), arachidonic acid (AA, 1 mmol/L), and collagen (4 mg/L). Each aggregation test was recorded for 5 min and reported as percent of maximal aggregation.

For platelet aggregation in whole blood by impedance method, citrated blood samples were diluted 1:1 with physiologic saline and the tests were performed in a Chrono-Log Whole Blood Aggregometer, Model 500 at a constant stirring of 1000 rpm. Aggregation was induced with ADP (20 μmol/L), collagen (4 mg/L) or AA (1 mmol/L) and was recorded for 8 min. The maximum increase in resistance, expressed in ohms, was calculated.

Reactive Oxygen Species (ROS) Assay

Intracellular ROS were evaluated in washed platelets by using the sensitive fluorescent indicator DCF-DA oxidized by H_2O_2 to the highly fluorescent DCF (Eruslanov and Kusmartsev, 2010). Washed platelets (6×10^7 ml^{-1}) were exposed to 10 μmol/L cell permeant reagent DCF-DA and DCF fluorescence was measured at basal and after stimulation with AA (100 μmol/L) added just before measuring fluorescence. To examine specific signaling in basal ROS generation, platelets were preincubated for 20 min with the NADPH-oxidase inhibitors APO (10 μmol/L) or DPI (10 μmol/L), or the cyclooxygenase-1 (COX-1) inhibitor indomethacin (INDO, 100 μmol/l) (Gerrits et al., 2010; Barale et al., 2017).

Fluorescence was measured over a 60-min period at 1-min intervals using a plate fluorometer (GloMax-Multi Detection System, Promega Corporation, Madison, WI, United States) fitted with 490 nm excitation and 520 nm emission filters. Fluorescence per minute was calculated for each sample.

Platelet S1P Assay

Washed platelets (500 μl for each sample containing 150×10^6 platelets) were used to measure S1P release both in the absence (resting platelets) and in the presence of a stir bar put into the cuvette (stirring platelets) (Lee et al., 2016). For samples subjected to stirring, the stir bar inside the sample is spun, thus stirring the washed platelets to a 1200 rpm speed at 37°C. An eight-channel optical aggregometer was used (Platelet Aggregation Profiler, Model PAP-8, BioData Corporation) at this end. After 8-min incubation with or without collagen (4 mg/l), all samples were submitted to repeated freeze-thaw cycles to let out the inside components, centrifuged at 3000 rpm for 20 min and supernatants were collected for S1P measurement.

S1P levels were determined by using an Enzyme-Linked Immuno-adsorbent Assay according to manufacturer instructions (Bioassay Technology Laboratory, Shanghai, China). Standard curve range was 5–1500 ng/l, the sensitivity of the kit was 2.34 ng/l, and intra- and inter-assay CV were <8% and <10%, respectively.

Western Blot Analysis in Platelets

To assess the activation state of platelets, we detected the phosphorylation/activation of phosphatidylinositol-3-kinases (PI3K) and extracellular signal-regulated kinases (ERK) in response to platelet agonists: washed platelets were stimulated by collagen (4 mg/L) or AA (100 μmol/L) for 8 min and the amounts of AKT, and pAKT, and ERK-2, pERK-1/2 were evaluated, respectively.

Cyclooxygenase-1 expression was also determined. Washed platelets samples were centrifuged and pellets solubilized in Laemmli buffer and processed as previously described (Russo et al., 2007). Membranes were incubated with rabbit anti-AKT, mouse anti-ERK-2 (Cell Signaling, Danvers, MA, United States), rabbit anti-phospho-Akt-Ser-473, mouse anti-phospho-ERK-1/2-Tyr-204, or mouse anti-COX-1 (Santa Cruz Biotechnology). As secondary antibodies, we used goat anti-mouse (Jackson Immuno Research Lab., West Grove, PA, United States) or goat anti-rabbit (Cell Signaling) antibodies conjugated to horseradish peroxidase. Blots were scanned and densitometrically analyzed by the image analyzer 1D Image Analysis software (Kodak, Rochester, NY, United States).

Animals

Male Wistar rats (n = 75; 4–5-month-old, body weight 400–450 g, Harlan Laboratories Udine, Italy) were used for the *ex vivo* experiments as specified below. Animals were housed under controlled conditions with free access to standard rat diet and tap water. Rats received humane care in compliance with the European Directive 2010/63/EU on the protection of animals used for scientific purposes. The animal protocols followed in this study were approved by the local "Animal Use and Care Committee." In this study, six hearts were discarded due to the very low left ventricular developed pressure or other technical issues after connection to the perfusion line.

Isolated Heart Preparations

Rats were anesthetized, heparinized (800 U/100 g b.w., i.m.), and hearts were rapidly excised, placed in an ice-cold buffer solution, and weighed. Isolated hearts were attached to the perfusion apparatus and retrogradely perfused with oxygenated Krebs–Henseleit buffer solution (KHS) containing (in mM): 127 NaCl, 5.1 KCl, 17.7 $NaHCO_3$, 1.26 $MgCl_4$, 1.5 $CaCl_2$, 11 D-glucose (pH 7.4; 37°C; 95% O_2/5% CO_2). Hearts were kept in a temperature-controlled chamber (37°C), electrically paced at 280 b.p.m. The hearts were perfused in constant-flow mode and to assess the preparation conditions, coronary perfusion pressure and left ventricular pressure were monitored during all experiments (Penna et al., 2005, 2012).

Experimental Groups

To verify the cardioprotective properties of washed PLTs derived from healthy subjects (healthy-PLTs) or diabetic patients (diabetic-PLTs), hearts were assigned to one of the experimental groups described below on the basis of availability of the platelet donor. In all groups, the hearts were subject to 30 min stabilization, and 30 min of normothermic global ischemia followed by 60 min reperfusion (I/R). Protocols are as follow (**Figure 1**):

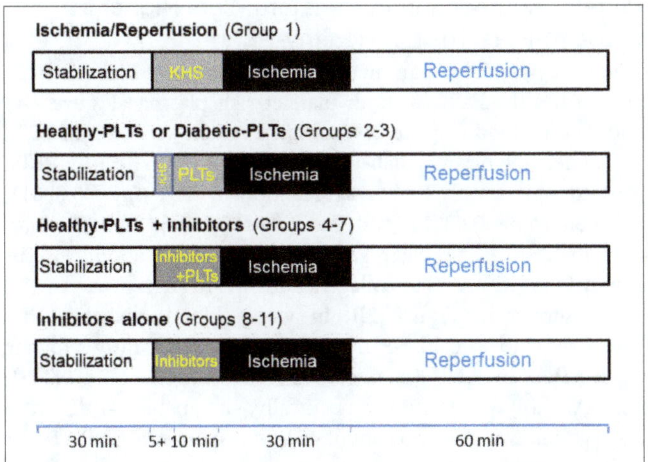

FIGURE 1 | Timeline of experimental protocols. Protocols of ischemia (black boxes) and reperfusion (white boxes) in isolated rat hearts. After stabilization (white boxes), Krebs-Henselite solution (KHS) was infused *via* a collateral line alone or with addition of washed PLTs and/or inhibitors (gray boxes). Washed platelets (PLTs) were given for 10 min before ischemia and inhibitors were given 5 min before PLTs and were stopped at the end of the 10 min of infusion of PLTs (total time infusion for inhibitors was 15 min). For further explanations, see the text.

(1) In the I/R group (n = 7), after stabilization, only the I/R protocol was performed (Bell et al., 2011);
(2) In the healthy-PLT group (n = 8) healthy subject washed platelets diluted in KHS (healthy-PLTs, 3×10^7 ml^{-1}) were infused to the heart, via a collateral line, for 10 min at a flow rate of 12 ml/h; then hearts were subjected to I/R protocol;
(3) In the diabetic-PLT group (n = 8) diabetic patient washed platelets diluted in KHS (diabetic-PLTs, 3×10^7 ml^{-1}) were infused to the heart, via a collateral line, for 10 min at a flow rate of 12 ml/h; then hearts were subjected to I/R protocol.

For groups 2 and 3, each rat heart was treated with the platelets from a single donor and the platelet concentration and time of infusion were similar to those used by Yang et al. (1993). This relatively low concentration of platelets reduces the risk of capillary plugging and loss of myocardial function.

Since only healthy-PLTs affected significantly infarct size (see section "Results"), the following healthy-PLT+inhibitors groups were studied. In these groups, hearts were subjected to infusion of inhibitor alone for 5 min, then a co-infusion with healthy-PLT, for 10 min as in group 2, was performed, and, finally, the hearts underwent I/R protocol. Therefore, inhibitors were infused for a total of 15 min:

(4) In the healthy-PLT+VPC group (n = 5), to ascertain the involvement of S1P receptors in healthy-PLT-induced cardioprotective mechanisms, we used the S1P receptor blocker VPC23019 (1×10^{-6} M) as S1P1/3 receptor antagonist (Davis et al., 2005; Vessey et al., 2009);
(5) In the healthy-PLT+U0126 group (n = 5), to ascertain the involvement of myocardial ERK1/2, we used the ERK1/2 antagonist, U0126 (60×10^{-6} M) (Mochizuki et al., 2013);
(6) In the healthy-PLT+LY group (n = 5), to ascertain the involvement of myocardial PI3K/AKT, we used the PI3K antagonist, LY294002 (5×10^{-5} M) (Penna et al., 2005);
(7) in the healthy-PLT+CHE group (n = 5), to ascertain the involvement of myocardial PKC, we used the PKC antagonist, Chelerythrine (1×10^{-6} M) (Penna et al., 2017);

Inhibitors were also tested alone at the same concentrations and for the same periods:

(8) In the VPC23019 group (n = 5): hearts were subjected to infusion of VPC23019 for 15 min; then hearts were subjected to I/R protocol;
(9) In the U0126 group (n = 4): hearts were subjected to infusion of U0126 for 15 min; then were subjected to I/R protocol;
(10) In the LY294002 group (n = 4): hearts were subjected to infusion of LY294002 for 15 min; then hearts were subjected to I/R protocol;
(11) In the Chelerythrine group (n = 4): hearts were subjected to infusion of Chelerythrine for 15 min; then hearts were subjected to I/R protocol.

Infarct Size Assessment

In order to assess infarct size extension, a gravimetric method was used in a blinded fashion. In briefly at the end of reperfusion, hearts were rapidly removed from perfusion apparatus and the left ventricular tissue was dissected into 2–3 mm circumferential slices. After 20 min of incubation at 37°C in 0.1% solution of nitro-blue tetrazolium in phosphate buffer, unstained necrotic tissue was carefully separated from stained viable tissue and weighed. The necrotic mass was expressed as a percentage of total left ventricular mass, which was considered as risk area (Penna et al., 2014, 2017).

Western Blot Analysis in Hearts

In additional experiments, immunoblot procedures and analyses were conducted as previously described (Penna et al., 2012, 2014, 2017). Immediately after the hearts had undergone I/R (n = 4) or PLT pretreatment (either healthy-PLTs, n = 8, or diabetic-PLTs n = 5), the cardiac specimens were frozen in liquid nitrogen before being stored at −80°C until protein extraction. Myocardial tissues of the above groups were homogenized in a frozen RIPA lysis buffer (Sigma-Aldrich, St. Louis, MO, United States) containing a mixture of protease inhibitors (1 mM of aprotinin, 20 mM of phenylmethylsulfonyl fluoride and 200 mM of sodium orthovanadate). Subsequently, myocardial homogenates were centrifuged at 15,000 × g for 25 min at 4°C for debris removal. Protein concentration was assessed using a Bradford reagent following the procedure described by the manufacturer (Sigma-Aldrich, St. Louis, MO, United States). Equivalent amounts of proteins (80 μg) were loaded and electrophoresed on SDS polyacrylamide gel and transferred to a polyvinylidene difluoride membrane. Membranes were then incubated overnight at 4°C with primary antibodies mouse anti-phospho-ERK-1/2-Tyr-204 (Santa Cruz Biotechnology) or mouse anti-ERK-1/2 (Cell Signaling, Danvers, MA, United States). As secondary antibody, we used goat anti-mouse (Jackson Immuno Research Lab., West Grove, PA, United States). Blots were scanned and densitometrically analyzed by the image analyzer ID Image Analysis software (Kodak, Rochester, NY, United States).

Chemicals

Collagen and arachidonic acid were purchased from Mascia Brunelli Spa (Monza, Milan, Italy). The sources of the specific antibodies are shown in the different sections. The other reagents were obtained from Sigma (St. Louis, MO, United States) if not differently specified.

Statistical Analysis

Data are expressed as mean ± SE. Statistical analysis was performed with one-way analysis of variance (ANOVA) followed by Student's t-test or Newman–Keuls multiple-range test depending on the experiments. P-value ≤ 0.05 was considered to be significant. A linear fit is assessed between ROS production and infarct size. A P-value < 0.05 was considered statistically significant.

RESULTS

The characteristics of study participants are shown in **Table 1**. Healthy volunteers and T2DM subjects were significantly different for BMI ($p < 0.0001$), HbA1c ($p < 0.0001$), fasting glucose ($p < 0.0001$), total cholesterol ($p < 0.0001$), triglycerides

TABLE 1 | Clinical characteristics, laboratory findings, and medications of healthy and T2DM subjects.

	Healthy subjects (n = 35)	T2DM subjects (n = 16)	p-value
M/F	17/18	7/9	
Age (years)	53.0 ± 1	57.1 ± 2	0.08
BMI (kg/m^2)	23.6 ± 0.2	31.6 ± 2	0.0001
HbAlc (%)	5.4 ± 0.1	11.3 ± 0.8	0.0001
Fasting glucose (mg/dl)	84.9 ± 2	320.5 ± 36	0.0001
Total cholesterol (mg/dl)	155.2 ± 4	193.9 ± 13	0.0001
HDL cholesterol (mg/dl)	52.0 ± 1	48.2 ± 2	0.074
Triglycerides (mg/dl)	105.0 ± 4	151.9 ± 22	0.005
LDL cholesterol (mg/dl)	85.7 ± 4	115.4 ± 10	0.002
SBP (mmHg)	120.6 ± 1	122.1 ± 8	0.786
DBP (mmHg)	78.5 ± 0.8	75.6 ± 2	0.093
Platelets (×l0^3/μl)	236.2 ± 5	243.9 ± 8	0.401
Insulin use	–	6 (38%)	
Oral antidiabetic medication use	–	9 (56%)	
Statin use	–	10 (63%)	
Antihypertensive drugs use	–	11 (69%)	

HDL, high-density lipoprotein; LDL, low-density lipoprotein; BMI, body mass index; SBP, systolic blood pressure; DBP, diastolic blood pressure.

($p < 0.005$), and LDL cholesterol ($p < 0.002$). There were no differences between the two groups with regard to age, HDL-cholesterol, platelet number, systolic and diastolic blood pressure.

Platelet Characteristics

We first analyzed platelet (PLT) characteristics in both T2DM and healthy subjects.

Platelet Aggregation Parameters Were Higher in Diabetic-PLTs Than in Healthy-PLTs

Platelet aggregation parameters were studied in diabetic-PLTs and in healthy-PLTs, in both platelet-rich plasma (**Figure 2A**) and whole blood (**Figure 2B**) samples. As shown in **Figure 2A**, in platelet-rich plasma, diabetic-PLTs, compared to healthy-PLTs, showed significantly higher aggregation to ADP ($p < 0.0001$), collagen ($p < 0.0001$), and AA ($p < 0.0001$). In particular, in diabetic-PLTs, the aggregation was higher by about 35% in response to ADP, 47% to collagen, and 30% to AA.

As shown in **Figure 2B**, in whole blood, diabetic-PLTs, compared to healthy-PLTs, showed significantly higher aggregation to ADP ($p < 0.0001$), to collagen ($p < 0.005$), and AA ($p < 0.0001$). Specifically, in diabetic-PLTs, the aggregation was higher by about 45% in response to ADP, 21% to collagen, and 53% to AA.

S1P Release Was Lower in Diabetic-PLTs Than in Healthy-PLTs

The release of S1P was measured in supernatants of washed platelets in *resting* and *stirring* conditions (**Figure 3**). In *resting* platelet samples, S1P levels did not differ significantly between healthy- and diabetic-PLTs both in the absence (149 ± 6 vs.

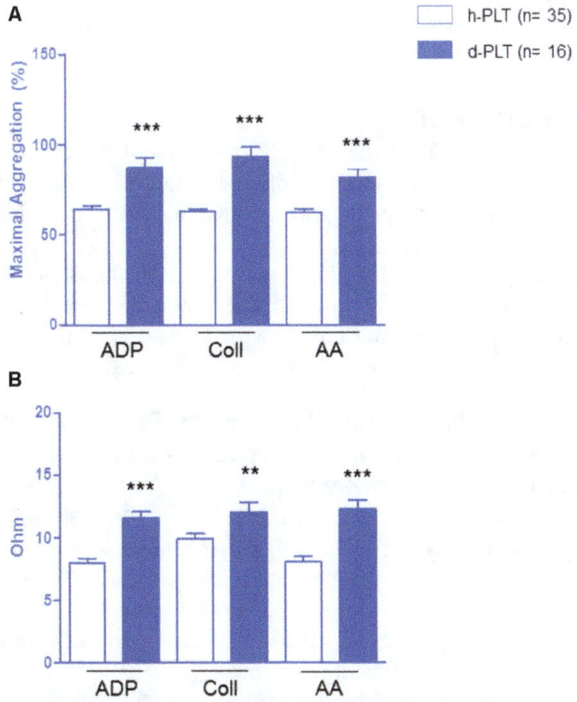

FIGURE 2 | Effect of platelet exposure to different pro-aggregating agents: ADP, collagen (Coll) and arachidonic acid (AA). Platelet aggregation parameters were higher in platelets of diabetic patients (d-PLT) than in those of healthy subjects (h-PLT), in both platelet-rich plasma **(A)** or washed platelets **(B)**. $^{**}p < 0.005$, $^{***}p < 0.0001$ vs. h-PLT (unpaired *t*-test).

112 ± 16 ng/l, p = ns) and in the presence of collagen (171 ± 3 vs. 132 ± 21 ng/l, p = ns).

When samples were subjected to *stirring*, a significant increase in S1P levels was observed in healthy-PLTs (from 149 ± 6 to 218 ± 10 ng/l, $p < 0.0001$) but not in diabetic-PLTs (from 112 ± 16 to 148 ± 13 ng/l, p = ns). Furthermore, S1P levels, in stirring samples, were lower in diabetic-PLTs than in healthy-ones both in the absence (148 ± 13 vs. 218 ± 10 ng/l, $p < 0.001$) and in the presence of collagen (199 ± 6 vs. 270 ± 7 ng/l, $p < 0.0001$).

ROS Levels Were Higher in Diabetic-PLTs Than in Healthy-PLTs

To ascertain whether higher aggregation parameters were associated with higher ROS levels, we used 2′,7′-dihydrodichlorofluoresceine diacetate (DCF-DA) oxidation to detect ROS intracellular concentration. As shown in **Figure 4A**, there was a significantly higher ROS level in resting, non-stimulated diabetic-PLTs than in controls ($p < 0.0001$).

To identify the origin of ROS, measurements were repeated after a 20-min pre-incubation with either apocynin (APO) or diphenyleneiodonium (DPI), two different NADPH-oxidase inhibitors, as well as the COX-1 inhibitor, Indomethacin (INDO). Data revealed that the basal ROS production in diabetic-PLTs is, at least in part, mediated by the activity of NADPH-oxidase and COX-1. In fact, with regard to baseline values, we observed a significant decrease of ROS production in the presence of NADPH-oxidase inhibitors, APO ($p < 0.001$) or DPI ($p < 0.005$), and COX-1 antagonist, INDO ($p < 0.001$). As expected, platelet stimulation with AA increased ROS levels in both healthy-PLTs and diabetic-PLTs (**Figure 4B**). Furthermore, diabetic-PLTs generated a significantly higher ROS amount after stimulation with AA (6 vs. 9 fold increase, $p < 0.0001$).

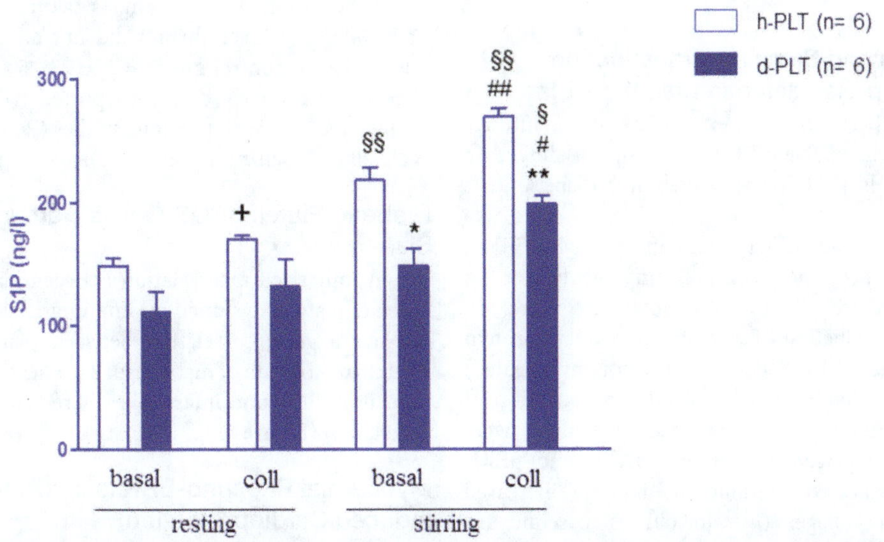

FIGURE 3 | S1P release in washed platelets, in resting and stirring conditions. In resting conditions, S1P levels were not different between platelets from T2DM patients (d-PLT) and platelets from healthy subjects (h-PLT). $+p < 0.05$ vs. resting basal. In stirring samples, S1P levels were lower in d-PLT than in h-PLT both in the absence and in the presence of collagen. $^{*}p < 0.001$, $^{**}p < 0.0001$ vs. healthy-PLT (unpaired *t*-test); $^{\#}p < 0.01$, $^{\#\#}p < 0.005$ vs. corresponding stirring basal; $^{\S}p < 0.005$, $^{\S\S}p < 0.001$ vs. corresponding resting conditions (Newman–Keuls multiple-range test).

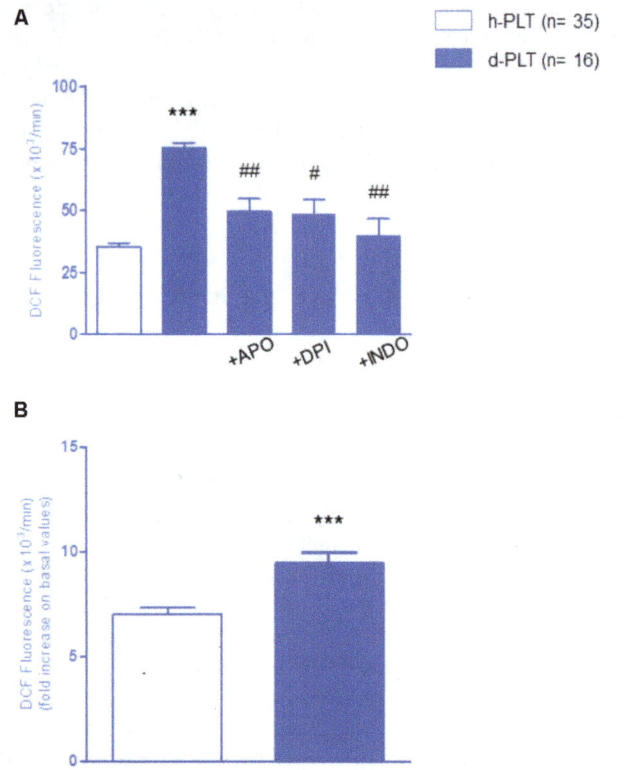

FIGURE 4 | Variation of the intra-platelet level of ROS measured by DCF fluorescence. **(A)** ROS level in resting platelets of diabetic patients (d-PLT) were higher than in resting platelets of healthy subjects (h-PLT). 20-min preincubation with apocynin (APO), diphenyleneiodonium (DPI), or indomethacin (INDO) reduced the levels of ROS produced by d-PLT. **(B)** PLT stimulation with arachidonic acid increased ROS levels in both h-PLTs and d-PLTs. ***$p < 0.0001$ vs. h-PLT; #$p < 0.005$, ##$p < 0.001$ vs. resting d-PLT (paired *t*-test).

COX-1 Expression and Signaling Transduction Molecules Were Up-Regulated in Diabetic-PLTs

We tested the hypothesis that the expression of constitutive COX-1 was higher in diabetic-PLTs. Indeed, as shown in **Figure 5A**, higher levels of COX-1 were present in diabetic-PLTs ($p < 0.0001$).

We argued that phospho-AKT (pAKT) and phospho-ERK-2 levels may be enhanced by the pro-aggregating agents more in diabetic-PLTs than in healthy-PLTs. As shown in **Figure 5B**, in healthy-PLTs and diabetic-PLTs, we found similar protein expression of AKT and ERK-2 (ERK-1 was not investigated) (Woulfe, 2010). To evaluate the agonist-induced activation of the PI-3K and ERK pathways, washed platelet samples were stimulated by either collagen or AA and pAKT and pERK level measured. As expected, the amount of pAKT increased in response to either collagen ($p < 0.0001$ vs. baseline, for both groups) or AA ($p < 0.0001$ vs. baseline for both groups). However, the increase was significantly greater in diabetic-PLTs than healthy-PLTs, for both collagen ($p < 0.01$) and AA ($p < 0.0001$). Similarly, the amount of pERK-2 increased in response to either collagen ($p < 0.0001$ vs. baseline for both groups) or AA ($p < 0.0001$ vs. baseline for both groups). Yet, the increase was greater in diabetic-PLTs than healthy-PLTs, for both collagen ($p < 0.05$) and AA ($p < 0.005$).

Isolated Hearts

Either healthy-PLTs or diabetic-PLTs were tested in isolated rat heart to verify their protective properties. Moreover, to ascertain the cardioprotective pathways activated by platelets, specific antagonists were used.

Of note, platelet infusion, as well as co-infusion with antagonists did not affect coronary perfusion pressure and left ventricular pressure (data not shown). These observations rule out impaired perfusion and plugged capillaries by platelets.

Infarct Size Was Reduced by Healthy-PLTs Pretreatment Only, via S1P Receptors and ERK/PI3K/PKC Pathways

After I/R, in control group infarct size was 59 ± 3% of the left ventricular mass. The 10 min pre-treatment with healthy-PLTs significantly ($p < 0.005$) reduced infarct size to 47 ± 2% of ventricular mass (**Figure 6A**). However, the 10 min pre-treatment with diabetic-PLTs did not reduce infarct size, which was 70 ± 2% of the left ventricular mass (Not Significant vs. I/R group; $p < 0.005$ vs. healthy-PLT group).

To study the role of myocardial S1P receptors and RISK pathway, healthy-PLTs were alternatively co-infused with one of the following compounds: VPC23019 to block cardiac S1P Receptors (types 1 and 3), U0126 to inhibit ERK1/2, LY294002 to inhibit PI3K, or Chelerythrine to block PKC. At the end of reperfusion, in these four inhibitor groups, infarct sizes (66 ± 2%, 61 ± 2%, 61 ± 3%, and 63 ± 3% of the ventricular mass, respectively) were similar to those observed in control I/R hearts, but significantly ($p < 0.005$ for all) higher than in healthy-PLTs group (**Figure 6B**).

The infusion of antagonists alone (VPC23019, U0126, LY294002, or Chelerythrine) did not affect infarct size, which was similar to control group (63 ± 2%, 59 ± 2%, 70 ± 5%, and 65 ± 3%, respectively, data not reported in the figure). These data are in agreement with previous studies (Penna et al., 2005; Vessey et al., 2009; Mochizuki et al., 2013).

Diabetic Platelet ROS Levels Correlate With Infarct Size

We hypothesized a correlation between platelet ROS levels (an index of platelet dysfunction) and infarct size. Indeed **Figure 6C** displays a good correlation between platelet ROS levels and infarct size for data of diabetic-PLTs, whereas between ROS levels in healthy-PLTs and infarct size there is a poor, not significant, correlation (**Figure 6D**).

Myocardial Phospho-ERK Is Involved in Healthy-PLT Induced Cardioprotection

To corroborate data obtained with inhibitors of survival kinases, we measured ERK-1/2 expression and phosphorylation in myocardial tissue of hearts treated with healthy-PLTs. The phosphorylation of ERK-1/2 was greater in hearts pre-treated with healthy-PLTs compared to hearts subjected to I/R

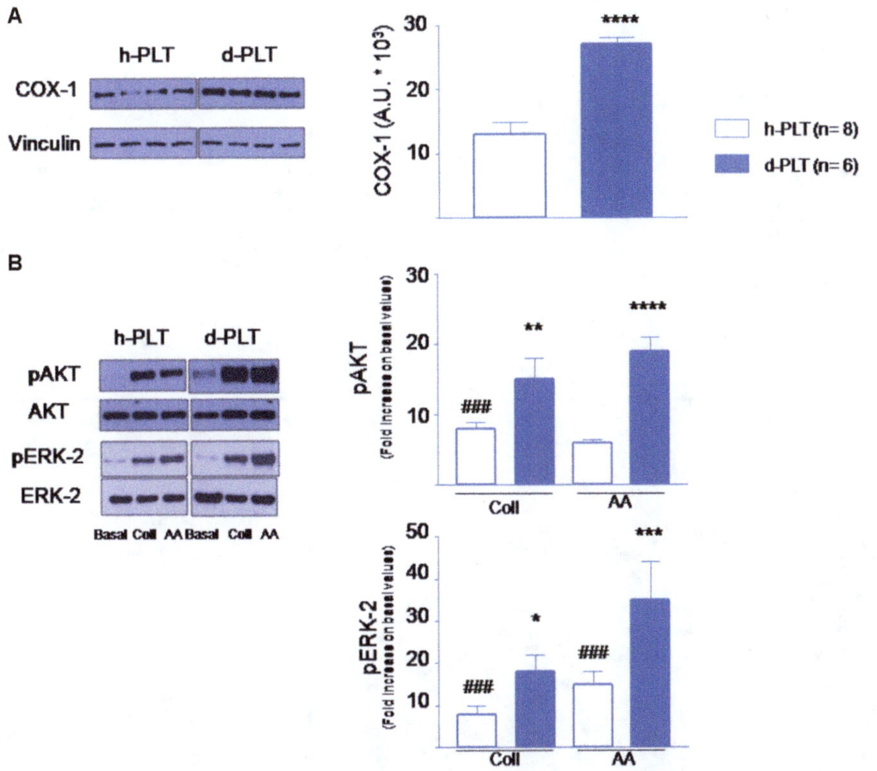

FIGURE 5 | Protein content in platelets determined by Western blot. **(A)** Cyclooxygenase-1 (COX-1) levels were higher in platelets of diabetic patients (d-PLT) than in those of healthy subjects (h-PLT). **(B)** Phosphorylated Protein Kinase B (pAKT) and Phosphorylated Extracellular Signal-regulated Kinase-2 (pERK-2) were increased by collagen (Coll) and arachidonic acid (AA) stimulation in both h-PLT and d-PLT. However, the increases were higher in d-PLTs than in h-PLTs. $^{###}p < 0.0001$ vs. basal level; $^{*}p < 0.05$, $^{**}p < 0.01$, $^{***}p < 0.005$, $^{****}p < 0.0001$ vs. h-PLT (unpaired *t*-test and Newman–Keuls multiple-range test).

($p < 0.0001$; **Figure 7**). A three–fourfold higher pERK/total ERK ratio was observed in healthy-PLT pretreated hearts compared to I/R hearts. In diabetic-PLT pretreated hearts the ratio was not different from that in I/R hearts.

DISCUSSION

The main novel findings of this study are: (1) the heart pretreatment with platelets of healthy humans (healthy-PLTs) reduces infarct size, (2) the cardioprotective properties of healthy-PLTs depend on myocardial S1P receptor and RISK (PI3K-ERK-1/2-PKC) pathway activation, (3) the cardioprotective properties are lost by platelets from T2DM patients (diabetic-PLTs), which release less S1P than healthy-PLTs after mechanical and chemical stimulation, *in vitro*, and (4) the higher is the ROS level in PLTs the higher is infarct size in hearts pretreated with diabetic PLTs.

Pretreatment With Healthy Human PLTs Reduces Infarct Size via S1P Receptor Activation

Pre-treatment with healthy human PLTs limits infarct size in the Langendorff isolated rat heart. Thus, platelets may interact with uninjured organ to trigger protection in hearts subsequently subjected to I/R *ex vivo*. Data are in agreement with previous studies showing that perfusion of isolated rat hearts with platelets from normal rats protects against myocardial dysfunction caused by I/R, improving both biochemical and dynamic cardiac parameters (Yang et al., 1993, 1994; Yang and Mehta, 1994; Mehta et al., 1999). Similar cardioprotection was observed in hearts perfused with platelet supernatant (Yang et al., 1998, 1999), thus suggesting an important role for factors released by platelets.

In our model, the treatment of hearts with VPC23019, an $S1PR_1$ and $S1PR_3$ antagonist (Davis et al., 2005), abrogates cardioprotection induced by healthy-PLTs. Therefore, it is likely that healthy human platelets protect the hearts against I/R injury *via* an S1P mediated mechanism. Indeed, S1P is a platelet factor whose release originates from two pools: one constitutively secreted and located at the plasma membrane, and the other rapidly phosphorylated upon stimulation and mobilized from granules (Yatomi et al., 1995; Tani et al., 2005). This release in the supernatant is influenced by mechanical (stirring) and chemical (collagen) stimuli *in vitro*.

Intriguingly, S1P is a crucial signal molecule abundantly stored in platelets, which displayed a variety of cellular functions, including cardioprotective properties (Chalfant and Spiegel, 2005; Cohen et al., 2016). S1P is stored within the platelets and is released in certain circumstances (Tani et al., 2005).

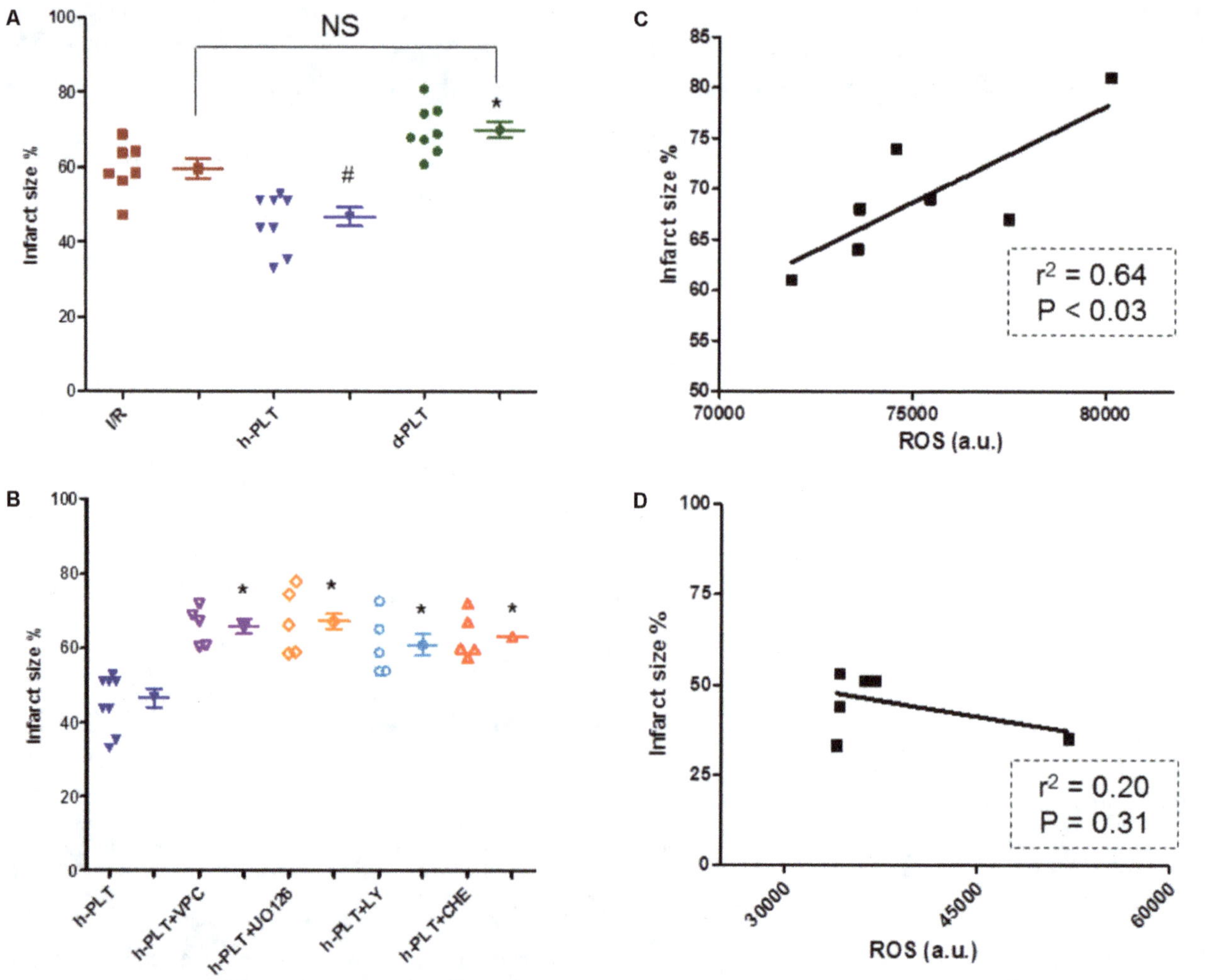

FIGURE 6 | Infarct size expressed as percent of area at risk **(A,B)**, and platelet ROS-infarct size correlations **(C,D)**. **(A)** Washed platelets derived from healthy subjects (h-PLT) limited infarct size. The infarct size in hearts treated with platelets derived from diabetic patients (d-PLT) was higher than that observed in hearts pretreated with h-PLT. **(B)** The infarct size limitation effects of h-PLTs was abrogated by the blocker of S1P receptors, VPC23019, the antagonist of ERK1/2, U0126, the inhibitor of PI3K, LY or the antagonist of PKC, CHE. *$p < 0.005$ vs. h-PLT; #$p < 0.005$ vs. I/R; NS, not significant (Newman–Keuls multiple-range test). **(C)** Correlation between ROS platelet levels and infarct size for the d-PLT group ($n = 7$; linear regression). **(D)** correlation between ROS platelet levels and infarct size for the h-PLT group ($n = 7$; linear regression).

Several studies performed in animal and *in vitro* models have proposed that S1P possesses cardioprotective effects (Kupperman et al., 2000; Jin et al., 2002; Zhang et al., 2007; Karliner, 2013; Maceyka and Spiegel, 2014). Moreover, S1P protects cultured rat neonatal cardiomyocytes from ischemia-induced cell death (Jin et al., 2002; Karliner, 2013). Since only $S1PR_1$, $S1PR_2$, and $S1PR_3$ are the receptor subtypes expressed in cardiac myocytes and endothelial cells (Peters and Alewijnse, 2007; Karliner, 2009; Means and Brown, 2009; Zhang et al., 2013), it is likely that these receptors play a major role in cardioprotection by healthy-PLT pretreatment. Indeed, in the heart binding of S1P to $S1PR_1$ leads to activation of ERK1/2 and binding to the $S1PR_3$ receptor promotes the activation of PI3K/AKT (Knapp, 2011; Somers et al., 2012). Nevertheless, it is likely that the cardioprotective effect of S1P is the result of a co-operation of the three receptors expressed by the heart (Means et al., 2007; Vessey et al., 2009; Cohen et al., 2016). That is why blocking both $S1PR_1$ and $S1PR_3$ with VPC23019, we blocked the platelet cardioprotective effects. It is unlikely that VPC23019 interfered with platelet S1P receptors because platelets express mainly $S1PR_2$ and $S1PR_4$ (Randriamboavonjy et al., 2009; Onuma et al., 2017) (see also below "Methodological considerations *and limitations of the study*").

Infarct Size Limitation by Healthy-PLTs Is Reversed by RISK (PI3K, ERK-1/2, and PKC) Pathway Inhibition

It has been reported that nitric oxide release may mediate cardioprotection by S1P (Egom et al., 2011). Since in the RISK pathway AKT is upstream to nitric oxide synthase, we verified whether inhibitors of RISK pathway may avoid

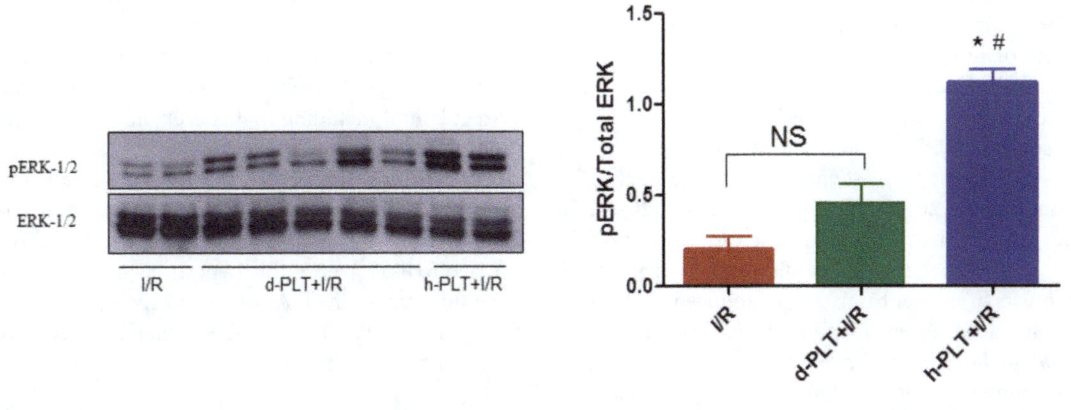

FIGURE 7 | Phosphorylation of extracellular signal-regulated kinases (ERK-1/2) in lysates from hearts subjected to I/R only (control) or pre-treated with d-PLTs (washed platelets derived from diabetic patients) or h-PLTs (washed platelets derived from healthy subjects). Representative western blot of ERK-1/2 phosphorylation and total ERK-1/2 of protein extract from control I/R ($n = 4$), d-PLTs ($n = 5$), and h-PLTs ($n = 8$) hearts. Histograms represent the ratio of phosphorylated over total ERK protein expression. Data suggest that pretreatment with h-PLTs induces an increase in ERK-1/2 phosphorylation with respect to I/R only. $^{*}P < 0.0001$ vs. *I/R*; $^{\#}P < 0.001$ vs. d-PLTs (Newman–Keuls multiple-range test).

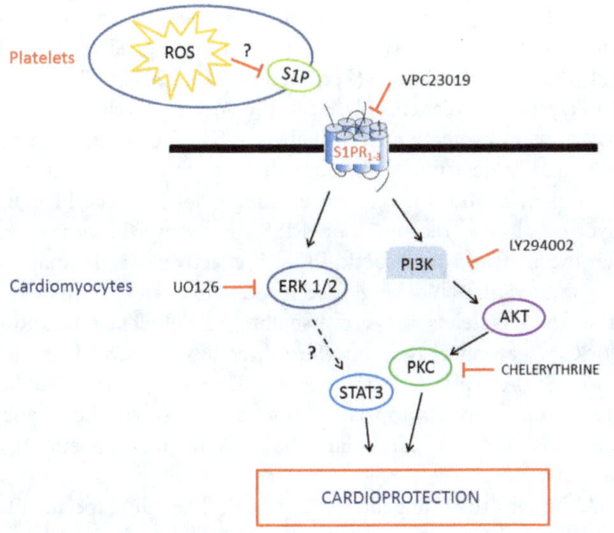

FIGURE 8 | Schematic representation of the intracellular pathway involved in the platelet/S1P cardioprotection.

platelet-induced cardioprotection. Indeed, healthy-PLT-induced cardioprotection was completely abolished by pre-treating the heart with LY294002 to block PI3K, or Chelerythrine to block PKC, as well as U0126 to inhibit ERK-1/2. Thus, suggesting a pivotal role of these survival kinases in the platelet-induced cardioprotection (**Figure 8**). A role which is corroborated by myocardial Western blot data, revealing elevated levels of *pERK-1/2* in healthy-PLT pretreated hearts only. This kinase phosphorylation is usually observed in conditioning treatments, with a peak of the pERK/total ERK ratio 10–15 min after the end of ischemia and a progressive reduction thereafter (Ferdinandy et al., 2014; Penna et al., 2014; Cohen and Downey, 2015). A three-fourfold higher pERK/total ERK ratios in hearts pretreated with healthy-PLTs is a strong indication of kinase involvement in protection, especially if we consider that healthy-PLT pretreated hearts have just a 30% more vital tissue than control I/R hearts.

Moreover, since STAT3 seems to be downstream to ERK (Knapp, 2011; Somers et al., 2012) in ongoing experiments we tested whether healthy or diabetic PLTs can activate myocardial STAT3. Indeed, we found that h-PLT treated hearts display a higher pSTAT3 level than d-PLT treated hearts (see **Supplementary Materials**).

However, it has been also shown that in some circumstances, platelets may contribute to initiation and propagation of I/R myocardial injury (Aiken et al., 1981; Vanhoutte and Houston, 1985; Yee et al., 1986; Patel et al., 2001; Seligmann et al., 2013). These apparently conflicting reports may reflect different experimental designs: platelets introduced into the coronary system of heart preparations not before but during or after ischemia, atherosclerotic coronary arteries or coronary endothelial barrier failure. In particular, it has been suggested that the deleterious effects of platelets on reperfused myocardium depend on their activation status, which is enhanced by the previous exposure to I/R injured myocardium (Mirabet et al., 2002). In other words, it seems that in I/R scenario platelet deleterious effects are due to interaction with injured tissues and/or platelet pre-activation. Therefore, we studied the "*hyperreactive*" diabetic-PLTs.

Cardioprotective Properties Are Lost by Diabetic-PLTs

The cardioprotective properties seen for healthy-PLTs are lost by diabetic-PLTs. In fact, infarct size after intracoronary pretreatment with diabetic-PLTs is significantly higher than that observed in hearts pre-treated with healthy-PLTs and not significantly different from the control I/R hearts. This is in agreement with the idea that activated platelets lose the cardioprotective properties (Mirabet et al., 2002).

Multiple factors may cause dysregulation of platelet signaling pathways leading to a hyper-reactive platelet phenotype. Indeed, diabetic subjects of our study were not only characterized by hyperglycemia and uncontrolled diabetes but also by other dysmetabolic conditions such as obesity and dyslipidemia, commonly associated with T2DM, and each of them may contribute to the diabetic-PLT hyper-reactivity observed in this population (Russo, 2012; Morange and Alessi, 2013). In this study, we confirm that, in comparison with healthy-PLTs, platelets from T2DM patients show: (a) higher aggregating response to agonists (b) higher basal and AA-induced production of ROS, (c) enhanced levels of COX-1 and (d) increased levels of *phospho-AKT* and *phospho-ERK-2* upon stimulation with agonists, more in diabetic than healthy platelets, thus confirming the hyper-reactivity of diabetic platelets. However, unlike myocardium, these two kinases are not linked to a survival signaling in platelets (Kovacsovics et al., 1995; Aharonovitz and Granot, 1996). Indeed, *following stimuli*, ERK and AKT regulate platelet activation and function, such as adhesion or secretory changes, and are actively involved in conveying signals from several pathways leading to platelet activation (Kovacsovics et al., 1995; Aharonovitz and Granot, 1996).

Our findings on platelet function in T2DM subjects fit into the general picture of the current research that describes platelet hyper-reactivity as responsible, at least in part, of the prothrombotic state in T2DM (Jung et al., 2015). We also demonstrate that higher ROS levels in diabetic-PLTs are, at least in part, due to enhanced production by NADPH-oxidase and COX-1 activity. Indeed, ROS generation in diabetic-PLTs is mostly produced by COX-1 activity, as shown by the significant reduction of ROS levels using the COX-1 inhibitor, INDO. A role is also played by the pro-oxidant enzyme NADPH-oxidase, as shown by the significant reduction of ROS levels when diabetic-PLTs were preincubated with two different NADPH-oxidase inhibitors, APO or DPI. Several reports have suggested that ROS represent a new modulator of platelet activity and ROS generated by platelets have a direct role in the control of their responsiveness (Vazzana et al., 2012).

The correlation between platelet ROS levels in diabetic platelets and the extension of infarct size suggests that the redox status in these platelets may play a pivotal role in influencing their cardiac effects. The absence of correlation for healthy platelets suggests that a certain threshold of ROS should be reached to affect protective properties. Of note, a complete prevention of the post-ischemic cardio-depressive effects by platelets – administrated during ischemia or reperfusion on isolated guinea pig hearts – was observed after platelet pretreatment with the NADPH-oxidase inhibitor, DPI (Seligmann et al., 2013). These data are in agreement with our data that ROS levels in hyperactive platelets are correlated to the extension of I/R injury and that platelet ROS derive, at least in part, from NADPH-oxidase. Nevertheless, correlation is not causality and our results need further studies to clarify the role of ROS.

Here, we show that diabetic platelets release less S1P when mechanically (*stirring*) or chemically (collagen) stimulated. Our findings are in line with the observation that diabetic platelets have a dysregulation of the S1P component ready to be mobilized (Książek et al., 2015). Moreover, the fact that S1P release is compromised is in agreement with the observation that diabetic platelets display higher expression of signs and factors of dysregulation, including higher ROS amount produced at basal condition and after stimulation with AA. In other words, the loss of protective properties observed in diabetic platelets could be linked to the altered redox and aggregatory conditions of these platelets that would alter the modality and/or quantity of released S1P. However, this hypothesis needs more experiments to be fully ascertained. Also, the consequences and mechanisms of S1P dysregulation in diabetic platelets need to be further investigated.

Methodological Considerations and Limitations of the Study

The main aim of the present study was to ascertain the mechanisms of platelet-induced cardioprotection. However, diabetic PLTs were not protective and it remains to ascertain the reasons for this ineffectiveness. Indeed, the use of a normal heart allowed us to rule out that the lack of protection is due to myocardial resistance to protection, typical of diabetes and other co-morbidities (Ferdinandy et al., 2014). The defect is likely within diabetic platelets: the impaired release of S1P may prevent protection from diabetic-PLTs. However, it cannot be so easily determined because these platelets are ineffective in influencing the infarct size in Langendorff hearts: blocking myocardial S1P receptors or RISK pathway will not reveal the mechanism of diabetic-PLTs ineffectiveness. It may be also argued that blocking ROS production with antioxidants in washed platelets may reverse the platelet defect but ROS blockers/scavengers may interfere directly with myocardial I/R injury and/or platelet S1P release. Therefore, future studies should envision appropriate protocols to solve these open questions and, in particular, the reasons for diabetic-PLTs ineffectiveness.

Although the Langendorff's model, like all experimental paradigms, has disadvantages and advantages, it is a useful paradigm for studying the role of cardioprotective procedures (Bell et al., 2011). Indeed, Langendorff's model allows to subjecting the heart to a "clean" test, and to remove unwanted interferences by blood cells, protein and other "confounding variables," such as temperature, perfusion, and neuro-hormonal influences. Indeed, experiments performed on Langendorff's murine model provided very strong data on the cardioprotective effect of S1P (Jin et al., 2002; Lecour et al., 2002; Vessey et al., 2006, 2008).

It is unlikely that the $S1PR_{1/3}$ antagonist, VPC23019, interfered with the capacity of platelets to release S1P. It has been reported that human platelets may express types 1, 2, and 4 of S1PRs (Hla et al., 2012; Urtz et al., 2015). However, Fleming and co-workers were able to detect $S1PR_2$, but not $S1PR_1$ on human platelets (Randriamboavonjy et al., 2009); in this study, $S1PR_2$ displayed a pro-aggregating role. In another study, it has been suggested that S1P suppresses collagen-induced aggregation *via* $S1PR_4$, but not through $S1PR_1$ in human platelets

(Onuma et al., 2017). Therefore, it seems that human platelets express $S1PR_2$ and $S1PR_4$, with a pro- and anti-aggregant role, respectively. Whether $S1PR_1$ is present and/or play a role seems controversial. Therefore, VPC23019 may not interfere with the principal receptors present on platelets, but it is specific for the receptors expressed by the cardiac tissues. Nevertheless, S1PRs are involved in platelet-induced cardioprotection.

We used a commercially available ELISA kit for the assessment of S1P release in washed platelets. This differs from protocol usually performed to measure S1P levels in serum or plasma samples where high-density lipoproteins are the major plasma carriers for S1P. Clearly, S1P values in our study are not comparable to those obtained in blood/plasma samples.

We used washed platelets, therefore it is unlikely that the S1P was already in the perfusate. Only the S1P released by circulating platelets may be involved in the cardioprotective effect. Indeed, stirring may simulate the circulating conditions that allow the release of larger quantities of S1P. Nevertheless, in future studies, it might be worthwhile to test whether platelet-derived supernatant can be protective *via* S1P mechanism.

In summary, three key observations regarding the platelet function and role in I/R scenario were made in this study: (1) S1P/S1PRs play important roles in determining healthy-platelet-induced cardioprotection *via* myocardial RISK pathway, in an isolated rat heart model, (2) these cardioprotective properties are lost by diabetic platelets, which produce higher levels of ROS and lower levels of S1P when stimulated *in vitro*, and (3) infarct size correlates with the amount of ROS produced by diabetic platelets.

CONCLUSION

Here we provide evidence that human healthy platelets exert cardioprotective effects *via* activation of an S1P related mechanism. It is likely that myocardial RISK pathway plays a pivotal role in platelet-induced cardioprotection. Our data also suggest that alterations in ROS production and in S1P release may be involved in the impairment of function and the loss of cardioprotective properties by diabetic platelets. Since plasma S1P concentration is reduced in patients with myocardial infarction (Knapp et al., 2009), its modulation by drugs targeting platelets might be very important and need to be better understood. Since exosomes greatly contribute to platelet activity, whether and how the platelet-induced cardioprotection is linked to the well-known exosome-induced cardioprotection (Barile et al., 2014, 2018) remain to be elucidated. Further studies in this direction are warranted.

AUTHOR CONTRIBUTIONS

CP, IR, and PP conception and design of the experiments. CB and IR performed the experiments on isolated platelets and western blot analyses for both platelets and myocardium. CP, FT, and SF performed the I/R experiments on isolated hearts. CB, CP, FC, FT, PP, IR, and SF analysis and interpretation of the data. CP, IR, SF, and PP drafted the article. CP, FC, PP, IR, SF, and SG revised the manuscript critically for important intellectual content.

FUNDING

This work was supported by the University of Turin, Ricerca Locale Ex-60% (Grants: PAGP_RIC_LOC_15_01; PAGP_RILO_16_01; RUSI_RILO_17_01).

ACKNOWLEDGMENTS

The authors thank Prof. Giuseppe Alloatti (University of Turin) for his help in the intellectual discussions regarding platelet factors and ischemia/reperfusion injury. This article is based upon work from COST Action EU-CARDIOPROTECTION CA16225 supported by COST (European Cooperation in Science and Technology).

FIGURE S1 | Expression of extracellular signal-regulated kinases (ERK-1/2) in lysates from hearts subjected to ischemia/reperfusion only (I/R) or pre-treated with platelets from healthy subjects (hPLT+IR).

FIGURE S2 | Phosphorylation of extracellular signal-regulated kinases (pERK-1/2) in lysates from hearts subjected to ischemia/reperfusion only (I/R) or pre-treated with platelets from healthy subjects (hPLT+IR).

FIGURE S3 | Expression of protein kinase B (AKT) in platelets from healthy and Type 2 Diabetes Mellitus (T2DM) subjects in the absence (basal) or in the presence of collagen (coll) or arachidonic acid (AA).

FIGURE S4 | Expression of ciclooxygenase-1 (COX-1) in platelets from healthy and Type 2 Diabetes Mellitus (T2DM) subjects.

FIGURE S5 | Expression of extracellular signal-regulated kinase-2 (ERK-2) in platelets from healthy and Type 2 Diabetes Mellitus (T2DM) subjects in the absence (basal) or in the presence of collagen (coll) or arachidonic acid (AA).

FIGURE S6 | Phosphorylation of protein kinase B (pAKT) in platelets from healthy and Type 2 Diabetes Mellitus (T2DM) subjects in the absence (basal) or in the presence of collagen (coll) or arachidonic acid (AA).

FIGURE S7 | Phosphorylation of extracellular signal-regulated kinases (pERK-1/2) in platelets from healthy and Type 2 Diabetes Mellitus (T2DM) subjects in the absence (basal) or in the presence of collagen (coll) or arachidonic acid (AA).

FIGURE S8 | Expression of vinculin in platelets from healthy and Type 2 Diabetes Mellitus (T2DM) subjects.

FIGURE S9 | Expression of extracellular signal-regulated kinases (ERK-1/2) in lysates from hearts subjected to ischemia/reperfusion only (I/R), pre-treated with platelets from Type 2 Diabetes Mellitus (T2DM) subjects (dPLT+IR) or healthy (hPLT+IR).

FIGURE S10 | Phosphorylation of extracellular signal-regulated kinases (pERK-1/2) in lysates from hearts subjected to ischemia/reperfusion only (I/R), pre-treated with platelets from Type 2 Diabetes Mellitus (T2DM) subjects (dPLT+IR) or healthy (hPLT+IR).

FIGURE S11 | Phosphorylation of STAT-3 (pSTAT-3) in lysates from hearts subjected to ischemia/reperfusion only (I/R), pre-treated with platelets from healthy (hPLT+IR) or Type 2 Diabetes Mellitus (T2DM) subjects (dPLT+IR).

REFERENCES

Aharonovitz, O., and Granot, Y. (1996). Stimulation of mitogen-activated protein kinase and Na+/H+ exchanger in human platelets. Differential effect of phorbol ester and vasopressin. *J. Biol. Chem.* 271, 16494–16499. doi: 10.1074/jbc.271.28.16494

Aiken, J. W., Shebuski, R. J., Miller, O. V., and Gorman, R. R. (1981). Endogenous prostacyclin contributes to the efficacy of a thromboxane synthetase inhibitor for preventing coronary artery thrombosis. *J. Pharmacol. Exp. Ther.* 219, 299–308.

Barale, C., Buracco, S., Cavalot, F., Frascaroli, C., Guerrasio, A., and Russo, I. (2017). Glucagon-like peptide 1-related peptides increase nitric oxide effects to reduce platelet activation. *Thromb. Haemost.* 117, 1115–1128. doi: 10.1160/TH16-07-0586

Barile, L., Cervio, E., Lionetti, V., Milano, G., Ciullo, A., and Biemmi, V., et al. (2018). Cardioprotection by cardiac progenitor cell-secreted exosomes:Role of pregnancy-associated plasma protein-A. *Cardiovasc. Res.* 114, 992–1005. doi: 10.1093/cvr/cvy055

Barile, L., Lionetti, V., Cervio, E., Matteucci, M., Gherghiceanu, M., Popescu, L. M., et al. (2014). Extracellular vesicles from human cardiac progenitor cells inhibit cardiomyocyte apoptosis and improve cardiac function after myocardial infarction. *Cardiovasc. Res.* 103, 530–541. doi: 10.1093/cvr/cvu167

Bell, R. M., Mocanu, M. M., and Yellon, D. M. (2011). Retrograde heart perfusion: the Langendorff technique of isolated heart perfusion. *J. Mol. Cell. Cardiol.* 50, 940–950. doi: 10.1016/j.yjmcc.2011.02.018

Bell, R. M., Sivaraman, V., Kunuthur, S. P., Cohen, M. V., Downey, J. M., and Yellon, D. M. (2015). Cardioprotective properties of the platelet P2Y12 receptor inhibitor, cangrelor: protective in diabetics and reliant upon the presence of blood. *Cardiovasc. Drugs Ther.* 29, 415–418. doi: 10.1007/s10557-015-6609-2

Born, G. V. (1962). Aggregation of blood platelets by adenosine diphosphate and its reversal. *Nature* 194, 927–929. doi: 10.1038/194927b0

Chalfant, C. E., and Spiegel, S. (2005). Sphingosine 1-phosphate and ceramide 1-phosphate: expanding roles in cell signaling. *J. Cell Sci.* 118, 4605–4612. doi: 10.1242/jcs.02637

Cohen, M. V., and Downey, J. M. (2014). Combined cardioprotectant and antithrombotic actions of platelet P2Y12 receptor antagonists in acute coronary syndrome: just what the doctor ordered. *J. Cardiovasc. Pharmacol. Ther.* 19, 179–190. doi: 10.1177/1074248413508465

Cohen, M. V., and Downey, J. M. (2015). Signalling pathways and mechanisms of protection in pre- and postconditioning: historical perspective and lessons for the future. *Br. J. Pharmacol.* 172, 1913–1932. doi: 10.1111/bph.12903

Cohen, M. V., Yang, X. M., White, J., Yellon, D. M., Bell, R. M., and Downey, J. M. (2016). Cangrelor-mediated cardioprotection requires platelets and sphingosine phosphorylation. *Cardiovasc. Drugs Ther.* 30, 229–232. doi: 10.1007/s10557-015-6633-2

Davis, M. D., Clemens, J. J., Macdonald, T. L., and Lynch, K. R. (2005). Sphingosine 1-phosphate analogs as receptor antagonists. *J. Biol. Chem.* 280, 9833–9341. doi: 10.1074/jbc.M412356200

Egom, E. E., Mohamed, T. M., Mamas, M. A., Shi, Y., Liu, W., Chirico, D., et al. (2011). Activation of Pak1/Akt/eNOS signaling following sphingosine-1-phosphate release as part of a mechanism protecting cardiomyocytes against ischemic cell injury. *Am. J. Physiol. Heart Circ. Physiol.* 301, H1487–H1495. doi: 10.1152/ajpheart.01003.2010

Eruslanov, E., and Kusmartsev, S. (2010). Identification of ROS using oxidized DCFDA and flow-cytometry. *Methods Mol. Biol.* 594, 57–72. doi: 10.1007/978-1-60761-411-1_4

Ferdinandy, P., Hausenloy, D. J., Heusch, G., Baxter, G. F., and Schulz, R. (2014). Interaction of risk factors, comorbidities, and comedications with ischemia/reperfusion injury and cardioprotection by preconditioning, postconditioning, and remote conditioning. *Pharmacol. Rev.* 66, 1142–1174. doi: 10.1124/pr.113.008300

Fox, T. E., Bewley, M. C., Unrath, K. A., Pedersen, M. M., Anderson, R. E., Jung, D. Y., et al. (2011). Circulating sphingolipid biomarkers in models of type 1 diabetes. *J. Lipid Res.* 52, 509–517. doi: 10.1194/jlr.M010595

Gerrits, A. J., Koekman, C. A., van Haeften, T. W., and Akkerman, J. W. (2010). Platelet tissue factor synthesis in type 2 diabetic patients is resistant to inhibition by insulin. *Diabetes* 59, 1487–1495. doi: 10.2337/db09-1008

Hla, T., Galvani, S., Rafii, S., and Nachman, R. (2012). S1P and the birth of platelets. *J. Exp. Med.* 209, 2137–2140. doi: 10.1084/jem.20122284

Jin, Z. Q., Zhou, H. Z., Zhu, P., Honbo, N., Mochly-Rosen, D., Messing, R. O., et al. (2002). Cardioprotection mediated by sphingosine-1-phosphate and ganglioside GM-1 in wild-type and PKC epsilon knockout mouse hearts. *Am. J. Physiol. Heart Circ. Physiol.* 282, H1970–H1977. doi: 10.1152/ajpheart.01029.2001

Jung, J. H., Tantry, U. S., Gurbel, P., and Jeong, Y. H. (2015). Current antiplatelet treatment strategy in patients with diabetes mellitus. *Diabetes Metab. J.* 39, 95–113. doi: 10.4093/dmj.2015.39.2.95

Karliner, J. S. (2009). Sphingosine kinase and sphingosine 1-phosphate in cardioprotection. *J. Cardiovasc. Pharmacol.* 53, 189–197. doi: 10.1097/FJC.0b013e3181926706

Karliner, J. S. (2013). Sphingosine kinase and sphingosine 1-phosphate in the heart: a decade of progress. *Biochim. Biophys. Acta* 1831, 203–212. doi: 10.1016/j.bbalip.2012.06.006

Knapp, M. (2011). Cardioprotective role of sphingosine-1-phosphate. *J. Physiol. Pharmacol.* 62, 601–207.

Knapp, M., Baranowski, M., Czarnowski, D., Lisowska, A., Zabielski, P., Górski, J., et al. (2009). Plasma sphingosine-1-phosphate concentration is reduced in patients with myocardial infarction. *Med. Sci. Monit.* 15, CR490–CR493.

Kovacsovics, T. J., Bachelot, C., Toker, A., Vlahos, C. J., Duckworth, B., Cantley, L. C., et al. (1995). Phosphoinositide 3-kinase inhibition spares actin assembly in activating platelets but reverses platelet aggregation. *J. Biol. Chem.* 270, 11358–11366. doi: 10.1074/jbc.270.19.11358

Książek, M., Chacińska, M., Chabowski, A., and Baranowski, M. (2015). Sources, metabolism, and regulation of circulating sphingosine-1-phosphate. *J. Lipid Res.* 56, 1271–1281. doi: 10.1194/jlr.R059543

Kulinski, J. M., Muńoz-Cano, R., and Olivera, A. (2016). Sphingosine-1-phosphate and other lipid mediators generated by mast cells as critical players in allergy and mast cell function. *Eur. J. Pharmacol.* 778, 56–67. doi: 10.1016/j.ejphar.2015.02.058

Kupperman, E., An, S., Osborne, N., Waldron, S., and Stainier, D. Y. (2000). A sphingosine-1-phosphate receptor regulates cell migration during vertebrate heart development. *Nature* 406, 192–195. doi: 10.1038/35018092

Lecour, S., Smith, R. M., Woodward, B., Opie, L. H., Rochette, L., and Sack, M. N. (2002). Identification of a novel role for sphingolipid signaling in TNF alpha and ischemic preconditioning mediated cardioprotection. *J. Mol. Cell Cardiol.* 34, 509–518. doi: 10.1006/jmcc.2002.1533

Lee, H., Kim, G., Lim, C., Lee, B., and Shin, S. (2016). A simple method for activating the platelets used in microfluidic platelet aggregation tests: stirring-induced platelet activation. *Biomicrofluidics* 10:064118. doi: 10.1063/1.4972077

Maceyka, M., and Spiegel, S. (2014). Sphingolipid metabolites in inflammatory disease. *Nature* 510, 58–67. doi: 10.1038/nature13475

Means, C. K., and Brown, J. H. (2009). Sphingosine-1-phosphate receptor signalling in the heart. *Cardiovasc. Res.* 82, 193–200. doi: 10.1093/cvr/cvp086

Means, C. K., Xiao, C. Y., Li, Z., Zhang, T., Omens, J. H., Ishii, I., et al. (2007). Sphingosine 1-phosphate S1P2 and S1P3 receptor-mediated Akt activation protects against in vivo myocardial ischemia-reperfusion injury. *Am. J. Physiol. Heart Circ. Physiol.* 292, H2944–H2951. doi: 10.1152/ajpheart.01331.2006

Mehta, J. L., Yang, B. C., Strates, B. S., and Mehta, P. (1999). Role of TGF-beta1 in platelet-mediated cardioprotection during ischemia-reperfusion in isolated rat hearts. *Growth Factors* 16, 179–190. doi: 10.3109/08977199909002128

Mirabet, M., Garcia-Dorado, D., Inserte, J., Barrabés, J. A., Lidón, R. M., Soriano, B., et al. (2002). Platelets activated by transient coronary occlusion exacerbate ischemia-reperfusion injury in rat hearts. *Am. J. Physiol. Heart Circ. Physiol.* 283, H1134–H1141. doi: 10.1152/ajpheart.00065.2002

Mochizuki, T., Jiang, Q., Katoh, T., Aoki, K., and Sato, S. (2013). Quality of cardiopulmonary resuscitation affects cardioprotection by induced hypothermia at 34 °C against ischemia/reperfusion injury in a rat isolated heart model. *Shock* 39, 527–532. doi: 10.1097/SHK.0b013e318294e259

Morange, P. E., and Alessi, M. C. (2013). Thrombosis in central obesity and metabolic syndrome: mechanisms and epidemiology. *Thromb. Haemost.* 110, 669–680. doi: 10.1160/TH13-01-0075

Ono, Y., Kurano, M., Ohkawa, R., Yokota, H., Igarashi, K., Aoki, J., et al. (2013). Sphingosine 1-phosphate release from platelets during clot formation: close correlation between platelet count and serum sphingosine 1-phosphate concentration. *Lipids Health Dis.* 12:20. doi: 10.1186/1476-511X-12-20

Onuma, T., Tanabe, K., Kito, Y., Tsujimoto, M., Uematsu, K., Enomoto, Y., et al. (2017). Sphingosine 1-phosphate (S1P) suppresses the collagen-induced activation of human platelets via S1P4 receptor. *Thromb. Res.* 156, 91–100. doi: 10.1016/j.thromres.2017.06.001

Pagliaro, P., and Penna, C. (2015). Redox signalling and cardioprotection: translatability and mechanism. *Br. J. Pharmacol.* 172, 1974–1995. doi: 10.1111/bph.12975

Patel, M. B., Kilgore, K. S., and Ortolano, G. A. (2001). Conditioned blood reperfusion during angioplasty (CoBRA) treatment of acute myocardial infarction. *Perfusion* 16(Suppl.), 39–49. doi: 10.1177/026765910101600i106

Penna, C., Alloatti, G., Cappello, S., Gattullo, D., Berta, G., Mognetti, B., et al. (2005). Platelet-activating factor induces cardioprotection in isolated rat heart akin to ischemic preconditioning: role of phosphoinositide 3-kinase and protein kinase C activation. *Am. J. Physiol. Heart Circ. Physiol.* 288, H2512–H2520. doi: 10.1152/ajpheart.00599.2004

Penna, C., Brancaccio, M., Tullio, F., Rubinetto, C., Perrelli, M. G., Angotti, C., et al. (2014). Overexpression of the muscle-specific protein, melusin, protects from cardiac ischemia/reperfusion injury. *Basic Res. Cardiol.* 109:418. doi: 10.1007/s00395-014-0418-9

Penna, C., Granata, R., Tocchetti, C. G., Gallo, M. P., Alloatti, G., and Pagliaro, P. (2015). Endogenous Cardioprotective Agents: role in Pre and Postconditioning. *Curr. Drug Targets* 16, 843–867. doi: 10.2174/138945011666615030911 5536

Penna, C., Pasqua, T., Perrelli, M. G., Pagliaro, P., Cerra, M. C., and Angelone, T. (2012). Postconditioning with glucagon like peptide-2 reduces ischemia/reperfusion injury in isolated rat hearts: role of survival kinases and mitochondrial KATP channels. *Basic Res. Cardiol.* 107:272. doi: 10.1007/s00395-012-0272-6

Penna, C., Tullio, F., Femminò, S., Rocca, C., Angelone, T., Cerra, M. C., et al. (2017). Obestatin regulates cardiovascular function and promotes cardioprotection through the nitric oxide pathway. *J. Cell Mol. Med.* 21, 3670–3678. doi: 10.1111/jcmm.13277

Peters, S. L., and Alewijnse, A. E. (2007). Sphingosine-1-phosphate signaling in the cardiovascular system. *Curr. Opin. Pharmacol.* 7, 186–192. doi: 10.1016/j.coph.2006.09.008

Randriamboavonjy, V., Badenhoop, K., Schmidt, H., Geisslinger, G., Fisslthaler, B., and Fleming, I. (2009). The S1P2 receptor expressed in human platelets is linked to the RhoA-Rho kinase pathway and is down regulated in type 2 diabetes. *Basic Res. Cardiol.* 104, 333–340. doi: 10.1007/s00395-008-0769-1

Russo, I. (2012). The prothrombotic tendency in metabolic syndrome: focus on the potential mechanisms involved in impaired haemostasis and fibrinolytic balance. *Scientifica* 2012:525374. doi: 10.6064/2012/525374

Russo, I., Del Mese, P., Doronzo, G., De Salve, A., Secchi, M., Trovati, M., et al. (2007). Platelet resistance to the antiaggregatory cyclic nucleotides in central obesity involves reduced phosphorylation of vasodilator-stimulated phosphoprotein. *Clin. Chem.* 53, 1053–1060. doi: 10.1373/clinchem.2006.076208

Russo, I., Penna, C., Musso, T., Popara, J., Alloatti, G., Cavalot, F., et al. (2017). Platelets, diabetes and myocardial ischemia/reperfusion injury. *Cardiovasc. Diabetol.* 16:71. doi: 10.1186/s12933-017-0550-6

Seligmann, C., Prechtl, G., Kusus-Seligmann, M., and Daniel, W. G. (2013). A myocardial ischemia- and reperfusion-induced injury is mediated by reactive oxygen species released from blood platelets. *Platelets* 24, 37–43. doi: 10.3109/09537104.2012.658107

Somers, S. J., Frias, M., Lacerda, L., Opie, L. H., and Lecour, S. (2012). Interplay between SAFE and RISK pathways in sphingosine-1-phosphate-induced cardioprotection. *Cardiovasc. Drugs Ther.* 26, 227–237. doi: 10.1007/s10557-012-6376-2

Tani, M., Sano, T., Ito, M., and Igarashi, Y. (2005). Mechanisms of sphingosine and sphingosine 1-phosphate generation in human platelets. *J. Lipid Res.* 46, 2458–2467. doi: 10.1194/jlr.M500268-JLR200

Ulrych, T., Böhm, A., Polzin, A., Daum, G., Nüsing, R. M., Geisslinger, G., et al. (2011). Release of sphingosine-1-phosphate from human platelets is dependent on thromboxane formation. *J. Thromb. Haemost.* 9, 790–798. doi: 10.1111/j.1538-7836.2011.04194.x

Urtz, N., Gaertner, F., von Bruehl, M. L., Chandraratne, S., Rahimi, F., Zhang, L., et al. (2015). Sphingosine 1-Phosphate produced by sphingosine kinase 2 intrinsically controls platelet aggregation in vitro and in vivo. *Circ. Res.* 117, 376–387. doi: 10.1161/CIRCRESAHA.115.306901

Vanhoutte, P. M., and Houston, D. S. (1985). Platelets, endothelium, and vasospasm. *Circulation* 72, 728–734. doi: 10.1161/01.CIR.72.4.728

Vazzana, N., Ranalli, P., Cuccurullo, C., and Davì, G. (2012). Diabetes mellitus and thrombosis. *Thromb. Res.* 129, 371–377. doi: 10.1016/j.thromres.2011.11

Vessey, D. A., Kelley, M., Li, L., Huang, Y., Zhou, H. Z., Zhu, B. Q., et al. (2006). Role of sphingosine kinase activity in protection of heart against ischemia reperfusion injury. *Med. Sci. Monit.* 12, BR318–BR324.

Vessey, D. A., Li, L., Honbo, N., and Karliner, J. S. (2009). Sphingosine 1-phosphate is an important endogenous cardioprotectant released by ischemic pre- and postconditioning. *Am. J. Physiol. Heart Circ. Physiol.* 297, H1429–H1435. doi: 10.1152/ajpheart.00358.2009

Vessey, D. A., Li, L., Kelley, M., and Karliner, J. S. (2008). Combined sphingosine, S1P and ischemic postconditioning rescue the heart after protracted ischemia. *Biochem. Biophys. Res. Commun.* 375, 425–429. doi: 10.1016/j.bbrc.2008.08.022

Vito, C. D., Hadi, L. A., Navone, S. E., Marfia, G., Campanella, R., Mancuso, M. E., et al. (2016). Platelet-derived sphingosine-1-phosphate and inflammation: from basic mechanisms to clinical implications. *Platelets* 27, 393–401. doi: 10.3109/09537104.2016.1144179

Watala, C., Boncler, M., and Gresner, P. (2005). Blood platelet abnormalities and pharmacological modulation of platelet reactivity in patients with diabetes mellitus. *Pharmacol. Rep.* 57(Suppl.), 42–58.

Woulfe, D. S. (2010). Akt signaling in platelets and thrombosis. *Expert Rev. Hematol.* 3, 81–91. doi: 10.1586/ehm.09.75

Yang, B., Mehta, P., and Mehta, J. L. (1998). Platelet-mediated cardioprotective effect against ischemia-reperfusion injury in isolated rat hearts: role of platelet number and contribution of supernatant of aggregated platelets. *J. Cardiovasc. Pharmacol. Ther.* 3, 23–28. doi: 10.1177/107424849800300103

Yang, B. C., Mehta, A., and Mehta, J. L. (1994). Cardioprotective effects of platelets against ischaemia-reperfusion injury are related in part to platelet glutathione redox cycle. *Cardiovasc. Res.* 28, 1586–1593. doi: 10.1093/cvr/28.10.1586

Yang, B. C., and Mehta, J. L. (1994). Platelet-derived adenosine contributes to the cardioprotective effects of platelets against ischemia-reperfusion injury in isolated rat heart. *J. Cardiovasc. Pharmacol.* 24, 779–785. doi: 10.1097/00005344-199424050-00013

Yang, B. C., Virmani, R., Nichols, W. W., and Mehta, J. L. (1993). Platelets protect against myocardial dysfunction and injury induced by ischemia and reperfusion in isolated rat hearts. *Circ. Res.* 72, 1181–1190. doi: 10.1161/01.RES.72.6.1181

Yang, B. C., Zander, D. S., and Mehta, J. L. (1999). Hypoxia-reoxygenation-induced apoptosis in cultured adult rat myocytes and the protective effect of platelets and transforming growth factor-beta(1). *J. Pharmacol. Exp. Ther.* 291, 733–738.

Yang, X. M., Cui, L., Alhammouri, A., Downey, J. M., and Cohen, M. V. (2013a). Triple therapy greatly increases myocardial salvage during ischemia/reperfusion in the in situ rat heart. *Cardiovasc. Drugs Ther.* 27, 403–412. doi: 10.1007/s10557-013-6474-9

Yang, X. M., Liu, Y., Cui, L., Yang, X., Liu, Y., Tandon, N., et al. (2013b). Two classes of anti-platelet drugs reduce anatomical infarct size in monkey hearts. *Cardiovasc. Drugs Ther.* 27, 109–115. doi: 10.1007/s10557-012-6436-7

Yatomi, Y., Ruan, F., Hakomori, S., and Igarashi, Y. (1995). Sphingosine-1-phosphate: a platelet-activating sphingolipid released from agonist-stimulated human platelets. *Blood* 86, 193–202.

Yee, E. S., Price, D. C., Aherne, T., and Ebert, P. A. (1986). Intracoronary platelet aggregation: pattern of deposition after ischemia, cardioplegia, and reperfusion. *J. Surg. Res.* 40, 499–503. doi: 10.1016/0022-4804(86)90222-2

Zhang, G., Yang, L., Kim, G. S., Ryan, K., Lu, S., O'Donnell, R. K., et al. (2013). Critical role of sphingosine-1-phosphate receptor 2 (S1PR2) in acute vascular inflammation. *Blood* 122, 443–455. doi: 10.1182/blood-2012-11-46 7191

Zhang, J., Honbo, N., Goetzl, E. J., Chatterjee, K., Karliner, J. S., and Gray, M. O. (2007). Signals from type 1 sphingosine 1-phosphate receptors enhance adult mouse cardiac myocyte survival during hypoxia. *Am. J. Physiol. Heart Circ. Physiol.* 293, H3150–H318. doi: 10.1152/ajpheart.00587.2006

3

Lack of Contribution of p66shc and its Mitochondrial Translocation to Ischemia-Reperfusion Injury and Cardioprotection by Ischemic Preconditioning

*Kerstin Boengler[1], Péter Bencsik[2,3], János Palóczi[2,3], Krisztina Kiss[2,3], Márton Pipicz[2,3], Judit Pipis[2], Péter Ferdinandy[2,3,4], Klaus-Dieter Schlüter[1] and Rainer Schulz[1]**

[1] Physiologisches Institut, Justus-Liebig-Universität, Giessen, Germany, [2] Pharmahungary Group, Szeged, Hungary, [3] Cardiovascular Research Group, Department of Biochemistry, University of Szeged, Szeged, Hungary, [4] Department of Pharmacology and Pharmacotherapy, Semmelweis University, Budapest, Hungary

Edited by:
Pasquale Pagliaro,
University of Turin, Italy

Reviewed by:
Tommaso Angelone,
University of Calabria, Italy
Carlo Gabriele Tocchetti,
Federico II University Hospital, Italy

***Correspondence:**
Rainer Schulz
rainer.schulz@physiologie.med.uni-giessen.de

Whereas high amounts of reactive oxygen species (ROS) contribute to cardiac damage following ischemia and reperfusion (IR), low amounts function as trigger molecules in the cardioprotection by ischemic preconditioning (IPC). The mitochondrial translocation and contribution of the hydrogen peroxide-generating protein p66shc in the cardioprotection by IPC is unclear yet. In the present study, we investigated the mitochondrial translocation of p66shc, addressed the impact of p66shc on ROS formation after IR, and characterized the role of p66shc in IR injury *per se* and in the cardioprotection by IPC. The amount of p66shc in subsarcolemmal (SSM) and interfibrillar mitochondria (IFM) isolated from wildtype mouse left ventricles (LV) was determined after 40 min normoxic perfusion and after 30 min ischemia and 10 min reperfusion without and with IPC. The p66shc content in SSM (in % of normoxic controls, $n = 5$) was 174 ± 16% ($n = 6$, $p < 0.05$) after IR, and was reduced to 128 ± 13% after IPC ($n = 6$, p = ns). In IFM, the amount of p66shc remained unchanged (IR: 81 ± 7%, $n = 6$; IPC: 110 ± 5%, $n = 6$, p = ns). IR induced an increase in ROS formation in SSM and IFM isolated from mouse wildtype LV, which was more pronounced in SSM than in IFM (1.18 ± 0.18 vs. 0.81 ± 0.16, $n = 6$, $p < 0.05$). In mitochondria from p66shc-knockout mice (p66shc-KO), the increase in ROS formation by IR was not different between SSM and IFM (0.90 ± 0.11 vs. 0.73 ± 0.08, $n = 6$, p = ns). Infarct size (in % of the left ventricle) was 51.7 ± 2.9% in wildtype and 59.7 ± 3.8% in p66shc-KO hearts *in vitro* and was significantly reduced to 35.8 ± 4.4% (wildtype) and 34.7 ± 5.6% (p66shc-KO) by IPC, respectively. *In vivo*, infarct size was 57.8 ± 2.9% following IR ($n = 9$) and was reduced to 40.3 ± 3.5% by IPC ($n = 11$, $p < 0.05$) in wildtype mice. In p66shc-knockout mice, infarct sizes were similar to those measured in wildtype animals (IR: 56.2 ± 4.3%, $n = 11$; IPC: 42.1 ± 3.9%, $n = 13$, $p < 0.05$). Taken together, the mitochondrial translocation of p66shc following IR and

IPC differs between mitochondrial populations. However, similar infarct sizes after IR and preserved infarct size reductions by IPC in p66shc-KO mice suggest that p66shc-derived ROS are not involved in the cardioprotection by IPC nor do they contribute to IR injury *per se*.

Keywords: ischemia/reperfusion, ischemic preconditioning, reactive oxygen species, mitochondria, p66shc

INTRODUCTION

An imbalance in the formation and removal of reactive oxygen species (ROS) leads to oxidative stress, which plays a role in the development of cardiovascular diseases, such as hypertension (Chen et al., 2017), hypertrophy (Dai et al., 2011; Sag et al., 2014), heart failure (Akhmedov A. T. et al., 2015), and myocardial injury following ischemia and reperfusion (IR) (Granger and Kvietys, 2015). During IR, a certain amount of ROS is generated during ischemia, whereas the majority of ROS is formed at the onset of reperfusion (Zweier et al., 1987; Bolli et al., 1989). High amounts of ROS contribute to myocardial injury and ultimately cell death via detrimental effects on proteins and lipids and also on the histone-free mitochondrial DNA. However, ROS do not only participate in myocardial damage, they also function as trigger molecules in the cardioprotection by ischemic preconditioning (IPC). Here, a modest ROS formation is suggested to activate signal transduction cascades which finally confer protection against the burst of ROS at reperfusion. Indeed, ROS scavenging during the preconditioning cycles of IR as well as prior to reperfusion abolish the infarct size reduction by IPC (Skyschally et al., 2003; Liu et al., 2008). It is generally accepted that mitochondria represent the predominant source of ROS. Within mitochondria, ROS are formed by the electron transport chain (ETC)—especially from ETC complexes I, II and III (Barja, 1999)—with around 0.2% of the oxygen consumed by the ETC used for ROS formation (St-Pierre et al., 2002). In addition to the ETC, mitochondrial ROS are also produced by monoamino oxidases (MAO), which transfer electrons from amine compounds to oxygen and thereby generate hydrogen peroxide.

Another protein contributing to mitochondrial ROS formation is p66shc, an ubiquitously expressed member of the spontaneous human combustion (shc) family. Together with p46shc and p52shc, p66shc represents an isoform encoded by the human shcA locus. The structure of p66shc includes an aminoterminal CH2 domain (collagen homology domain), followed by a phosphotyrosine binding (PTB) domain, another collagen-homology (CH1) domain, and a carboxyterminal src-homology (SH2) domain. The PTB domain allows the interaction with tyrosine-containing peptides, the CH1 domain of p66shc contains two major tyrosine phosphorylation sites, whereas the SH2 domain is important for protein-protein interactions. The important phosphorylation site serine 36 is located in the CH2 domain of p66shc. Under basal conditions, the majority of p66shc resides in the cytosol, but translocates into the mitochondria upon stress signals (Pinton et al., 2007). For this translocation, the phosphorylation of p66shc at serine 36 by protein kinase C beta (PKCβ) is important (Pinton et al., 2007). Within mitochondria, p66shc is present in the intermembrane space. Here, p66shc oxidizes reduced cytochrome c and thereby catalyzes the reduction of oxygen to hydrogen peroxide (Giorgio et al., 2005). Accordingly, p66shc-deficient cells have decreased levels of ROS (Trinei et al., 2002; Carpi et al., 2009). The reduced ROS formation in p66shc-deficient mice has been suggested to prolong the life span of these animals (Migliaccio et al., 1999), however, when the mice are housed under more natural conditions this effect is abolished (Giorgio et al., 2012). p66shc-mediated ROS formation is linked to cardiovascular pathologies such as hypertrophy (Graiani et al., 2005) and heart failure (Rota et al., 2006) (for review see Di Lisa et al., 2017). Also, heart-rupture is reduced in p66shc-deficient mice following myocardial infarction (Baysa et al., 2015). The measurement of myocardial damage following IR in wildtype and p66shc-knockout mice shows conflicting results: whereas in one study the ablation of p66shc elicits cardiac protection (Carpi et al., 2009), another study displays larger infarcts in p66shc-deficient mice following IR (Akhmedov A. et al., 2015). Studies on the role of p66shc in the cardioprotection by IPC *in vivo* are still lacking.

In the present study, we investigated the translocation of the protein into mitochondrial subpopulations after IR and IPC. Also, the p66shc-mediated ROS formation induced by IR was studied. In addition, we characterized the impact of p66shc on the cardioprotection by IPC in mouse hearts *in vitro* and *in vivo*.

MATERIALS AND METHODS

Animals

The present study conforms to the Guide for the Care and Use of Laboratory Animals published by the US National Institutes of Health (NIH publication No. 85–23, revised 1996) and was approved by the animal welfare office of the Justus-Liebig-University Giessen as well as the National Scientific Ethical Committee on Animal Experimentation, Budapest, Hungary. In the study, 12–22 weeks old male and female C57Bl6/J mice (25–30 g, Janvier, Le Genest-Saint-Isles, France) and p66shc knockout (p66shc-KO) mice were used. Mice were kept in dark/light cycles of 12 h each and had free access to standard chow and drinking water.

Ischemia/Reperfusion *in Vitro*

Mice were anesthetized with 5% isoflurane and killed by cervical dislocation. Thereafter, hearts were rapidly excised and the aorta was cannulated for retrograde perfusion with an Aortic Cannula for mouse hearts (Ø 1 mm, Hugo Sachs Elektronik-Harvard Apparatus, March, Germany) connected to a Langendorff perfusion system. Hearts were perfused with 37°C warm modified Krebs Henseleit buffer (containing in mM:

NaCl 118, KCl 4.7, $MgSO_4$ 0.8, KH_2PO_4 1.2, glucose 5, $CaCl_2$ 2.5, $NaHCO_3$ 25, pyruvate 1.9, continuously gased with 95% O_2, 5% CO_2, pH 7.4) at a constant perfusion pressure of 70 mmHg (transduced by a Replacement Transducer Head for APT300 Pressure Transducer, Hugo Sachs Elektronik-Harvard Apparatus). A balloon was inserted into the left ventricle and was connected to a pressure transducer (Combitrans 1-fach Set Mod.II University Giessen, B. Braun, Melsungen, Germany) for assessment of ventricular performance. The balloon was inflated to yield a left ventricular end-diastolic pressure of 12–14 mmHg, which was kept constant thereafter. Hearts were paced during measurements at 600 bpm. Left ventricular developed pressure (LVDP, systolic pressure—diastolic pressure) was recorded. Perfused hearts were left to stabilize for 5 min. Ischemia was induced by stopping flow and pacing. The following protocols were performed:

a) p66shc translocation and ROS formation
Normoxia: 40 min normoxia
IR: 30 min ischemia, 10 min reperfusion
IPC: Three times 3 min ischemia, 5 min reperfusion, followed by 30 min ischemia and 10 min reperfusion
At the end of the protocol, hearts were used to isolate mitochondria
b) Infarct size determination
IR: 45 min ischemia, 120 min reperfusion
IPC: Three times 3 min ischemia, 5 min reperfusion, followed by 45 min ischemia and 120 min reperfusion
After 120 min of reperfusion, the hearts were removed from the perfusion apparatus and frozen at −20°C for 30 min. Subsequently, hearts were cut in 7–8 slices and incubated in 1.2% triphenyl-tetrazolium chloride for 20 min at 37°C. Heart slices were then fixated in 7% formalin at room temperature overnight. Digital images were taken from both sides of the heart slices with a M60 microscope (Leica, Wetzlar, Germany) at 2.5-fold magnification. Infarct size was determined by planimetrie using the Leica Application Suite LAS version 4.6 (Leica).

The use of either 30 or 45 min ischemia was due to the necessity to compare data of p66shc translocation with previous studies (were 30 min ischemia were analyzed, Yang et al., 2014) and to induce substantial myocardial infarction in order to demonstrate effective cardioprotection by IPC (45 min ischemia).

Ischemia/Reperfusion *in Vivo*

Mice were weighed (weight range 22.1 ± 1.0–24.7 ± 1.1 g, p = ns between groups) and anesthetized with sodium pentobarbital (Euthasol, Produlab Pharma b.v., Raamsdonksveer, The Netherlands; 90 mg/kg bolus dose followed by 15–20 mg/kg when required during the experiment). The hair in the neck and chest area was removed by using a depilatory cream. Maintenance of body core temperature was assisted using a constant temperature heating pad. The trachea was intubated with a plastic cannula connected to a rodent ventilator (Model Minivent 845, Harvard Apparatus, Holliston, MA). The animals were ventilated with room air, volume and rate set-ups accorded to the recommendation of the manufacturer (100–240 μL, 120–150 breath/min according to the weight of the animal). Surface-lead ECG and body core temperature were monitored throughout the experiments to ensure the stability of the preparation (Haemosys data acquisition system, Experimetria, Budapest, Hungary). The heart rates ranged from 429 ± 17 to 451 ± 20 bpm and were not significantly different between groups. The chest was opened at the 4th intercostal space and an 8-0 Prolene suture was placed around the middle portion of the left anterior descending branch (LAD) of the left coronary artery. Then the suture was looped and a piece of PE-10 cannula was placed into the loop. For coronary artery occlusion and reperfusion, both strands of the suture were pulled and fixed thereby pressing the plastic cannula onto the surface of the heart directly above the coronary artery, and then released. Mice were subjected to 45 min occlusion of the left coronary artery (test ischemia) and then released to develop acute myocardial infarction. In IPC groups, mice were subjected to 5 min ischemia/5 min reperfusion in four cycles prior to test ischemia. To ensure recanalization of the occluded vessel, sodium heparin was administered i.p. at 100 U/kg dose three times during the surgeries: 45 min before test ischemia; 5 min before the onset of reperfusion, and at the 115th min of reperfusion.

After 120 min of reperfusion, risk area was re-occluded, and mice were injected with 0.4 ml of 2% Evans blue dye through the apex of the left ventricle. Following Evans staining, hearts were isolated, right ventricle was removed and left ventricles (LV) were cut into seven transversal slices. Heart slices were washed in PBS buffer for 1 min to remove excess dye and then incubated in 1% triphenyl-tetrazolium-chloride for 10 min at 37°C followed by formalin fixation for 10 min. Digital images were taken from both surface of heart slices by a Nikon DSLR camera (Nikon Corporation, Tokyo, Japan). Planimetric evaluation was carried out to determine infarct size using InfarctSize™ software version 2.5, (Pharmahungary, Szeged, Hungary).

Isolation of Mitochondria

Subsarcolemmal (SSM) and interfibrillar mitochondria (IFM) were isolated as previously described (Boengler et al., 2009). All steps were performed at 4°C. Hearts were washed in buffer A (100 mM KCl, 50 mM 3-[N-Morpholino]-propanesulfonic acid (MOPS), 5 mM MgSO4, 1 mM ATP, 1 mM EGTA, pH 7.4), weighed, the tissue was minced in 10 ml/g buffer A with scissors and was then disrupted with a Potter-Elvejhem tissue homogenizer. The homogenate was centrifuged for 10 min at 800 g. The resulting supernatant, which contained the SSM, was centrifuged for 10 min at 8,000 g. The sedimented mitochondria were washed in buffer A and were resuspended in a small volume of buffer A. The sediment of the first centrifugation, which contained the IFM, was resuspended in buffer A (10 ml/g tissue). The protease nagarse was added (Bacterial type XXIV, Sigma, 8 U/g), incubated at 4°C for 1 min and the samples were then disrupted using a Potter-Elvejhem tissue homogenizer. Subsequently, samples were centrifuged for 10 min at 800 g, and IFM were collected by centrifugation of the supernatant for 10 min at 8,000 g. The sedimented IFM were washed by resuspension in buffer A and centrifugation (8,000 g for 10 min), and were finally resuspended in buffer A. These mitochondrial preparations were used to study ROS formation. To analyse the amount of p66shc in SSM and IFM by Western blot, mitochondria were further purified by layering them on top of a 30% Percoll solution in isolation buffer (in mM: sucrose 250; HEPES 10; EGTA 1; pH 7.4) and subsequent ultracentrifugation at 35,000 g for 30 min at 4°C. The mitochondrial band was collected, washed twice in isolation buffer by centrifugation at 8,000 g for 5 min, and the purified mitochondria were stored at −80°C.

ROS Formation

ROS formation was measured as described previously (Boengler et al., 2017). Fifty microgram mitochondria (SSM and IFM) isolated after normoxia or IR were transferred to incubation buffer supplemented with 5 mM glutamate and 2.5 mM malate, 50 μM Amplex UltraRed (Invitrogen, Eugene, OR), and 0.1 U/ml horseradish peroxidase. The fluorescence was measured continuously for 4 min with a Cary Eclipse spectrophotometer (Agilent Technologies, Santa Clara, CA) at the excitation/emission wavelengths of 565/581 nm, respectively. As positive control served control mitochondria supplemented with 2 μM of the complex I inhibitor rotenone. Background fluorescence of the buffer without mitochondria was subtracted and the slope fluorescence in arbitrary units/time (4 min) was calculated.

Western Blot Analysis

Isolated SSM, IFM, or left ventricular tissue sections were lysed in 1 × Cell Lysis buffer (25 mM Tris, 150 mM NaCl, 1 mM EDTA, 1% NP-40, 5% glycerol, pH 7.4) supplemented with 1X PhosStop and Complete inhibitors (Roche, Basel, Switzerland) as well as 1 μM neocuproine. Protein concentration was determined using the Lowry assay. Thirty microgram proteins were electrophoretically separated on 10% Bis/Tris gels and proteins were transferred to nitrocellulose membranes. After blocking, membranes were incubated with rabbit polyclonal anti-human/rat SHC antibodies (BD Biosciences), rabbit polyclonal anti-human voltage dependent anion channel (VDAC, Acris, Rockville MD), or rabbit polyclonal anti-human manganese superoxide dismutase antibodies (MnSOD, Merck Millipore, Darmstadt, Germany). After washing and incubation with the respective secondary antibodies, immunoreactive signals were detected by chemiluminescence (SuperSignal West Femto or SuperSignal West Pico Chemiluminescent Substrate, ThermoFisher) and quantified using Scion Image software (Frederick, MD). The purity of the mitochondrial preparations was determined as the absence of immunoreactivity for Na^+/K^+-ATPase (sarcolemma), sarcoplasmic/endoplasmic reticulum calcium ATPase (sarcoplasmic reticulum), histone deacetylase 2 (nucleus), and glycerinaldehyde-3-phosphate dehydrogenase (cytosol), data not shown.

Statistics

Data are shown as mean ± SEM and a $p < 0.05$ is considered to indicate a significant difference. Data on the mitochondrial content of p66shc in SSM and IFM (basal, following IR and IPC) were compared by non-parametric Rank Sum test. Data on ROS formation, EDP, LVDP, the recovery of LVDP, area at risk *in vivo*, as well as on infarct size determination *in vitro* and *in vivo* were analyzed by two-way ANOVA, following Bonferroni corrections. The program SigmaStat 3.5 (Systat, Software GmbH, Erkrath, Germany) was used for statistical analysis.

RESULTS

To study the mitochondrial translocation of p66shc, isolated mouse hearts were perfused under normoxic conditions or subjected to IR (30 min ischemia, 10 min reperfusion) without and with IPC. SSM and IFM were isolated and analyzed for their p66shc content by Western blot (**Figure 1**). In SSM, IR induced an increased translocation of p66shc into the mitochondria, however, following IPC the p66shc content was reduced to that of normoxic controls. In contrast to SSM, the amount of p66shc in IFM was not affected by IR or IPC.

To investigate whether or not the mitochondrial amount of p66shc correlates with the ROS formation following IR, isolated hearts from wildtype (WT) or p66shc-KO mice underwent normoxia or IR. Subsequently, SSM and IFM were isolated and ROS formation was measured as the increase in the Amplex UltraRed fluorescence (**Figure 2**). Under normoxic conditions, ROS formation tended to be higher in SSM compared to IFM isolated from both WT and p66shc-KO hearts without reaching statistical significance. Following IR, ROS formation increased in both SSM and IFM from WT and p66shc-KO hearts, however, the raise in ROS formation in SSM compared to IFM was more pronounced in WT than in p66shc-KO mitochondria. When ROS formation was stimulated by the addition of rotenone, there were no differences in the slope of the Amplex UltraRed fluorescence (in arbitrary units/min) between SSM and IFM isolated from WT (SSM Nx: 1.6 ± 0.2; SSM IR: 1.8 ± 0.2; IFM Nx: 2.3 ± 0.5; IFM IR: 1.9 ± 0.3, $n = 6$, $p =$ ns) and p66shc-KO hearts (SSM Nx: 2.16 ± 0.3; SSM IR: 2.2 ± 0.2; IFM Nx: 1.9 ± 0.3; IFM IR: 2.5 ± 0.3, $n = 6$, $p =$ ns).

The impact of p66shc on left ventricular function was determined in isolated WT and p66shc-KO hearts subjected to IR without or with IPC. Under baseline conditions (i.e., at the end of the stabilization period), end-diastolic pressure and LVDP were not different between groups (**Table 1**). The recovery of the LVDP at the end of reperfusion was more pronounced in WT hearts undergoing IPC than in p66shc-KO hearts (**Figure 3A**, **Table 1**). However, the improved functional recovery was not a consequence of altered infarct size, since IPC induced a similar infarct size reduction in WT and in p66shc-KO hearts *in vitro* (**Figure 3B**). Myocardial infarction after IR alone was not different between WT and p66shc-KO hearts.

To study the role of p66shc in the cardioprotection by IPC *in vivo*, the LAD branch of the left coronary artery was reversibly occluded in WT and p66shc-KO mice to induce IR without and with IPC. The area at risk (in % of the left ventricle) was not different between groups (WT, IR: 23.2 ± 2.4, $n = 9$; WT IPC: 34.5 ± 5.2, $n = 11$; p66shc-KO IR: 26.9 ± 2.5, $n = 11$; p66shc-KO IPC: 27.9 ± 2.7, $n = 13$, $p =$ ns). Also, there was no significant difference in infarct size after IR between WT and p66shc-KO mice (**Figure 4**). However, with IPC infarct size was significantly reduced in both WT and p66shc-KO mice

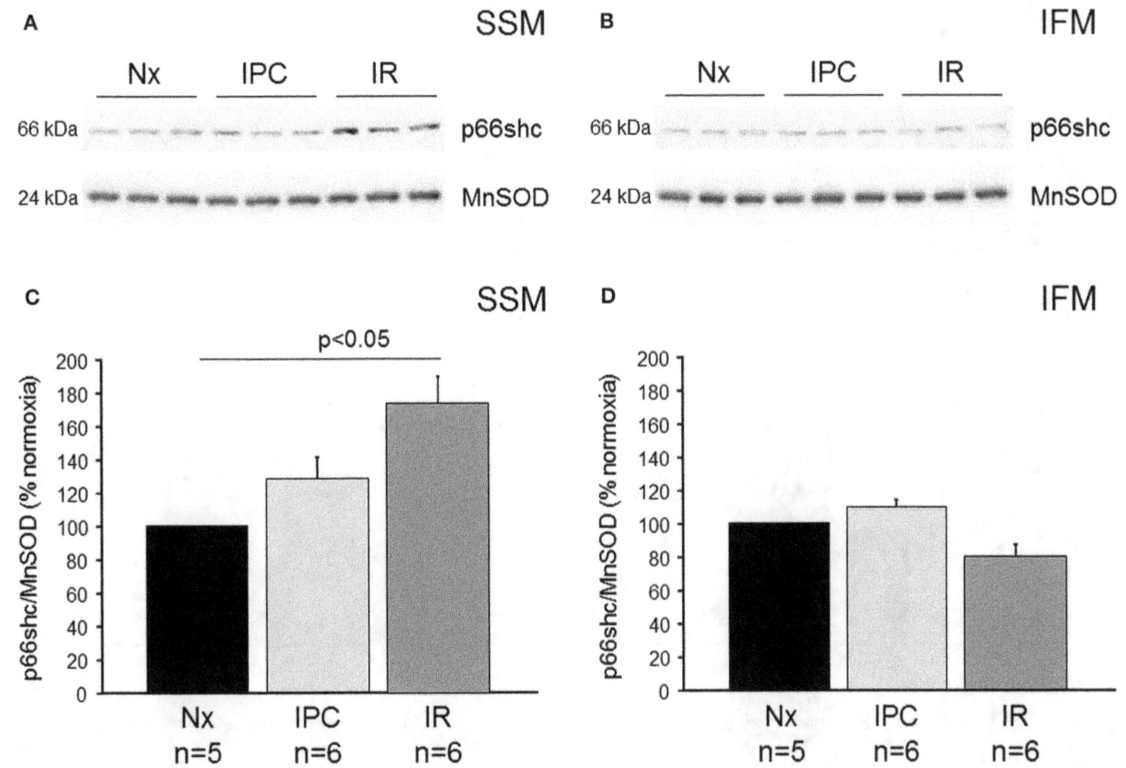

FIGURE 1 | Mitochondrial p66shc translocation following ischemia/reperfusion or ischemic preconditioning. Western blot analysis was performed for p66shc and the mitochondrial marker protein MnSOD (manganese superoxide dismutase) on SSM **(A)** and IFM **(B)** isolated from wildtype mice undergoing normoxia (Nx), ischemia/reperfusion (IR) or IR with ischemic preconditioning (IPC). Bar graphs represent the ratios of p66shc over MnSOD in SSM **(C)** and IFM **(D)** isolated after Nx, IR, or IPC.

demonstrating effective cardioprotection not only in WT but also in p66shc-KO mice *in vivo* (**Figure 4**).

DISCUSSION

The present study demonstrates that the translocation of p66shc after IR or IPC differs between mitochondrial subpopulations. An increase in the mitochondrial level of p66shc in SSM is associated with enhanced ROS formation after IR. However, the altered mitochondrial amounts of p66shc after IR or IPC had no consequences for infarct development *per se* or the cardioprotection, since p66shc knockout hearts showed an effective infarct size reduction by IPC both *in vitro* and *in vivo*.

The presence of p66shc has been described in mitochondria of several cell types, including mouse embryonic fibroblasts (Nemoto et al., 2006), human endothelial cells (Paneni et al., 2015; Spescha et al., 2015; Zhu et al., 2015), and mitochondria isolated from cardiac tissue (Yang et al., 2014). Cardiomyocytes contain at least two mitochondrial subpopulations, the SSM and IFM, which differ in form and function (Palmer et al., 1977, 1986; Boengler et al., 2009). When analyzing the presence of p66shc in mitochondria of ventricular origin, only SSM have been studied so far (Yang et al., 2014). In the present study, we detected p66shc not only in cardiac SSM but also in IFM. Under basal conditions, the majority of p66shc resides in the cytosol and a translocation of the protein into the mitochondrial intermembrane space occurs under stress conditions, among them IR (Giorgio et al., 2005; Zhu et al., 2015). A previous study demonstrates that the translocation of p66shc into SSM is dependent on the duration of IR in guinea pig hearts (Yang et al., 2014). Here, 30 min of ischemia were not sufficient to increase the mitochondrial amount of p66shc, whereas 30 min ischemia and 10 min reperfusion enhanced the mitochondrial content of the protein. In the present study, the increased mitochondrial amount of p66shc after 30 min ischemia and 10 min reperfusion in SSM was confirmed, but this translocation was specific for SSM since the mitochondrial amounts of p66shc in IFM was not affected by IR.

The import of p66shc into mitochondria requires the phosphorylation at serine 36 by protein kinase C beta (PKCβ), and the subsequent prolyl-isomerization by peptidyl-prolyl cis-trans isomerase 1 (Pin1) is important. Indeed, it has already been shown that 30 min IR induces the activation/phosphorylation of PKCβ and simultaneously that of p66shc at serine 36, and that the inhibition of PKCβ decreases p66shc phosphorylation and the mitochondrial translocation of the protein (Kong et al., 2008; Yang et al., 2014). However, serine 36 phosphorylation of p66shc may also require c-Jun terminal kinase activity (Khalid et al., 2016). In human umbilical vein endothelial cells, hypoxia/reoxygenation

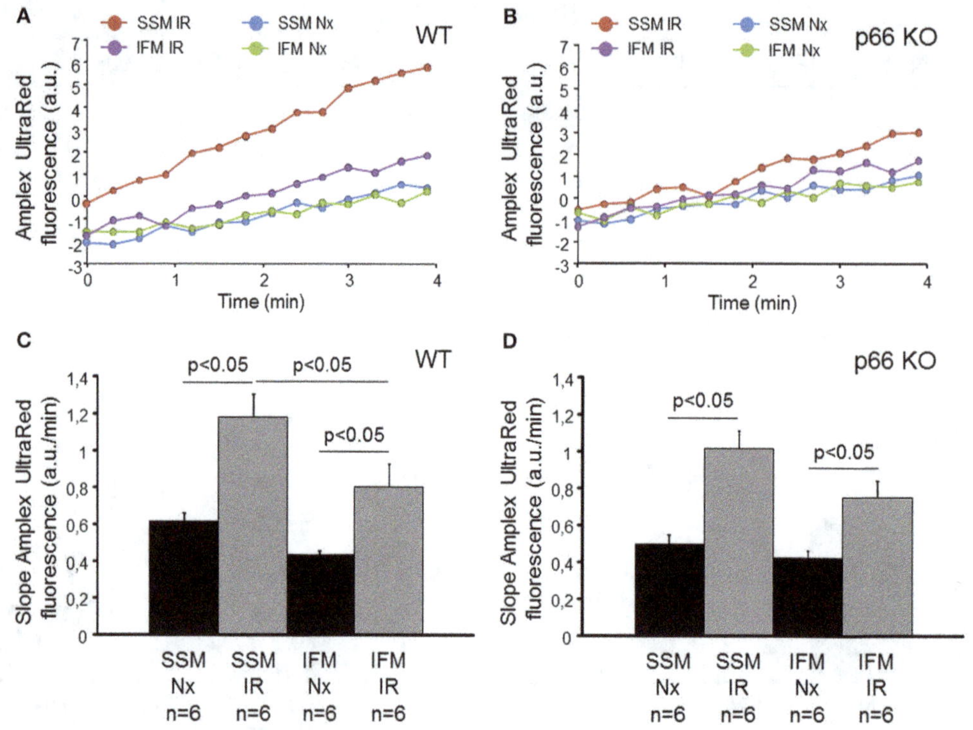

FIGURE 2 | ROS formation in SSM and IFM isolated from mouse hearts following normoxia or ischemia/reperfusion *in vitro*. Original traces showing Amplex UltraRed fluorescence in SSM and IFM isolated after normoxia (Nx) or ischemia/reperfusion (IR) in wildtype (WT, **A**) or p66shc knockout (p66 KO, **B**) hearts *in vitro*. Bar graphs represent the slope of the Amplex UltraRed fluorescence measured for 4 min in WT **(C)** and p66 KO **(D)** mitochondria.

TABLE 1 | Summary of the baseline parameters and hemodynamic data throughout ischaemia-reperfusion protocols *in vitro*.

Genotype	Protocol	n-value	Body weight (g)	Heart weight/body weight (mg/g)	EDP (mm Hg)			LVDP (mm Hg)		
					basal	10 min reperfusion	End of reperfusion	basal	10 min reperfusion	End of reperfusion
WT	IR *in vitro*	7	28.9 ± 1.2	6.25 ± 0.27	12.8 ± 0.4	51.4 ± 6.1	26.3 ± 4.1	107.0 ± 3.7	59.8 ± 11.9	56.7 ± 2.8
WT	IPC *in vitro*	7	27.7 ± 1.5	6.51 ± 0.24	11.1 ± 0.7	25.7 ± 2.5*	14.2 ± 0.9*	101.8 ± 7.7	67.5 ± 4.2	59.5 ± 6.4
p66 KO	IR *in vitro*	5	25.2 ± 0.5	6.91 ± 0.51	12.0 ± 1.0	62.7 ± 11.3	31.0 ± 4.4	90.6 ± 10.5	32.7 ± 8.3*	36.0 ± 2.7*
p66 KO	IPC *in vitro*	5	26.0 ± 0.9	6.30 ± 0.48	11.6 ± 0.9	33.8 ± 16.0	19.0 ± 7.4	95.4 ± 10.3	31.0 ± 8.1**	38.7 ± 3.5**

*Enddiastolic pressure (EDP) and left ventricular developed pressure (LVDP) in wildtype and p66shc knockout (p66 KO) hearts undergoing IR without and with ischemic preconditioning (IPC). Basal data were collected at the end of the stabilization period. *p < 0.05 vs. I/R WT, **p < 0.05 vs. IPC WT.*

is associated with increased phosphorylation and mitochondrial translocation of p66shc (Zhu et al., 2015). Here, the increased p66shc phosphorylation is attributed to decreased activity of phosphatase 2A rather than to increased activity of PKCβ. The mitochondrial translocation of p66shc after intestinal IR injury is abrogated following the inhibition of Pin1 leading to improved survival (Feng et al., 2017). Under high glucose conditions, the phosphorylation and mitochondrial translocation of p66shc is facilitated by a Sirtuin 1-regulated lysine acetylation (Kumar et al., 2017). Although we tried to measure serine 36 phosphorylation of p66shc by Western blot and immunoprecipitation in the present study, but were unable to detect specific signals with available antibodies (data not shown), we cannot correlate p66shc phosphorylation with the mitochondrial amount of the protein.

The ablation of p66shc is associated with a reduced ROS formation after IR in the brain (Spescha et al., 2013) as well as in the heart (Carpi et al., 2009). However, one study also shows that the deletion of p66shc (via siRNA or by genetic ablation) has no influence on myocardial ROS formation following IR (Spescha et al., 2015). In our study, we found an increase in ROS formation after IR compared to normoxia in SSM and IFM of wildtype and p66shc-deficient mice. In wildtype mice, this increase was more pronounced in SSM than in IFM and therefore correlated with the mitochondrial translocation of p66shc. However,

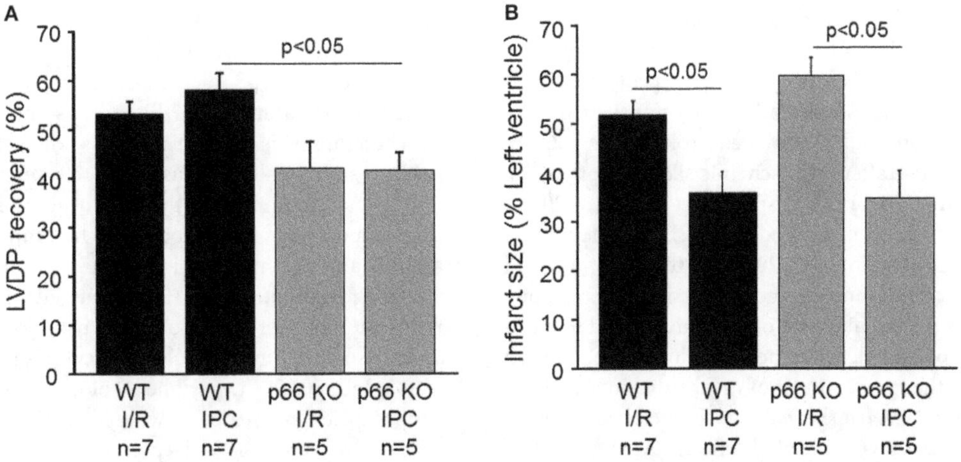

FIGURE 3 | Influence of p66shc on myocardial function, IR injury and cardioprotection *in vitro*. **(A)** Left ventricular developed pressure (LVDP) at the end of reperfusion in % of that at the end of the stabilization period in wildtype (WT) and p66shc knockout (p66 KO) mice undergoing ischemia/reperfusion (IR) or ischemic preconditioning (IPC). **(B)** Infarct size (in % of left ventricle) in WT and p66shc-KO mice subjected to IR or IPC.

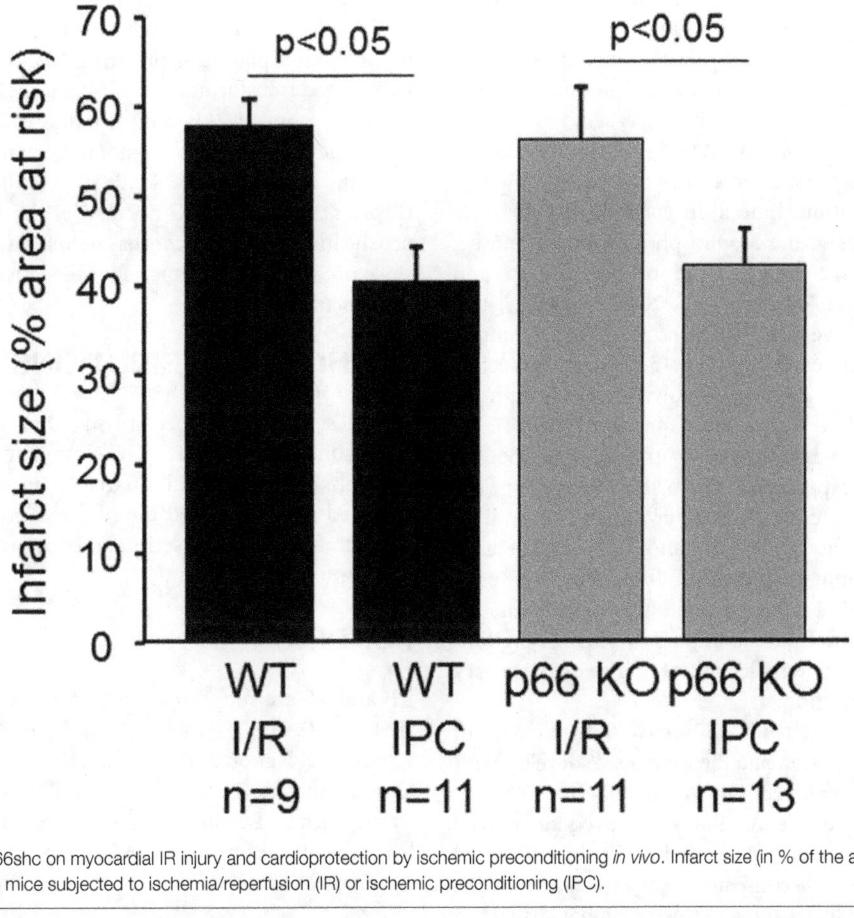

FIGURE 4 | Influence of p66shc on myocardial IR injury and cardioprotection by ischemic preconditioning *in vivo*. Infarct size (in % of the area at risk) in WT and p66shc knockout (p66 KO) mice subjected to ischemia/reperfusion (IR) or ischemic preconditioning (IPC).

in mitochondria isolated from p66shc-deficient mice ROS formation was not different in SSM and IFM after IR indicating that p66shc contributes sufficient amounts to the ROS formation induced by myocardial IR.

Since ROS are known to contribute to either myocardial damage or protection—depending on their timing and their amount—p66shc represents an interesting target to be studied in IR and protection from it. p66shc induces opening of the mitochondrial permeability transition pore, which leads to swelling of the organelle, rupture of the outer mitochondrial membrane and finally cell death (Giorgio et al., 2005). Therefore, the deletion of p66shc has been suggested to be protective in IR injury, and indeed IR in the brain induced by transient middle cerebral artery occlusion results in reduced stroke size in p66shc-KO mice or in WT mice after post-ischemic silencing of p66shc compared to that in control mice (Spescha et al., 2013, 2015). Also, muscle fiber necrosis is reduced in p66shc-deficient mice after hindlimb IR (Zaccagnini et al., 2004). In the heart, the data on the role of p66shc in IR injury are controversial. Whereas, one study demonstrates the maintenance of cell viability and reduced oxidative stress in p66shc-deficient hearts following IR *in vitro* (Carpi et al., 2009), the measurement of myocardial infarction in p66shc-deficient mice *in vivo* shows larger infarct sizes after IR compared to that in wildtype mice (Akhmedov A. et al., 2015). However, myocardial infarction is untypically small in this study, and the increase in myocardial damage is only evident after short term ischemia (30 min), whereas with the prolongation of ischemia to 45 or 60 min no differences in infarct sizes occur between wildtype and p66shc-deficient mice. In the present study, we determined the infarct sizes of wildtype and p66shc-deficient mice undergoing IR (with 45 min of ischemia) *in vitro* and *in vivo* and we observed similar myocardial infarction in both genotypes indicating that p66shc—and the p66shc-induced ROS formation—does not contribute to IR injury *per se*.

Due to the important role of ROS in IR injury and in the protection by IPC, p66shc represents a putative target of such protective intervention. Indeed, in cortical cells chemical preconditioning induces serine 36 phosphorylation of p66shc, subsequent mitochondrial translocation of the protein and finally reduces cell death (Brown et al., 2010). Whereas, this study suggests a protective role of p66shc in preconditioning, another study demonstrates that IPC in the liver is protective against IR injury via a pathway involving the Sirtuin 1-mediated downregulation of p66shc (Yan et al., 2014). In the present study, we measured the translocation of p66shc into mitochondria after perfusion of isolated wildtype hearts under normoxic control conditions, after IR and as well as after IPC and found that whereas IR and IPC did not alter the mitochondrial amount of p66shc in IFM, the IR-induced increase of p66shc in SSM was abrogated after IPC. Thus, the inhibition of mitochondrial p66shc import by IPC may reduce myocardial ROS formation to such amounts which are necessary for triggering cardioprotection.

In addition, the present study addressed the influence of p66shc on myocardial function and the infarct size development following IR without and with IPC *in vitro* and *in vivo*.

Whereas the recovery of the LVDP was improved in wildtype compared to p66shc-deficient mice after IPC, the enhanced functional recovery was not a consequence of altered myocardial infarction, since IPC reduced infarct sizes to similar extents in both genotypes *in vitro*. Comparable results were obtained in the *in vivo* situation where IPC was equally cardioprotective in wildtype and in p66shc-deficient mice. Therefore, despite the putative normalization of the IR-induced increase of ROS by IPC in SSM, p66shc-mediated ROS formation is no prerequisite for the cardioprotection by IPC. The role of p66shc in IPC in the heart has previously been investigated in one study only (Carpi et al., 2009). Here, myocardial damage was assessed as the release of lactate dehydrogenase (LDH) from isolated hearts *in vitro*. Compared to wildtype mice, LDH release was already reduced in p66shc-deficient mice after IR and was not further affected by IPC. Therefore, it is difficult to assess whether or not IPC was capable to additionally decrease LDH release.

Our data demonstrate that in healthy hearts p66shc is of no importance for myocardial I/R injury and that the protein is also not involved in the cardioprotection by classical ischemic preconditioning. However, alterations in p66shc expression/phosphorylation occur in pathological conditions in humans, such as in muscular pericytes of diabetic patients (Vono et al., 2016), in peripheral blood monocytes and renal tissue biopsies of patients with diabetic nephropathy (Xu et al., 2016), and also in peripheral blood monocytes of patients with acute coronary syndrome, but not with stable coronary artery disease (Franzeck et al., 2012). Since such risk factors and co-morbidities may abrogate the cardioprotection by preconditioning (Ferdinandy et al., 2014), it remains to be elucidated whether p66shc contributes toward cardioprotection under pathological conditions.

Taken together, our study demonstrates that within cardiac mitochondria p66shc is present in SSM as well as in IFM. The IR-induced translocation of p66shc into SSM correlates with the ROS formation in this mitochondrial subpopulation. However, ROS generation by p66shc is not important for myocardial injury, since the ablation of p66shc does not influence infarct size after IR *per se*. Whereas, IPC normalizes the IR-induced increase of p66shc in SSM, this process has no relevance for cardioprotection since p66shc-deficient mice show effective infarct size reduction *in vitro* and *in vivo*.

AUTHOR CONTRIBUTIONS

KB designed and performed the research on isolated mitochondria; PB, JaP, KK, MP, and JuP performed the research on myocardial infarction *in vivo*; PF, KS, and RS designed and supervised the research. All authors analyzed the data, drafted the manuscript, and approved the final version of the manuscript.

FUNDING

KB and RS are supported by the German Research Foundation (BO-2955/2-1, SCHU 843/9-1, and CRC1213-B05) and PF and PB by the National Research, Development, and Innovation Office, Hungary (NVKP 16-1-2016-0017). KS and RS are funded by the German Research Foundation SFB1213. PB was supported by the János Bolyai Research Scholarship of the Hungarian Academy of Sciences.

ACKNOWLEDGMENTS

The authors would like to thank Anna Reis, Elvira Ungefug, and Nadine Woitasky for excellent technical assistance and Marco Giorgio (Milan, Italy) for kindly providing the p66shc-KO mice.

REFERENCES

Akhmedov, A., Montecucco, F., Braunersreuther, V., Camici, G. G., Jakob, P., Reiner, M. F., et al. (2015). Genetic deletion of the adaptor protein p66Shc increases susceptibility to short-term ischaemic myocardial injury via intracellular salvage pathways. *Eur. Heart J.* 36, 516–526a. doi: 10.1093/eurheartj/ehu400

Akhmedov, A. T., Rybin, V., and Marin-Garcia, J. (2015). Mitochondrial oxidative metabolism and uncoupling proteins in the failing heart. *Heart Fail. Rev.* 20, 227–249. doi: 10.1007/s10741-014-9457-4

Barja, G. (1999). Mitochondrial oxygen radical generation and leak: sites of production in states 4 and 3, organ specificity, and relation to aging and longevity. *J. Bioenerg. Biomembr.* 31, 347–366. doi: 10.1023/A:1005427919188

Baysa, A., Sagave, J., Carpi, A., Zaglia, T., Campesan, M., Dahl, C. P., et al. (2015). The p66ShcA adaptor protein regulates healing after myocardial infarction. *Basic Res. Cardiol.* 110:13. doi: 10.1007/s00395-015-0470-0

Boengler, K., Bulic, M., Schreckenberg, R., Schluter, K. D., and Schulz, R. (2017). The gap junction modifier ZP1609 decreases cardiomyocyte hypercontracture following ischaemia/reperfusion independent from mitochondrial connexin 43. *Br. J. Pharmacol.* 174, 2060–2073. doi: 10.1111/bph.13804

Boengler, K., Stahlhofen, S., Van De Sand, A., Gres, P., Ruiz-Meana, M., Garcia-Dorado, D., et al. (2009). Presence of connexin 43 in subsarcolemmal, but not in interfibrillar cardiomyocyte mitochondria. *Basic Res. Cardiol.* 104, 141–147. doi: 10.1007/s00395-009-0007-5

Bolli, R., Jeroudi, M. O., Patel, B. S., Dubose, C. M., Lai, E. K., Roberts, R., et al. (1989). Direct evidence that oxygen-derived free radicals contribute to postischemic myocardial dysfunction in the intact dog. *Proc. Natl. Acad. Sci. U.S.A.* 86, 4695–4699. doi: 10.1073/pnas.86.12.4695

Brown, J. E., Zeiger, S. L., Hettinger, J. C., Brooks, J. D., Holt, B., Morrow, J. D., et al. (2010). Essential role of the redox-sensitive kinase p66shc in determining energetic and oxidative status and cell fate in neuronal preconditioning. *J. Neurosci.* 30, 5242–5252. doi: 10.1523/JNEUROSCI.6366-09.2010

Carpi, A., Menabo, R., Kaludercic, N., Pelicci, P., Di Lisa, F., and Giorgio, M. (2009). The cardioprotective effects elicited by p66(Shc) ablation demonstrate the crucial role of mitochondrial ROS formation in ischemia/reperfusion injury. *Biochim. Biophys. Acta* 1787, 774–780. doi: 10.1016/j.bbabio.2009.04.001

Chen, Q., Wang, Q., Zhu, J., Xiao, Q., and Zhang, L. (2017). Reactive oxygen species: key regulators in vascular health and diseases. *Br. J. Pharmacol.* doi: 10.1111/bph.13828. [Epub ahead of print].

Dai, D. F., Johnson, S. C., Villarin, J. J., Chin, M. T., Nieves-Cintron, M., Chen, T., et al. (2011). Mitochondrial oxidative stress mediates angiotensin II-induced cardiac hypertrophy and Galphaq overexpression-induced heart failure. *Circ. Res.* 108, 837–846. doi: 10.1161/CIRCRESAHA.110.232306

Di Lisa, F., Giorgio, M., Ferdinandy, P., and Schulz, R. (2017). New aspects of p66Shc in ischaemia reperfusion injury and other cardiovascular diseases. *Br. J. Pharmacol.* 174, 1690–1703. doi: 10.1111/bph.13478

Feng, D., Yao, J., Wang, G., Li, Z., Zu, G., Li, Y., et al. (2017). Inhibition of p66Shc-mediated mitochondrial apoptosis via targeting prolyl-isomerase Pin1 attenuates intestinal ischemia/reperfusion injury in rats. *Clin. Sci.* 131, 759–773. doi: 10.1042/CS20160799

Ferdinandy, P., Hausenloy, D. J., Heusch, G., Baxter, G. F., and Schulz, R. (2014). Interaction of risk factors, comorbidities, and comedications with ischemia/reperfusion injury and cardioprotection by preconditioning, postconditioning, and remote conditioning. *Pharmacol. Rev.* 66, 1142–1174. doi: 10.1124/pr.113.008300

Franzeck, F. C., Hof, D., Spescha, R. D., Hasun, M., Akhmedov, A., Steffel, J., et al. (2012). Expression of the aging gene p66Shc is increased in peripheral blood monocytes of patients with acute coronary syndrome but not with stable coronary artery disease. *Atherosclerosis* 220, 282–286. doi: 10.1016/j.atherosclerosis.2011.10.035

Giorgio, M., Berry, A., Berniakovich, I., Poletaeva, I., Trinei, M., Stendardo, M., et al. (2012). The p66Shc knocked out mice are short lived under natural condition. *Aging Cell* 11, 162–168. doi: 10.1111/j.1474-9726.2011.00770.x

Giorgio, M., Migliaccio, E., Orsini, F., Paolucci, D., Moroni, M., Contursi, C., et al. (2005). Electron transfer between cytochrome c and p66Shc generates reactive oxygen species that trigger mitochondrial apoptosis. *Cell* 122, 221–233. doi: 10.1016/j.cell.2005.05.011

Graiani, G., Lagrasta, C., Migliaccio, E., Spillmann, F., Meloni, M., Madeddu, P., et al. (2005). Genetic deletion of the p66Shc adaptor protein protects from angiotensin II-induced myocardial damage. *Hypertension* 46, 433–440. doi: 10.1161/01.HYP.0000174986.73346.ba

Granger, D. N., and Kvietys, P. R. (2015). Reperfusion injury and reactive oxygen species: the evolution of a concept. *Redox Biol.* 6, 524–551. doi: 10.1016/j.redox.2015.08.020

Khalid, S., Drasche, A., Thurner, M., Hermann, M., Ashraf, M. I., Fresser, F., et al. (2016). cJun N-terminal kinase (JNK) phosphorylation of serine 36 is critical for p66Shc activation. *Sci. Rep.* 6:20930. doi: 10.1038/srep20930

Kong, L., Andrassy, M., Chang, J. S., Huang, C., Asai, T., Szabolcs, M. J., et al. (2008). PKCβ modulates ischemia-reperfusion injury in the heart. *Am. J. Physiol. Heart Circ. Physiol.* 294, H1862–H1870. doi: 10.1152/ajpheart.01346.2007

Kumar, S., Kim, Y. R., Vikram, A., Naqvi, A., Li, Q., Kassan, M., et al. (2017). Sirtuin1-regulated lysine acetylation of p66Shc governs diabetes-induced vascular oxidative stress and endothelial dysfunction. *Proc. Natl. Acad. Sci. U.S.A.* 114, 1714–1719. doi: 10.1073/pnas.1614112114

Liu, Y., Yang, X. M., Iliodromitis, E. K., Kremastinos, D. T., Dost, T., Cohen, M. V., et al. (2008). Redox signaling at reperfusion is required for protection from ischemic preconditioning but not from a direct PKC activator. *Basic Res. Cardiol.* 103, 54–59. doi: 10.1007/s00395-007-0683-y

Migliaccio, E., Giorgio, M., Mele, S., Pelicci, G., Reboldi, P., Pandolfi, P. P., et al. (1999). The p66shc adaptor protein controls oxidative stress response and life span in mammals. *Nature* 402, 309–313. doi: 10.1038/46311

Nemoto, S., Combs, C. A., French, S., Ahn, B. H., Fergusson, M. M., Balaban, R. S., et al. (2006). The mammalian longevity-associated gene product p66shc regulates mitochondrial metabolism. *J. Biol. Chem.* 281, 10555–10560. doi: 10.1074/jbc.M511626200

Palmer, J. W., Tandler, B., and Hoppel, C. L. (1977). Biochemical properties of subsarcolemmal and interfibrillar mitochondria isolated from rat cardiac muscle. *J. Biol. Chem.* 252, 8731–8739.

Palmer, J. W., Tandler, B., and Hoppel, C. L. (1986). Heterogeneous response of subsarcolemmal heart mitochondria to calcium. *Am. J. Physiol.* 250, H741–H748.

Paneni, F., Costantino, S., Castello, L., Battista, R., Capretti, G., Chiandotto, S., et al. (2015). Targeting prolyl-isomerase Pin1 prevents mitochondrial oxidative stress and vascular dysfunction: insights in patients with diabetes. *Eur. Heart J.* 36, 817–828. doi: 10.1093/eurheartj/ehu179

Pinton, P., Rimessi, A., Marchi, S., Orsini, F., Migliaccio, E., Giorgio, M., et al. (2007). Protein kinase C beta and prolyl isomerase 1 regulate mitochondrial effects of the life-span determinant p66Shc. *Science* 315, 659–663. doi: 10.1126/science.1135380

Rota, M., Lecapitaine, N., Hosoda, T., Boni, A., De Angelis, A., Padin-Iruegas, M. E., et al. (2006). Diabetes promotes cardiac stem cell aging and heart failure, which are prevented by deletion of the p66shc gene. *Circ. Res.* 99, 42–52. doi: 10.1161/01.RES.0000231289.63468.08

Sag, C. M., Santos, C. X., and Shah, A. M. (2014). Redox regulation of cardiac hypertrophy. *J. Mol. Cell. Cardiol.* 73, 103–111. doi: 10.1016/j.yjmcc.2014.02.002

Skyschally, A., Schulz, R., Gres, P., Korth, H. G., and Heusch, G. (2003). Attenuation of ischemic preconditioning in pigs by scavenging of free oxyradicals with ascorbic acid. *Am. J. Physiol. Heart Circ. Physiol.* 284, H698–H703. doi: 10.1152/ajpheart.00693.2002

Spescha, R. D., Klohs, J., Semerano, A., Giacalone, G., Derungs, R. S., Reiner, M. F., et al. (2015). Post-ischaemic silencing of p66Shc reduces ischaemia/reperfusion brain injury and its expression correlates to clinical outcome in stroke. *Eur. Heart J.* 36, 1590–1600. doi: 10.1093/eurheartj/ehv140

Spescha, R. D., Shi, Y., Wegener, S., Keller, S., Weber, B., Wyss, M. M., et al. (2013). Deletion of the ageing gene p66(Shc) reduces early stroke size following ischaemia/reperfusion brain injury. *Eur. Heart J.* 34, 96–103. doi: 10.1093/eurheartj/ehs331

St-Pierre, J., Buckingham, J. A., Roebuck, S. J., and Brand, M. D. (2002). Topology of superoxide production from different sites in the mitochondrial electron transport chain. *J. Biol. Chem.* 277, 44784–44790. doi: 10.1074/jbc.M207217200

Trinei, M., Giorgio, M., Cicalese, A., Barozzi, S., Ventura, A., Migliaccio, E., et al. (2002). A p53-p66Shc signalling pathway controls intracellular redox status, levels of oxidation-damaged DNA and oxidative stress-induced apoptosis. *Oncogene* 21, 3872–3878. doi: 10.1038/sj.onc.1205513

Vono, R., Fuoco, C., Testa, S., Pirro, S., Maselli, D., Ferland Mccollough, D., et al. (2016). Activation of the pro-oxidant PKCβII-p66Shc signaling pathway contributes to pericyte dysfunction in skeletal ischemia muscles of patients with diabetes with critical limb. *Diabetes* 65, 3691–3704. doi: 10.2337/db16-0248

Xu, X., Zhu, X., Ma, M., Han, Y., Hu, C., Yuan, S., et al. (2016). p66Shc: a novel biomarker of tubular oxidative injury in patients with diabetic nephropathy. *Sci. Rep.* 6:29302. doi: 10.1038/srep29302

Yan, H., Jihong, Y., Feng, Z., Xiaomei, X., Xiaohan, Z., Guangzhi, W., et al. (2014). Sirtuin 1-mediated inhibition of p66shc expression alleviates liver ischemia/reperfusion injury. *Crit. Care Med.* 42, e373–e381. doi: 10.1097/CCM.0000000000000246

Yang, M., Stowe, D. F., Udoh, K. B., Heisner, J. S., and Camara, A. K. (2014). Reversible blockade of complex I or inhibition of PKCβ reduces activation and mitochondria translocation of p66Shc to preserve cardiac function after ischemia. *PLoS ONE* 9:e113534. doi: 10.1371/journal.pone.0113534

Zaccagnini, G., Martelli, F., Fasanaro, P., Magenta, A., Gaetano, C., Di Carlo, A., et al. (2004). p66ShcA modulates tissue response to hindlimb ischemia. *Circulation* 109, 2917–2923. doi: 10.1161/01.CIR.0000129309.58874.0F

Zhu, M., Ding, J., Jiang, H., Kong, L., Sun, Z., Chen, J., et al. (2015). Propofol ameliorates endothelial inflammation induced by hypoxia/reoxygenation in human umbilical vein endothelial cells: role of phosphatase A2. *Vascul. Pharmacol.* 73, 149–157. doi: 10.1016/j.vph.2015.06.002

Zweier, J. L., Flaherty, J. T., and Weisfeldt, M. L. (1987). Direct measurement of free radical generation following reperfusion of ischemic myocardium. *Proc. Natl. Acad. Sci. U.S.A.* 84, 1404–1407. doi: 10.1073/pnas.84.5.1404

4

Loss of *Akap1* Exacerbates Pressure Overload-Induced Cardiac Hypertrophy and Heart Failure

*Gabriele G. Schiattarella[1], Nicola Boccella[1], Roberta Paolillo[1], Fabio Cattaneo[1,2], Valentina Trimarco[3], Anna Franzone[1,4], Stefania D'Apice[1], Giuseppe Giugliano[1], Laura Rinaldi[2], Domenica Borzacchiello[2], Alessandra Gentile[5], Assunta Lombardi[5], Antonio Feliciello[2], Giovanni Esposito[1] and Cinzia Perrino[1]**

[1] Department of Advanced Biomedical Sciences, University of Naples Federico II, Naples, Italy, [2] Department of Molecular Medicine and Medical Biotechnologies, University of Naples Federico II, Naples, Italy, [3] Department of Neuroscience, Reproductive Science and Odontostomatology, University of Naples Federico II, Naples, Italy, [4] Department of Cardiology, Inselspital, Universitätsspital Bern, Bern, Switzerland, [5] Department of Biology, University of Naples Federico II, Naples, Italy

Edited by:
Pasquale Pagliaro,
Università degli Studi di Torino, Italy

Reviewed by:
Alfredo Criollo,
Universidad de Chile, Chile
Wang Wang,
University of Washington,
United States

***Correspondence:**
Cinzia Perrino
perrino@unina.it

Left ventricular hypertrophy (LVH) is a major contributor to the development of heart failure (HF). Alterations in cyclic adenosine monophosphate (cAMP)-dependent signaling pathways participate in cardiomyocyte hypertrophy and mitochondrial dysfunction occurring in LVH and HF. cAMP signals are received and integrated by a family of cAMP-dependent protein kinase A (PKA) anchor proteins (AKAPs), tethering PKA to discrete cellular locations. AKAPs encoded by the *Akap1* gene (mitoAKAPs) promote PKA mitochondrial targeting, regulating mitochondrial structure and function, reactive oxygen species production, and cell survival. To determine the role of mitoAKAPs in LVH development, in the present investigation, mice with global genetic deletion of *Akap1* (*Akap1*$^{-/-}$), *Akap1* heterozygous (*Akap1*$^{+/-}$), and their wild-type (*wt*) littermates underwent transverse aortic constriction (TAC) or SHAM procedure for 1 week. In *wt* mice, pressure overload induced the downregulation of AKAP121, the major cardiac mitoAKAP. Compared to *wt*, *Akap1*$^{-/-}$ mice did not display basal alterations in cardiac structure or function and cardiomyocyte size or fibrosis. However, loss of *Akap1* exacerbated LVH and cardiomyocyte hypertrophy induced by pressure overload and accelerated the progression toward HF in TAC mice, and these changes were not observed upon prevention of AKAP121 degradation in seven *in absentia* homolog 2 (*Siah2*) knockout mice (*Siah2*$^{-/-}$). Loss of *Akap1* was also associated to a significant increase in cardiac apoptosis as well as lack of activation of Akt signaling after pressure overload. Taken together, these results demonstrate that *in vivo* genetic deletion of *Akap1* enhances LVH development and accelerates pressure overload-induced cardiac dysfunction, pointing at *Akap1* as a novel repressor of pathological LVH. These results confirm and extend the important role of mitoAKAPs in cardiac response to stress.

Keywords: heart failure, Akt, cardiac hypertrophy, cardiomyocytes, pressure overload

INTRODUCTION

Pathological left ventricular hypertrophy (LVH) is a hallmark feature of a number cardiovascular diseases (Hill and Olson, 2008; Schiattarella and Hill, 2015; Schiattarella et al., 2017) and is strongly associated with increased risk of developing heart failure (HF; Levy et al., 1990). In response to stress, such as hypertension and pressure overload, several cellular and sub-cellular modifications lead to cardiac remodeling (Perrino and Rockman, 2007; Burchfield et al., 2013). Despite the critical role of LVH in the development of cardiac dysfunction, the mechanisms underlying cardiomyocyte hypertrophy in response to pressure overload still remain not completely understood.

Members of a family of cyclic adenosine monophosphate (cAMP)-dependent protein kinase A (PKA) anchor proteins (AKAPs) have been identified as potential regulators of cardiac responses to pathological stimuli including pressure overload-induced LVH (Perrino et al., 2010; Diviani et al., 2011; Rababa'h et al., 2014). By anchoring PKA to membranes and cellular organelles, AKAPs play a key role in the intracellular propagation of cAMP/PKA signals (Feliciello et al., 2001; Carlucci et al., 2008b). Several AKAPs are expressed in cardiomyocytes, regulating crucial cellular functions (Diviani et al., 2011). Among these, mAKAP has been shown to regulate hypertrophy of neonatal cardiomyocytes through mitogen-activated protein kinases (MAPKs) signaling pathways (Rababa'h et al., 2014). Moreover, AKAP-Lbc also regulates cardiomyocytes hypertrophy forming a complex with other protein kinases (Carnegie et al., 2008).

Mitochondria are the major energy source for contraction and relaxation in cardiomyocytes. LVH and ultimately HF are characterized by mitochondrial dysfunction leading to reduced ATP production and increased generation of mitochondrial reactive oxygen species (ROS; Torrealba et al., 2017). A sub-family of AKAPs deriving from the alternative splicing of the *Akap1* gene amplifies signals to mitochondria (mitoAKAPs), and has been shown to be critical under several pathological conditions (Carlucci et al., 2008a; Perrino et al., 2010; Scorziello et al., 2013; Schiattarella et al., 2016). We have previously demonstrated that the absence of *Akap1* exacerbates cardiac injury following myocardial infarction in mice, promoting mitochondrial dysfunction, enhancing ROS production and infarct size, and ultimately reducing survival (Schiattarella et al., 2016). Using a rat model of LVH, we have shown that degradation of AKAP121, the most abundant *Akap1* product in muscle cells, occurs early in response to pressure overload, and is associated with impaired mitochondrial function and reduced cell survival (Perrino et al., 2010). Degradation of AKAP121 is mediated, in part, by the E3 ubiquitin ligase seven *in absentia* homolog 2 (*Siah2*; Carlucci et al., 2008a). Previous studies in our laboratory and others have also shown that AKAP121 degradation upon ischemia is reduced in *Siah2* knockout mice (*Siah2*$^{-/-}$; Kim et al., 2011; Schiattarella et al., 2016), and that *Siah2* deletion reduces cardiac susceptibility to ischemia due to loss of *Akap1* (Schiattarella et al., 2016). Although the potential role of AKAP121 in the hypertrophic growth of cardiomyocytes has been suggested by *in vitro* studies (Abrenica et al., 2009), basal cardiac mass, structure, and function of *Akap1*$^{-/-}$ mice were not significantly different compared to their *wt* littermates. Thus, whether *Akap1* plays a causal role during the development of LVH *in vivo* remains unknown. In the present investigation, we hypothesized that loss of *Akap1* exacerbates cardiac hypertrophy in response to pressure overload, leading to an accelerated progression toward HF.

MATERIALS AND METHODS

Experimental Animals

All experiments involving animals in this study were conformed to the Guide for the Care and Use of Laboratory Animals published by the US National Institutes of Health (NIH Publication 8th edition, update 2011), and were approved by the animal welfare regulation of University of Naples Federico II, Naples, Italy, and by the Ministry of Health, Italy. *Akap*1 knockout mice (*Akap*1$^{-/-}$, C57BL/6 background) and *Akap1* heterozygous mice (*Akap*$^{+/-}$, C57BL/6 background) were kindly donated by McKnight G. S. and have been previously described (Newhall et al., 2006; Schiattarella et al., 2016). *Siah2* knockout mice (*Siah2*$^{-/-}$, C57BL/6 background) were kindly donated by Bowtell D. Wild-type (*wt*, C57BL/6 background) *Akap*1$^{+/-}$ and *Akap*1$^{-/-}$ mice of either gender (8–9 weeks old) were included in the study and maintained under identical conditions of temperature (21 ± 1°C), humidity (60 ± 5%), and light/dark cycle, and had free access to normal mouse chow.

Mouse Model of Pressure Overload-Induced Cardiac Hypertrophy and Heart Failure

Pressure overload was induced in adult *Akap1*$^{+/-}$, *Akap*1$^{-/-}$, and *Siah2*$^{-/-}$ mice and their *wt* littermates by transverse aortic constriction (TAC) as previously described (Esposito et al., 2011; Angrisano et al., 2014). Briefly, mice were anesthetized by intraperitoneal injection of 0.1 ml/kg of mixture of 50% Tiletamine and 50% Zolazepam (Zoletil 100) and Xylazine 5 mg/kg (Sigma-Aldrich) and a surgical suture was passed across the aortic arch between left common carotid artery and innominate artery. Another group of animals underwent a left thoracotomy without aortic constriction (sham). Mice from all the groups were sacrificed 1 week (1w) after surgery to perform molecular analyses. Only TAC animals with systolic pressure gradients >40 mmHg were included in the study.

Transthoracic Echocardiography

Cardiac function was non-invasively monitored by transthoracic echocardiography using the Vevo 770 high-resolution imaging system equipped with a 30-MHz RMV-707B scanning head (Visual-Sonics, Toronto, ON, Canada) 1w after sham or TAC operation in mice of all genotypes as previously described (Esposito et al., 2011; Perrino et al., 2013).

Protein Extraction and Immunoblotting

Heart and cellular samples were homogenized in a buffer containing 150 mmol/L NaCl, 50 mmol/L Tris-HCl (pH 8.5), 2 mmol/L EDTA, 1% v/v NP-40, 0.5% w/v deoxycholate, 10 mmol/L NaF, 10 mM sodium pyrophosphate, 2 mmol/L PMSF, 2 heart leupeptin, 2 heart aprotinin, pH 7.4, using the program Protein_1 on a GentleMACS tissue Dissociator (Miltenyi Biotec; Esposito et al., 2015; Cattaneo et al., 2016). Protein concentration in all lysates was measured by using a dye-binding protein assay kit (Bio-Rad) and a SmartSpec Plus spectrophotometer (Bio-Rad) reading at a wavelength of 595 nm. Immunoblotting was performed by using commercially available antibodies: anti-Akt (rabbit polyclonal, Santa Cruz Biotechnology), anti-pAkt (Ser473, rabbit polyclonal, Cell Signaling), anti-cleaved Caspase-3 (rabbit polyclonal, Cell Signaling), anti-AKAP121 (Carlucci et al., 2008a; rabbit polyclonal), anti-caspase-9 (rabbit polyclonal, Santa Cruz Biotechnology), anti-IDH2 (goat polyclonal, Santa Cruz Biotechnology), anti-phosphoPKA substrates (rabbit polyclonal, Cell Signaling), anti-GAPDH (mouse monoclonal, Santa Cruz Biotechnology), and anti-tubulin (mouse monoclonal, Sigma-Aldrich). Secondary antibodies were purchased from Amersham Life Sciences (GE Healthcare). Bands were visualized by enhanced chemiluminescence (ECL; Amersham Life Sciences) according to the manufacturer's instructions, and were quantified by using densitometry (Chemidoc, Bio-Rad). Each experiment and densitometric quantification was separately repeated at least three times.

RNA Isolation and Real-Time PCR

Total RNA was prepared using TRIzol (Invitrogen, Eugene, OR, United States), according to the manufacturer's instruction. Oligo-dT first strand cDNA was synthesized using the SuperScript VILO cDNA Synthesis Kit (Invitrogen, Life technologies) according to the manufacturer's instructions. mRNA expression was determined in cardiac samples from different experimental groups by real-time quantitative PCR (RT-PCR) using a IQ-5 Multicolor Real-Time PCR Detection System (BIORAD). The primers used were: β-MHC: forward 5′-GAGACGACTGTGGCCTCC-3′, reverse 5′-GCAT GATGGCGCCTGTCAG-3′; Collagen IA1: forward 5′-GGAGAC AGGTCAGACCTGTGTG-3′, reverse 5′-CAGCTGGATAGC GACATCGGC-3′; Collagen III: forward 5′-ATATCAAACACGC AAGGC-3′, reverse 5′-GATTAAAGCAAGAGGAACAC-3′; Fibronectin: forward 5′- ACCGTGTCAGGCTTCCGG-3′, reverse 5′- ACGGAAGTGGCCGTGCTT-3′; and GAPDH: forward 5′-TGCAGTGGCAAAGTGGAGATT-3′, reverse 5′-TC GCTCCTGGAAGATGGTGAT-3′.

Mitochondria Isolation and Evaluation of Respiratory Parameters

Mitochondria were isolated from cardiac samples and respiration rate was detected on isolated mitochondria as previously described (Perrino et al., 2013; Schiattarella et al., 2016). Briefly, hearts were gently homogenized in a buffer containing 220 mM mannitol, 70 mM sucrose, 20 mM Tris·HCl, 1 mM EDTA, and 5 mM EGTA (pH 7.4) and then centrifuged at 8,000 *g* for 10 min at 4°C. The supernatant was further centrifuged and the mitochondrial pellet was either use for immunoblot analysis or to measure mitochondrial respiration (Perrino et al., 2013; Schiattarella et al., 2016).

Adult Ventricular Murine Myocytes Isolation

Adult ventricular myocytes were isolated from murine adult hearts using a modified heart retrograde perfusion-based method. Briefly, mice were injected with heparin and anesthetized with an intraperitoneal injection of 0.1 ml/kg of mixture of 50% Tiletamine and 50% Zolazepam (Zoletil 100) and Xylazine 5 mg/kg (Sigma-Aldrich). The heart was quickly excised, and the aorta was cannulated for retrograde perfusion in a Langendorff apparatus at a constant flow rate of 1.5 ml/min at 37°C. The heart was perfused for 9–10 min with isolation buffer [NaCl 120 mM, KCl 4.4 mM, $MgCl_2$ 1 M, NaH_2PO_4 1.2 mM, $NaHCO_3$ 20 mM, glucose 5 mM, 2,3-butanedione monoxime (BDM) 1.25 mM, and taurine 5 mM, pH 7.4], bubbling the isolation solution with 95% O_2 – 5% CO_2, followed by digestion for 13 min with collagenase II (350 U/ml; Worthington) in isolation buffer. After digestion, myocytes were suspended in isolation buffer, filtered with a mesh (100 μm), gently spin down (300 g for 1 min), and resuspended for stepwise Ca^{2+} reintroduction from 25 μmol/L to 1.0 mmol/L. Myocytes were than lyzed in a buffer containing Tris 1 M, 1% v/v Nonidet P-40, NaCl 5 M, 10% w/v deoxycholate, $NaVO_3$ 100 mM, and NaF 100 mM to extract protein as described above.

Histology

Mouse heart specimens were fixed in 4% formaldehyde and embedded in paraffin. After de-paraffinization and re-hydratation, 4-μm-thick sections were prepared and mounted on glass slides. An even number of cardiac cross sections per group were stained with wheat germ agglutinin (WGA) or Picosirius red as previously described (Schiattarella et al., 2016). Briefly, thin cardiac sections were analyzed using Nikon light microscope and NIS Elements Basic Research software (Nikon). For assessment of cardiomyocyte cross sectional area, mean area was evaluated by measuring 400–500 cells per heart (n = 4–5 animals/group). Fibrotic regions (6–8 fields/section, n = 4–5 animals/group) were measured as percent of collagen-stained area/total myocardial area and averaged using a computer-assisted image analysis software (Image J software, National Institutes of Health).

TUNEL Staining

Cardiac DNA nicks were assayed by an *in situ* Apoptosis Detection kit or ApopTag Fluorescein Direct *in situ* Apoptosis Detection kit (Chemicon) according to manufacturer's instructions as previously described (Esposito et al., 2015; Schiattarella et al., 2016). TUNEL staining was visualized by specific green fluorescence and nuclei by 4′-6-diamidino-2-phenylindole (DAPI). TUNEL-positive cardiomyocytes nuclei identified were normalized by total nuclei stained in the same sections by DAPI (n = 7–8 animals/group). An even numbers of slides were analyzed for each group.

Statistical Analysis

All data presented are representative of three or more independent experiments and are expressed as mean ± SEM. Comparisons between two groups were performed using the unpaired Student's t-test. For experiments including three or more experimental groups, comparisons were made by one-way analysis of variance (ANOVA) or 2-way ANOVA, and p values shown indicate the effect of genotype response. Correction for multiple comparisons was made using the Student–Newman–Keuls method. A minimum value of $p < 0.05$ was considered statistically significant. All statistical analyses were conducted with Prism statistical software.

RESULTS

Akap1 Deletion Enhances Cardiac Hypertrophy After Transverse Aortic Constriction in Mice

We have previously demonstrated that myocardial levels of AKAP121 decrease in a rat model of LVH induced by ascending aortic banding (Perrino et al., 2010), suggesting a role for this adaptor protein in the transmission of hypertrophic signals in the myocardium. However, the effects of *Akap1* genetic deletion on cardiac remodeling in response to pressure overload are currently unknown. Consistent with our previous results, AKAP121 cardiac levels were significantly decreased in *wt* mice subjected to 1w TAC compared to sham-operated littermates (**Figure 1A**), and these results were associated with the impairment of mitochondrial PKA signaling (Supplementary Figure S1). Importantly, AKAP121 downregulation was also observed in adult ventricular myocytes isolated from *wt* TAC hearts (Supplementary Figure S2), demonstrating that AKAP121 downregulation in LVH occurs in cardiomyocytes. Interestingly, after TAC, both *Akap1*$^{+/-}$ and *Akap1*$^{-/-}$ mice exhibited a significant further increase in LVW/BW compared to *wt* TAC mice (**Figure 1B** and **Table 1**), coupled with an increase in cardiomyocytes cross-sectional area measured by WGA staining (**Figure 1C**) and in β-myosin heavy chain (β-MHC) mRNA abundance (**Figure 1D**). No differences were found among the three different genotypes in cardiac interstitial fibrosis, measured by Picrosirius red staining (**Figure 2A**), as well as in the mRNA abundance of the most common fibrotic markers: collagen type I, type III, and fibronectin (**Figures 2B–D**). Collectively, these data suggest that loss of *Akap1* exacerbates cardiac hypertrophy induced by pressure overload without affecting the fibrotic response.

Genetic Deletion of *Akap1* Precipitates Heart Failure Induced by Pressure Overload

Chronic pressure overload inevitably leads to impairment in LV systolic function and ultimately HF (Esposito et al., 2011; Schiattarella and Hill, 2015). As expected, after 1w TAC, *wt* mice exhibited a mild but significant reduction in % FS compared to sham-operated animals (**Figures 3A,B** and **Table 1**). Reduction in % FS in *wt* mice was mainly due to the increase in LV end-systolic diameter (LVESd, **Figure 3C**) without significant changes in LV end-diastolic diameter (LVEDd, **Figure 3D**). In *Akap1*$^{+/-}$ and *Akap1*$^{-/-}$ mice, TAC operation caused a significant further decrease of % FS compared to TAC *wt* mice (**Figures 3A,B**). Reduction in % FS observed in *Akap1*$^{+/-}$ and *Akap1*$^{-/-}$ after TAC, resulted by increase in both LVESd and LVEDd (**Figures 3C,D**). The differences in LV systolic function between *wt* and *Akap1*-deficient mice after stress suggest that *Akap1* plays an important role in the progression toward HF after chronic pressure overload.

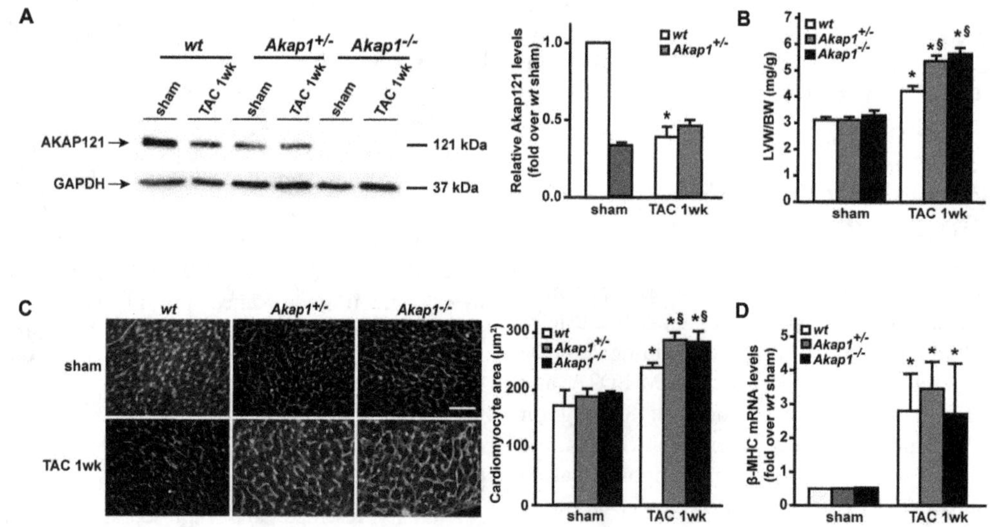

FIGURE 1 | *Akap1* deficiency exacerbates pressure overload-induced cardiac hypertrophy. **(A)** Representative immunoblot (left) and densitometric analysis (right) of AKAP121 protein levels in hearts from sham ($n = 5$) and 1 week transverse aortic constriction (TAC 1w; $n = 7$) operated *wt*, *Akap1*$^{+/-}$, and *Akap1*$^{-/-}$ mice. GAPDH was used as control of loading sample (*$p < 0.05$ vs. *wt* sham). **(B)** Bar graphs showing cumulative data of left ventricular weight (LVW) to body weight (BW) 1 week after sham or TAC procedures in *wt*, *Akap1*$^{+/-}$, and *Akap1*$^{-/-}$ mice (*$p < 0.05$ vs. sham; $^{\S}p < 0.05$ vs. *wt* TAC 1w; $n = 7$ hearts/group). **(C)** (Left) Representative images of wheat germ agglutinin (WGA) staining of cardiac transversal sections from *wt*, *Akap1*$^{+/-}$, and *Akap1*$^{-/-}$ mice 1 week after sham or TAC procedure. DAPI was used as nuclei counterstaining. Scale bar: 20 μm. (Right) Bar graphs showing cumulative data of multiple independent experiments analyzing cardiomyocytes cross-sectional area (*$p < 0.05$ vs. sham; $^{\S}p < 0.05$ vs. *wt* TAC 1w; $n = 5$ hearts/group). **(D)** mRNA levels of β-myosin heavy chain (β-MHC) in cardiac samples from *wt*, *Akap1*$^{+/-}$, and *Akap1*$^{-/-}$ mice 1 week after sham or TAC procedure (*$p < 0.05$ vs. sham; $n = 5$ hearts/group).

TABLE 1 | Echocardiographic and morphometric analysis in the different experimental groups of mice.

	wt		*Akap1*$^{+/-}$		*Akap1*$^{-/-}$	
	Sham (*n* = 8)	**TAC 1w (*n* = 12)**	**Sham (*n* = 6)**	**TAC 1w (*n* = 13)**	**Sham (*n* = 6)**	**TAC 1w (*n* = 9)**
Morphometry						
BW (g)	27.3 ± 1.4	23.0 ± 0.7*	23.3 ± 0.8	23.6 ± 0.9	23.4 ± 1.1	23.0 ± 0.5
LVW (mg)	84.9 ± 4.9	100.4 ± 5.9*	73.6 ± 3.3	124.0 ± 4.4*$	76.9 ± 7.0	99.6 ± 5.3*#
HW (mg)	112.5 ± 7.0	131.8 ± 7.8	95.8 ± 4.7	154.6 ± 4.7*$	105.8 ± 10.2	135.1 ± 7.3*#
LVW/BW (mg/g)	3.1 ± 0.1	4.2 ± 0.2*	3.1 ± 0.1	5.4 ± 0.2*$	3.3 ± 0.2	5.7 ± 0.6*$
HW/BW (mg/g)	4.9 ± 0.1	5.6 ± 0.3*	4.1 ± 0.1	6.6 ± 0.2*	4.5 ± 0.3	5.9 ± 0.3*
Echocardiography						
LVEDd (mm)	3.0 ± 0.1	3.1 ± 0.1	3.0 ± 0.1	4.0 ± 0.1*$	3.2 ± 0.1	3.6 ± 0.1*$
LVESd (mm)	1.2 ± 0.1	1.6 ± 0.1*	1.2 ± 0.1	2.7 ± 0.1*$	1.3 ± 0.1	2.4 ± 0.2*$
IVS,d (mm)	0.7 ± 0.0	1.1 ± 0.0*	0.8 ± 0.0	1.0 ± 0.0*	0.8 ± 0.0	1.0 ± 0.0*
PW,d (mm)	0.8 ± 0.0	0.9 ± 0.0*	0.8 ± 0.0	1.0 ± 0.0*	0.8 ± 0.0	0.9 ± 0.1
FS (%)	60.6 ± 1.8	50.3 ± 2.3*	60.0 ± 1.2	32.5 ± 2.8*$	58.6 ± 2.3	33.5 ± 3.4*$
HR (bpm)	573 ± 11	583 ± 17	595 ± 30	584 ± 23	681 ± 19	661 ± 16

BW, body weight; LVW, left ventricle weight; HW, heart weight; LVEDd, left ventricular end-diastolic diameter; LVESd, left ventricular end-systolic diameter; IVS,d interventricular septum end-diastolic diameter; PW,d posterior wall end-diastolic diameter; FS, fractional shortening; HR, heart rate ($p < 0.05$ vs. correspondent sham; $^{\$}p < 0.05$ vs. wt TAC 1w; and $^{\#}p < 0.05$ vs. Akap1$^{+/-}$ TAC 1w).*

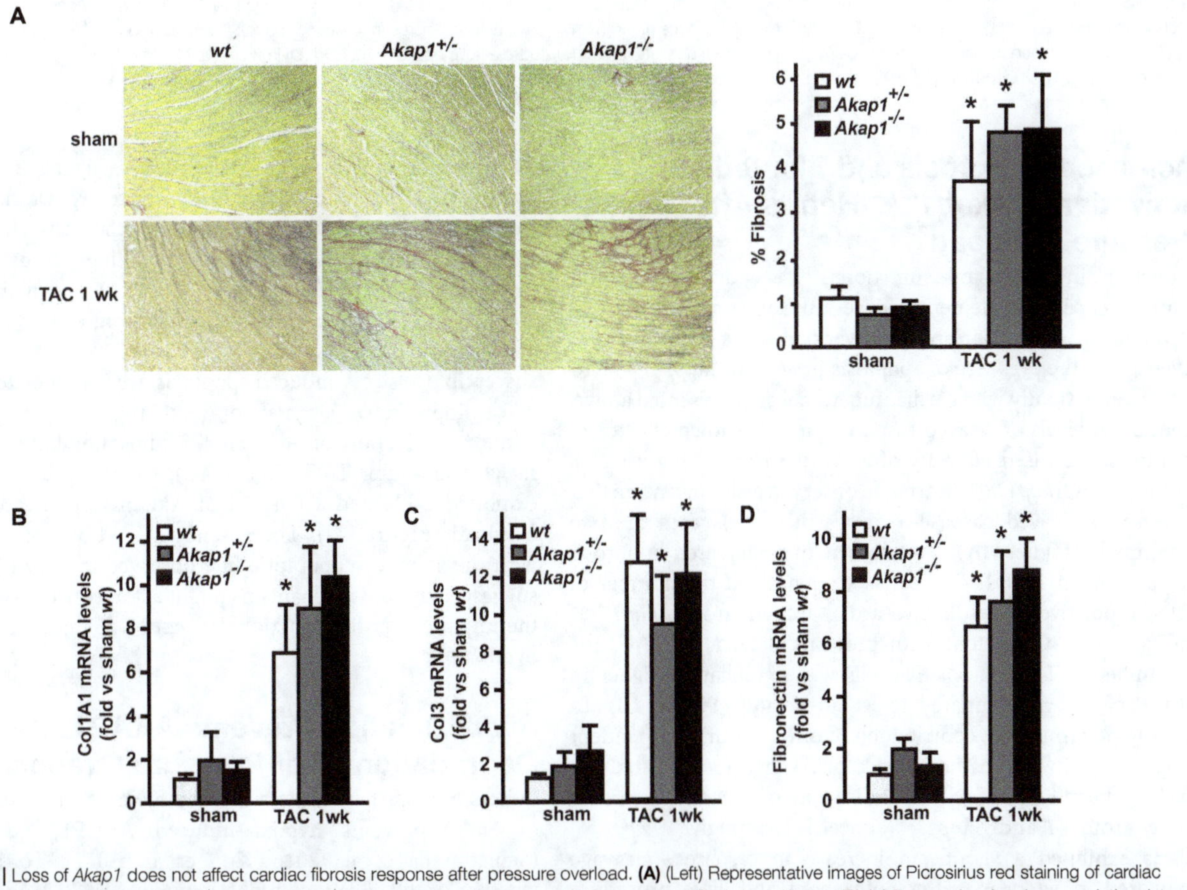

FIGURE 2 | Loss of *Akap1* does not affect cardiac fibrosis response after pressure overload. **(A)** (Left) Representative images of Picrosirius red staining of cardiac transversal sections from *wt*, *Akap1*$^{+/-}$, and *Akap1*$^{-/-}$ mice 1 week after sham or TAC procedure. Scale bar: 40 μm. (Right) Bar graphs showing cumulative data of multiple independent experiments analyzing percentage of fibrosis (*$p < 0.05$ vs. sham *wt*; $n = 5$ hearts/group). mRNA levels of collagen I (Col1A1, **B**), collagen III (Col3; **C**), and fibronectin **(D)** in cardiac samples from *wt*, *Akap1*$^{+/-}$, and *Akap1*$^{-/-}$ mice 1 week after sham or TAC procedure (*$p < 0.05$ vs. sham; $n = 5$ hearts/group).

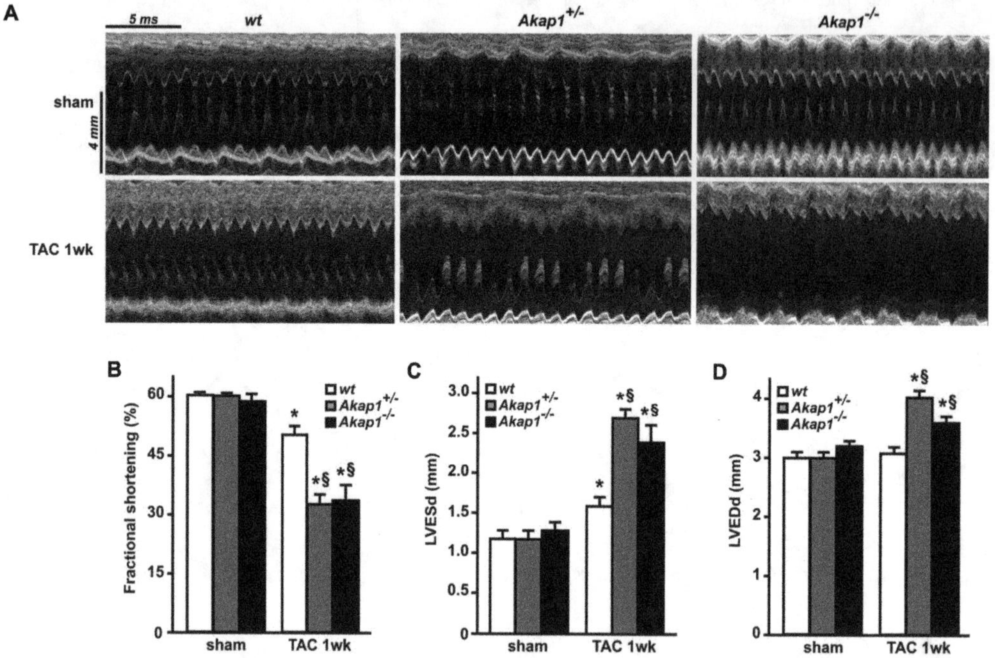

FIGURE 3 | Genetic deletion of *Akap1* accelerates the progression toward heart failure in TAC mice **(A)**. Representative left ventricular (LV) M-mode echocardiographic tracings from *wt*, *Akap1*$^{+/-}$ and *Akap1*$^{-/-}$ mice after sham or TAC 1w procedures ($n = 7$ mice/group). Cumulative data of % fractional shortening **(B)**, left ventricular end-systolic diameter (LVESd; **C**) and left ventricular end-diastolic diameter (LVEDd; **D**) in *wt*, *Akap1*$^{+/-}$ and *Akap1*$^{-/-}$ mice 1 week after sham or TAC procedure ($^{*}p < 0.05$ vs. sham; $^{\S}p < 0.05$ vs. TAC 1w *wt*; $n = 5$ hearts/group).

Increased Apoptosis and Blunted *Akt* Activation in *Akap1*$^{-/-}$ Hearts After Pressure Overload

Reduction in LV systolic function is dependent on loss of contractile cellular elements, since cardiomyocytes apoptosis occurs in the context of pressure overload stress. Thus, we next investigated the presence of apoptosis in *wt* and *Akap1*$^{-/-}$ TAC hearts. Consistently with cardiac functional data presented above, myocardial levels of cleaved caspase-3, a well-known effector of apoptosis, increased after 1w of TAC in *wt* mice (**Figure 4A**). Strikingly, in *Akap1*$^{-/-}$ hearts, we observed a significant further increase in cleaved caspase-3 myocardial levels compared to *wt* animals (**Figure 4A**). To confirm that increased apoptosis was present in *Akap1*$^{-/-}$ hearts, we quantified the number of TUNEL-positive nuclei in myocardial sections from *Akap1*$^{-/-}$ and *wt* mice. Consistent with previous data, after TAC, the % number of TUNEL-positive cells was significantly higher in *Akap1*$^{-/-}$ hearts compared to *wt* littermates (**Figure 4B**). In order to determine the contribution of mitochondrial-dependent apoptotic pathways in the absence of *Akap1*, we evaluated the levels of the mitochondrial apoptotic protein caspase-9 in cardiac lysates from *wt* and *Akap1*$^{-/-}$ mice. Interestingly, *Akap1*$^{-/-}$ hearts exhibited a significant increase in caspase-9 cleavage compared to *wt* hearts after both sham and TAC procedure (Supplementary Figure S3). These data indicate that loss of *Akap1*$^{-/-}$ increased the susceptibility to pressure overload-induced apoptosis, which is, at least in part, dependent by activation of mitochondrial pro-apoptotic pathways.

Activation of Akt-dependent protective signals is a hallmark of HF (Chaanine and Hajjar, 2011). Recently, we have shown that loss of *Akap1* in vascular endothelial cells (ECs) blunts ischemia-induced Akt activation resulting in dysfunctional behavior of ECs (Schiattarella et al., 2018). Given the fact the *Akap1*$^{-/-}$ mice have an accelerated progression toward HF after pressure overload and that *Akap1*$^{-/-}$ hearts are more susceptible to stress-induced apoptosis, we hypothesized that loss of cardioprotective signals from Akt might play a role in this context. Activation of Akt (Ser473 phosphorylation) occurred in *wt* hearts after TAC (**Figure 4C**), whereas *Akap1*$^{-/-}$ hearts exhibited a blunted activation of Akt in response to pressure overload (**Figure 4C**). The absence of Akt activation together with the enhanced apoptotic rate observed in *Akap1*$^{-/-}$ hearts suggests that both mechanisms might act in concert to determine the impaired cardiac function of *Akap1*$^{-/-}$ mice after pressure overload.

Siah2 Deletion Prevents AKAP121 Degradation After Pressure Overload

Others and we have previously demonstrated that the absence of *Siah2* prevents hypoxia-induced AKAP121 degradation (Schiattarella et al., 2016; Kim et al., 2011). To investigate whether *Siah2* deletion might prevent AKAP121 degradation in response to pressure overload, *Siah2*$^{-/-}$ mice underwent the TAC procedure. One week after surgery, downregulation of AKAP121 cardiac levels was significantly inhibited in *Siah2*$^{-/-}$ mice compared to *wt* littermates (**Figure 5A**). Interestingly,

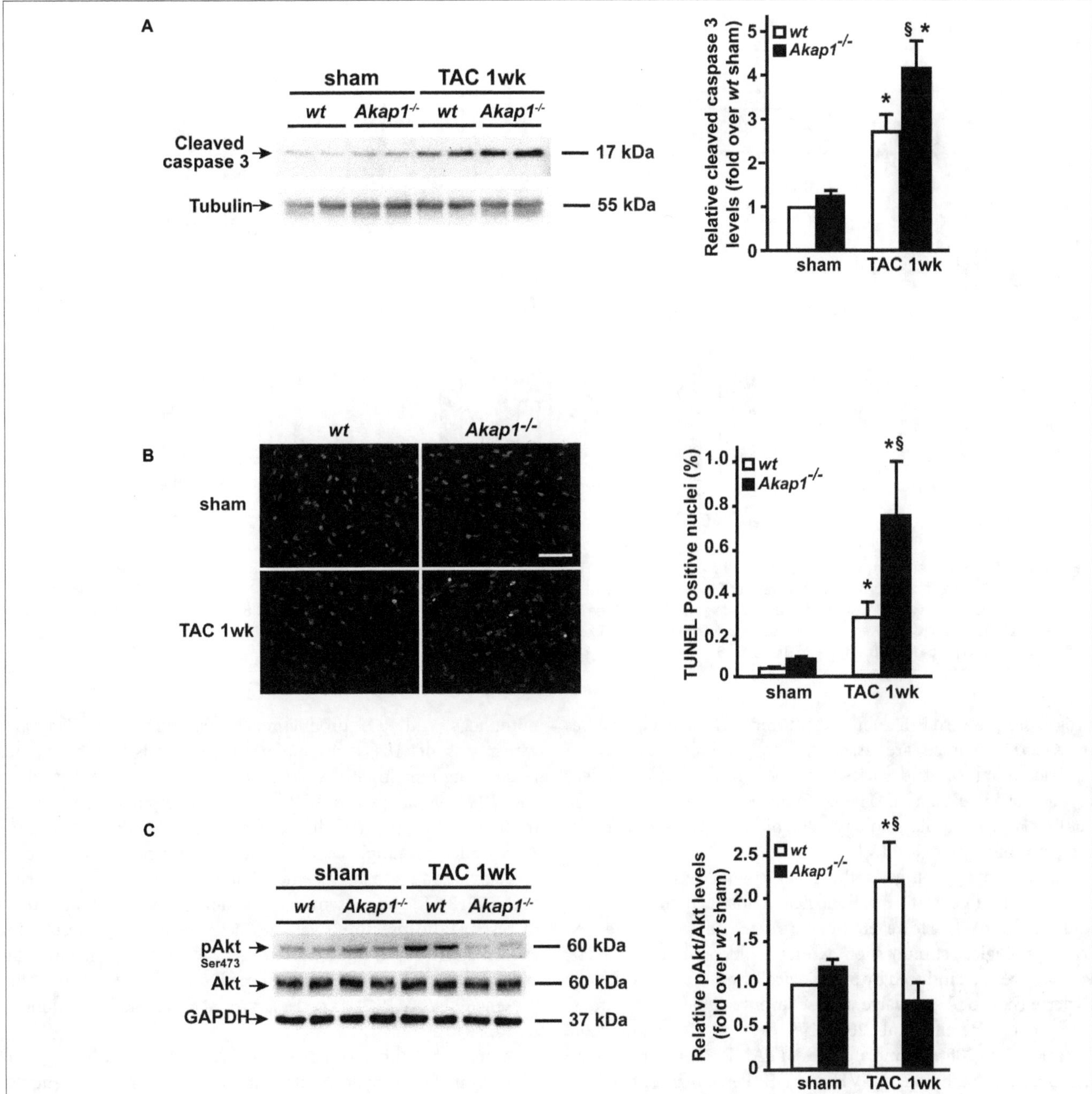

FIGURE 4 | Increased cardiac apoptosis and lack of Akt activation in *Akap1*$^{-/-}$ mice after TAC. **(A)** Representative immunoblot (left) and densitometric analysis (right) of cleaved caspase-3 protein levels in *wt* and *Akap1*$^{-/-}$ hearts 1 week after sham or TAC procedure (*$p < 0.05$ vs. sham; $^{\S}p < 0.05$ vs. *wt* TAC 1w; $n = 5$ hearts/group). Tubulin was used as control of loading sample. **(B)** (Left) Representative DAPI and TUNEL staining of cardiac sections from *wt*, *Akap1*$^{+/-}$, and *Akap1*$^{-/-}$ mice 1 week after sham or TAC procedure. Positive nuclei appear green. Scale bar: 20 μm. (Right) Bar graphs showing cumulative data of multiple independent experiments evaluating TUNEL-positive cells (*$p < 0.05$ vs. sham; $^{\S}p < 0.05$ vs. *wt* TAC 1w; $n = 5$ hearts/group). **(C)** Representative immunoblot (left) and densitometric analysis (right) of Akt Ser 473 phosphorylation (pAkt) and Akt in *wt* and *Akap1*$^{-/-}$ hearts 1 week after sham or TAC procedure. GAPDH was used as control of loading sample (*$p < 0.05$ vs. sham; $^{\S}p < 0.05$ vs. *Akap1*$^{-/-}$ TAC 1w; $n = 5$ hearts/group).

Siah2$^{-/-}$ mice exhibited the same extent of cardiac hypertrophy estimated by LVW/BW compared to *wt* controls (**Figure 5B**), as well as similar deterioration of cardiac function investigated by means of FS% (**Figure 5C**), LVESd (**Figure 5D**), and LVEDd (**Figure 5E**).

DISCUSSION

In the present study, we demonstrate for the first time that *in vivo* genetic deletion of *Akap1* exacerbates pressure overload-induced cardiac hypertrophy development and accelerates the

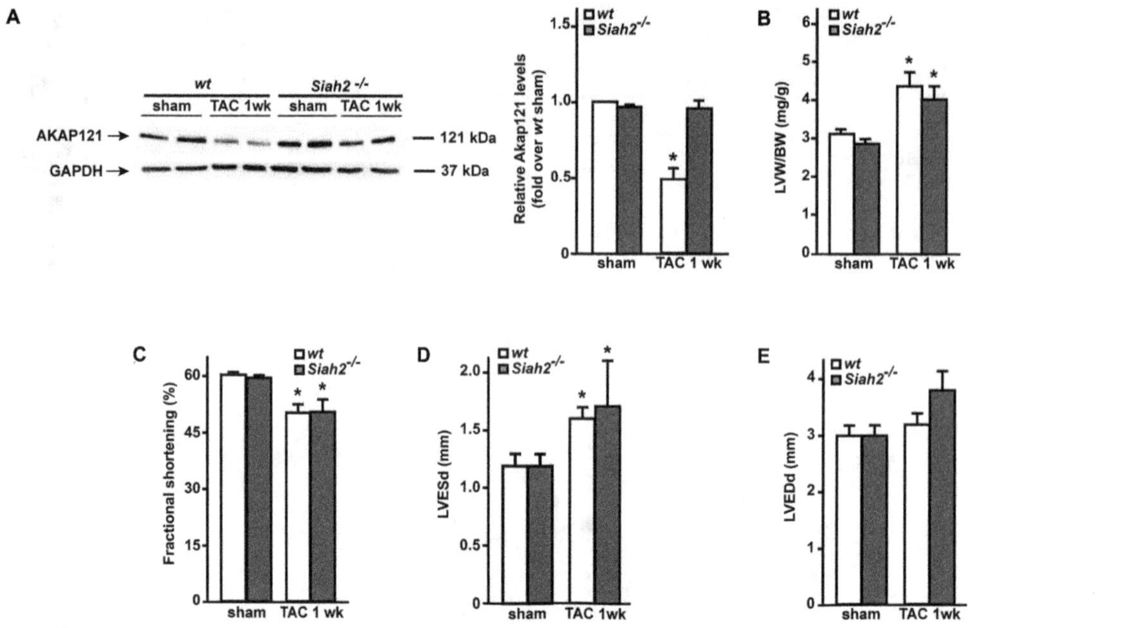

FIGURE 5 | Siah2 deficiency prevents AKAP121 degradation after TAC. **(A)** Representative immunoblot (left) and densitometric analysis (right) of AKAP121 protein levels in *wt* and *Siah2*$^{-/-}$ hearts 1 week after sham or TAC procedure. GAPDH was used as control of loading sample (*$p < 0.05$ vs. *wt* sham). **(B)** Bar graphs showing cumulative data of LVW/ BW 1 week after sham or TAC procedures in *wt* and *Siah2*$^{-/-}$ mice (*$p < 0.05$ vs. sham; $n = 6$ hearts/group). Cumulative data of % fractional shortening **(C)**, left ventricular end-systolic diameter (LVESd; **D**), and left ventricular end-diastolic diameter (LVEDd; **E**) in *wt* and *Siah2*$^{-/-}$ mice 1 week after sham or TAC procedure (*$p < 0.05$ vs. sham; $n = 6$ hearts/group).

progression toward HF after TAC in mice. These abnormalities in *Akap1*$^{-/-}$ mice are associated to an increased rate of cardiac apoptosis and lack of activation of Akt-dependent cardioprotective signals. These results extend the knowledge about *Akap1* in cardiac biology, and confirm its role as a critical mediator of pathological LVH.

Cardiac hypertrophy is the first, general response of the heart to physiological or pathological loads (Chien, 1999; Frey and Olson, 2003). However, while cardiac adaptations induced by physiological stimuli such as exercise do not result in HF, cardiac overload induced by pathological stimuli, such as chronic hypertension or heart valve disease, eventually leads to cardiac dysfunction (Berenji et al., 2005; Heineke and Molkentin, 2006; Perrino et al., 2006). Abnormalities in cAMP/PKA signaling are a hallmark of pathological LVH and HF (Perrino and Rockman, 2007). AKAPs scaffold proteins compartmentalize PKA activity into subcellular domains (e.g., mitochondria), thus allowing a tight-controlled spatial and temporal regulation of cellular responses (Feliciello et al., 2001; Newhall et al., 2006).

The transmission of cAMP signaling to mitochondria is reached by a family of mitoAKAPs that have been shown to play an important role in cardiac response to stress (Perrino et al., 2010; Diviani et al., 2011). In particular, others and we have shown that AKAP121 is critical for cardiomyocytes response to ischemic injury (Kim et al., 2011; Schiattarella et al., 2016). Genetic deletion of *Akap1* results in larger infarct size, worse LV systolic function, and increased mortality after myocardial infarction (Schiattarella et al., 2016). Although the absence of *Akap1* was associated to increased mitochondrial dysfunction, mitophagy, and ROS production, the specific mechanisms by which loss of *Akap1* results in worse post-ischemic cardiac remodeling remain elusive. More recently, we have shown that AKAP121 also regulates ECs behavior in response to ischemia through Akt signaling (Schiattarella et al., 2018). In ECs, lack of *Akap1* affects multiple cellular functions and results in reduced Akt activation upon angiogenic stimuli or hypoxia (Schiattarella et al., 2018). In the present investigation, we demonstrated that in response to pressure overload, deletion of *Akap1* results in exacerbated LVH in the absence of Akt activation, confirming in a different experimental model of cardiovascular disease that the presence of AKAP121 is necessary to achieve Akt activation in response to stress.

A previous study has shown that AKAP121 acts as a repressor of cardiomyocytes hypertrophy (Abrenica et al., 2009). Silencing of AKAP121 *in vitro* resulted in increased cardiomyocytes cell size in the absence of any pro-hypertrophic stimulus (Abrenica et al., 2009). Although our data confirm the role of AKAP121 as a brake of cardiomyocytes growth, others and we repetitively observed the absence of any basal cardiac alterations in *Akap1*$^{-/-}$ mice (Newhall et al., 2006; Schiattarella et al., 2016, 2018). In-depth characterization of cardiac structure and function in *Akap1*$^{-/-}$ mice revealed that absence of *Akap1* did not cause LVH and HF over time. In addition, we have previously demonstrated that *in vivo* administration of synthetic peptides displacing AKAP121 from mitochondria increased cardiac ROS and apoptotic cell death, but is was not sufficient to induce cardiac hypertrophy, even if we observed increased nuclear localization of nuclear factor of activated T-cells (NFAT), the main effector of the calcineurin-dependent pro-hypertrophic signaling pathway (Perrino et al., 2010). However, when subjected to pressure overload, *Akap1*-deficient mice develop a more robust hypertrophic response and an accelerated progression toward HF, confirming that *Akap1* acts as a repressor of cardiomyocytes hypertrophy. The fact that, only if stressed, *Akap1*$^{-/-}$ hearts exhibit pronounced cardiac hypertrophy might be in contrast with the previous notion that knockdown of AKAP121 *in vitro* affects *per se* cardiomyocyte size. However, this apparent discrepancy can be explained by the fact that, *in vivo*, Rab32, a mitochondria-targeted AKAP-like protein, might exert compensatory effects in the absence of *Akap1* (Alto et al., 2002; Bui et al., 2010). The pivotal role of AKAP121 in the regulation of HF development was also confirmed by the evidence that while *Akap1*-deficient mice underwent rapid deterioration of cardiac function in response to pressure overload, and this process was not observed in *Siah2*-deficient mice.

The absence of *Akap1* has been variously associated with increased ROS production and mitochondrial dysfunction in several models of cardio- and cerebrovascular diseases as well as in cancer (Feliciello et al., 1998; Scorziello et al., 2013; Schiattarella et al., 2016; Rinaldi et al., 2017). For example, despite no basal differences were found in mitochondrial respiration between *Akap1*$^{-/-}$ and *wt* hearts, following myocardial infarction, *Akap1*$^{-/-}$ mice exhibited increase levels of cardiac ROS and more prominent alterations in mitochondrial morphology compared to *wt* controls (Schiattarella et al., 2016). After 1w-TAC, no differences were observed between *Akap1*$^{-/-}$ and *wt* mice in cardiac mitochondrial respiratory function (Supplementary Figure S4). However, we cannot exclude that alterations in mitochondrial function might occur at a later time point in *Akap1*$^{-/-}$ hearts in the context of pressure overload. These results suggest that mitochondrial morphological and functional alterations induced by the absence of *Akap1* might be influenced by the nature and/or duration of stress that triggers cardiac dysfunction.

As mentioned above, the absence of *Akap1* leads to lack of Akt activation in hypertrophic hearts, and we speculate that Akt could mediate the effects of *Akap1* deletion on hypertrophic growth. Akt is at the crossroad of signaling pathways regulating cardiac growth and contractile function (Aoyagi and Matsui, 2011; Chaanine and Hajjar, 2011). Being downstream of insulin/insulin-like growth factor (IGF), Akt activation has been associated to physiological LVH development (Ellison et al., 2012). However, Akt phosphorylation has also been found increased in pathological LVH as an initial response to afterload stress (Chaanine and Hajjar, 2011). Therefore, Akt activation in TAC has been recognized as a pro-survival adaptation signal, required for the activation of protein synthesis in cardiomyocytes (Matsui et al., 1999; Fujio et al., 2000; Cannavo et al., 2013). Consistent with this notion, *Akap1*$^{-/-}$ mice subjected to TAC exhibited increased cardiac cell death and an accelerated progression toward HF coupled with lack of Akt activation. A number of signaling molecules are placed downstream of Akt. Among these, the mechanistic target of rapamycin (mTOR) plays a central role in cardiomyocyte hypertrophy (Morales et al., 2016). Recently, *Akap1* has been shown to control mTOR regulating cancer cells growth (Rinaldi et al., 2017). However, the mechanisms by which *Akap1* influences Akt/mTOR signaling pathway remain poorly understood. Akt localizes to diverse sub-cellular compartments, including mitochondria, where it contributes to phosphorylation of key mitochondrial targets (Bijur and Jope, 2003; Miyamoto et al., 2008; Lim et al., 2016). The absence of *Akap1* leads to reduction in Akt phosphorylation in LVH as well as in vascular dysfunction (Schiattarella et al., 2018), suggesting that mitoAKAPs might also contribute to Akt subcellular distribution to promote cell survival. Hence, it is possible to hypothesize that mitoAKAPs might act as a signaling platform contributing to stabilize Akt mitochondrial localization to preserve mitochondrial function and promote survival. Further studies will be necessary to clarify the precise mechanism(s) by which loss of *Akap1* prevents Akt activation upon different stressors.

CONCLUSION

Our findings support the critical role of mitoAKAPs in cardiac responses to pressure overload, identifying Akt as potential mediator of their anti-hypertrophic effects.

AUTHOR CONTRIBUTIONS

GS, NB, RP, FC, VT, AFr, SD'A, GG, LR, DB, and AG performed the experiments and made the analyses. GS and CP wrote the manuscript. AL, AFe, and GE contributed to the experimental design and manuscript preparation. CP conceived the project.

FUNDING

This work was supported, in part, by Ministero della Salute (GR-1004 2009-1596220), Ministero dell'Istruzione, Università e Ricerca Scientifica (RBFR124FEN; 2015583WMX) grants to CP and Associazione Italiana Ricerca sul Cancro grant (IG-15264) to AFe. This research was also carried out in the frame of Program STAR, financially supported by University of Naples Federico II (Unina) and Compagnia di San Paolo (grant to CP).

ACKNOWLEDGMENTS

We gratefully thank Prof. Stanley McKnight (Department of Pharmacology, University of Washington, United States) for kindly providing us with *Akap1*$^{-/-}$ mice and Prof. David Bowtell Ph.D. (Peter MacCallum Cancer Centre, Melbourne, Australia) for kindly providing us with *Siah2*$^{-/-}$ mice.

REFERENCES

Abrenica, B., Alshaaban, M., and Czubryt, M. P. (2009). The A-kinase anchor protein AKAP121 is a negative regulator of cardiomyocyte hypertrophy. *J. Mol. Cell Cardiol.* 46, 674–681. doi: 10.1016/j.yjmcc.2009.01.018

Alto, N. M., Soderling, J., and Scott, J. D. (2002). Rab32 is an A-kinase anchoring protein and participates in mitochondrial dynamics. *J. Cell Biol.* 158, 659–668. doi: 10.1083/jcb.200204081

Angrisano, T., Schiattarella, G. G., Keller, S., Pironti, G., Florio, E., Magliulo, F., et al. (2014). Epigenetic switch at atp2a2 and myh7 gene promoters in pressure overload-induced heart failure. *PLoS One* 9:e106024. doi: 10.1371/journal.pone.0106024

Aoyagi, T., and Matsui, T. (2011). Phosphoinositide-3 kinase signaling in cardiac hypertrophy and heart failure. *Curr. Pharm. Des.* 17, 1818–1824. doi: 10.2174/138161211796390976

Berenji, K., Drazner, M. H., Rothermel, B. A., and Hill, J. A. (2005). Does load-induced ventricular hypertrophy progress to systolic heart failure? *Am. J. Physiol. Heart Circ. Physiol.* 289, H8–H16. doi: 10.1152/ajpheart.01303.2004

Bijur, G. N., and Jope, R. S. (2003). Rapid accumulation of Akt in mitochondria following phosphatidylinositol 3-kinase activation. *J. Neurochem.* 87, 1427–1435. doi: 10.1046/j.1471-4159.2003.02113.x

Bui, M., Gilady, S. Y., Fitzsimmons, R. E., Benson, M. D., Lynes, E. M., Gesson, K., et al. (2010). Rab32 modulates apoptosis onset and mitochondria-associated membrane (MAM) properties. *J. Biol. Chem.* 285, 31590–31602. doi: 10.1074/jbc.M110.101584

Burchfield, J. S., Xie, M., and Hill, J. A. (2013). Pathological ventricular remodeling: mechanisms: part 1 of 2. *Circulation* 128, 388–400. doi: 10.1161/CIRCULATIONAHA.113.001878

Cannavo, A., Rengo, G., Liccardo, D., Pironti, G., Scimia, M. C., Scudiero, L., et al. (2013). Prothymosin alpha protects cardiomyocytes against ischemia-induced apoptosis via preservation of Akt activation. *Apoptosis* 18, 1252–1261. doi: 10.1007/s10495-013-0876-9

Carlucci, A., Adornetto, A., Scorziello, A., Viggiano, D., Foca, M., Cuomo, O., et al. (2008a). Proteolysis of AKAP121 regulates mitochondrial activity during cellular hypoxia and brain ischaemia. *EMBO J.* 27, 1073–1084. doi: 10.1038/emboj.2008.33

Carlucci, A., Lignitto, L., and Feliciello, A. (2008b). Control of mitochondria dynamics and oxidative metabolism by cAMP, AKAPs and the proteasome. *Trends Cell Biol.* 18, 604–613. doi: 10.1016/j.tcb.2008.09.006

Carnegie, G. K., Soughayer, J., Smith, F. D., Pedroja, B. S., Zhang, F., Diviani, D., et al. (2008). AKAP-Lbc mobilizes a cardiac hypertrophy signaling pathway. *Mol. Cell* 32, 169–179. doi: 10.1016/j.molcel.2008.08.030

Cattaneo, F., Parisi, M., Fioretti, T., Sarnataro, D., Esposito, G., and Ammendola, R. (2016). Nuclear localization of Formyl-Peptide Receptor 2 in human cancer cells. *Arch. Biochem. Biophys.* 603, 10–19. doi: 10.1016/j.abb.2016.05.006

Chaanine, A. H., and Hajjar, R. J. (2011). AKT signalling in the failing heart. *Eur. J. Heart Fail.* 13, 825–829. doi: 10.1093/eurjhf/hfr080

Chien, K. R. (1999). Stress pathways and heart failure. *Cell* 98, 555–558. doi: 10.1016/S0092-8674(00)80043-4

Diviani, D., Dodge-Kafka, K. L., Li, J., and Kapiloff, M. S. (2011). A-kinase anchoring proteins: scaffolding proteins in the heart. *Am. J. Physiol. Heart Circ. Physiol.* 301, H1742–H1753. doi: 10.1152/ajpheart.00569.2011

Ellison, G. M., Waring, C. D., Vicinanza, C., and Torella, D. (2012). Physiological cardiac remodelling in response to endurance exercise training: cellular and molecular mechanisms. *Heart* 98, 5–10. doi: 10.1136/heartjnl-2011-300639

Esposito, G., Perrino, C., Cannavo, A., Schiattarella, G. G., Borgia, F., Sannino, A., et al. (2011). EGFR trans-activation by urotensin II receptor is mediated by beta-arrestin recruitment and confers cardioprotection in pressure overload-induced cardiac hypertrophy. *Basic Res. Cardiol.* 106, 577–589. doi: 10.1007/s00395-011-0163-2

Esposito, G., Schiattarella, G. G., Perrino, C., Cattaneo, F., Pironti, G., Franzone, A., et al. (2015). Dermcidin: a skeletal muscle myokine modulating cardiomyocyte survival and infarct size after coronary artery ligation. *Cardiovasc. Res.* 107, 431–441. doi: 10.1093/cvr/cvv173

Feliciello, A., Gottesman, M. E., and Avvedimento, E. V. (2001). The biological functions of A-kinase anchor proteins. *J. Mol. Biol.* 308, 99–114. doi: 10.1006/jmbi.2001.4585

Feliciello, A., Rubin, C. S., Avvedimento, E. V., and Gottesman, M. E. (1998). Expression of a kinase anchor protein 121 is regulated by hormones in thyroid and testicular germ cells. *J. Biol. Chem.* 273, 23361–23366. doi: 10.1074/jbc.273.36.23361

Frey, N., and Olson, E. N. (2003). Cardiac hypertrophy: the good, the bad, and the ugly. *Annu. Rev. Physiol.* 65, 45–79. doi: 10.1146/annurev.physiol.65.092101.142243

Fujio, Y., Nguyen, T., Wencker, D., Kitsis, R. N., and Walsh, K. (2000). Akt promotes survival of cardiomyocytes in vitro and protects against ischemia-reperfusion injury in mouse heart. *Circulation* 101, 660–667. doi: 10.1161/01.CIR.101.6.660

Heineke, J., and Molkentin, J. D. (2006). Regulation of cardiac hypertrophy by intracellular signalling pathways. *Nat. Rev. Mol. Cell Biol.* 7, 589–600. doi: 10.1038/nrm1983

Hill, J. A., and Olson, E. N. (2008). Cardiac plasticity. *N. Engl. J. Med.* 358, 1370–1380. doi: 10.1056/NEJMra072139

Kim, H., Scimia, M. C., Wilkinson, D., Trelles, R. D., Wood, M. R., Bowtell, D., et al. (2011). Fine-tuning of Drp1/Fis1 availability by AKAP121/Siah2 regulates mitochondrial adaptation to hypoxia. *Mol. Cell* 44, 532–544. doi: 10.1016/j.molcel.2011.08.045

Levy, D., Garrison, R. J., Savage, D. D., Kannel, W. B., and Castelli, W. P. (1990). Prognostic implications of echocardiographically determined left ventricular mass in the Framingham Heart Study. *N. Engl. J. Med.* 322, 1561–1566. doi: 10.1056/NEJM199005313222203

Lim, S., Smith, K. R., Lim, S. T., Tian, R., Lu, J., and Tan, M. (2016). Regulation of mitochondrial functions by protein phosphorylation and dephosphorylation. *Cell Biosci.* 6:25. doi: 10.1186/s13578-016-0089-3

Matsui, T., Li, L., Del Monte, F., Fukui, Y., Franke, T. F., Hajjar, R. J., et al. (1999). Adenoviral gene transfer of activated phosphatidylinositol 3′-kinase and Akt inhibits apoptosis of hypoxic cardiomyocytes in vitro. *Circulation* 100, 2373–2379. doi: 10.1161/01.CIR.100.23.2373

Miyamoto, S., Murphy, A. N., and Brown, J. H. (2008). Akt mediates mitochondrial protection in cardiomyocytes through phosphorylation of mitochondrial hexokinase-II. *Cell Death Differ.* 15, 521–529. doi: 10.1038/sj.cdd.4402285

Morales, C. R., Li, D. L., Pedrozo, Z., May, H. I., Jiang, N., Kyrychenko, V., et al. (2016). Inhibition of class I histone deacetylases blunts cardiac hypertrophy through TSC2-dependent mTOR repression. *Sci. Signal.* 9:ra34. doi: 10.1126/scisignal.aad5736

Newhall, K. J., Criniti, A. R., Cheah, C. S., Smith, K. C., Kafer, K. E., Burkart, A. D., et al. (2006). Dynamic anchoring of PKA is essential during oocyte maturation. *Curr. Biol.* 16, 321–327. doi: 10.1016/j.cub.2005.12.031

Perrino, C., Feliciello, A., Schiattarella, G. G., Esposito, G., Guerriero, R., Zaccaro, L., et al. (2010). AKAP121 downregulation impairs protective cAMP signals, promotes mitochondrial dysfunction, and increases oxidative stress. *Cardiovasc. Res.* 88, 101–110. doi: 10.1093/cvr/cvq155

Perrino, C., Naga Prasad, S. V., Mao, L., Noma, T., Yan, Z., Kim, H. S., et al. (2006). Intermittent pressure overload triggers hypertrophy-independent cardiac dysfunction and vascular rarefaction. *J. Clin. Invest.* 116, 1547–1560. doi: 10.1172/JCI25397

Perrino, C., and Rockman, H. A. (2007). Reversal of cardiac remodeling by modulation of adrenergic receptors: a new frontier in heart failure. *Curr. Opin. Cardiol.* 22, 443–449. doi: 10.1097/HCO.0b013e3282294d72

Perrino, C., Schiattarella, G. G., Sannino, A., Pironti, G., Petretta, M. P., Cannavo, A., et al. (2013). Genetic deletion of uncoupling protein 3 exaggerates apoptotic cell death in the ischemic heart leading to heart failure. *J. Am. Heart Assoc.* 2:e000086. doi: 10.1161/JAHA.113.000086

Rababa'h, A., Singh, S., Suryavanshi, S. V., Altarabsheh, S. E., Deo, S. V., and Mcconnell, B. K. (2014). Compartmentalization role of A-kinase anchoring proteins (AKAPs) in mediating protein kinase A (PKA) signaling and cardiomyocyte hypertrophy. *Int. J. Mol. Sci.* 16, 218–229. doi: 10.3390/ijms16010218

Rinaldi, L., Sepe, M., Delle Donne, R., Conte, K., Arcella, A., Borzacchiello, D., et al. (2017). Mitochondrial AKAP1 supports mTOR pathway and tumor growth. *Cell Death Dis.* 8:e2842. doi: 10.1038/cddis.2017.241

Schiattarella, G. G., Cattaneo, F., Carrizzo, A., Paolillo, R., Boccella, N., Ambrosio, M., et al. (2018). Akap1 regulates vascular function and endothelial cells behavior. *Hypertension* 71, 507–517. doi: 10.1161/HYPERTENSIONAHA.117.10185

Schiattarella, G. G., Cattaneo, F., Pironti, G., Magliulo, F., Carotenuto, G., Pirozzi, M., et al. (2016). Akap1 deficiency promotes mitochondrial aberrations and exacerbates cardiac injury following permanent coronary ligation via enhanced mitophagy and apoptosis. *PLoS One* 11:e0154076. doi: 10.1371/journal.pone.0154076

Schiattarella, G. G., and Hill, J. A. (2015). Inhibition of hypertrophy is a good therapeutic strategy in ventricular pressure overload. *Circulation* 131, 1435–1447. doi: 10.1161/CIRCULATIONAHA.115.013894

Schiattarella, G. G., Hill, T. M., and Hill, J. A. (2017). Is load-induced ventricular hypertrophy ever compensatory? *Circulation* 136, 1273–1275. doi: 10.1161/CIRCULATIONAHA.117.030730

Scorziello, A., Savoia, C., Sisalli, M. J., Adornetto, A., Secondo, A., Boscia, F., et al. (2013). NCX3 regulates mitochondrial Ca(2+) handling through the AKAP121-anchored signaling complex and prevents hypoxia-induced neuronal death. *J. Cell Sci.* 126, 5566–5577. doi: 10.1242/jcs.129668

Torrealba, N., Aranguiz, P., Alonso, C., Rothermel, B. A., and Lavandero, S. (2017). Mitochondria in structural and functional cardiac remodeling. *Adv. Exp. Med. Biol.* 982, 277–306. doi: 10.1007/978-3-319-55330-6_15

5

Mitochondria in Cardiac Postconditioning

Pasquale Pagliaro, Saveria Femminò, Jasmin Popara and Claudia Penna**

Department of Clinical and Biological Sciences, University of Turin, Turin, Italy

Edited by:
Mariarosaria Santillo,
University of Naples Federico II, Italy

Reviewed by:
Giulio Agnetti,
Johns Hopkins University,
United States
Kerstin Boengler,
Justus Liebig Universität Gießen,
Germany

***Correspondence:**
Pasquale Pagliaro
pasquale.pagliaro@unito.it
Claudia Penna
claudia.penna@unito.it

Mitochondria play a pivotal role in cardioprotection. Here we report some fundamental studies which considered the role of mitochondrial components (connexin 43, mitochondrial KATP channels and mitochondrial permeability transition pore) in postconditioning cardioprotection. We briefly discuss the role of mitochondria, reactive oxygen species and gaseous molecules in postconditioning. Also the effects of anesthetics—used as cardioprotective substances—is briefly considered in the context of postconditioning. The role of mitochondrial postconditioning signaling in determining the limitation of cell death is underpinned. Issues in clinical translation are briefly considered. The aim of the present mini-review is to discuss in a historical perspective the role of main mitochondria mechanisms in cardiac postconditioning.

Keywords: cardioprotection, ischemia/reperfusion, reactive oxygen species, redox signaling, mitochondria, connexin 43

INTRODUCTION

Mitochondria are fundamental as sources of energy, but also to sustain life being elements involved in cell survival and death. Mitochondrial dysfunction is a critical element of many diseases including ischemia/reperfusion (I/R) and subsequent development of ventricular systolic dysfunction and possible compensatory heart hypertrophy. This article outlines the role of mitochondria as targets for reducing I/R damage in myocardial postconditioning.

Cardiac postconditioning has been defined by the seminal work of Vinten-Johansen's group as "repetitive ischemia applied during early reperfusion" (Zhao et al., 2003). The name postconditioning was proposed in comparison with the previously discovered ischemic preconditioning. It soon became clear that intramyocardial mechanisms are responsible for both pre and postconditioning cardioprotection and that mitochondria may play a pivotal role (Pagliaro et al., 2004; Tsang et al., 2004; Hausenloy and Yellon, 2016).

Postconditioning attracted the interest of researchers as it allows an easier approach in humans. Indeed, it has been tested several times, both with a mechanical (brief ischemia) or pharmacological approach to target mitochondria in animals and humans. Also, inhibition of mitochondrial permeability transition to limit the so-called "post-cardiac arrest syndrome," observed in patients resuscitated from cardiac arrest, has been tested in a pre-clinical study (Cour et al., 2011). The results with both approaches are contradictory and have been reviewed elsewhere (Gomez et al., 2009; Penna et al., 2013a; Dongworth et al., 2014). The main purpose of the present article is a diachronic approach to studies that considered mitochondria mechanisms involvement in postconditioning.

MITOCHONDRIA AND HEART POSTCONDITIONING

Searching on Pubmed for "Mitochondria* [title] and heart and postconditioning" with a publication date limit from 2003/01/01 to 2017/12/31 we found 82 articles.

In this series of article, the first report which hypothesized and confirmed an important role for mitochondria in postconditioning was the article by Argaud et al. (2005). These authors confirmed a role for the *mitochondrial permeability transition pore* (mPTP) in lethal reperfusion injury and suggested that this pore is modulated by postconditioning. The study was conducted in anesthetized open-chest rabbits. Mitochondria were isolated from the risk area of myocardium, and calcium-induced mPTP opening was determined using a potentiometric method. Postconditioning inhibited the opening of the mPTP and provided a robust anti-ischemic protection. Later, the same group demonstrated that mitochondrial calcium decreased in pre-conditioning, but increased significantly either in postconditioning or after inhibition of mPTP (Argaud et al., 2008). These data have suggested that Ca^{2+} retention within mitochondria may clarify the limitation of reperfusion damage in postconditioned hearts (but not in preconditioned). The involvement of mitochondria in postconditioning protection has been confirmed in several studies, for Reviews see ((Boengler et al., 2011a, 2013; Di Lisa et al., 2011)).

The mPTP, whose nature is still controversial (**Figure 1**), plays a pivotal role in the shift from life to death (Bernardi et al., 2015; Kwong and Molkentin, 2015). Already in 2006 Ovize's group reviewed the evidence for an important role of the mPTP in postconditioning (Gateau-Roesch et al., 2006). It was soon evident that mPTP priming occurs during ischemia and early reperfusion, and that mPTP opens at the time of full reperfusion, leading to cell death, whereas pre- and postconditioning prevent the pore formation. Also, modulation of electron transport has emerged as a mechanism responsible for cardiac mitochondria protection, which decreases myocardial injury during ischemia and early reperfusion (Chen et al., 2006). In 2007 Gomez et al. confirmed that inhibition of mPTP at reperfusion not only limits infarct size but also improves functional recovery and mice survival (Gomez et al., 2007). Then, in a dog model of myocardial I/R, Mykytenko et al. demonstrated that the beneficial effects of postconditioning and effects on mitochondrial function persisted 24 h after the ischemic event (Mykytenko et al., 2008). In particular, postconditioning reduced infarct size and decreased CK activity after prolonged reperfusion and the protection was attributable to the opening of mitochondrial KATP channels (mKATP) and inhibition of mPTP opening. Nevertheless, mPTP physiology is complex and its transient opening during preconditioning is protective (Dongworth et al., 2014; Hausenloy and Yellon, 2016).

It is likely that the *signal transducer and activator of transcription 3* (STAT3) contributes to cardioprotection by stimulation of respiration and inhibition of mPTP opening (Boengler et al., 2010; Heusch et al., 2011). We confirmed the role of STAT3 in ischemic postconditioning but as a component upstream to mitochondrial ROS (Reactive Oxygen Species) signaling (Penna et al., 2013b). In cardiac cells, two main types of mitochondria are present: interfibrillar (IFM) and subsarcolemmal (SSM) with different biochemical and morphological properties (e.g., lower oxidation potential and lower enzyme activities of complex I, succinate dehydrogenase, in SSM than IFM) (Palmer et al., 1977). In cardiac cells, STAT3 was principally present in the matrix of SSM and IFM. STAT1 was also found in mitochondria under physiological conditions, but this does not occur for STAT5 (Boengler et al., 2010; Heusch et al., 2011).

Mitochondrial *connexin 43* and postconditioning protection were studied several times (Penna et al., 2009; He et al., 2010; Boengler et al., 2011a; Di Lisa et al., 2011). The mitochondrial location of connexin 43 being central for cardioprotection has been proposed by Schulz and co-workers (Boengler et al., 2011a). It is clear that mitochondrial connexin 43 has a role in postconditioning-induced ROS-signaling, but its precise function is not clear. Recently, Tu et al. (2017) have described a role for mitochondrial connexin 43 in hypoxic postconditioning. However, postconditioning (unlike preconditioning) effectively reduces infarct size in heterozygous connexin 43-deficient ($Cx43^{+/-}$) mice *in vivo* (Heusch et al., 2006), questioning the role of connexin 43 in this cardioprotective intervention. Nevertheless, a difference exists between IFM and SSM in terms of connexin 43 presence and function. The role of these subpopulations of mitochondria deserves more studies.

The *mitochondrial ATP-sensitive* K^+ *channels* (mKATP) have a putative important role in postconditioning cardioprotection (Garlid and Halestrap, 2012; Jin et al., 2012). It has also been suggested that the mitochondrial calcium uniporter is involved in the mechanisms of ischemic postconditioning (Yu et al., 2011).

MITOCHONDRIA AND ROS

Serviddio et al. suggested that mitochondria play a pivotal role in H_2O_2 production and redox stress during reperfusion and are important for the cardioprotective effect of postconditioning (Serviddio et al., 2005). These authors used isolated perfused rat hearts in which they compared an early normoxic reperfusion with a hypoxic reperfusion. They found out that mitochondria carbonyl proteins are somewhat lower in hypoxic than in the normoxic group at the end of reperfusion and concluded that hypoxic reperfusion at its onset limits myocardial injury and the amount of mitochondrial H_2O_2 production. Although this was not a real postconditioning, as defined by Vinten-Johansen's group (Zhao et al., 2003), it was the first study to hypothesize some changes in redox aspects within mitochondria in early reperfusion after a protective intervention.

We were the first to show that in order to induce cardioprotection by postconditioning in isolated perfused rat hearts, a signaling through a mKATP activation and redox-sensitive mechanism is required (Penna et al., 2006). It is likely that postconditioning procedures reduce the production of ROS in early reperfusion, but if ROS are completely removed in the initial minutes of reperfusion the heart cannot be protected by the "repetitive ischemia applied during early reperfusion." Our observation was confirmed several times by different laboratories. The same year Bopassa et al. confirmed the involvement of mPTP and suggested that *phosphatidylinositol 3-kinase* (PI3K) regulates mPTP in isolated perfused rat hearts subjected to a postconditioning protocol (Bopassa et al., 2006). We then demonstrated that targeting of specific cellular sites such as

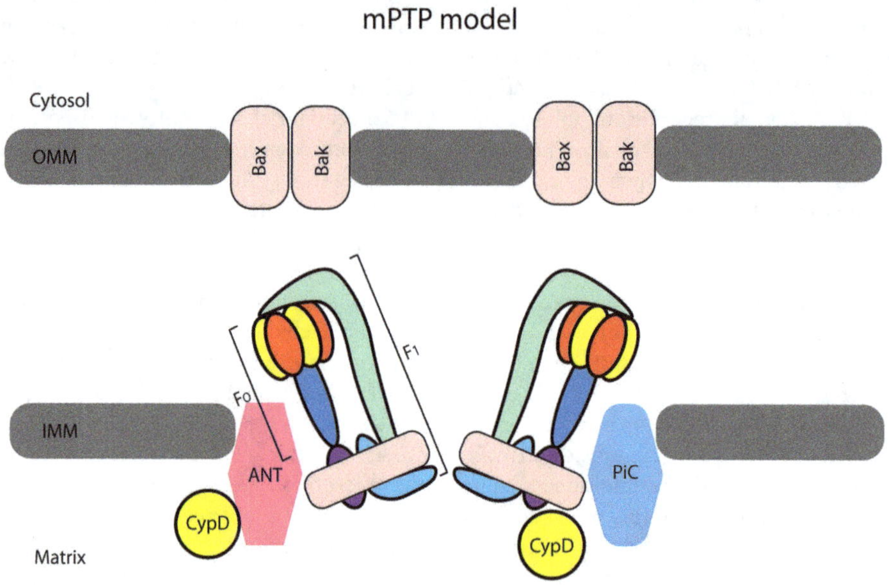

FIGURE 1 | The most accepted model considers ATP synthase subunits as central elements of the mitochondrial permeability transition pore (mPTP). Indeed, the F1FO ATP synthase has been suggested by Bernardi et al. (2015) to be a pore component for the inner mitochondrial membrane (IMM) forming a unit of the mPTP. It has been suggested that adenine nucleotide translocase (ANT) and cyclophilin-D (CypD), together with mitochondrial phosphate carrier (PiC) form a complex that acts as pore regulator. The pro-apoptotic proteins Bax/Bak located in the outer mitochondrial membrane (OMM) favor swelling and subsequently, mitochondria rupture once the IMM complex opens (Kwong and Molkentin, 2015).

bradykinin B2 receptors and mKATP channels during early reperfusion elicits postconditioning-like protection through ROS signaling and ROS compartmentalization (Penna et al., 2007). Very recently Boengler et al. (2017) have shown that p66shc is present in both SSM and in IFM. However, it seems that ROS formation by p66shc is not involved in determining myocardial injury.

MITOCHONDRIA AND GASEOUS CARDIOPROTECTIVE SUBSTANCES

Hydrogen sulfide (H_2S), carbon monoxide (CO) and Nitric Oxide (NO) are recognized as three gaseous mediators for cardioprotection. All these molecules have potential cardioprotective effects in the heart. In particular, the beneficial actions were demonstrated against myocardial I/R injury, including infarction, arrhythmia, hypertrophy, fibrosis, and heart failure. These protective effects were mediated by complex pathway and the effects included: anti-oxidative action, anti-inflammatory responses, reduction of apoptosis, angiogenic actions, and regulation of ion channel (Mancardi et al., 2009; Andreadou et al., 2015; Penna et al., 2015). Since these gasses may be produced within mitochondria and may profoundly affect the function of these organelles, here we discuss briefly their role in the context of cardioprotection. The enzymatic production of NO is mediated by three isoforms of NOS isoforms: neuronal (nNOS or NOS I), inducible (iNOS or NOS II), and endothelial (eNOS or NOS III). A specific mitochondrial NOS isoform has been also proposed. NOS activity is governed by different factors (co-factors and substrate availability, and endogenous inhibitors) and the NO can induce post-transcriptional, post-translational and transcriptional modulations in specific subcellular compartments. Importantly, during ischemia, when pH becomes acidic and oxygen-dependent NOS activity may be impaired, the formation of NO can also derive from the non-enzymatic reduction of nitrite/nitrate, which can be dietary and endogenous in origin (Andreadou et al., 2015).

Also, the activation of the NO/cGMP pathway, with augmentation of cGMP and NO levels, has been observed after postconditioning maneuvers in different cardiac models. During postconditioning, the activation of eNOS and Akt pathway converge on Glycogen Synthase Kinase-3β (GSK-3β) and inhibits mPTP opening (Correa et al., 2015). Different concentrations of NO induce different action in the mitochondria. In particular, high NO concentration open the mPTP with the formation of peroxynitrite and disulphide bonds formation, while physiological NO levels favor mPTP closure with post-translational modification of protein S-nitrosylation (Correa et al., 2015 and references therein). In early reperfusion, a temporary interruption of respiration may prevent exaggerated generation of superoxide anion (O_2^-) and $ONOO^-$ and reduce the thiol oxidation with permanent inactivation of metabolic enzymes or inhibition of mPTP opening (Piantadosi, 2012).

Hydrogen sulfide (H_2S) is produced by several enzymes, within and outside mitochondria. It seems that H_2S produced by cystathionine-gamma-lyase (CSE) from L-cysteine can readily scavenge the ROS and may induced protection with two mechanisms, one reperfusion injury salvage kinase (RISK)-dependent and the other RISK-independent. Therefore, H_2S as

NO has important antioxidant properties, but in contrast to NO, H_2S cannot directly form radicals (Mancardi et al., 2009). An interesting and recent paper by Banu et al. (2016) reports that both postconditioning maneuvers and H_2S postconditioning significantly restores the complex I activity to near normal level, particularly in IFM. The preserved IFM activity was evidenced by the improvement in electron transport chain enzyme activities and mitochondrial respiration.

Endogenous carbon monoxide (CO) is synthesized by hemoxygenases (HO-1 and HO-2) as a consequence of the catabolism of haem and is an important bioactive molecule. It has been observed that CO induces the mitochondrial production of O_2^-, which is transformed by superoxide dismutase to H_2O_2, and then a subsequent Akt activation by H_2O_2 limits apoptosis after I/R (Kondo-Nakamura et al., 2010). Moreover, the anti-apoptotic effects of CO are related to the inhibition of mPTP. In isolated mitochondria, CO inhibited mPTP opening, loss of potential, cytochrome c release and swelling (Queiroga et al., 2010). Further details on the role of NO, H_2S, and CO in cardioprotection can be found on Andreadou et al. (2015).

MITOCHONDRIA AND ANESTHETICS

Agents targeting mitochondria with prominent postconditioning effects are anesthetics. The volatile anesthetic *sevoflurane* given for 2 min at the beginning of reperfusion-induced myocardial protection against myocardial I/R injury. This sevoflurane-postconditioning is mediated, at least in part, by mKATP-channels (Obal et al., 2005). Almost simultaneously, in a similar model, Feng et al. have published that another volatile anesthetic, *isoflurane*, induces postconditioning preventing the opening of the mPTP *via* inhibition of GSK-3β (Feng et al., 2005). It was also demonstrated, *in vivo*, that the antiapoptotic protein B cell lymphoma-2 (Bcl-2) mediates myocardial postconditioning protection by isoflurane, thus indirectly modulating mPTP activity (Wang et al., 2006; Pravdic et al., 2010).

Propofol, another anesthetic, also displayed cardioprotective effect against cardiac I/R injury associated with inhibition of mPTP opening. Intriguingly, compared to propofol, sevoflurane induces more beneficial effects on functional recovery and infarct size (He et al., 2008). Another study suggested that sevoflurane postconditioning protects isolated rat hearts through the involvement of the ROS-ERK 1/2-mPTP signaling cascade (Yao et al., 2010). Moreover, sevoflurane postconditioning protects infarcted rat hearts against I/R damage by inhibiting mPTP opening through the involvement of PKB/Akt and ERK1/2 (Yao et al., 2009). Nevertheless, sevoflurane-induced postconditioning, as other conditioning protocols, results impaired by the presence of hyperglycemia. This impairment of protection was reversed by the mPTP inhibition with cyclosporine A (Huhn et al., 2008) or by inhibition of excess mitochondrial fission with dynamin-related protein 1 inhibitor (Yu et al., 2017). Lim et al. have confirmed that the mPTP plays an essential role in in the cardioprotection induced by ischemic and pharmacological preconditioning and by postconditioning (Lim et al., 2007). Yet, pharmacological postconditioning may be limited by a "ceiling effect of protection," but, this ceiling effect may be reversed by simultaneous inhibition of GSK-3β *via* the opening of mKATP channels (Couvreur et al., 2009). GSK-3β modulates mitochondrial function and Gomez et al.confirmed that GSK-3β inhibition *via* its S9-phosphorylation is required for postconditioning and that this phosphorylation likely works by inhibiting the opening of the mPTP (Gomez et al., 2008). Indeed, it has been suggested that the phosphorylation/inactivation of GSK-3β is involved in the inhibition of mPTP opening *via* the interaction with several elements of the mPTP regulatory complex and subsequent increase in mPTP-ROS threshold (Tanno et al., 2014). Finally, it is of note that *morphine,* an opiate often given to patients who have undergone surgery and anesthesia, may induce postconditioning *via* delta-1 opioid receptors activation and mPTP modulation (Kim et al., 2011).

MITOCHONDRIAL POSTCONDITIONING SIGNALING AND LIMITATION OF CELL DEATH

Postconditioning signaling converges on mitochondria, thus limiting all forms of cell death. We have suggested that postconditioning or perfusion of the heart with bradykinin may activate cellular signaling leading to the opening of mKATP channels, increasing ROS production, inhibiting the mPTP and inducing cardioprotection (Penna et al., 2006). It has been suggested that the cooperation between bradykinin and bradykinin-receptor may favor the assembly of a caveolar signaling platform (*signalosome*). The receptors with ligands migrate to caveolae, where signaling elements are scaffolded into signalosomes that translocate to mitochondria. The signalosome-mitochondria interaction then initiates mKATP channels, increases ROS production, which favors mitochondrial protein kinase C epsilon activation and mPTP inhibition, thus decreasing myocardial injury (Quinlan et al., 2008). It has been suggested that postconditioning similarly to adenosine may induce HSP90-dependent translocation of PKCε to mitochondria, likely *via* mitochondrial import machinery TOM70 (Yang et al., 2012). These results suggest an important implication of cytosolic protein translocation within mitochondria in ischemic postconditioning (Boengler et al., 2011b).

Mitochondria are important players in many types of *apoptotic* and necrotic cell death (Murphy and Steenbergen, 2011). We were among the first to demonstrate that postconditioning increases the levels of anti-apoptotic markers, including the phospho-GSK-3β and Pim-1 kinases, while decreasing the pro-apoptotic markers, namely cytochrome c, thus preserving the mitochondrial morphology (Penna et al., 2009). Fang et al. confirmed that postconditioning attenuates cardiomyocyte injury and apoptosis by blocking mPTP (Fang et al., 2008). Subsequently, Li et al. suggested that the cardioprotective effect of postconditioning is mediated by apoptosis repressor with caspase recruitment domain (ARC) (Li et al., 2009). Dong et al. also showed that postconditioning may protect cardiomyocytes from apoptosis *via* an interaction between PKCε and calcium-sensing receptors to inhibit endoplasmic and sarcoplasmic reticulum-mitochondria crosstalk (Dong et al., 2010).

The influence of mitochondrial dynamics in I/R and cardioprotection, and their potential as targets in treating cardiovascular disease, are also emerging (Boengler et al., 2011a; Ong and Hausenloy, 2017). Finally, experimental studies highlighted the importance of exosomes and vesicles in local and distant intercellular communication mechanisms after myocardial infarction. Exosomes and vesicles are potentially useful as cell-free therapeutic candidates (Lai et al., 2010; Bell et al., 2012; Chen et al., 2013; Barile et al., 2014; Giricz et al., 2014; Ibrahim et al., 2014; Yellon and Davidson, 2014; de Couto et al., 2017; Sluijter et al., 2018). However, caution must be used and extensive studies are necessary because their mechanisms of protection are still unknown.

TRANSLATION ISSUES

Pharmacological and mechanical ischemic postconditioning can be therapeutic options (Pagliaro and Penna, 2015). For instance, blocking the mPTP could be beneficial, but mPTP blockers have yielded mostly neutral effects in both myocardial infarction and heart failure patients. Also, mechanical ischemic postconditioning yielded contradictory results. In animal models, postconditioning resulted in an increase in myocardial salvage (about 30 % in rats, 35% in dogs, 50% in pigs, and 65% in rabbits) (Zhao et al., 2003; Mykytenko et al., 2008; Sun et al., 2010). However, in humans studies of postconditioning effects on markers of myocardial injury have obtained conflicting results (Lønborg, 2015; Pagliaro and Penna, 2015). Several authors (Staat et al., 2005; Thibault et al., 2007; Xue et al., 2010) reported a decrease in enzyme leakage. Lønborg et al. (2010) using magnetic resonance imaging found an increase in myocardial salvage ratio. Yet authors (Sörensson et al., 2010; Freixa et al., 2012; Hahn et al., 2013) do not observe any effect of postconditioning in humans with myocardial infarction. Thus, additional studies with adequately sized and designed randomized trials are necessary. Hope comes from a recent trial which reports a significant increase in myocardial salvage when classical postconditioning has been combined with remote ischemic conditioning (Eitel et al., 2015).

CONCLUSIONS

In conclusion, here we have reported several studies which have shown that different signal transduction pathways are switched on or switched off both by ischemic postconditioning and by pharmacological postconditioning. These signaling pathways converge on mitochondria where different components are affected preserving many of the mitochondrial functions after ischemia/reperfusion. Within mitochondria, a central role is played by connexin 43, mKATP channels and mPTP. Mitochondrial dynamics are also of fundamental importance in I/R and cardioprotection (Boengler et al., 2011a; Ong and Hausenloy, 2017). Many other factors and consequently several other studies are not considered and we apologize to authors of those studies. However, the core aim of the present mini-review was to report the main steps which allow us to understand the role of these organelles in postconditioning and it may represent a starting point to deepen the understanding of mitochondria role in cardioprotection. Future researches and developments in this field should rely on appropriate animal models (with comorbidities and co-medication) that can allow identifying candidates for future clinical trials and, 1 day, discovery the appropriate strategies to eradicate myocardial infarction and its sequela.

AUTHOR CONTRIBUTIONS

CP and PP drafted the first version and supervised the manuscript. All authors evaluated retrieved papers and their reference lists to identify additional relevant articles. JP and SF made the figure. All authors revised the manuscript and approved the final version of the manuscript.

FUNDING

This study was funded by the University of Turin, Ricerca Locale Ex-60% (Grants: PAGP_RILO_16_01).

ACKNOWLEDGMENTS

The authors of this work were supported by the University of Turin.

REFERENCES

Andreadou, I., Iliodromitis, E. K., Rassaf, T., Schulz, R., Papapetropoulos, A., and Ferdinandy, P. (2015). The role of gasotransmitters NO, H_2S and CO in myocardial ischaemia/reperfusion injury and cardioprotection by preconditioning, postconditioning and remote conditioning. *Br. J. Pharmacol.* 172, 1587–1606. doi: 10.1111/bph.12811

Argaud, L., Gateau-Roesch, O., Augeul, L., Couture-Lepetit, E., Loufouat, J., Gomez, L., et al. (2008). Increased mitochondrial calcium coexists with decreased reperfusion injury in postconditioned (but not preconditioned) hearts. *Am. J. Physiol. Heart Circ. Physiol.* 294, H386–H391. doi: 10.1152/ajpheart.01035.2007

Argaud, L., Gateau-Roesch, O., Raisky, O., Loufouat, J., Robert, D., and Ovize, M. (2005). Postconditioning inhibits mitochondrial permeability transition. *Circulation* 111, 194–197. doi: 10.1161/01.CIR.0000151290.04952.3B

Banu, S. A., Ravindran, S., and Kurian, G. A. (2016). Hydrogen sulfide post-conditioning preserves interfibrillar mitochondria of rat heart during ischemia reperfusion injury. *Cell Stress Chaperones* 21, 571–582. doi: 10.1007/s12192-016-0682-8

Barile, L., Lionetti, V., Cervio, E., Matteucci, M., Gherghiceanu, M., Popescu, L. M., et al. (2014). Extracellular vesicles from human cardiac progenitor cells inhibit cardiomyocyte apoptosis and improve cardiac function after myocardial infarction. *Cardiovasc. Res.* 103, 530–541. doi: 10.1093/cvr/cvu167

Bell, R., Beeuwkes, R., Bøtker, H. E., Davidson, S., Downey, J., Garcia-Dorado, D., et al. (2012). Trials, tribulations and speculation! Report from the 7th Biennial Hatter Cardiovascular Institute Workshop. *Basic Res. Cardiol.* 107, 300. doi: 10.1007/s00395-012-0300-6

Bernardi, P., Rasola, A., Forte, M., and Lippe, G. (2015). The mitochondrial permeability transition pore: channel formation by F-ATP synthase, integration in signal transduction, and role in pathophysiology. *Physiol. Rev.* 95, 1111–1155. doi: 10.1152/physrev.00001.2015

Boengler, K., Bencsik, P., Palóczi, J., Kiss, K., Pipicz, M., Pipis, J., et al. (2017). Lack of contribution of p66shc and its mitochondrial translocation to ischemia-reperfusion injury and cardioprotection by ischemic preconditioning. *Front. Physiol.* 8:733. doi: 10.3389/fphys.2017.00733

Boengler, K., Heusch, G., and Schulz, R. (2011a). Mitochondria in postconditioning. *Antioxid. Redox Signal.* 14, 863–880. doi: 10.1089/ars.2010.3309

Boengler, K., Heusch, G., and Schulz, R. (2011b). Nuclear-encoded mitochondrial proteins and their role in cardioprotection. *Biochim. Biophys. Acta Mol. Cell Res.* 1813, 1286–1294. doi: 10.1016/j.bbamcr.2011.01.009

Boengler, K., Hilfiker-Kleiner, D., Heusch, G., and Schulz, R. (2010). Inhibition of permeability transition pore opening by mitochondrial STAT3 and its role in myocardial ischemia/reperfusion. *Basic Res. Cardiol.* 105, 771–785. doi: 10.1007/s00395-010-0124-1

Boengler, K., Ungefug, E., Heusch, G., and Schulz, R. (2013). The STAT3 inhibitor stattic impairs cardiomyocyte mitochondrial function through increased reactive oxygen species formation. *Curr. Pharm. Des.* 19, 6890–6895. doi: 10.2174/138161281939131127115940

Bopassa, J. C., Ferrera, R., Gateau-Roesch, O., Couture-Lepetit, E., and Ovize, M. (2006). PI 3-kinase regulates the mitochondrial transition pore in controlled reperfusion and postconditioning. *Cardiovasc. Res.* 69, 178–185. doi: 10.1016/j.cardiores.2005.07.014

Chen, L., Wang, Y., Pan, Y., Zhang, L., Shen, C., Qin, G., et al. (2013). Cardiac progenitor-derived exosomes protect ischemic myocardium from acute ischemia/reperfusion injury. *Biochem. Biophys. Res. Commun.* 431, 566–571. doi: 10.1016/j.bbrc.2013.01.015

Chen, Q., Camara, A. K., Stowe, D. F., Hoppel, C. L., and Lesnefsky, E. J. (2006). Modulation of electron transport protects cardiac mitochondria and decreases myocardial injury during ischemia and reperfusion. *Am. J. Physiol. Cell Physiol.* 292, C137–C147. doi: 10.1152/ajpcell.00270.2006

Correa, F., Buelna-Chontal, M., Chagoya, V., García-Rivas, G., Vigueras, R. M., Pedraza-Chaverri, J., et al. (2015). Inhibition of the nitric oxide/cyclic guanosine monophosphate pathway limited the cardioprotective effect of post-conditioning in hearts with apical myocardial infarction. *Eur. J. Pharmacol.* 765, 472–481. doi: 10.1016/j.ejphar.2015.09.018

Cour, M., Loufouat, J., Paillard, M., Augeul, L., Goudable, J., Ovize, M., et al. (2011). Inhibition of mitochondrial permeability transition to prevent the post-cardiac arrest syndrome: a pre-clinical study. *Eur. Heart J.* 32, 226–235. doi: 10.1093/eurheartj/ehq112

Couvreur, N., Tissier, R., Pons, S., Chenoune, M., Waintraub, X., Berdeaux, A., et al. (2009). The ceiling effect of pharmacological postconditioning with the phytoestrogen genistein is reversed by the GSK3β inhibitor SB 216763 [3-(2,4-dichlorophenyl)–4(1-methyl-1H-indol-3-yl)-1H-pyrrole-2,5-dione] through mitochondrial ATP-dependent potassium chan. *J. Pharmacol. Exp. Ther.* 329, 1134–1141. doi: 10.1124/jpet.109.152587

de Couto, G., Gallet, R., Cambier, L., Jaghatspanyan, E., Makkar, N., et al. (2017). Exosomal MicroRNA transfer into macrophages mediates cellular postconditioning. *Circulation* 136, 200–214. doi: 10.1161/CIRCULATIONAHA.116.024590

Di Lisa, F., Canton, M., Carpi, A., Kaludercic, N., Menabò, R., Menazza, S., et al. (2011). Mitochondrial injury and protection in ischemic pre- and postconditioning. *Antioxid. Redox Signal.* 14, 881–891. doi: 10.1089/ars.2010.3375

Dong, S., Teng, Z., Lu, F. H., Zhao, Y. J., Li, H., Ren, H., et al. (2010). Post-conditioning protects cardiomyocytes from apoptosis via PKC(epsilon)-interacting with calcium-sensing receptors to inhibit endo(sarco)plasmic reticulum-mitochondria crosstalk. *Mol. Cell. Biochem.* 341, 195–206. doi: 10.1007/s11010-010-0450-5

Dongworth, R. K., Hall, A. R., Burke, N., and Hausenloy, D. J. (2014). Targeting mitochondria for cardioprotection: examining the benefit for patients. *Future Cardiol.* 10, 255–272. doi: 10.2217/fca.14.6

Eitel, I., Stiermaier, T., Rommel, K. P., Fuernau, G., Sandri, M., Mangner, N., et al. (2015). Cardioprotection by combined intrahospital remote ischaemic perconditioning and postconditioning in ST-elevation myocardial infarction: the randomized LIPSIA CONDITIONING trial. *Eur. Heart J.* 36, 3049–3057. doi: 10.1093/eurheartj/ehv463

Fang, J., Wu, L., and Chen, L. (2008). Postconditioning attenuates cardiocyte ultrastructure injury and apoptosis by blocking mitochondrial permeability transition in rats. *Acta Cardiol.* 63, 377–387. doi: 10.2143/AC.63.3.1020316

Feng, J., Lucchinetti, E., Ahuja, P., Pasch, T., Perriard, J. C., and Zaugg, M. (2005). Isoflurane postconditioning prevents opening of the mitochondrial permeability transition pore through inhibition of glycogen synthase kinase 3β. *Anesthesiology* 103, 987–995. doi: 10.1097/00000542-200511000-00013

Freixa, X., Bellera, N., Ortiz-Pérez, J. T., Jiménez, M., Paré, C., Bosch, X., et al. (2012). Ischaemic postconditioning revisited: lack of effects on infarct size following primary percutaneous coronary intervention. *Eur. Heart J.* 33, 103–112. doi: 10.1093/eurheartj/ehr297

Garlid, K. D., and Halestrap, A. P. (2012). The mitochondrial KATP channel—Fact or fiction? *J. Mol. Cell. Cardiol.* 52, 578–583. doi: 10.1016/j.yjmcc.2011.12.011

Gateau-Roesch, O., Argaud, L., and Ovize, M. (2006). Mitochondrial permeability transition pore and postconditioning. *Cardiovasc. Res.* 70, 264–273. doi: 10.1016/j.cardiores.2006.02.024

Giricz, Z., Varga, Z. V., Baranyai, T., Sipos, P., Pálóczi, K., Kittel, Á., et al. (2014). Cardioprotection by remote ischemic preconditioning of the rat heart is mediated by extracellular vesicles. *J. Mol. Cell. Cardiol.* 68, 75–78. doi: 10.1016/j.yjmcc.2014.01.004

Gomez, L., Li, B., Mewton, N., Sanchez, I., Piot, C., Elbaz, M., et al. (2009). Inhibition of mitochondrial permeability transition pore opening: translation to patients. *Cardiovasc. Res.* 83, 226–233. doi: 10.1093/cvr/cvp063

Gomez, L., Paillard, M., Thibault, H., Derumeaux, G., and Ovize, M. (2008). Inhibition of GSK3β by postconditioning is required to prevent opening of the mitochondrial permeability transition pore during reperfusion. *Circulation* 117, 2761–2768. doi: 10.1161/CIRCULATIONAHA.107.755066

Gomez, L., Thibault, H., Gharib, A., Dumont, J. M., Vuagniaux, G., and Scalfaro, P. (2007). Inhibition of mitochondrial permeability transition improves functional recovery and reduces mortality following acute myocardial infarction in mice. *Am. J. Physiol. Heart Circ. Physiol.* 293, H1654–H1661. doi: 10.1152/ajpheart.01378.2006

Hahn, J. Y., Song, Y. B., Kim, E. K., Yu, C. W., Bae, J. W., Chung, W. Y., et al. (2013). Ischemic postconditioning during primary percutaneous coronary intervention: the effects of postconditioning on myocardial reperfusion in patients with ST-segment elevation myocardial infarction (POST) randomized trial. *Circulation* 128, 1889–1896. doi: 10.1161/CIRCULATIONAHA.113.001690

Hausenloy, D. J., and Yellon, D. M. (2016). Ischaemic conditioning and reperfusion injury. *Nat. Rev. Cardiol.* 13, 193–209. doi: 10.1038/nrcardio.2016.5

He, W., Zhang, F. J., Wang, S. P., Chen, G., Chen, C. C., and Yan, M. (2008). Postconditioning of sevoflurane and propofol is associated with mitochondrial permeability transition pore. *J. Zhejiang Univ. Sci. B* 9, 100–108. doi: 10.1631/jzus.B0710586

He, Y., Zeng, Z. Y., Zhong, G. Q., Li, J. Y., Li, W. K., and Li, W. (2010). Mitochondrial connexin43 and postconditioning protection in rabbits underwent myocardial ischemia/reperfusion injury. *Zhonghua Xin Xue Guan Bing Za Zhi* 38, 357–362. doi: 10.3760/cma.j.issn.0253-3758.2010.04.020

Heusch, G., Büchert, A., Feldhaus, S., and Schulz, R. (2006). No loss of cardioprotection by postconditioning in connexin 43-deficient mice. *Basic Res. Cardiol.* 101, 354–356. doi: 10.1007/s00395-006-0589-0

Heusch, G., Musiolik, J., Gedik, N., and Skyschally, A. (2011). Mitochondrial STAT3 activation and cardioprotection by ischemic postconditioning in pigs with regional myocardial ischemia/reperfusion. *Circ. Res.* 109, 1302–1308. doi: 10.1161/CIRCRESAHA.111.255604

Huhn, R., Heinen, A., Weber, N. C., Hollmann, M. W., Schlack, W., and Preckel, B. (2008). Hyperglycaemia blocks sevoflurane-induced postconditioning in the rat heart *in vivo*: cardioprotection can be restored by blocking the mitochondrial permeability transition pore. *Br. J. Anaesth.* 100, 465–471. doi: 10.1093/bja/aen022

Ibrahim, A. G., Cheng, K., and Marbán, E. (2014). Exosomes as critical agents of cardiac regeneration triggered by cell therapy. *Stem Cell Rep.* 2, 606–619. doi: 10.1016/j.stemcr.2014.04.006

Jin, C., Wu, J., Watanabe, M., Okada, T., and Iesaki, T. (2012). Mitochondrial K^+ channels are involved in ischemic postconditioning in rat hearts. *J. Physiol. Sci.* 62, 325–332. doi: 10.1007/s12576-012-0206-y

Kim, J. H., Chun, K. J., Park, Y. H., Kim, J., Kim, J. S., Jang, Y. H., et al. (2011). Morphine-induced postconditioning modulates mitochondrial permeability transition pore opening via delta-1 opioid receptors activation in isolated rat hearts. *Korean J. Anesthesiol.* 61, 69–74. doi: 10.4097/kjae.2011.61.1.69

Kondo-Nakamura, M., Shintani-Ishida, K., Uemura, K., and Yoshida, K. (2010). Brief exposure to carbon monoxide preconditions cardiomyogenic cells against apoptosis in ischemia-reperfusion. *Biochem. Biophys. Res. Commun.* 393, 449–454. doi: 10.1016/j.bbrc.2010.02.017

Kwong, J. Q., and Molkentin, J. D. (2015). Physiological and pathological roles of the mitochondrial permeability transition pore in the heart. *Cell Metab.* 21, 206–214. doi: 10.1016/j.cmet.2014.12.001

Lai, R. C., Arslan, F., Lee, M. M., Sze, N. S., Choo, A., Chen, T. S., et al. (2010). Exosome secreted by MSC reduces myocardial ischemia/reperfusion injury. *Stem Cell Res.* 4, 214–222. doi: 10.1016/j.scr.2009.12.003

Li, Y., Ge, X., and Liu, X. (2009). The cardioprotective effect of postconditioning is mediated by ARC through inhibiting mitochondrial apoptotic pathway. *Apoptosis* 14, 164–172. doi: 10.1007/s10495-008-0296-4

Lim, S. Y., Davidson, S. M., Hausenloy, D. J., and Yellon, D. M. (2007). Preconditioning and postconditioning: the essential role of the mitochondrial permeability transition pore. *Cardiovasc. Res.* 75, 530–535. doi: 10.1016/j.cardiores.2007.04.022

Lønborg, J., Kelbaek, H., Vejlstrup, N., Jørgensen, E., Helqvist, S., Saunamäki, K., et al. (2010). Cardioprotective effects of ischemic postconditioning in patients treated with primary percutaneous coronary intervention, evaluated by magnetic resonance. *Circ. Cardiovasc. Interv.* 3, 34–41. doi: 10.1161/CIRCINTERVENTIONS.109.905521

Lønborg, J. T., (2015). Targeting reperfusion injury in the era of primary percutaneous coronary intervention: hope or hype? *Heart* 101, 1612–1618. doi: 10.1136/heartjnl-2015-307804

Mancardi, D., Penna, C., Merlino, A., Del Soldato, P., Wink, D. A., and Pagliaro, P. (2009). Physiological and pharmacological features of the novel gasotransmitter: hydrogen sulfide. *Biochim. Biophys. Acta* 1787, 864–872. doi: 10.1016/j.bbabio.2009.03.005

Murphy, E., and Steenbergen, C. (2011). What makes the mitochondria a killer? Can we condition them to be less destructive? *Biochim. Biophys. Acta* 1813, 1302–1308. doi: 10.1016/j.bbamcr.2010.09.003

Mykytenko, J., Reeves, J. G., Kin, H., Wang, N. P., Zatta, A. J., Jiang, R., et al. (2008). Persistent beneficial effect of postconditioning against infarct size: role of mitochondrial KATP channels during reperfusion. *Basic Res. Cardiol.* 103, 472–484. doi: 10.1007/s00395-008-0731-2

Obal, D., Dettwiler, S., Favoccia, C., Scharbatke, H., Preckel, B., and Schlack, W. (2005). The influence of mitochondrial KATP-channels in the cardioprotection of preconditioning and postconditioning by sevoflurane in the rat *in vivo*. *Anesth. Analg.* 101, 1252–1260. doi: 10.1213/01.ANE.0000181336.96511.32

Ong, S. B., and Hausenloy, D. J. (2017). Mitochondrial dynamics as a therapeutic target for treating cardiac diseases. *Handb. Exp. Pharmacol.* 240, 251–279 doi: 10.1007/164_2016_7

Pagliaro, P., and Penna, C. (2015). Redox signalling and cardioprotection: translatability and mechanism. *Br. J. Pharmacol.* 172, 1974–1995. doi: 10.1111/bph.12975

Pagliaro, P., Rastaldo, R., Penna, C., Mancardi, D., Cappello, S., and Losano, G. (2004). Nitric oxide (NO)-cyclic guanosine monophosphate (cGMP) pathway is involved in ischemic postconditioning in the isolated rat heart. *Circulation* 110:136.

Palmer, J. W., Tandler, B., and Hoppel, C. L. (1977). Biochemical properties of subsarcolemmal and interfibrillar mitochondria isolated from rat cardiac muscle. *J. Biol. Chem.* 252, 8731–8739.

Penna, C., Granata, R., Tocchetti, C. G., Gallo, M. P., Alloatti, G., and Pagliaro, P. (2015). Endogenous cardioprotective agents: role in pre and postconditioning. *Curr. Drug Targets* 16, 843–867. doi: 10.2174/1389450116666150309115536

Penna, C., Mancardi, D., Rastaldo, R., Losano, G., and Pagliaro, P. (2007). Intermittent activation of bradykinin B2 receptors and mitochondrial KATP channels trigger cardiac postconditioning through redox signaling. *Cardiovasc. Res.* 75, 168–177. doi: 10.1016/j.cardiores.2007.03.001

Penna, C., Perrelli, M. G., and Pagliaro, P. (2013a). Mitochondrial pathways, permeability transition pore, and redox signaling in cardioprotection: therapeutic implications. *Antioxid. Redox Signal.* 18, 556–599. doi: 10.1089/ars.2011.4459

Penna, C., Perrelli, M. G., Raimondo, S., Tullio, F., Merlino, A., Moro, F., et al. (2009). Postconditioning induces an anti-apoptotic effect and preserves mitochondrial integrity in isolated rat hearts. *Biochim. Biophys. Acta* 1787, 794–801. doi: 10.1016/j.bbabio.2009.03.013

Penna, C., Perrelli, M. G., Tullio, F., Angotti, C., Camporeale, A., Poli, V., et al. (2013b). Diazoxide postconditioning induces mitochondrial protein S-Nitrosylation and a redox-sensitive mitochondrial phosphorylation/translocation of RISK elements: No role for SAFE. *Basic Res. Cardiol.* 108, 371. doi: 10.1007/s00395-013-0371-z

Penna, C., Rastaldo, R., Mancardi, D., Raimondo, S., Cappello, S., and Gattullo, D. (2006). Post-conditioning induced cardioprotection requires signaling through a redox-sensitive mechanism, mitochondrial ATP-sensitive K^+ channel and protein kinase C activation. *Basic Res. Cardiol.* 101, 180–189. doi: 10.1007/s00395-006-0584-5

Piantadosi, C. A. (2012). Regulation of mitochondrial processes by protein S-nitrosylation. *Biochim. Biophys. Acta* 1820, 712–721. doi: 10.1016/j.bbagen.2011.03.008

Pravdic, D., Mio, Y., Sedlic, F., Pratt, P. F., Warltier, D. C., Bosnjak, Z. J., et al. (2010). Isoflurane protects cardiomyocytes and mitochondria by immediate and cytosol-independent action at reperfusion. *Br. J. Pharmacol.* 160, 220–232. doi: 10.1111/j.1476-5381.2010.00698.x

Queiroga, C. S., Almeida, A. S., Martel, C., Brenner, C., Alves, P. M., and Vieira, H. L. (2010). Glutathionylation of adenine nucleotide translocase induced by carbon monoxide prevents mitochondrial membrane permeabilization and apoptosis. *J. Biol. Chem.* 285, 17077–17088. doi: 10.1074/jbc.M109.065052

Quinlan, C. L., Costa, A. D., Costa, C. L., Pierre, S. V., Dos Santos, P., and Garlid, K. D. (2008). Conditioning the heart induces formation of signalosomes that interact with mitochondria to open mitoKATP channels. *Am. J. Physiol. Hear Circ. Physiol.* 295, H953–H961. doi: 10.1152/ajpheart.00520.2008

Serviddio, G., Di Venosa, N., Federici, A., D'Agostino, D., Rollo, T., and Prigigallo, F. (2005). Brief hypoxia before normoxic reperfusion (postconditioning) protects the heart against ischemia-reperfusion injury by preventing mitochondria peroxyde production and glutathione depletion. *FASEB J.* 19, 354–361. doi: 10.1096/fj.04-2338com

Sluijter, J. P. G., Davidson, S. M., Boulanger, C. M., Buzás, E. I., de Kleijn, D. P. V., Engel, F. B., et al. (2018). Extracellular vesicles in diagnostics and therapy of the ischaemic heart: position paper from the working group on cellular biology of the heart of the European Society of Cardiology. *Cardiovasc. Res.* 114, 19–34. doi: 10.1093/cvr/cvx211

Sörensson, P., Saleh, N., Bouvier, F., Böhm, F., Settergren, M., Caidahl, K., et al. (2010). Effect of postconditioning on infarct size in patients with ST elevation myocardial infarction. *Heart* 96, 1710–1715. doi: 10.1136/hrt.2010.199430

Staat, P., Rioufol, G., Piot, C., Cottin, Y., Cung, T. T., L'Huillier, I., et al. (2005). Postconditioning the human heart. *Circulation* 112, 2143–2148. doi: 10.1161/CIRCULATIONAHA.105.558122

Sun, H., Guo, T., Liu, L., Yu, Z., Xu, W., Chen, W., et al. (2010). Ischemic postconditioning inhibits apoptosis after acute myocardial infarction in pigs. *Heart Surg. Forum* 13, E305–E310. doi: 10.1532/HSF98.20101013

Tanno, M., Kuno, A., Ishikawa, S., Miki, T., Kouzu, H., Yano, T., et al. (2014). Translocation of Glycogen Synthase Kinase-3β (GSK-3β), a trigger of permeability transition, is kinase activity-dependent and mediated by interaction with Voltage-dependent Anion Channel 2 (VDAC2). *J. Biol. Chem.* 289, 29285–29296. doi: 10.1074/jbc.M114.563924

Thibault, H., Piot, C., and Ovize, M. (2007). Postconditioning in man. *Heart Fail. Rev.* 12, 245–248. doi: 10.1007/s10741-007-9033-2

Tsang, A., Hausenloy, D. J., Mocanu, M. M., and Yellon, D. M. (2004). Postconditioning: a form of "modified reperfusion" protects the myocardium by activating the phosphatidylinositol 3-kinase-Akt pathway. *Circ. Res.* 95, 230–232. doi: 10.1161/01.RES.0000138303.76488.fe

Tu, R. H., Li, Q. J., Huang, Z., He, Y., Meng, J. J., Zheng, H. L., et al. (2017). Novel functional role of heat shock protein 90 in mitochondrial connexin 43-mediated hypoxic postconditioning. *Cell. Physiol. Biochem.* 44, 982–997. doi: 10.1159/000485399

Wang, C., Neff, D. A., Krolikowski, J. G., Weihrauch, D., Bienengraeber, M., Warltier, D. C., et al. (2006). The influence of B-cell lymphoma 2 protein, an antiapoptotic regulator of mitochondrial permeability transition, on isoflurane-induced and ischemic postconditioning in rabbits. *Anesth. Analg.* 102, 1355–1360. doi: 10.1213/01.ane.0000202463.28618.64

Xue, F., Yang, X., Zhang, B., Zhao, C., Song, J., Jiang, T., et al. (2010). Postconditioning the human heart in percutaneous coronary intervention. *Clin. Cardiol.* 33, 439–444. doi: 10.1002/clc.20796

Yang, Z., Sun, W., and Hu, K. (2012). Molecular mechanism underlying adenosine receptor-mediated mitochondrial targeting of protein kinase C. *Biochim. Biophys. Acta* 1823, 950–958. doi: 10.1016/j.bbamcr.2011.12.012

Yao, Y., Li, L., Li, L., Gao, C., and Shi, C. (2009). Sevoflurane postconditioning protects chronically-infarcted rat hearts against ischemia-reperfusion injury by activation of pro-survival kinases and inhibition of mitochondrial permeability transition pore opening upon reperfusion. *Biol. Pharm. Bull.* 32, 1854–1861. doi: 10.1248/bpb.32.1854

Yao, Y. T., Li, L. H., Chen, L., Wang, W. P., Li, L. B., and Gao, C. Q. (2010). Sevoflurane postconditioning protects isolated rat hearts against ischemia-reperfusion injury: the role of radical oxygen species, extracellular signal-related kinases 1/2 and mitochondrial permeability transition pore. *Mol. Biol. Rep.* 37, 2439–2446. doi: 10.1007/s11033-009-9755-4

Yellon, D. M., and Davidson, S. M. (2014). Exosomes: nanoparticles involved in cardioprotection? *Circ. Res.* 114, 325–332. doi: 10.1161/CIRCRESAHA.113.300636

Yu, J., Maimaitili, Y., Xie, P., Wu, J. J., Wang, J., Yang, Y. N., et al. (2017). High glucose concentration abrogatessevoflurane post-conditioning cardioprotection by advancing mitochondrial fission but dynamin-related protein 1 inhibitor restores these effects. *Acta Physiol.* 220, 83–98. doi: 10.1111/apha.12812

Yu, T. N., Hong, H., Yang, J. Q., Gao, Q., and Xia, Q. (2011). Role of mitochondrial calcium uniporter in cardioprotection induced by ischemic postconditioning in isolated rat heart. *Zhejiang Da Xue Xue Bao Yi Xue Ban* 40, 304–308.

Zhao, Z. Q., Corvera, J. S., Halkos, M. E., Kerendi, F., Wang, N. P., Guyton, R. A., et al. (2003). Inhibition of myocardial injury by ischemic postconditioning during reperfusion: comparison with ischemic preconditioning. *Am. J. Physiol. Hear Circ. Physiol.* 285, H579–H588. doi: 10.1152/ajpheart.01064.2002

6

Antineoplastic Drug-Induced Cardiotoxicity: A Redox Perspective

Gilda Varricchi[1,2*], Pietro Ameri[3], Christian Cadeddu[4], Alessandra Ghigo[5], Rosalinda Madonna[6,7], Giancarlo Marone[8,9], Valentina Mercurio[1], Ines Monte[10], Giuseppina Novo[11], Paolo Parrella[1], Flora Pirozzi[1], Antonio Pecoraro[1], Paolo Spallarossa[3], Concetta Zito[12], Giuseppe Mercuro[4], Pasquale Pagliaro[13] and Carlo G. Tocchetti[1*]

[1] Department of Translational Medical Sciences, University of Naples Federico II, Naples, Italy, [2] Department of Translational Medical Sciences, Center for Basic and Clinical Immunology Research, University of Naples Federico II, Naples, Italy, [3] Clinic of Cardiovascular Diseases, IRCCS San Martino IST, Genova, Italy, [4] Department of Medical Sciences and Public Health, University of Cagliari, Cagliari, Italy, [5] Department of Molecular Biotechnology and Health Sciences, Molecular Biotechnology Center, University of Turin, Turin, Italy, [6] Institute of Cardiology, Center of Excellence on Aging, Università degli Studi "G. d'Annunzio" Chieti – Pescara, Chieti, Italy, [7] Department of Internal Medicine, Texas Heart Institute and Center for Cardiovascular Biology and Atherosclerosis Research, University of Texas Health Science Center, Houston, TX, United States, [8] Section of Hygiene, Department of Public Health, University of Naples Federico II, Naples, Italy, [9] Monaldi Hospital Pharmacy, Naples, Italy, [10] Department of General Surgery and Medical-Surgery Specialities, University of Catania, Catania, Italy, [11] U.O.C. Magnetic Resonance Imaging, Fondazione Toscana G. Monasterio C.N.R., Pisa, Italy, [12] Division of Clinical and Experimental Cardiology, Department of Medicine and Pharmacology, Policlinico "G. Martino" University of Messina, Messina, Italy, [13] Department of Clinical and Biological Sciences, University of Turin, Turin, Italy

Edited by:
Gerald A. Meininger, University of Missouri, United States

Reviewed by:
Francesco Moccia, University of Pavia, Italy
Michele Samaja, Università degli Studi di Milano, Italy

***Correspondence:**
Gilda Varricchi
gilda.varricchi@unina.it
Carlo G. Tocchetti
carlogabriele.tocchetti@unina.it

Antineoplastic drugs can be associated with several side effects, including cardiovascular toxicity (CTX). Biochemical studies have identified multiple mechanisms of CTX. Chemoterapeutic agents can alter redox homeostasis by increasing the production of reactive oxygen species (ROS) and reactive nitrogen species RNS. Cellular sources of ROS/RNS are cardiomyocytes, endothelial cells, stromal and inflammatory cells in the heart. Mitochondria, peroxisomes and other subcellular components are central hubs that control redox homeostasis. Mitochondria are central targets for antineoplastic drug-induced CTX. Understanding the mechanisms of CTX is fundamental for effective cardioprotection, without compromising the efficacy of anticancer treatments. Type 1 CTX is associated with irreversible cardiac cell injury and is typically caused by anthracyclines and conventional chemotherapeutic agents. Type 2 CTX, associated with reversible myocardial dysfunction, is generally caused by biologicals and targeted drugs. Although oxidative/nitrosative reactions play a central role in CTX caused by different antineoplastic drugs, additional mechanisms involving directly and indirectly cardiomyocytes and inflammatory cells play a role in cardiovascular toxicities. Identification of cardiologic risk factors and an integrated approach using molecular, imaging, and clinical data may allow the selection of patients at risk of developing chemotherapy-related CTX. Although the last decade has witnessed intense research related to the molecular and biochemical mechanisms of CTX of antineoplastic drugs, experimental and clinical studies are urgently needed to balance safety and efficacy of novel cancer therapies.

Keywords: chemotherapy, HER-2 inhibitors, oxidative/nitrosative stress, vascular endothelial growth factor, tyrosine kinase inhibitors

INTRODUCTION

Antineoplastic treatments have improved overall survival and progression-free survival in the treatment of an increasing number of malignancies (Jemal et al., 2011). However, different antineoplastic drugs can cause a wide spectrum of cardiovascular (CV) toxicities (CTX), particularly in long-term cancer survivors (Oeffinger et al., 2006; Tocchetti et al., 2013; Moslehi and Deininger, 2015; Mercurio et al., 2016; Zamorano et al., 2016; Armenian et al., 2017). CTX include vasospastic and thromboembolic ischemia, hypertension, dysrhythmia, myocarditis and left ventricular (LV) dysfunction, leading to heart failure (Yeh and Bickford, 2009; Ky et al., 2013; Suter and Ewer, 2013; Zamorano et al., 2016). **Figure 1** schematically illustrates the wide spectrum of cardiovascular toxicities associated with different antineoplastic drugs in patients with cancer. Anthracyclines (ANTs) can cause irreversible type 1 CTX through the production of reactive oxygen species (ROS) and reactive nitrogen species (RNS) (Ewer and Lenihan, 2008; Ewer and Ewer, 2010; Scott et al., 2011). Intracellular signaling inhibitors (e.g., tyrosine kinase inhibitors) block pathways that are main regulators of myocardial function, especially under conditions of cardiac stress, such as hypertension or hypertrophy (Suter and Ewer, 2013). The toxicity induced by biological drugs (e.g., trastuzumab) is often reversible, and has been classified as type 2 CTX (Ewer and Lippman, 2005; Ewer et al., 2005). However, these two forms of CTX may overlap. For example, trastuzumab, a monoclonal antibody anti-HER-2 (Shinkai et al., 1999), can cause irreversible LV dysfunction in patients previously treated with ANTs (Timolati et al., 2006; Suter and Ewer, 2013; Zamorano et al., 2016). More recently, immune myocarditis has entered as a novel challenge in the cardio-oncologic arena, due to a growing number of patients treated with immune checkpoint inhibitors (Swain and Vici) that unleash immune responses (Johnson et al., 2016; Varricchi et al., 2017d).

Here, we review the cellular and molecular mechanisms of CTX of antineoplastic drugs from a redox perspective, since plenty of evidence supports the importance of redox homeostasis for the maintainance of cardiovascular health, while anticancer drugs can disrupt such delicate balance in the myocardium and in the endothelium (Ferroni et al., 2011; Vincent et al., 2013; Zamorano et al., 2016).

OXIDATIVE AND NITROSATIVE STRESS IN CARDIOVASCULAR TOXICITY

ROS is a collective term that includes oxygen radicals, like superoxide ($O_2^{-\bullet}$) and hydroxyl radicals ($OH^{\bullet}$), and other non-radicals such as hydrogen peroxide (H_2O_2), singlet oxygen ($^1O_2$), etc. (Del Río, 2015). The term RNS includes radicals like nitric oxide ($NO^{\bullet}$) and nitric dioxide ($NO_2^{\bullet}$), as well as non-radicals such as nitrous acid (HNO_2) and dinitrogen tetroxide (N_2O_4), among others. Redox stress, resulting from overproduction of ROS and RNS, may directly or indirectly induce cardiac injury (Nediani et al., 2011; Willis and Patterson, 2013).

Physiological levels of ROS and RNS are fundamental for the regulation of many cellular functions (Egea et al., 2017). For example, H_2O_2 is an endothelium-derived vasodilator of the coronary vessels (Saitoh et al., 2007). In pathological conditions (e.g., cancer growth) there is a deregulation of homeostatic control of ROS production leading to DNA damage, inhibition of cellular repair mechanisms and abnormal cell proliferation. ROS/RNS contribute to dysregulation of gene expression and genome stability, but also influence epigenetic pathways affecting the functions/expression of histone and DNA modifying enzymes (Mikhed et al., 2015; Niu et al., 2015). Several antineoplastic drugs induce CTX through an unbalanced generation of ROS/RNS, leading to the so-called oxidative/nitrosative stress. ROS/RNS imbalance derives from increased production or inactivation of endogenous antioxidant enzymes by antineoplastic drugs. **Figure 2** schematically illustrates the transition from the homeostatic role of ROS/RNS in healthy subjects to the pathological role in cancer patients and during chemotherapy or radiotherapy.

The heart is particularly vulnerable to ROS/RNS injury because antioxidant resources are lower than other tissues (e.g., liver) (Minotti et al., 2004, 2010). High levels of ROS/RNS, by exhausting endogeneous antioxidant defenses, can hamper cellular signaling pathways in the CV system. Oxidative stress and low grade inflammation are interdependent processes implicated in cardiovascular diseases and cancer (Galdiero et al., 2016; Varricchi et al., 2017a). Tissue resident (e.g., macrophages, mast cells) and circulating inflammatory cells (e.g., neutrophils, monocytes) can also release ROS increasing oxidative stress (Varricchi et al., 2017a), interestingly ROS can initiate intracellular signaling increasing proinflammatory gene expression (Biswas, 2016).

High levels of ROS/RNS induce membrane lipid peroxidation and membrane damage, DNA damage and trigger death cell and apoptosis, leading to cardiomyocyte death and replacement by connective tissue, which results in irreversible cardiac damage (Li and Singal, 2000; Menna et al., 2008, 2012; Zang et al., 2012; Ky et al., 2013; Suter and Ewer, 2013; Hahn et al., 2014; Salvatorelli et al., 2015; Mercurio et al., 2016).

The major intracellular sources of ROS include the mitochondrial electron transport and the NADPH oxidase family (NOXs) (Lassègue and Griendling, 2010; Zhang et al., 2013). Mitochondria are key organelles for the regulation of redox signaling and redox homeostasis (Egea et al., 2017). Mitochondria function as a central hub that directly and indirectly controls redox homeostasis by hosting several redox-active complexes and enzymes that generate ROS and RNS. Mitochondria represent ≅35% of the myocyte volume and produce ≅90% of the cellular energy. Therefore, impairment of mitochondrial function is critical in cardiomyocytes (Pagliaro et al., 2011; Pagliaro and Penna, 2015; Tocchetti et al., 2015b). At present, the NOX family is composed of five isoforms (NOX1, NOX2, NOX3, NOX4, and NOX5). Cardiomyocytes (Varga et al., 2013) and macrophages (Moon et al., 2016) express NOX4. Mitochondrial and extramitochondrial NOX4 is a source of ROS and can be affected by anticancer drugs. Activated myocardial NOX2 produces $O_2^{\bullet -}$, whereas NOX4 generates

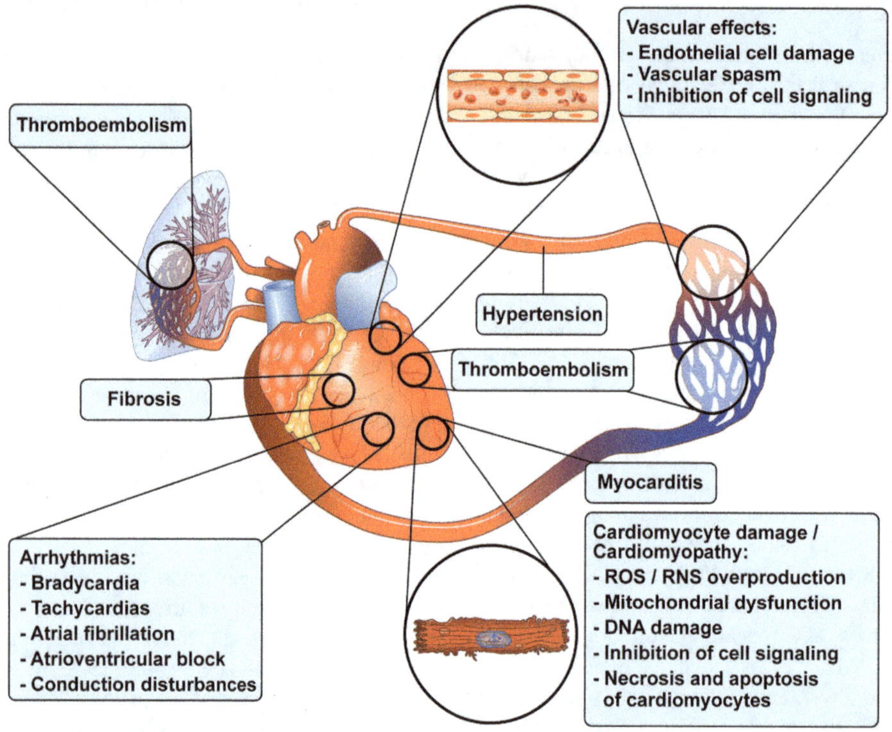

FIGURE 1 | Schematic representation of some of the cardiovascular toxicities associated with antineoplastic drugs in patients with cancer. Modified with permission from Albini et al. (2010).

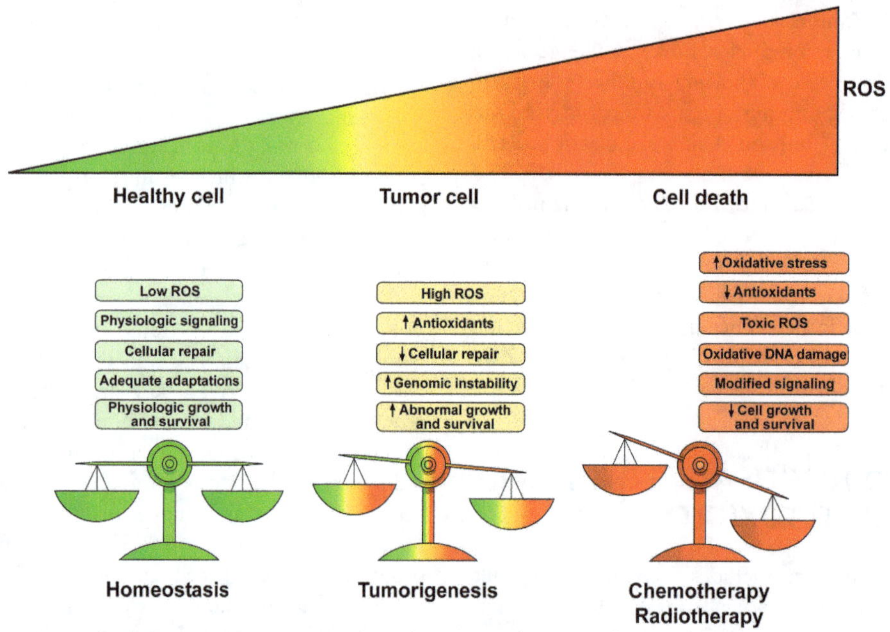

FIGURE 2 | Schematic representation of the homeostatic role of ROS and their pathologic role in tumor growth and cell death. Low production of ROS and balanced antioxidant activity play a fundamental role in cellular signaling and repair resulting in controlled growth and survival. Proliferation of tumor cells yields elevated ROS concentrations enhancing cell survival and proliferation leading to DNA damage and genetic instability causing cell dysfunction. Chemotherapeutic agents and radiotherapy increase ROS production to toxic concentrations resulting in irreparable damage to the cell, inadequate adaptations and eventually cell death. The heart is particularly vulnerable to ROS/RNS injury because antioxidant resources are lower than other tissues. Modified with permission from Moloney and Cotter (2017).

H_2O_2. Moreover, superoxide dismutases (SODs) convert $O_2^{\bullet-}$ to H_2O_2. In mitochondria, H_2O_2 may be converted to O_2 and H_2O by catalase and by glutathione peroxidase (GPx). In the presence of iron complexes, these ROS may be converted to the more toxic $OH^{\bullet}$ within and outside mitochondria (Zhao et al., 2010; Pagliaro et al., 2011; Penna et al., 2014; Pagliaro and Penna, 2015; Tocchetti et al., 2015a). Interestingly, mitochondrial ROS are involved in the modulation of immune cells, including human neutrophils (Vorobjeva et al., 2017).

Peroxisomes, cytoplasmic organelles specialized for carrying out oxidative reactions, also play a role in ROS production/regulation in cardiomyocytes. Several substrates (i.e., amino acids, uric acid, and fatty acids) are broken down by oxidative reactions in peroxisomes. Fatty acid metabolism is very active in cardiomyocytes and peroxisomes are critical for processing long carbon chain fatty acids. The contribution of peroxisomes in the mechanism of CTX is largely unknown (Zanardelli et al., 2014).

Nitric oxide (NO) is a key regulator of cellular functions. It is a redox species with both oxidant and antioxidant properties (Takimoto and Kass, 2007; Pagliaro and Penna, 2015; Tocchetti et al., 2015a) produced produced from the metabolism of the amino acid, L-arginine by three isoforms of nitric oxide synthase (NOS): the endothelial (eNOS or NOS3) and neuronal (nNOS or NOS1) NOSs, constitutively expressed in cardiomyocytes, and the inducible NOS2 (iNOS), which is induced by pro-inflammatory mediators or by ischemia (Pagliaro and Penna, 2015; Tocchetti et al., 2015a). NO is also produced by other reactions termed "non-NOS" processes (Penna et al., 2014; Pagliaro and Penna, 2015). ROS can react with NO to form different RNS, thus amplifying the production of oxidant compounds, and NOS itself may produce ROS (Fogli et al., 2004; Penna et al., 2014; Pagliaro and Penna, 2015; Tocchetti et al., 2015b). NO together with RNS has an important role in mediating proteotoxic stress and modifications of mitochondrial activities, resulting in cytotoxicity and cell necrosis (Lala and Chakraborty, 2001). S-nitrosylation (SNO) is the covalent attachment of a NO moiety to a protein thiol group. SNO is a redox-dependent modification that exerts an antioxidant effect, shielding critical cysteine residues from oxidation and affecting protein functions (Penna et al., 2014; Pagliaro and Penna, 2015).

ANTHRACYCLINES

The production of ROS/RNS is central in the CTX of several anti-cancer drugs. Some agents alter the activity of redox enzymes within and outside the mitochondria, including NOSs, respiratory complexes, the Krebs cycle, oxidative phosphorylation, and β-oxidation (Tocchetti et al., 2017). This impairment results in oxidative/nitrosative stress, a reduction in antioxidant capacity, and induction of cell death (Fogli et al., 2004; Albini et al., 2010; Mele et al., 2016a,b).

ANTs (doxorubicin, epirubicin and daunorubicin), widely used as anticancer agents, are recognized as prototype of type 1 CTX since the 1960s (Tan et al., 1967). ANTs can induce LV dysfunction, leading to HF in up to 9% of patients (Cardinale et al., 2015). ANT can cause CTX *via* a series of many cellular and molecular mechanisms (Zhang et al., 2012; Zamorano et al., 2016). **Figure 3** schematically illustrates the complex interplay of the major mechanisms by which ANTs can induce injury to cardiac cells. The administration of ANTs can alter redox homeostasis in cardiomyocytes and tissue resident (e.g., fibroblasts, endothelial cells, mast cells, macrophages) and circulating inflammatory cells (e.g., neutrophils, eosinophils) in the heart by producing ROS and RNS (Pagliaro and Penna, 2015; Ghigo et al., 2016; Tocchetti et al., 2017).

A basic mechanism by which ANTs can cause CTX is the interaction with topoisomerase 2 (TOP2) A and -B highly expressed in cardiomyocytes (Lyu et al., 2007). The former is present in rapidly dividing cells, such as cancer cells, and forms the ternary TOP2-doxorubicin-DNA complex, inducing cell apoptosis. TOP2B, highly expressed in human cardiomyocytes, forms the TOP2B-doxorubicin-DNA complex, which causes DNA damage leading to cell apoptosis. The tumor suppressor protein p53, a pivotal enzyme for activating DNA repair proteins, can cause mitochondrial dysfunction and metabolic failure (Sawyer, 2013). The metabolic alterations caused by doxorubicin-activated p53 damage mitochondria in the cardiomyocytes, result in enhanced ROS/RNS generation and ultimately cell death. Collectively, these results indicate that oxidative reactions play a central role in ANT-induced LV dysfunction. Therefore, drugs that interfere with molecules involved in heart metabolism (e.g., p53) may represent a potential approach in limiting LV dysfunction (Sawyer, 2013; Mercurio et al., 2016).

Besides directly damaging cardiomyocytes, doxorubicin induces apoptosis of immune (e.g., macrophages) and cancer cells releasing high mobility group box 1 (HMGB1) which, in turn, triggers toll-like receptor (TLR)-2 and-4 (Ma et al., 2012; Yao et al., 2012). TLR-2 and TLR-4 are found in cardiomyocytes and inflammatory cells and their engagement induces the release of proinflammatory cytokines (i.e., IL-6, IL-1β, TNF-α). Overall, these findings emphasize the contribution of TLRs in mediating ANT-induces inflammation and CTX and envisage the possibility of targeting this pathway for therapeutic purposes.

A better characterization of the multiple molecular mechanisms of ANT-related toxicity of blood vessels and cardiomyocytes appears fundamental to select the best approach to prevent and treat CTX (Van Cutsem et al., 2002; Scott et al., 2011; Madonna et al., 2015a,b; Cadeddu et al., 2016).

As mentioned in a previous section, mitochondrial ROS (mtROS) represent a prominent source (≅80%) of ROS, expecially in the heart (Russell and Cotter, 2015). mtROS play a pivotal role in ANT-induced CTX (Minotti et al., 2004, 2010). Doxorubicin binds with high affinity to the mitochondrial phospholipid cardiolipin, inhibits its function, stimulates ROS/RNS production, inhibits oxidative phosphorylation, and causes mitochondrial DNA damage (Pereira et al., 2016). ANTs also cause mitochondrial calcium accumulation, leading to mitochondrial injury (Pereira, Pereira et al., 2016). ANTs can also affect cardiac progenitor cells following myocardial injury (Huang et al., 2010; Oliveira et al., 2013).

The production of ROS is a central event in ANT-induced CTX. ROS are effectors of membrane lipid peroxidation,

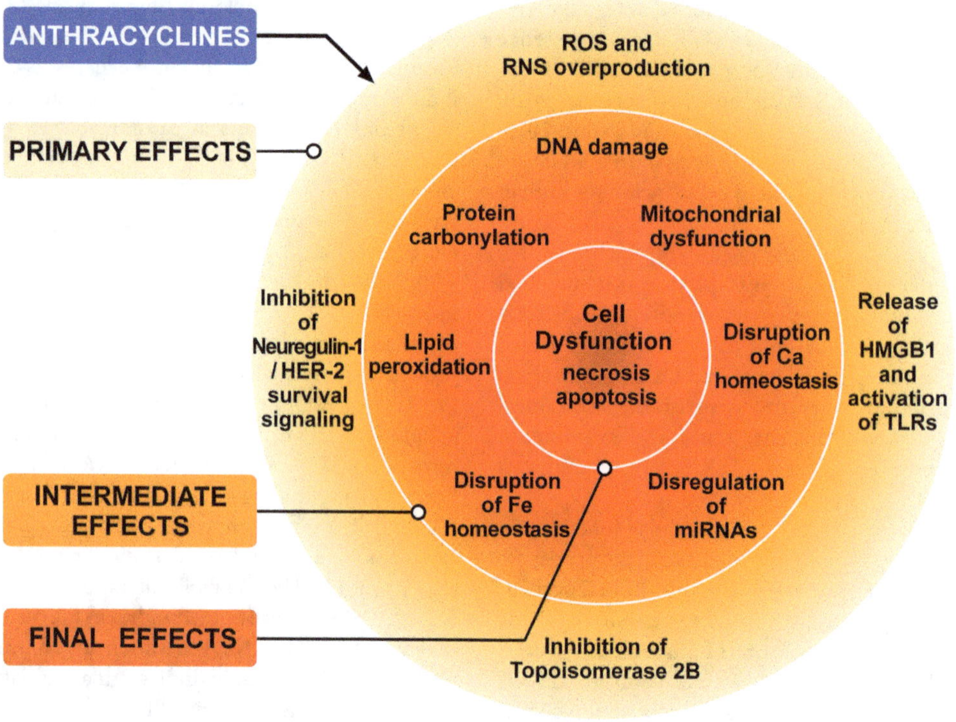

FIGURE 3 | Schematic representation of the main mechanisms of anthracycline-induced injury to cardiac cells. The classic model of anthracycline (ANT) cardiotoxicity involves the generation of ROS by the quinone moiety common to all anthracyclines. ROS and RNS hyperproduction results in damage to DNA, protein carbonylation and lipid peroxidation leading to cellular dysfunction and cardiomyocyte death. ANTs can also bind and block the functions of both topoisomerases 2A (TOP2A) and 2B (TOP2B). Tumor cells express high levels of TOP2A, whereas TOP2B is ubiquitously expressed. Cardiomyocytes express TOP2B, but not TOP2A. ANTs form a complex with TOP2B inhibiting its enzymatic activity. Without functional TOP2B, DNA breaks accrue, leading to the activation of p53 tumor-suppressor protein, mitochondrial dysfunction, and the generation of ROS that result in cardiomyocyte death. Another mechanism underlying doxorubicin-dependent oxidative stress is linked to the ability of the drug to directly interfere with the activity of NADPH oxidase and nitric oxide synthase (NOS). Both NADPH oxidase and NOS can transfer electron from NADPH to doxorubicin, causing the formation of semiquinone doxorubicin (SQ-DOX). SQ-DOX in turn transfers electron to O_2 and generates O_2^-. In the NOS compartment, O_2^- can react with NO to form peroxynitrite ($ONOO^-$), a powerful oxidant that can generate free radicals. An alternative mechanism by which ANTs exert their cardiotoxic effects is the inhibition of neuregulin-1 (NRG-1)-HER-2 in cardiomyocytes. Doxorubicin also induces necrosis of immune (i.e., macrophages) and cancer cells releasing HMGB1 which activates TLR-2 and TLR-4 in cardiomyocytes and inflammatory cells inducing the release of proinflammatory cytokines. These primary effects induce a plethora of secondary effects in cardiomyocytes (e.g., DNA damage, lipid peroxidation, mitochondrial dysfunction, etc.,) which result in cell dysfunction and death. Modified with permission from Tocchetti et al. (2017).

irreversible damage, and myocyte replacement by connective tissue (Menna et al., 2008, 2012; Zhang et al., 2012; Ky et al., 2013; Suter and Ewer, 2013; Salvatorelli et al., 2015). ROS generated by ANTs affect mitochondrial enzymes, NOSs, NAD(P)H oxidases, and catalase, leading to oxidative stress and cell injury. ANTs are metabolized to unstable compounds (such as doxorubicin-semiquinone), which react with O_2, producing H_2O_2 and $O_2^{\bullet-}$.

ANTs chelate free intracellular iron, forming iron-doxorubicin complexes. ANTs also interfere with iron-transporting and -binding proteins (Gammella et al., 2014; Ghigo et al., 2016). Ardehali and collaborators found that doxorubicin impairs a mitochondrial iron exporter with consequent iron accumulation and subsequent ROS generation (Ichikawa et al., 2014). Cardiac dysfunction following ANT treatment is associated with high mitochondrial iron levels compared with normal hearts (Ichikawa et al., 2014). Collectively, these findings indicate that oxidative stress and mitochondrial iron accumulation play a key role in ANT-induced CTX.

ANTs interact with cardiolipin leading to concentration of the drug in mitochondrial membrane phospholipids (Goormaghtigh et al., 1990). In mitochondria, the drug exerts adverse effects (e.g., ROS generation, inhibition of oxidative phosphorylation, and mitochondrial DNA damage). ROS cause peroxidation of cardiolipin, which induces the release of mitochondrial factors, such as cytochrome c, which in turn triggers cardiolipin peroxidation. This cycle exacerbates ANT-induced injury. NO inhibits both the peroxidase activity of cytochrome c and cardiolipin oxidation. NO, which possesses antioxidant properties, may counteract the toxic effects of ANTs (Vlasova et al., 2006; Gonzalvez and Gottlieb, 2007; Pointon et al., 2010).

Enzymes located outside the mitochondria also able to produce ROS. A nonexhaustive list includes NADPH oxidases (NOXs), xanthine oxidase (XO), and monoamine oxidase. Xanthine oxidase and NADPH, may be targeted by ANTs. Doxorubicin deoxyaglycone can be obtained by a reduction process and accumulates in membranes, altering the function of NADH dehydrogenase in mitochondria or the NOXs in the plasma membrane (Thorn et al., 2011). Among other mechanisms involved in cardiotoxicity caused by ANTs, recent studies have highlighted the role of altered myocardial energetics, expressed by a lower phosphocreatine/adenosine triphosphate (ATP) ratio, which precedes LV dysfunction (Maslov et al., 2010). Indeed, ANTs can oxidize sulfhydryl groups of creatine kinase (CK), reducing its function, thus impairing myocardial energetics (Maslov et al., 2010), hence causing LV dysfunction. More studies on such an interesting mechanism could be helpful in order to identify new protective therapeutic strategies. Indeed, overexpression of myofibrillar CK in mice with HF induced by transverse aortic constriction increased heart function (Gupta et al., 2012) supporting a role for CK in HF prevention and treatment. Accordingly, the same group demonstrated that CK overexpression also ameliorated myocardial energetics, contractile function, and survival in murine anthracyclines cardiotoxicity (Gupta et al., 2013). These results provide novel strategies for limitation of anthracycline-related cardiotoxicity.

ANTs are also able to alter cardiac energy metabolism by lowering the level of 5′ AMP-activated protein kinase (AMPK, activated in the response to energy stress) and phosphorylation of anti-acetyl-CoA carboxylase, leading to impairment of fatty acid oxidation (Tokarska-Schlattner et al., 2005).The mechanisms underlying inhibition of AMPK need to be fur-ther elucidated (Mercurio et al., 2016).

Importantly, along with ANTs (Menna et al., 2012; Sawyer, 2013; Sterba et al., 2013; Ghigo et al., 2016), redox abnormalities are central in the pathophysiology of cardiotoxicity caused by other anticancer drugs, among which are new biologic antineoplastic agents, such as intracellular signaling inhibitors, that are increasingly being used (Tocchetti et al., 2017). Such agents may cause cardiotoxicity, since they block pathways important for the modulation of myocardial function, especially under conditions of cardiac stress, such as hypertension or hypertrophy (Suter and Ewer, 2013), with mechanisms of action that often involve redox dysregulation as well.

ANTIMETABOLITES

Fluoropyrimidines [i.e., 5-fluorouracil (5-FU), capecitabine, and gemcitabine] are used in the treatment of several tumors. 5-FU administered intravenously has a short half-life, but active metabolites concentrate in cardiac and cancer cells, resulting in a prolonged exposure to the drug (Kosmas et al., 2008; Miura et al., 2010; Lestuzzi et al., 2011). Capecitabine is converted into its active form preferentially within tumors (Ng et al., 2005; Aprile et al., 2009; Khan et al., 2014; Petrelli et al., 2016). 5-FU and its main metabolite can induce CTX after few days of treatment (Jensen and Sorensen, 2006; Jensen and Sørensen, 2012). The enzyme involved in the conversion of capecitabine to 5-FU is expressed in both atherosclerotic plaques and cancer cells, explaining the CTX in patients with coronary artery disease. The incidence of CTX caused by 5-FU ranges from 0 to 35%, with a mortality rate between 2 and 13%. Myocardial ischemia is the strongest risk factors for fluoropyrimidine-induced CTX (Koca et al., 2011; Polk et al., 2013, 2014). Silent ischemia due to cardiac stress test has been reported in 6–7% of 5-FU-treated patients (Lestuzzi et al., 2014). The mechanisms involved in the CTX of 5-FU and its metabolites involve inhibition of NO (Cianci et al., 2003; Shoemaker et al., 2004), enhanced generation of ROS/RNS (Lamberti et al., 2014), higher endothelial thrombogenicity (Kalam and Marwick, 2013) and senescence (Altieri et al., 2017), and DNA and RNA damage. 5-FU can induce oxidative stress in cardiomyocytes and endothelial cells. This drug causes eNOS dysregulation, endothelin 1 upregulation and the activation of protein kinase C. These effects lead to endothelium-dependent and -independent vasoconstriction, and eventually to coronary spasm (Alter et al., 2006; Sorrentino et al., 2012).

HER-2 INHIBITORS

Epidermal growth factor receptor 2 (ErbB2) (also called HER-2), ErbB1, ErbB3, and ErbB4 are members of the human epidermal growth factor receptor family. When activated by their ligands, these transmembrane receptors homodimerize or heterodimerize and are phosphorylated, initiating several cellular responses (Force et al., 2007). HER-2, present on human heart and overexpressed in approximately 30% of breast cancers, can interact with HER-1 and HER-3, independently from ligand stimulation, thus triggering signaling pathways that stimulate tumor growth (Slamon et al., 1987). Trastuzumab, a humanized mAb that binds the extracellular domain IV of HER-2 (Force et al., 2007; Suter et al., 2007), can cause type 2 CTX (Ewer and Lippman, 2005; Ewer et al., 2005) in approximately 30% of patients when combined with ANTs (Slamon et al., 2001; Suter et al., 2007; De Keulenaer et al., 2010).

Several oral small molecules inhibiting tyrosine kinase (TK) associated with HER are clinically used or under development (De Keulenaer et al., 2010; Ades et al., 2014). Lapatinib and neratinib are novel HER-2/HER-4 TK inhibitors undergoing clinical development in HER-2^+ breast cancer. Their cardiac safety data show a favorable profile (Ades et al., 2014). Several clinical trials have demonstrated that lapatinib is less toxic than trastuzumab (Ades et al., 2014). Pertuzumab is a humanized mAb blocking domain II of the extracellular part of HER-2, thus stopping HER-2/HER-3 homo-heterodimeration. Several clinical trials have assessed the cardiac toxicity of pertuzumab (Bowles et al., 2012; Molinaro et al., 2015). Pertuzumab causes a modest (≅10%) reduction of LVSD in patients with HER-2^+ breast cancer (Baselga et al., 2012; Gianni et al., 2012; Swain et al., 2013).

Importantly, in breast cancer treatment, the co-administration of trastuzumab with ANTs enhances the latter's toxicity and is now avoided. In fact, anti-HER-2 mAbs block the protective mechanisms of HER-2, exhacerbating the oxidative damage caused by doxorubicin (Ewer and Ewer, 2010). Indeed, redox mechanisms have also been advocated for the neuregulin/ErbB2 pathway. This pathway can modulate the increase in ROS caused by doxorubicin in animal models (Timolati et al., 2006), suggesting that cardiotoxicity from ErbB2 blockade can also involve a dysregulation of redox homeostasis (Gordon et al., 2009; Mercurio et al., 2016).

In the heart, endothelial cells release neoregulin 1 (NRG-1), especially the NRG-1β isoform (Lim et al., 2015), which triggers HER-4/HER-4 homodimerization and HER-4/HER-2 heterodimerization on cardiomyocytes to activate protective pathways in response to stress (De Keulenaer et al., 2010; Odiete et al., 2012; Lim et al., 2015; **Figure 4**). The HER-2 pathway mediates cell survival and possibly regeneration (D'Uva et al., 2015) and is stimulated when the heart experiences stress, including hypertension (de Korte et al., 2007; Ewer and Ewer, 2010) and ANT therapy (Gabrielson et al., 2007). Anti-HER-2 agents interfere with the NRG-1/HER-4/HER-2 axis and can cause cardiomyocyte damage. This hypothesis is corroborated by ErbB2 KO-mice that present with LV dilation and increased susceptibility to ANT-induced cardiac damage (Crone et al., 2002; Ozcelik et al., 2002), supporting a fundamental role of HER-2 in the heart. Conversely, cardiac ErbB2 overexpressed mice exhibited reduced levels of ROS in mitochondria, with lower ROS levels and less cell death after treatment of neonatal cardiomyocytes isolated from ErbB2 (Bosch et al., 2013) hearts with anthracyclines. This was due to higher levels of glutathione peroxidase 1 (GPx1) protein and GPx activity, with increased levels of two known GPx activators, c-Abl and Arg (Belmonte et al., 2015; Tocchetti et al., 2017).

HER-2 and HER-4 receptor expression and activation/phosphorylation are lower in failing human myocardium, a condition characterized by increased oxidative stress (Rohrbach et al., 1999). Dogs with HF showed increased phosphorylation of ErbB4 and ErbB2 (Doggen et al., 2009). NRG-1 expression is enhanced in HF (Rohrbach et al., 1999; Doggen et al., 2009). Collectively, these results indicate that NRG-1/HER-4/HER-2 activity is involved in the pathophysiology of HF (Mercurio et al., 2016). (Mercurio et al., 2016). Importantly, NRG-1 exerts a lusitropic effect on isolated cardiac muscle preparations via a NO-dependent mechanism (Lemmens et al., 2004): this requires a functional NO synthase, with preserved NO bioavailability, a condition which can be hampered by the increased oxidative stress in HF (Nediani et al., 2011; Arcaro et al., 2016).

Based on cardioprotective properties of NRG-1 *via* HER-4/HER-2, the neuregulin-HER pathway is currently being assessed in clinical studies for HF treatment (Galindo et al., 2014a,b). NRG-1β increases LV function and reduces cardiac dimensions in experimental failing hearts (Liu et al., 2006; Li et al., 2011; Galindo et al., 2014a,b; Mercurio et al., 2016). NRG-1 also inhibits cardiac fibroblasts and prevents fibrosis (Galindo et al., 2014a,b). NRG-1 administration after myocardial infarction is able to blunt remodeling of the damaged heart (Liu et al., 2006; Galindo et al., 2014a,b). Clinical trials have shown that NRG-1 is well-tolerated and ameliorates heart dimensions and LVEF up to 3 months after treatment (Gao et al., 2010; Jabbour et al., 2011). However, NRG-1 may be a growth factor for cancer cells, and further studies are necessary to assess the safety

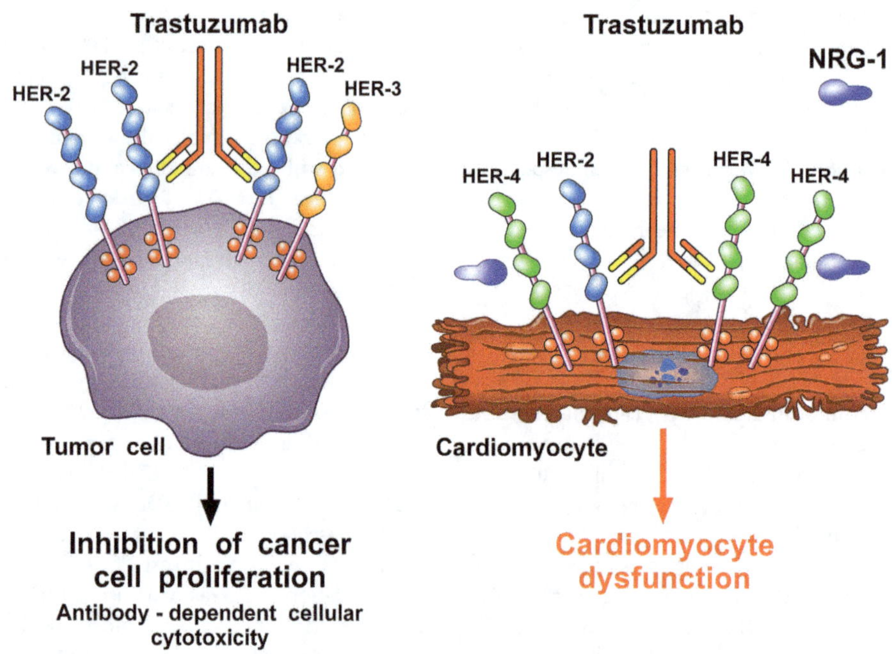

FIGURE 4 | Schematic representation of the mechanism of action of trastuzumab and pathogenesis of its cardiotoxicity. Trastuzumab is a mAb that binds the extracellular domain IV of HER-2. It is used to treat breast cancer patients (≅30%) in which HER-2 is overexpressed and spontaneously homodimerizes or forms heterodimers with other HER receptors, especially HER-3. This ligand-independent activation of HER-2 promotes proliferation and survival of tumor cells. Trastuzumab blocks the interaction HER-2/HER-3 and downstream signaling halting the growth of tumor cells. Moreover, trastuzumab induces the antibody-dependent immune cell-mediated cytotoxicity of cancer cells **(left side)**. In the heart, neuregulin-1 (NRG-1) triggers HER-4/HER-4 homodimerization and HER-4/HER-2 heterodimerization on cardiomyocytes to induce protective pathways in response to stress. Blockade of cardiac HER-2 by trastuzumab results in the disruption of NRG-1-dependent signaling and consequently in alterations of structure and functions that cause cardiomyocyte death **(right side)**.

and efficacy of NRG-1 in HF (Lim et al., 2015; Mercurio et al., 2016).

INHIBITORS OF VASCULAR ENDOTHELIAL GROWTH FACTOR (VEGF) SIGNALING

Vascular endothelial growth factors (VEGF-A, VEGF-B, VEGF-C, VEGF-D. and PlGF) activate specific tyrosine kinase (TK) receptors (VEGFR-1, VEGFR-2, and VEGFR-3) on blood endothelial cells (Loffredo et al., 2016; Staiano et al., 2016) and on endothelial colony forming cells (Dragoni et al., 2011) and have a major role in myocardial angiogenesis at rest and in pressure-overload hearts (Oka et al., 2014). Inhibitors of VEGF signaling (i.e., mAbs anti-VEGF-A and "specific" TK inhibitors) are used for the treatment of several malignancies (Hurwitz et al., 2004; Sandler et al., 2006). VEGFs also regulate several myocardial functions and the integrity of coronary and systemic blood vessels (Folkman, 2007; Eschenhagen et al., 2011; Curigliano et al., 2012; Tocchetti et al., 2013; Marone and Granata, 2014), hence, not surprisingly, beside fighting cancer proliferation by inhibiting angiogenesis, VEGF antagonists may produce different forms of CTX, mainly hypertension, thromboembolism, LV dysfunction, and HF (Gressett and Shah, 2009; Nazer et al., 2011; Welti et al., 2013).

Bevacizumab (anti-VEGF mAb), sunitinib and sorafenib (TK inhibitors: TKIs) are used for the treatment of different types of cancer (Hurwitz et al., 2004; Sandler et al., 2006). Bevacizumab can induce hypertension and cardiac dysfunction in 1–3% patients undergoing chemotherapy (Miller et al., 2005). Regorafenib is a multi-target TKI that inhibits VEGFR1, endothelial-specific receptor tyrosine kinase (trk2), PDGFR, fibroblast growth factor receptor (FGFR), KIT, and RET. Regorafenib, used in therapeutic protocolos for gastrointestinal tumors, can induce hypertension (Brinda et al., 2016) and less frequently cardiac ischemia and myocardial infarction (Bronte et al., 2015). Treatment with pazopanib and axitinib (inhibitors of VEGFRs, PDGFRA and B, and KIT) can lead to hypertension (Motzer et al., 2013). 40% of patients treated with axitinib can experience hypertension (Hutson et al., 2013). Novel anti-angiogenic drugs such as cediranib, vatalanib and nintedanib also exhibit a potential risk of hypertension and HF (Goss et al., 2010; Van Cutsem et al., 2011; Reck et al., 2014).

Sunitinib and sorafenib are not selective TKIs and inhibit several kinases other than VEGFR (Cheng and Force, 2010). Sunitinib inhibits more than 30 TKs, including platelet-derived growth factor receptor (PDGFR), KIT, and colony-stimulating factor 1 receptor (CSF1R) (Force et al., 2007; Cheng and Force, 2010; Hasinoff and Patel, 2010). All these kinases are regulators of CV functions (Lévy, 2006; Anisimov et al., 2009). Up to 28% of patients can develop cardiac dysfunction from sunitinib (Chu et al., 2007; Motzer et al., 2007; Khakoo et al., 2008; Telli et al., 2008). The CTX induced by sunitinib is also due to interference with ribosomal S6 kinase (Tokarska-Schlattner et al., 2005) that then triggers apoptosis (Force et al., 2007; Kerkela et al., 2009). Sunitinib prolongs opening of the mitochondrial permeability transition pore (mPTP) and mitochondrial swelling in myocytes from heart subjected to pressure overload (Chu et al., 2007). Also, treatment of different myocardial preparations with sunitinib produces a dose-dependent negative inotropic effect, paralleled by a decline in intracellular Ca^{2+} and increase of ROS production (Rainer et al., 2012; Tocchetti et al., 2013). Interestingly, our preliminary data show that CK might play a role in the regulation of sunitinib cardiac effects (Tocchetti et al., 2015b). In addition, sutinitib can harm pericytes in cardiac vessels (Chintalgattu et al., 2013). Sorafenib inhibits at least 15 kinases, including the VEGFR, PDGFR, and KIT (Force et al., 2007; Cheng and Force, 2010; Tocchetti et al., 2013).

In conclusion, cardiac dysfunction can be induced by many mechanisms in patients treated with mAbs anti-VEGF and TKIs including alterations of mitochontrial function and energy production with increase in ROS generation, as well as induction of arterial hypertension (Mourad and Levy, 2011). Bevacizumab and sunitinib can cause hypertension because of functional (inactivation of endothelial NO synthase and production of vasoconstrictors such as endothelin-1) and anatomic modifications, bringing to vasoconstriction and to an increase in peripheral vascular resistance (Ku et al., 1993; Mourad and Levy, 2011; Nazer et al., 2011; Hahn et al., 2014). Arterial and venous thrombosis is due to reduction of NO synthesis, endothelial dysfunction, and plaque instability.

ANTIOXIDANT PROPERTIES OF CARDIOVASCULAR DRUGS: A USEFUL TOOL FOR THE PROTECTION FROM CARDIOTOXICITY OF ANTINEOPLASTIC DRUGS

It has been suggested that drugs with antioxidant properties can prevent CTX induced by an increase in ROS (Swain et al., 1997; Li and Singal, 2000; Spallarossa et al., 2004; Cadeddu et al., 2010; Lipshultz et al., 2012; Dessí et al., 2013; Broeyer et al., 2014). Dexrazoxane, an iron-chelating drug, is a cardioprotective agent approved by the FDA for ANT-induced CTX. It is a pro-drug that enters the cardiomyocyte, is rapidly metabolized into its active form, and inhibits the formation of ANT-iron complexes and the production of ROS (Simunek et al., 2009). Its efficacy in several types of tumors has been demonstrated in clinical trials and two pooled analyses (Swain et al., 1997; Seymour et al., 1999; Swain and Vici, 2004; Lipshultz et al., 2012). Other iron chelators have not shown any cardioprotective effect suggesting that dexrazoxane exerts its effects by means of additional protective mechanisms (Simunek et al., 2009). Dexrazoxane changes the Top2β configuration preventing its interface with ANTs, thereby impeding the formation of the Top2-DNA complexes (Lyu et al., 2007; Lencova-Popelova et al., 2016). Stěrba and coworkers have shown that the cardioprotective effects of dexrazoxane are due to its interaction with Top2-β, rather than to its iron chelating activity (Sterba et al., 2013). Derivatives of dexrazoxane lacking effects on Top2β were found not to be protective in models of ANT-induced CTX (Martin et al., 2009; Tocchetti et al., 2017) suggesting the relevance of Top2β in the cardioprotective mechanism.

ANTIOXIDANT PROPERTIES OF BETA BLOCKERS: BEYOND THE ANTIADRENERGIC EFFECTS

β-blockers are cornerstone treatments for patients with low LVEF (Ponikowski et al., 2016), and there is evidence to encourage their use in asymptomatic ANT-related LV dysfunction (Curigliano et al., 2012; Cadeddu et al., 2016). The rationale for β blocker utilization in ANT-induced CTX is based on clinical and experimental results. Alterations of β-adrenergic receptor (β-AR) signaling are present in LV dysfunction caused by ANTs and in other types of dilated cardiomyopathies (Fu et al., 1994). Furthermore, a positive effect of β-AR blockage in reducing oxidative stress and myocardial calcium overload (Nakamura et al., 2002; Asanuma et al., 2004) has been shown in experimental models. New-generation β blockers (i.e., carvedilol and nebivolol) have been taken into consideration for their cardioprotective properties. Carvedilol, a non-selective β- and α1-AR antagonist with strong antioxidant properties, was compared to atenolol, a β blocker devoid of antioxidant properties. Only carvedidol conferred protection from ANT-induced LV-dysfunction and such effect has been attributed to its antioxidant properties rather than to the β-AR blocking action (Matsui et al., 1999). Carvedilol inhibits ANT-induced ROS release, cardiomyocyte apoptosis (Spallarossa et al., 2004), and mitochondrial alterations (Santos et al., 2002). In a small clinical trial evaluating the cardioprotective effect of carvedilol in patients treated with ANTs a reduced incidence of LV dysfunction was reported (Kalay et al., 2006). More studies are needed in order to confirm this cardioprotective effect.

In an experimental model of ANT-induced CTX, nebivolol, a cardio-selective β blocker with limited vasodilating properties, improved LV function, while enhancing NO levels and lowering oxidative stress (de Nigris et al., 2008; Tocchetti et al., 2015a). In a small clinical trial the prophylactic use of nebivolol in patients undergoing ANT-based treatments was associated with lower incidence of LV dilatation and systolic dysfunction in the nebivolol group compared to the placebo group (Kaya et al., 2013).

Interestingly, β blockers have been associated with reduced risk of cardiac dysfunction in patients on trastuzumab, ANTs, or both (Seicean et al., 2013). More recently, β blockers such as bisoprolol (Pituskin et al., 2017) and metoprolol have not shown promising results in the prevention of trastuzumab-induced LV dysfunction, suggesting that blockade of β1 alone is not cardioprotective (Gulati et al., 2016). This supports the use of non-selective β1 and β2 blockers (Sysa-Shah et al., 2016).

THE REDOX ROLE OF RENIN-ANGIOTENSIN-ALDOSTERONE SYSTEM ANTAGONISTS

The renin-angiotensin-aldosterone system (RAAS) is a key player in ANT-induced CTX (Arnolda et al., 1985). Angiotensin-converting enzyme inhibitors (ACE-Is) and angiotensin II receptor blockers (ARBs) can reduce the progression of heart dysfunction and prevent HF in high-risk patients (Ponikowski et al., 2016). Experimental studies have shown the efficacy of ACE-Is in fighting ANT-induced CTX (Abd El-Aziz et al., 2001; Boucek et al., 2003). ACE-Is can confer protection from ANT-related CTX by reducing ROS damage, intracellular calcium overload and fibrosis, and by enhancing mitochondrial respiration and cardiomyocyte metabolism (Abd El-Aziz et al., 2001; Boucek et al., 2003). Enalapril, captopril, and lisinopril can improve acute and chronic ANT-induced cardiotoxicity in experimental models (Abd El-Aziz et al., 2001). In ANTs-treated patients, enalapril reduced the incidence of LV dysfunction compared to placebo (Cardinale et al., 2015). Candesartan modulates experimental cardiotoxicity induced by ANTs (Soga et al., 2006). Pre- and post-treatment with telmisartan protects against acute doxorubicin-induced LV dysfunction in rats (Iqbal et al., 2008). Telmisartan affects the bioavailability of NO and inhibits the production of interleukin-6 (IL-6) and tumor necrosis factor-α (TNF-α) (Yamagishi and Takeuchi, 2005). In a small prospective study, telmisartan blunted subclinical cardiotoxic effects of epirubicin (EPI) (Cadeddu et al., 2010). Telmisartan reversed early EPI-induced myocardial dysfunction and maintained a normal systolic function up to the 18-month follow-up (Dessí et al., 2011, 2013). Valsartan exerted a cardioprotective effect in patients treated with ANTs (Nakamae et al., 2005).

The combination of ACE-Is (enalapril) and β blockers (carvedidol) seems to be beneficial in treating ANT-induced CTX (Bosch et al., 2013). Several clinical trials have evaluated the role of ACE-Is and ARBs as cardiopreventive agents in patients undergoing chemotherapy (Lim et al., 2015; Molinaro et al., 2015). A recent meta-analysis showed that the prophylactic administration of ACE-Is and ARBs in patients treated with ANTs reduced the risk of developing CTX compared with placebo (Kalam and Marwick, 2013). Unfortunately, recent studies have failed to show promising results about prevention of cardiotoxicity with beta blockers or ACE-Is or ARBs (Boekhout et al., 2016; Gulati et al., 2016; Pituskin et al., 2017).

Non-dihydropyridine calcium channel blockers are not indicated in patients with anti-angiogenic drug-induced hypertension, due to the pharmacokinetic interaction of sorafenib and sunitinib with CYP3A4 (Maitland et al., 2010; Cadeddu et al., 2016). Experimental and clinical studies should evaluate the safety and efficacy of the combination of ACE-Is and β blockers in preventing sunitinib-induced CTX.

EXPERIMENTAL ANTIOXIDANT DRUGS IN CARDIOPROTECTION AGAINST CARDIOTOXIC EFFECTS OF ANTHRACYCLINES

Several drugs (e.g., ranolazine, statins, and phosphodiesterase-5 inhibitors) have been assessed in counteracting ANT-induced CTX. The efficacy of different statins in preventing ANT-induced CTX is so far unproven, due to controversial data. Statins (i.e., lovastatin and fluvastatin) were cardioprotective in cellular studies performed on proliferating H9c2 cell line, but not on cardiomyocytes (Riad et al., 2009; Huelsenbeck et al., 2011). Lovastatin did not modify LV dysfunction induced by doxorubicin (Henninger et al., 2015). Small clinical studies have reported protective/marginal effects of statins in patients treated with ANTs (Seicean et al., 2012; Chotenimitkhun et al., 2015). Hence, several experimental models of cardiac dysfunction have suggested a cardioprotective effect with ranolazine (Sabbah et al., 2002; Rastogi et al., 2008; Coppini et al., 2013, 2017). Ranolazine can preserve cardiac function in mice treated with ANTs by reducing oxidative stress (Tocchetti et al., 2014; Cappetta et al., 2017). Ranolazine can prevent calcium overload and the occurrence of oxidative damage by suppressing ROS production (Kohlhaas et al., 2010). Although the INTERACT study indicated that ranolazine was a promising agent for the prevention of DOX-induced cardiotoxicity, more studies are needed to confirm such evidence (Minotti, 2013).

Sildenafil, a phosphodiesterase-5 inhibitor, seems to protect from ANT-induced cardiac dysfunction by opening mitochondrial K_{ATP} channels, preserving mitochondrial membrane potential and myofibrillar integrity, and preventing cardiomyocyte apoptosis (Fisher et al., 2005). Tadalafil blunted ANT-induced LV dysfunction through NO-mediated rises in cGMP levels (Koka et al., 2010; Jin et al., 2013).

Hydrogen sulfide (H_2S), a redox compound, also attracted the interest of cardio-oncologists. Cystathionine gamma-lyase, a key enzyme in the synthesis of H_2S, is involved in ANT-induced CTX in cardiomyocytes and exogenous H_2S has been shown to protect against CTX (Papapetropoulos et al., 2015; Cadeddu et al., 2016; Mele et al., 2016b). Further experimental research and randomized trials will be needed to assess the safety and efficacy of H_2S.

Experimental data show that VEGF-B favors coronary artheriogenesis, physiological cardiac hyperthrophy, and resistance to ischemia (Bry et al., 2010; Kivelä et al., 2014). Furthermore, VEGF-B has been proposed as a candidate for the therapy of dilated cardiomyophaty (Kivelä et al., 2014; Woitek et al., 2015). There is preliminary evidence that VEGF-B gene therapy can inhibit doxorubicin-induced CTX (Räsänen et al., 2016).

BEYOND PHARMACOLOGIC APPROACHES

Nutritional supplementation and exercise training may also exert antioxidant properties (Andreadou et al., 2009; Haykowsky et al., 2009; Scott et al., 2011, 2013; Kirkham and Davis, 2015; Stefani et al., 2015; Singh et al., 2016). While in experimental models, dietary supplementation of antioxidants can mitigate LV dysfunction induced by ANTs (Rephaeli et al., 2007; Andreadou et al., 2009; Xi et al., 2012), evidence suggesting that antioxidant supplementation may modulate ANT-induced CTX in cancer patients is still scant (Fuchs-Tarlovsky, 2013).

Exercise has a positive impact on CV risk factors (e.g., hypertension, high cholesterol and lipids, overweight and diabetes; Kirkham and Davis, 2015) and it has been hypothesized that aerobic exercise can reduce ROS production and restore calcium cycling, thus improving myocardial energetics (Scott et al., 2011). There is some evidence that physical exercise can be beneficial to cancer patients (Stefani et al., 2015). Preliminary studies showed a role for aerobic exercise in combating ANT- (Schermuly et al., 2005) and trastuzumab-induced CTX (Haykowsky et al., 2009). Further studies will be necessary to assess the effects of exercise on CTX caused by anticancer agents (Scott et al., 2013).

REDOX-RELATED BIOMARKERS OF CARDIOTOXICITY

One of the main obstacles that renders difficult the prevention of several types of CTX is their complex pathogenesis and lack of reliable biomarkers. Biomarkers ideally should be simple to measure, widely available, low-cost, and used in other pathological conditions. Rather than using single biomarkers, the complexity of CTX is likely to be captured by the association of two or more biomarkers or by modern high-throughout "omics" platform (Chen et al., 2012). At the moment, troponins (Oztop et al., 2004; Suter and Ewer, 2013; Zamorano et al., 2016), brain natriuretic peptide (BNP) and its N-terminal fragment (NT-proBNP), mainly released from cardiomyocytes may be used as biomarkers of CTX in clinical practice (Cardinale et al., 2015; Novo et al., 2016b).

In the setting of cardiac toxicity induced by redox alterations from anticancer drugs, most ROS/RNS are very unstable, with half-lives of 10^{-6}–10^{-9}s. Also more long-lasting ROS, such as H_2O_2, have a half-life of less than a millisecond (Garcia-Garcia et al., 2012). Hence, it is still difficult to assess ROS/RNS generation due to limitations that affect their detection. Therefore, there is a need to identify alternative biomarkers of oxidative/nitrosative CTX. The metabolomic identification of acetate and succinate can be used as a redox-biomarker (Andreadou et al., 2009). Decrease in NAD(P)H:quinone oxidoreductase 1 activity and increased ROS production by NAD(P)H oxidases have been proposed as early biomarkers of LV dysfunction due to ANTs (Novo et al., 2016b). An increase of IL-6 and its soluble receptor (sIL-6R), has been correlated with an early alteration in systolic function in patients treated with EPI (Dessí et al., 2011, 2013). Other potential redox-related biomarkers are high-sensitivity C-reactive protein (CRP), heart-type fatty acid-binding protein (H-FABP), and glycogen phosphorylase BB (GPBB), while some miRNAs that could be used in the assessment of acute coronary syndromes (Novo et al., 2016b) may also be helpful in early detection of CTX (Horacek et al., 2010; Horie et al., 2010; Wang et al., 2013).

CONCLUSIONS AND PERSPECTIVES

Novel anticancer drugs (e.g., targeted therapies and immune checkpoint inhibitors) have revolutioned the management of a wide spectrum of malignancies (Johnson et al., 2016; Menzies et al., 2017; Varricchi et al., 2017b). However, CTX caused by both conventional and novel antineoplastic drugs remains a critical issue (Tocchetti et al., 2013; Ghigo et al., 2016).

Chemotherapeutics such as doxorubicin are the prototype of drugs causing CTX (Ghigo et al., 2016). Targeted therapies, initially thought to be safer, can also be responsible of some degree of CTX. Moreover, there is increasing evidence that immune checkpoint inhibitors (i.e., mAbs blocking CTLA-4, PD-1, and PD-L1 on immune cells) can also produce a spectrum of immune-related adverse events, including CTX (Varricchi et al., 2017c,d). Importantly, certain drugs used to prevent cardiovascular complications can even contribute to cancer induction (De Caterina, 2015). Several strategies have been proposed to prevent CTX from antineoplastic agents. None of these is completely safe and satisfactory. This is, at least in part, due to the complexity of different types of CTX. Moreover, it is important to note that heart dysfunction can also manifest years after cancer therapy, making it difficult to evaluate preventive and treatment strategies. It is important to understand the biochemical and molecular mechanisms by which anticancer agents affect cardiomyocytes and immune cells for implementing optimal drug design.

Although oxidative and nitrosative stress elicited by chemotherapeutic agents can harm the heart, indiscriminate elimination of ROS and RNS by antioxidant drugs may not provide beneficial effect, and may even impair physiological cellular functions (Aon et al., 2010; Cortassa et al., 2014; Nickel et al., 2014; Münzel et al., 2015; Arcaro et al., 2016). Indeed, anti-oxidants have been shown to fight LV remodeling and ameliorate contractility in many HF experimental models. Nevertheless, when translated to the clinical arena, these therapeutic approaches did not lead to much benefit or even worsened mortality (Kirk and Paolocci, 2014; Arcaro et al., 2016), when the antioxidant effect was not coupled to other pharmaceutical and biological properties (Fonarow, 2009). Importantly, the site of generation of ROS can determine their biological effects on cardiomyocytes. Hence, more specific, targeted, and "compartmentalized" antioxidant strategies that blunt local ROS/RNS production might be more successful than broad indiscriminate approaches.

In conclusion, although in the last decade research implicating ROS/RNS in antineoplastic drug-induced CTX has greatly advanced, experimental studies and clinical trials are needed to close several gaps in our knowledge of molecular and clinical aspects of CTX in order to balance safety and efficacy of cancer therapy.

AUTHOR CONTRIBUTIONS

All authors listed have made a substantial, direct and intellectual contribution to the work, and approved it for publication.

FUNDING

The authors are supported by Regione Campania CISI-Lab, CRÈME Project and TIMING Project (GV and CT), the University of Cagliari (CC and GM), and MeccaSaric of the University of Turin (PasP).

ACKNOWLEDGMENTS

We would like to thank Prof. Gianni Marone for his invaluable intellectual inputs, and the Italian Society of Cardiovascular Research and the Working Group on Drug Cardiotoxicity and Cardioprotection of the Italian Society of Cardiology for having made possible the meeting of scientists who participated in the drafting of this manuscript. The authors thank Dr. Gjada Criscuolo for critical reading of the manuscript and Fabrizio Fiorbianco for the elaboration of the figures.

REFERENCES

Abd El-Aziz, M. A., Othman, A. I., Amer, M., and El-Missiry, M. A. (2001). Potential protective role of angiotensin-converting enzyme inhibitors captopril and enalapril against adriamycin-induced acute cardiac and hepatic toxicity in rats. *J. Appl. Toxicol.* 21, 469–473. doi: 10.1002/jat.782

Ades, F., Zardavas, D., Pinto, A. C., Criscitiello, C., Aftimos, P., and de Azambuja, E. (2014). Cardiotoxicity of systemic agents used in breast cancer. *Breast* 23, 317–328. doi: 10.1016/j.breast.2014.04.002

Albini, A., Pennesi, G., Donatelli, F., Cammarota, R., De Flora, S., and Noonan, D. M. (2010). Cardiotoxicity of anticancer drugs: the need for cardio-oncology and cardio-oncological prevention. *J. Natl. Cancer Inst.* 102, 14–25. doi: 10.1093/jnci/djp440

Alter, P., Herzum, M., Soufi, M., Schaefer, J. R., and Maisch, B. (2006). Cardiotoxicity of 5-fluorouracil. *Cardiovasc. Hematol. Agents Med. Chem.* 4, 1–5. doi: 10.2174/187152506775268785

Altieri, P., Murialdo, R., Barisione, C., Lazzarini, E., Garibaldi, S., Fabbi, P., et al. (2017). 5-fluorouracil causes endothelial cell senescence: potential protective role of glucagon-like peptide 1. *Br. J. Pharmacol.* 174, 3713–3726. doi: 10.1111/bph.13725

Andreadou, I., Papaefthimiou, M., Zira, A., Constantinou, M., Sigala, F., Skaltsounis, A. L., et al. (2009). Metabonomic identification of novel biomarkers in doxorubicin cardiotoxicity and protective effect of the natural antioxidant oleuropein. *NMR Biomed.* 22, 585–592. doi: 10.1002/nbm.1370

Anisimov, A., Alitalo, A., Korpisalo, P., Soronen, J., Kaijalainen, S., Leppänen, V. M., et al. (2009). Activated forms of VEGF-C and VEGF-D provide improved vascular function in skeletal muscle. *Circ. Res.* 104, 1302–1312. doi: 10.1161/CIRCRESAHA.109.197830

Aon, M. A., Cortassa, S., and O'Rourke, B. (2010). Redox-optimized ROS balance: a unifying hypothesis. *Biochim. Biophys. Acta* 1797, 865–877. doi: 10.1016/j.bbabio.2010.02.016

Aprile, G., Mazzer, M., Moroso, S., and Puglisi, F. (2009). Pharmacology and therapeutic efficacy of capecitabine: focus on breast and colorectal cancer. *Anticancer. Drugs* 20, 217–229. doi: 10.1097/CAD.0b013e3283293fd4

Arcaro, A., Pirozzi, F., Angelini, A., Chimenti, C., Crotti, L., Giordano, C., et al. (2016). Novel perspectives in redox biology and pathophysiology of failing myocytes: modulation of the intramyocardial redox milieu for therapeutic interventions-a review article from the working group of cardiac cell biology, italian society of cardiology. *Oxid. Med. Cell. Longev.* 2016:6353469. doi: 10.1155/2016/6353469

Armenian, S. H., Lacchetti, C., Barac, A., Carver, J., Constine, L. S., Denduluri, N., et al. (2017). Prevention and monitoring of cardiac dysfunction in survivors of adult cancers: american society of clinical oncology clinical practice guideline. *J. Clin. Oncol.* 35, 893–911. doi: 10.1200/JCO.2016.70.5400

Arnolda, L., McGrath, B., Cocks, M., Sumithran, E., and Johnston, C. (1985). Adriamycin cardiomyopathy in the rabbit: an animal model of low output cardiac failure with activation of vasoconstrictor mechanisms. *Cardiovasc. Res.* 19, 378–382. doi: 10.1093/cvr/19.6.378

Asanuma, H., Minamino, T., Sanada, S., Takashima, S., Ogita, H., Ogai, A., et al. (2004). Beta-adrenoceptor blocker carvedilol provides cardioprotection via an adenosine-dependent mechanism in ischemic canine hearts. *Circulation* 109, 2773–2779. doi: 10.1161/01.CIR.0000130917.12959.04

Baselga, J., Cortés, J., Kim, S. B., Im, S. A., Hegg, R., Im, Y. H., et al. (2012). Pertuzumab plus trastuzumab plus docetaxel for metastatic breast cancer. *N. Engl. J. Med.* 366, 109–119. doi: 10.1056/NEJMoa1113216

Belmonte, F., Das, S., Sysa-Shah, P., Sivakumaran, V., Stanley, B., Guo, X., et al. (2015). ErbB2 overexpression upregulates antioxidant enzymes, reduces basal levels of reactive oxygen species, and protects against doxorubicin cardiotoxicity. *Am. J. Physiol. Heart Circ. Physiol.* 309, H1271–H1280. doi: 10.1152/ajpheart.00517.2014

Biswas, S. K. (2016). Does the Interdependence between Oxidative Stress and Inflammation Explain the Antioxidant Paradox? *Oxid. Med. Cell. Longev.* 2016:5698931. doi: 10.1155/2016/5698931

Boekhout, A. H., Gietema, J. A., Milojkovic Kerklaan, B., van Werkhoven, E. D., Altena, R., Honkoop, A., et al. (2016). Angiotensin II-receptor inhibition with candesartan to prevent trastuzumab-related cardiotoxic effects in patients with early breast cancer: a randomized clinical trial. *JAMA Oncol.* 2, 1030–1037. doi: 10.1001/jamaoncol.2016.1726

Bosch, X., Rovira, M., Sitges, M., Doménech, A., Ortiz-Pérez, J. T., de Caralt, T. M., et al. (2013). Enalapril and carvedilol for preventing chemotherapy-induced left ventricular systolic dysfunction in patients with malignant hemopathies: the OVERCOME trial (preventiOn of left Ventricular dysfunction with Enalapril and caRvedilol in patients submitted to intensive ChemOtherapy for the treatment of Malignant hEmopathies). *J. Am. Coll. Cardiol.* 61, 2355–2362. doi: 10.1016/j.jacc.2013.02.072

Boucek, R. J. Jr., Steele, A., Miracle, A., and Atkinson, J. (2003). Effects of angiotensin-converting enzyme inhibitor on delayed-onset doxorubicin-induced cardiotoxicity. *Cardiovasc. Toxicol.* 3, 319–329. doi: 10.1385/CT:3:4:319

Bowles, E. J., Wellman, R., Feigelson, H. S., Onitilo, A. A., Freedman, A. N., Delate, T., et al. (2012). Risk of heart failure in breast cancer patients after anthracycline and trastuzumab treatment: a retrospective cohort study. *J. Natl. Cancer Inst.* 104, 1293–1305. doi: 10.1093/jnci/djs317

Brinda, B. J., Viganego, F., Vo, T., Dolan, D., and Fradley, M. G. (2016). Anti-VEGF-induced hypertension: a review of pathophysiology and treatment options. *Curr. Treat. Options Cardiovasc. Med.* 18, 33. doi: 10.1007/s11936-016-0452-z

Broeyer, F. J., Osanto, S., Suzuki, J., de Jongh, F., van Slooten, H., Tanis, B. C., et al. (2014). Evaluation of lecithinized human recombinant super oxide dismutase as cardioprotectant in anthracycline-treated breast cancer patients. *Br. J. Clin. Pharmacol.* 78, 950–960. doi: 10.1111/bcp.12429

Bronte, G., Bronte, E., Novo, G., Pernice, G., Lo Vullo, F., Musso, E., et al. (2015). Conquests and perspectives of cardio-oncology in the field of tumor angiogenesis-targeting tyrosine kinase inhibitor-based therapy. *Expert Opin. Drug Saf.* 14, 253–267. doi: 10.1517/14740338.2015.986092

Bry, M., Kivela, R., Holopainen, T., Anisimov, A., Tammela, T., Soronen, J., et al. (2010). Vascular endothelial growth factor-B acts as a coronary growth factor in transgenic rats without inducing angiogenesis, vascular leak, or inflammation. *Circulation* 122, 1725–1733. doi: 10.1161/CIRCULATIONAHA.110.957332

Cadeddu, C., Mercurio, V., Spallarossa, P., Nodari, S., Triggiani, M., Monte, I., et al. (2016). Preventing antiblastic drug-related cardiomyopathy: old and new therapeutic strategies. *J. Cardiovasc. Med. (Hagerstown)* 17(Suppl. 1), e64–e75. doi: 10.2459/JCM.0000000000000382

Cadeddu, C., Piras, A., Mantovani, G., Deidda, M., Dessì, M., Madeddu, C., et al. (2010). Protective effects of the angiotensin II receptor blocker telmisartan on epirubicin-induced inflammation, oxidative stress, and early ventricular impairment. *Am. Heart J.* 160, e481–e487. doi: 10.1016/j.ahj.2010.05.037

Cappetta, D., Esposito, G., Coppini, R., Piegari, E., Russo, R., Ciuffreda, L. P., et al. (2017). Effects of ranolazine in a model of doxorubicin-induced left ventricle diastolic dysfunction. *Br. J. Pharmacol.* 174, 3696–3712. doi: 10.1111/bph.13791

Cardinale, D., Colombo, A., Bacchiani, G., Tedeschi, I., Meroni, C. A., Veglia, F., et al. (2015). Early detection of anthracycline cardiotoxicity and improvement with heart failure therapy. *Circulation* 131, 1981–1988. doi: 10.1161/CIRCULATIONAHA.114.013777

Chen, R., Mias, G. I., Li-Pook-Than, J., Jiang, L., Lam, H. Y., Miriami, E., et al. (2012). Personal omics profiling reveals dynamic molecular and medical phenotypes. *Cell* 148, 1293–1307. doi: 10.1016/j.cell.2012.02.009

Cheng, H., and Force, T. (2010). Molecular mechanisms of cardiovascular toxicity of targeted cancer therapeutics. *Circ. Res.* 106, 21–34. doi: 10.1161/CIRCRESAHA.109.206920

Chintalgattu, V., Rees, M. L., Culver, J. C., Goel, A., Jiffar, T., Zhang, J., et al. (2013). Coronary microvascular pericytes are the cellular target of sunitinib malate-induced cardiotoxicity. *Sci. Transl. Med.* 5:187ra169. doi: 10.1126/scitranslmed.3005066

Chotenimitkhun, R., D'Agostino, R. Jr., Lawrence, J. A., Hamilton, C. A., Jordan, J. H., Vasu, S., et al. (2015). Chronic statin administration may attenuate early anthracycline-associated declines in left ventricular ejection function. *Can. J. Cardiol.* 31, 302–307. doi: 10.1016/j.cjca.2014.11.020

Chu, T. F., Rupnick, M. A., Kerkela, R., Dallabrida, S. M., Zurakowski, D., Nguyen, L., et al. (2007). Cardiotoxicity associated with tyrosine kinase inhibitor sunitinib. *Lancet* 370, 2011–2019. doi: 10.1016/S0140-6736(07)61865-0

Cianci, G., Morelli, M. F., Cannita, K., Morese, R., Ricevuto, E., Di Rocco, Z. C., et al. (2003). Prophylactic options in patients with 5-fluorouracil-associated cardiotoxicity. *Br. J. Cancer* 88, 1507–1509. doi: 10.1038/sj.bjc.6600967

Coppini, R., Ferrantini, C., Yao, L., Fan, P., Del Lungo, M., Stillitano, F., et al. (2013). Late sodium current inhibition reverses electromechanical dysfunction in human hypertrophic cardiomyopathy. *Circulation* 127, 575–584. doi: 10.1161/CIRCULATIONAHA.112.134932

Coppini, R., Mazzoni, L., Ferrantini, C., Gentile, F., Pioner, J. M., Laurino, A., et al. (2017). Ranolazine prevents phenotype development in a mouse model of hypertrophic cardiomyopathy. *Circ. Heart Fail.* 10. doi: 10.1161/CIRCHEARTFAILURE.116.003565

Cortassa, S., O'Rourke, B., and Aon, M. A. (2014). Redox-optimized ROS balance and the relationship between mitochondrial respiration and ROS. *Biochim. Biophys. Acta* 1837, 287–295. doi: 10.1016/j.bbabio.2013.11.007

Crone, S. A., Zhao, Y. Y., Fan, L., Gu, Y., Minamisawa, S., Liu, Y., et al. (2002). ErbB2 is essential in the prevention of dilated cardiomyopathy. *Nat. Med.* 8, 459–465. doi: 10.1038/nm0502-459

Curigliano, G., Cardinale, D., Suter, T., Plataniotis, G., de Azambuja, E., Sandri, M. T., et al. (2012). Cardiovascular toxicity induced by chemotherapy, targeted agents and radiotherapy: ESMO Clinical Practice Guidelines. *Ann Oncol.* 23(Suppl. 7), vii155–vii166. doi: 10.1093/annonc/mds293

De Caterina, R. (2015). Cancer after intense and prolonged antiplatelet therapies–fact or fiction? *Thromb. Haemost.* 114, 1100–1103. doi: 10.1160/TH15-11-0842

De Keulenaer, G. W., Doggen, K., and Lemmens, K. (2010). The vulnerability of the heart as a pluricellular paracrine organ: lessons from unexpected triggers of heart failure in targeted ErbB2 anticancer therapy. *Circ. Res.* 106, 35–46. doi: 10.1161/CIRCRESAHA.109.205906

de Korte, M. A., de Vries, E. G., Lub-de Hooge, M. N., Jager, P. L., Gietema, J. A., van der Graaf, W. T. et al. (2007). 111Indium-trastuzumab visualises myocardial human epidermal growth factor receptor 2 expression shortly after anthracycline treatment but not during heart failure: a clue to uncover the mechanisms of trastuzumab-related cardiotoxicity. *Eur. J. Cancer* 43, 2046–2051. doi: 10.1016/j.ejca.2007.06.024

Del Río, L. A. (2015). ROS and RNS in plant physiology: an overview. *J. Exp. Bot.* 66, 2827–2837. doi: 10.1093/jxb/erv099

de Nigris, F., Rienzo, M., Schiano, C., Fiorito, C., Casamassimi, A., and Napoli, C. (2008). Prominent cardioprotective effects of third generation beta blocker nebivolol against anthracycline-induced cardiotoxicity using the model of isolated perfused rat heart. *Eur. J. Cancer* 44, 334–340. doi: 10.1016/j.ejca.2007.12.010

Dessí, M., Madeddu, C., Piras, A., Cadeddu, C., Antoni, G., Mercuro, G., et al. (2013). Long-term, up to 18 months, protective effects of the angiotensin II receptor blocker telmisartan on Epirubin-induced inflammation and oxidative stress assessed by serial strain rate. *Springerplus* 2:198. doi: 10.1186/2193-1801-2-198

Dessí, M., Piras, A., Madeddu, C., Cadeddu, C., Deidda, M., Massa, E., et al. (2011). Long-term protective effects of the angiotensin receptor blocker telmisartan on epirubicin-induced inflammation, oxidative stress and myocardial dysfunction. *Exp. Ther. Med.* 2, 1003–1009. doi: 10.3892/etm.2011.305

Doggen, K., Ray, L., Mathieu, M., Mc Entee, K., Lemmens, K., and De Keulenaer, G. W. (2009). Ventricular ErbB2/ErbB4 activation and downstream signaling in pacing-induced heart failure. *J. Mol. Cell. Cardiol.* 46, 33–38. doi: 10.1016/j.yjmcc.2008.10.010

Dragoni, S., Laforenza, U., Bonetti, E., Lodola, F., Bottino, C., Berra-Romani, R., et al. (2011). Vascular endothelial growth factor stimulates endothelial colony forming cells proliferation and tubulogenesis by inducing oscillations in intracellular Ca^{2+} concentration. *Stem Cells.* 29, 1898–1907. doi: 10.1002/stem.734

D'Uva, G., Aharonov, A., Lauriola, M., Kain, D., Yahalom-Ronen, Y., Carvalho, S., et al. (2015). ERBB2 triggers mammalian heart regeneration by promoting cardiomyocyte dedifferentiation and proliferation. *Nat. Cell Biol.* 17, 627–638. doi: 10.1038/ncb3149

Egea, J., Fabregat, I., Frapart, Y. M., Ghezzi, P., Görlach, A., Kietzmann, T., et al. (2017). European contribution to the study of ROS: a summary of the findings and prospects for the future from the COST action BM1203 (EU-ROS). *Redox Biol.* 13, 94–162. doi: 10.1016/j.redox.2017.05.007

Eschenhagen, T., Force, T., Ewer, M. S., de Keulenaer, G. W., Suter, T. M., Anker, S. D., et al. (2011). Cardiovascular side effects of cancer therapies: a position statement from the heart failure association of the european society of cardiology. *Eur. J. Heart Fail.* 13, 1–10. doi: 10.1093/eurjhf/hfq213

Ewer, M. S., and Ewer, S. M. (2010). Troponin I provides insight into cardiotoxicity and the anthracycline-trastuzumab interaction. *J. Clin. Oncol.* 28, 3901–3904. doi: 10.1200/JCO.2010.30.6274

Ewer, M. S., and Lenihan, D. J. (2008). Left ventricular ejection fraction and cardiotoxicity: is our ear really to the ground? *J. Clin. Oncol.* 26, 1201–1203. doi: 10.1200/JCO.2007.14.8742

Ewer, M. S., and Lippman, S. M. (2005). Type II chemotherapy-related cardiac dysfunction: time to recognize a new entity. *J. Clin. Oncol.* 23, 2900–2902. doi: 10.1200/JCO.2005.05.827

Ewer, M. S., Vooletich, M. T., Durand, J. B., Woods, M. L., Davis, J. R., Valero, V., et al. (2005). Reversibility of trastuzumab-related cardiotoxicity: new insights based on clinical course and response to medical treatment. *J. Clin. Oncol.* 23, 7820–7826. doi: 10.1200/JCO.2005.13.300

Ferroni, P., Della-Morte, D., Palmirotta, R., McClendon, M., Testa, G., Abete, P., et al. (2011). Platinum-based compounds and risk for cardiovascular toxicity in the elderly: role of the antioxidants in chemoprevention. *Rejuvenat. Res.* 14, 293–308. doi: 10.1089/rej.2010.1141

Fisher, P. W., Salloum, F., Das, A., Hyder, H., and Kukreja, R. C. (2005). Phosphodiesterase-5 inhibition with sildenafil attenuates cardiomyocyte apoptosis and left ventricular dysfunction in a chronic model of doxorubicin cardiotoxicity. *Circulation* 111, 1601–1610. doi: 10.1161/01.CIR.0000160359.49478.C2

Fogli, S., Nieri, P., and Breschi, M. C. (2004). The role of nitric oxide in anthracycline toxicity and prospects for pharmacologic prevention of cardiac damage. *FASEB J.* 18, 664–675. doi: 10.1096/fj.03-0724rev

Folkman, J. (2007). Angiogenesis: an organizing principle for drug discovery? *Nat. Rev. Drug Discov.* 6, 273–286. doi: 10.1038/nrd2115

Fonarow, G. C. (2009). Role of carvedilol controlled-release in cardiovascular disease. *Expert Rev. Cardiovasc. Ther.* 7, 483–498. doi: 10.1586/erc.09.15

Force, T., Krause, D. S., and Van Etten, R. A. (2007). Molecular mechanisms of cardiotoxicity of tyrosine kinase inhibition. *Nat. Rev. Cancer* 7, 332–344. doi: 10.1038/nrc2106

Fu, M., Matoba, M., Liang, Q. M., Sjögren, K. G., and Hjalmarson, A. (1994). Properties of G-protein modulated receptor-adenylyl cyclase system in myocardium of spontaneously hypertensive rats treated with adriamycin. *Int. J. Cardiol.* 44, 9–18. doi: 10.1016/0167-5273(94)90061-2

Fuchs-Tarlovsky, V. (2013). Role of antioxidants in cancer therapy. *Nutrition* 29, 15–21. doi: 10.1016/j.nut.2012.02.014

Gabrielson, K., Bedja, D., Pin, S., Tsao, A., Gama, L., Yuan, B., et al. (2007). Heat shock protein 90 and ErbB2 in the cardiac response to doxorubicin injury. *Cancer Res.* 67, 1436–1441. doi: 10.1158/0008-5472.CAN-06-3721

Galdiero, M. R., Varricchi, G., and Marone, G. (2016). The immune network in thyroid cancer. *Oncoimmunology* 5:e1168556. doi: 10.1080/2162402X.2016.1168556

Galindo, C. L., Kasasbeh, E., Murphy, A., Ryzhov, S., Lenihan, S., Ahmad, F. A., et al. (2014a). Anti-remodeling and anti-fibrotic effects of the neuregulin-1β glial growth factor 2 in a large animal model of heart failure. *J. Am. Heart Assoc.* 3:e000773. doi: 10.1161/JAHA.113.000773

Galindo, C. L., Ryzhov, S., and Sawyer, D. B. (2014b). Neuregulin as a heart failure therapy and mediator of reverse remodeling. *Curr. Heart Fail. Rep.* 11, 40–49. doi: 10.1007/s11897-013-0176-2

Gammella, E., Maccarinelli, F., Buratti, P., Recalcati, S., and Cairo, G. (2014). The role of iron in anthracycline cardiotoxicity. *Front. Pharmacol.* 5:25. doi: 10.3389/fphar.2014.00025

Gao, R., Zhang, J., Cheng, L., Wu, X., Dong, W., Yang, X., et al. (2010). A Phase II, randomized, double-blind, multicenter, based on standard therapy, placebo-controlled study of the efficacy and safety of recombinant human neuregulin-1 in patients with chronic heart failure. *J. Am. Coll. Cardiol.* 55, 1907–1914. doi: 10.1016/j.jacc.2009.12.044

Garcia-Garcia, A., Rodriguez-Rocha, H., Madayiputhiya, N., Pappa, A., Panayiotidis, M. I., and Franco, R. (2012). Biomarkers of protein oxidation in human disease. *Curr. Mol. Med.* 12, 681–697. doi: 10.2174/156652412800792543

Ghigo, A., Li, M., and Hirsch, E. (2016). New signal transduction paradigms in anthracycline-induced cardiotoxicity. *Biochim. Biophys. Acta* 1863, 1916–1925. doi: 10.1016/j.bbamcr.2016.01.021

Gianni, L., Pienkowski, T., Im, Y. H., Roman, L., Tseng, L. M., Liu, M. C., et al. (2012). Efficacy and safety of neoadjuvant pertuzumab and trastuzumab in women with locally advanced, inflammatory, or early HER2-positive breast cancer (NeoSphere): a randomised multicentre, open-label, phase 2 trial. *Lancet Oncol.* 13, 25–32. doi: 10.1016/S1470-2045(11)70336-9

Gonzalvez, F., and Gottlieb, E. (2007). Cardiolipin: setting the beat of apoptosis. *Apoptosis* 12, 877–885. doi: 10.1007/s10495-007-0718-8

Goormaghtigh, E., Huart, P., Praet, M., Brasseur, R., and Ruysschaert, J. M. (1990). Structure of the adriamycin-cardiolipin complex. Role in mitochondrial toxicity. *Biophys. Chem.* 35, 247–257. doi: 10.1016/0301-4622(90)80012-V

Gordon, L. I., Burke, M. A., Singh, A. T., Prachand, S., Lieberman, E. D., Sun, L., et al. (2009). Blockade of the erbB2 receptor induces cardiomyocyte death through mitochondrial and reactive oxygen species-dependent pathways. *J. Biol. Chem.* 284, 2080–2087. doi: 10.1074/jbc.M804570200

Goss, G. D., Arnold, A., Shepherd, F. A., Dediu, M., Ciuleanu, T. E., Fenton, D., et al. (2010). Randomized, double-blind trial of carboplatin and paclitaxel with either daily oral cediranib or placebo in advanced non-small-cell lung cancer: NCIC clinical trials group BR24 study. *J. Clin. Oncol.* 28, 49–55. doi: 10.1200/JCO.2009.22.9427

Gressett, S. M., and Shah, S. R. (2009). Intricacies of bevacizumab-induced toxicities and their management. *Ann. Pharmacother.* 43, 490–501. doi: 10.1345/aph.1L426

Gulati, G., Heck, S. L., Ree, A. H., Hoffmann, P., Schulz-Menger, J., Fagerland, M. W., et al. (2016). Prevention of cardiac dysfunction during adjuvant breast cancer therapy (PRADA): a 2 x 2 factorial, randomized, placebo-controlled, double-blind clinical trial of candesartan and metoprolol. *Eur. Heart J.* 37, 1671–1680. doi: 10.1093/eurheartj/ehw022

Gupta, A., Akki, A., Wang, Y., Leppo, M. K., Chacko, V. P., Foster, D. B., et al. (2012). Creatine kinase-mediated improvement of function in failing mouse hearts provides causal evidence the failing heart is energy starved. *J. Clin. Invest.* 122, 291–302. doi: 10.1172/JCI57426

Gupta, A., Rohlfsen, C., Leppo, M. K., Chacko, V. P., Wang, Y., Steenbergen, C., et al. (2013). Creatine kinase-overexpression improves myocardial energetics, contractile dysfunction and survival in murine doxorubicin cardiotoxicity. *PLoS ONE* 8:e74675. doi: 10.1371/journal.pone.0074675

Hahn, V. S., Lenihan, D. J., and Ky, B. (2014). Cancer therapy-induced cardiotoxicity: basic mechanisms and potential cardioprotective therapies. *J. Am. Heart Assoc.* 3:e000665. doi: 10.1161/JAHA.113.000665

Hasinoff, B. B., and Patel, D. (2010). The lack of target specificity of small molecule anticancer kinase inhibitors is correlated with their ability to damage myocytes *in vitro*. *Toxicol. Appl. Pharmacol.* 249, 132–139. doi: 10.1016/j.taap.2010.08.026

Haykowsky, M. J., Mackey, J. R., Thompson, R. B., Jones, L. W., and Paterson, D. I. (2009). Adjuvant trastuzumab induces ventricular remodeling despite aerobic exercise training. *Clin. Cancer Res.* 15, 4963–4967. doi: 10.1158/1078-0432.CCR-09-0628

Henninger, C., Huelsenbeck, S., Wenzel, P., Brand, M., Huelsenbeck, J., Schad, A., et al. (2015). Chronic heart damage following doxorubicin treatment is alleviated by lovastatin. *Pharmacol. Res.* 91, 47–56. doi: 10.1016/j.phrs.2014.11.003

Horacek, J. M., Vasatova, M., Tichy, M., Pudil, R., Jebavy, L., and Maly, J. (2010). The use of cardiac biomarkers in detection of cardiotoxicity associated with conventional and high-dose chemotherapy for acute leukemia. *Exp. Oncol.* 32, 97–99.

Horie, T., Ono, K., Nishi, H., Nagao, K., Kinoshita, M., Watanabe, S., et al. (2010). Acute doxorubicin cardiotoxicity is associated with miR-146a-induced inhibition of the neuregulin-ErbB pathway. *Cardiovasc. Res.* 87, 656–664. doi: 10.1093/cvr/cvq148

Huang, C., Zhang, X., Ramil, J. M., Rikka, S., Kim, L., Lee, Y., et al. (2010). Juvenile exposure to anthracyclines impairs cardiac progenitor cell function and vascularization resulting in greater susceptibility to stress-induced myocardial injury in adult mice. *Circulation* 121, 675–683. doi: 10.1161/CIRCULATIONAHA.109.902221

Huelsenbeck, J., Henninger, C., Schad, A., Lackner, K. J., Kaina, B., and Fritz, G. (2011). Inhibition of Rac1 signaling by lovastatin protects against anthracycline-induced cardiac toxicity. *Cell Death Dis.* 2:e190. doi: 10.1038/cddis.2011.65

Hurwitz, H., Fehrenbacher, L., Novotny, W., Cartwright, T., Hainsworth, J., Heim, W., et al. (2004). Bevacizumab plus irinotecan, fluorouracil, and leucovorin for metastatic colorectal cancer. *N. Engl. J. Med.* 350, 2335–2342. doi: 10.1056/NEJMoa032691

Hutson, T. E., Lesovoy, V., Al-Shukri, S., Stus, V. P., Lipatov, O. N., Bair, A. H., et al. (2013). Axitinib versus sorafenib as first-line therapy in patients with metastatic renal-cell carcinoma: a randomised open-label phase 3 trial. *Lancet Oncol.* 14, 1287–1294. doi: 10.1016/S1470-2045(13)70465-0

Ichikawa, Y., Ghanefar, M., Bayeva, M., Wu, R., Khechaduri, A., Naga Prasad, S. V., et al. (2014). Cardiotoxicity of doxorubicin is mediated through mitochondrial iron accumulation. *J. Clin. Invest.* 124, 617–630. doi: 10.1172/JCI72931

Iqbal, M., Dubey, K., Anwer, T., Ashish, A., and Pillai, K. K. (2008). Protective effects of telmisartan against acute doxorubicin-induced cardiotoxicity in rats. *Pharmacol. Rep.* 60, 382–390.

Jabbour, A., Hayward, C. S., Keogh, A. M., Kotlyar, E., McCrohon, J. A., England, J. F., et al. (2011). Parenteral administration of recombinant human neuregulin-1 to patients with stable chronic heart failure produces favourable acute and chronic haemodynamic responses. *Eur. J. Heart Fail.* 13, 83–92. doi: 10.1093/eurjhf/hfq152

Jemal, A., Bray, F., Center, M. M., Ferlay, J., Ward, E., and Forman, D. (2011). Global cancer statistics. *CA Cancer J. Clin.* 61, 69–90. doi: 10.3322/caac.20107

Jensen, S. A., and Sorensen, J. B. (2006). Risk factors and prevention of cardiotoxicity induced by 5-fluorouracil or capecitabine. *Cancer Chemother. Pharmacol.* 58, 487–493. doi: 10.1007/s00280-005-0178-1

Jensen, S. A., and Sørensen, J. B. (2012). 5-fluorouracil-based therapy induces endovascular injury having potential significance to development of clinically overt cardiotoxicity. *Cancer Chemother. Pharmacol.* 69, 57–64. doi: 10.1007/s00280-011-1669-x

Jin, Z., Zhang, J., Zhi, H., Hong, B., Zhang, S., Guo, H., et al. (2013). Beneficial effects of tadalafil on left ventricular dysfunction in doxorubicin-induced cardiomyopathy. *J. Cardiol.* 62, 110–116. doi: 10.1016/j.jjcc.2013.03.018

Johnson, D. B., Balko, J. M., Compton, M. L., Chalkias, S., Gorham, J., Xu, Y., et al. (2016). Fulminant Myocarditis with Combination Immune Checkpoint Blockade. *N. Engl. J. Med.* 375, 1749–1755. doi: 10.1056/NEJMoa1609214

Kalam, K., and Marwick, T. H. (2013). Role of cardioprotective therapy for prevention of cardiotoxicity with chemotherapy: a systematic review and meta-analysis. *Eur. J. Cancer* 49, 2900–2909. doi: 10.1016/j.ejca.2013.04.030

Kalay, N., Basar, E., Ozdogru, I., Er, O., Cetinkaya, Y., Dogan, A., et al. (2006). Protective effects of carvedilol against anthracycline-induced cardiomyopathy. *J. Am. Coll. Cardiol.* 48, 2258–2262. doi: 10.1016/j.jacc.2006.07.052

Kaya, M. G., Ozkan, M., Gunebakmaz, O., Akkaya, H., Kaya, E. G., Akpek, M., et al. (2013). Protective effects of nebivolol against anthracycline-induced cardiomyopathy: a randomized control study. *Int. J. Cardiol.* 167, 2306–2310. doi: 10.1016/j.ijcard.2012.06.023

Kerkela, R., Woulfe, K. C., Durand, J. B., Vagnozzi, R., Kramer, D., Chu, T. F., et al. (2009). Sunitinib-induced cardiotoxicity is mediated by off-target inhibition of AMP-activated protein kinase. *Clin. Transl. Sci.* 2, 15–25. doi: 10.1111/j.1752-8062.2008.00090.x

Khakoo, A. Y., Kassiotis, C. M., Tannir, N., Plana, J. C., Halushka, M., Bickford, C., et al. (2008). Heart failure associated with sunitinib malate: a multitargeted receptor tyrosine kinase inhibitor. *Cancer.* 112, 2500–2508. doi: 10.1002/cncr.23460

Khan, M. F., Gottesman, S., Boyella, R., and Juneman, E. (2014). Gemcitabine-induced cardiomyopathy: a case report and review of the literature. *J. Med. Case Rep.* 8:220. doi: 10.1186/1752-1947-8-220

Kirk, J. A., and Paolocci, N. (2014). New redox-related arrows in the arsenal of cardiac disease treatment. *Antioxid. Redox Signal.* 21, 1945–1948. doi: 10.1089/ars.2014.6124

Kirkham, A. A., and Davis, M. K. (2015). Exercise prevention of Cardiovascular disease in breast cancer survivors. *J. Oncol.* 2015:917606. doi: 10.1155/2015/917606

Kivelä, R., Bry, M., Robciuc, M. R., Räsänen, M., Taavitsainen, M., Silvola, J. M., et al. (2014). VEGF-B-induced vascular growth leads to metabolic reprogramming and ischemia resistance in the heart. *EMBO Mol. Med.* 6, 307–321. doi: 10.1002/emmm.201303147

Koca, D., Salman, T., Unek, I. T., Oztop, I., Ellidokuz, H., Eren, M., et al. (2011). Clinical and electrocardiography changes in patients treated with capecitabine. *Chemotherapy* 57, 381–387. doi: 10.1159/000331645

Kohlhaas, M., Liu, T., Knopp, A., Zeller, T., Ong, M. F., Böhm, M., et al. (2010). Elevated cytosolic Na^+ increases mitochondrial formation of reactive oxygen species in failing cardiac myocytes. *Circulation.* 121, 1606–1613. doi: 10.1161/CIRCULATIONAHA.109.914911

Koka, S., Das, A., Zhu, S. G., Durrant, D., Xi, L., and Kukreja, R. C. (2010). Long-acting phosphodiesterase-5 inhibitor tadalafil attenuates doxorubicin-induced cardiomyopathy without interfering with chemotherapeutic effect. *J. Pharmacol. Exp. Ther.* 334, 1023–1030. doi: 10.1124/jpet.110.170191

Kosmas, C., Kallistratos, M. S., Kopterides, P., Syrios, J., Skopelitis, H., Mylonakis, N., et al. (2008). Cardiotoxicity of fluoropyrimidines in different schedules of administration: a prospective study. *J. Cancer Res. Clin. Oncol.* 134, 75–82. doi: 10.1007/s00432-007-0250-9

Ku, D. D., Zaleski, J. K., Liu, S., and Brock, T. A. (1993). Vascular endothelial growth factor induces EDRF-dependent relaxation in coronary arteries. *Am. J. Physiol.* 265, H586–H592. doi: 10.1152/ajpheart.1993.265.2.H586

Ky, B., Vejpongsa, P., Yeh, E. T., Force, T., and Moslehi, J. J. (2013). Emerging paradigms in cardiomyopathies associated with cancer therapies. *Circ. Res.* 113, 754–764. doi: 10.1161/CIRCRESAHA.113.300218

Lala, P. K., and Chakraborty, C. (2001). Role of nitric oxide in carcinogenesis and tumour progression. *Lancet Oncol.* 2, 149–156. doi: 10.1016/S1470-2045(00)00256-4

Lamberti, M., Porto, S., Zappavigna, S., Addeo, E., Marra, M., Miraglia, N., et al. (2014). A mechanistic study on the cardiotoxicity of 5-fluorouracil *in vitro* and clinical and occupational perspectives. *Toxicol. Lett.* 227, 151–156. doi: 10.1016/j.toxlet.2014.03.018

Lassègue, B., and Griendling, K. K. (2010). NADPH oxidases: functions and pathologies in the vasculature. *Arterioscler. Thromb. Vasc. Biol.* 30, 653–661. doi: 10.1161/ATVBAHA.108.181610

Lemmens, K., Fransen, P., Sys, S. U., Brutsaert, D. L., and De Keulenaer, G. W. (2004). Neuregulin-1 induces a negative inotropic effect in cardiac muscle: role of nitric oxide synthase. *Circulation* 109, 324–326. doi: 10.1161/01.CIR.0000114521.88547.5E

Lencová-Popelová, O., Jirkovský, E., Jansová, H., Jirkovská-Vavrová, A., Vostatková-Tichotová, L., Mazurová, Y., et al. (2016). Cardioprotective effects of inorganic nitrate/nitrite in chronic anthracycline cardiotoxicity: comparison with dexrazoxane. *J. Mol. Cell. Cardiol.* 91, 92–103. doi: 10.1016/j.yjmcc.2015.12.021

Lestuzzi, C., Tartuferi, L., and Corona, G. (2011). Capecitabine (and 5 fluorouracil) cardiotoxicity. Metabolic considerations. *Breast J.* 17, 564–565. doi: 10.1111/j.1524-4741.2011.01120.x

Lestuzzi, C., Vaccher, E., Talamini, R., Lleshi, A., Meneguzzo, N., Viel, E., et al. (2014). Effort myocardial ischemia during chemotherapy with 5-fluorouracil: an underestimated risk. *Ann. Oncol.* 25, 1059–1064. doi: 10.1093/annonc/mdu055

Lévy, B. I. (2006). Microvascular plasticity and experimental heart failure. *Hypertension* 47, 827–829. doi: 10.1161/01.HYP.0000215283.53943.39

Li, B., Zheng, Z., Wei, Y., Wang, M., Peng, J., Kang, T., et al. (2011). Therapeutic effects of neuregulin-1 in diabetic cardiomyopathy rats. *Cardiovasc. Diabetol.* 10:69. doi: 10.1186/1475-2840-10-69

Li, T., and Singal, P. K. (2000). Adriamycin-induced early changes in myocardial antioxidant enzymes and their modulation by probucol. *Circulation* 102, 2105–2110. doi: 10.1161/01.CIR.102.17.2105

Lim, S. L., Lam, C. S., Segers, V. F., Brutsaert, D. L., and De Keulenaer, G. W. (2015). Cardiac endothelium-myocyte interaction: clinical opportunities for new heart failure therapies regardless of ejection fraction. *Eur. Heart J.* 36, 2050–2060. doi: 10.1093/eurheartj/ehv132

Lipshultz, S. E., Miller, T. L., Lipsitz, S. R., Neuberg, D. S., Dahlberg, S. E., Colan, S. D., et al. (2012). Continuous versus bolus infusion of doxorubicin in children with all: long-term cardiac outcomes. *Pediatrics* 130, 1003–1011. doi: 10.1542/peds.2012-0727

Liu, X., Gu, X., Li, Z., Li, X., Li, H., Chang, J., et al. (2006). Neuregulin-1/erbB-activation improves cardiac function and survival in models of ischemic, dilated, and viral cardiomyopathy. *J. Am. Coll. Cardiol.* 48, 1438–1447. doi: 10.1016/j.jacc.2006.05.057

Loffredo, S., Bova, M., Suffritti, C., Borriello, F., Zanichelli, A., Petraroli, A., et al. (2016). Elevated plasma levels of vascular permeability factors in C1 inhibitor-deficient hereditary angioedema. *Allergy* 71, 989–996. doi: 10.1111/all.12862

Lyu, Y. L., Kerrigan, J. E., Lin, C. P., Azarova, A. M., Tsai, Y. C., Ban, Y., et al. (2007). Topoisomerase IIbeta mediated DNA double-strand breaks: implications in doxorubicin cardiotoxicity and prevention by dexrazoxane. *Cancer Res.* 67, 8839–8846. doi: 10.1158/0008-5472.CAN-07-1649

Ma, Y., Zhang, X., Bao, H., Mi, S., Cai, W., Yan, H., et al. (2012). Toll-like receptor (TLR) 2 and TLR4 differentially regulate doxorubicin induced cardiomyopathy in mice. *PLoS ONE* 7:e40763. doi: 10.1371/journal.pone.0040763

Madonna, R., Cadeddu, C., Deidda, M., Giricz, Z., Madeddu, C., Mele, D., et al. (2015a). Cardioprotection by gene therapy: a review paper on behalf of the working group on drug cardiotoxicity and cardioprotection of the Italian Society of Cardiology. *Int. J. Cardiol.* 191, 203–210. doi: 10.1016/j.ijcard.2015.04.232

Madonna, R., Cadeddu, C., Deidda, M., Mele, D., Monte, I., Novo, G., et al. (2015b). Improving the preclinical models for the study of chemotherapy-induced cardiotoxicity: a Position Paper of the Italian Working Group on Drug Cardiotoxicity and Cardioprotection. *Heart Fail. Rev.* 20, 621–631. doi: 10.1007/s10741-015-9497-4

Maitland, M. L., Bakris, G. L., Black, H. R., Chen, H. X., Durand, J. B., Elliott, W. J., et al. (2010). Initial assessment, surveillance, and management of blood pressure in patients receiving vascular endothelial growth factor signaling pathway inhibitors. *J. Natl. Cancer Inst.* 102, 596–604. doi: 10.1093/jnci/djq091

Marone, G., and Granata, F. (2014). Angiogenesis, lymphangiogenesis and clinical implications. Preface. *Chem. Immunol. Allergy* 99, XI–XII. doi: 10.1159/000352074

Martin, E., Thougaard, A. V., Grauslund, M., Jensen, P. B., Bjorkling, F., Hasinoff, B. B., et al. (2009). Evaluation of the topoisomerase II-inactive bisdioxopiperazine ICRF-161 as a protectant against doxorubicin-induced cardiomyopathy. *Toxicology* 255, 72–79. doi: 10.1016/j.tox.2008.10.011

Maslov, M. Y., Chacko, V. P., Hirsch, G. A., Akki, A., Leppo, M. K., Steenbergen, C., et al. (2010). Reduced *in vivo* high-energy phosphates precede adriamycin-induced cardiac dysfunction. *Am. J. Physiol. Heart Circ. Physiol.* 299, H332–337. doi: 10.1152/ajpheart.00727.2009

Matsui, H., Morishima, I., Numaguchi, Y., Toki, Y., Okumura, K., and Hayakawa, T. (1999). Protective effects of carvedilol against doxorubicin-induced cardiomyopathy in rats. *Life Sci.* 65, 1265–1274. doi: 10.1016/S0024-3205(99)00362-8

Mele, D., Nardozza, M., Spallarossa, P., Frassoldati, A., Tocchetti, C. G., Cadeddu, C., et al. (2016a). Current views on anthracycline cardiotoxicity. *Heart Fail. Rev.* 21, 621–634. doi: 10.1007/s10741-016-9564-5

Mele, D., Tocchetti, C. G., Pagliaro, P., Madonna, R., Novo, G., Pepe, A., et al. (2016b). Pathophysiology of anthracycline cardiotoxicity. *J Cardiovasc Med (Hagerstown).* 17(Suppl. 1), e3–e11. doi: 10.2459/JCM.0000000000000378

Menna, P., Paz, O. G., Chello, M., Covino, E., Salvatorelli, E., and Minotti, G. (2012). Anthracycline cardiotoxicity. *Expert Opin. Drug Saf.* 11(Suppl. 1), S21–S36. doi: 10.1517/14740338.2011.589834

Menna, P., Salvatorelli, E., and Minotti, G. (2008). Cardiotoxicity of antitumor drugs. *Chem. Res. Toxicol.* 21, 978–989. doi: 10.1021/tx800002r

Menzies, A. M., Johnson, D. B., Ramanujam, S., Atkinson, V. G., Wong, A. N. M., Park, J. J., et al. (2017). Anti-PD-1 therapy in patients with advanced melanoma and preexisting autoimmune disorders or major toxicity with ipilimumab. *Ann. Oncol.* 28, 368–376. doi: 10.1093/annonc/mdw443

Mercurio, V., Pirozzi, F., Lazzarini, E., Marone, G., Rizzo, P., Agnetti, G., et al. (2016). Models of heart failure based on the cardiotoxicity of anticancer drugs. *J. Card. Fail.* 22, 449–458. doi: 10.1016/j.cardfail.2016.04.008

Mikhed, Y., Görlach, A., Knaus, U. G., and Daiber, A. (2015). Redox regulation of genome stability by effects on gene expression, epigenetic pathways and DNA damage/repair. *Redox Biol.* 5, 275–289. doi: 10.1016/j.redox.2015.05.008

Miller, K. D., Chap, L. I., Holmes, F. A., Cobleigh, M. A., Marcom, P. K., Fehrenbacher, L., et al. (2005). Randomized phase III trial of capecitabine compared with bevacizumab plus capecitabine in patients with previously treated metastatic breast cancer. *J. Clin. Oncol.* 23, 792–799. doi: 10.1200/JCO.2005.05.098

Minotti, G. (2013). Pharmacology at work for cardio-oncology: ranolazine to treat early cardiotoxicity induced by antitumor drugs. *J. Pharmacol. Exp. Ther.* 346, 343–349. doi: 10.1124/jpet.113.204057

Minotti, G., Menna, P., Salvatorelli, E., Cairo, G., and Gianni, L. (2004). Anthracyclines: molecular advances and pharmacologic developments in antitumor activity and cardiotoxicity. *Pharmacol. Rev.* 56, 185–229. doi: 10.1124/pr.56.2.6

Minotti, G., Salvatorelli, E., and Menna, P. (2010). Pharmacological foundations of cardio-oncology. *J. Pharmacol. Exp. Ther.* 334, 2–8. doi: 10.1124/jpet.110.165860

Miura, K., Kinouchi, M., Ishida, K., Fujibuchi, W., Naitoh, T., Ogawa, H., et al. (2010). 5-fu metabolism in cancer and orally-administrable 5-fu drugs. *Cancers* 2, 1717–1730. doi: 10.3390/cancers2031717

Molinaro, M., Ameri, P., Marone, G., Petretta, M., Abete, P., Di Lisa, F., et al. (2015). Recent advances on pathophysiology, diagnostic and therapeutic insights in cardiac dysfunction induced by antineoplastic drugs. *Biomed Res. Int.* 2015:138148. doi: 10.1155/2015/138148

Moloney, J. N., and Cotter, T. G. (2017). ROS signalling in the biology of cancer. *Semin. Cell Dev. Biol.* doi: 10.1016/j.semcdb.2017.05.023. [Epub ahead of print].

Moon, J. S., Nakahira, K., Chung, K. P., DeNicola, G. M., Koo, M. J., Pabón, M. A., et al. (2016). NOX4-dependent fatty acid oxidation promotes NLRP3 inflammasome activation in macrophages. *Nat. Med.* 22, 1002–1012. doi: 10.1038/nm.4153

Moslehi, J. J., and Deininger, M. (2015). Tyrosine Kinase Inhibitor-Associated Cardiovascular Toxicity in Chronic Myeloid Leukemia. *J. Clin. Oncol.* 33, 4210–4218. doi: 10.1200/JCO.2015.62.4718

Motzer, R. J., Hutson, T. E., Cella, D., Reeves, J., Hawkins, R., Guo, J., et al. (2013). Pazopanib versus sunitinib in metastatic renal-cell carcinoma. *N. Engl. J. Med.* 369, 722–731. doi: 10.1056/NEJMoa1303989

Motzer, R. J., Hutson, T. E., Tomczak, P., Michaelson, M. D., Bukowski, R. M., Rixe, O., et al. (2007). Sunitinib versus interferon alfa in metastatic renal-cell carcinoma. *N. Engl. J. Med.* 356, 115–124. doi: 10.1056/NEJMoa065044

Mourad, J. J., and Levy, B. I. (2011). Mechanisms of antiangiogenic-induced arterial hypertension. *Curr. Hypertens. Rep.* 13, 289–293. doi: 10.1007/s11906-011-0206-y

Münzel, T., Gori, T., Keaney, J. F. Jr., Maack, C., and Daiber, A. (2015). Pathophysiological role of oxidative stress in systolic and diastolic heart failure and its therapeutic implications. *Eur. Heart J.* 36, 2555–2564. doi: 10.1093/eurheartj/ehv305

Nakamae, H., Tsumura, K., Terada, Y., Nakane, T., Nakamae, M., Ohta, K., et al. (2005). Notable effects of angiotensin II receptor blocker, valsartan, on acute cardiotoxic changes after standard chemotherapy with cyclophosphamide, doxorubicin, vincristine, and prednisolone. *Cancer* 104, 2492–2498. doi: 10.1002/cncr.21478

Nakamura, K., Kusano, K., Nakamura, Y., Kakishita, M., Ohta, K., Nagase, S., et al. (2002). Carvedilol decreases elevated oxidative stress in human failing myocardium. *Circulation* 105, 2867–2871. doi: 10.1161/01.CIR.0000018605.14470.DD

Nazer, B., Humphreys, B. D., and Moslehi, J. (2011). Effects of novel angiogenesis inhibitors for the treatment of cancer on the cardiovascular system: focus on hypertension. *Circulation* 124, 1687–1691. doi: 10.1161/CIRCULATIONAHA.110.992230

Nediani, C., Raimondi, L., Borchi, E., and Cerbai, E. (2011). Nitric oxide/reactive oxygen species generation and nitroso/redox imbalance in heart failure: from molecular mechanisms to therapeutic implications. *Antioxid. Redox Signal.* 14, 289–331. doi: 10.1089/ars.2010.3198

Ng, M., Cunningham, D., and Norman, A. R. (2005). The frequency and pattern of cardiotoxicity observed with capecitabine used in conjunction with oxaliplatin in patients treated for advanced colorectal cancer (CRC). *Eur. J. Cance.* 41, 1542–1546. doi: 10.1016/j.ejca.2005.03.027

Nickel, A., Kohlhaas, M., and Maack, C. (2014). Mitochondrial reactive oxygen species production and elimination. *J. Mol. Cell. Cardiol.* 73, 26–33. doi: 10.1016/j.yjmcc.2014.03.011

Niu, Y., DesMarais, T. L., Tong, Z., Yao, Y., and Costa, M. (2015). Oxidative stress alters global histone modification and DNA methylation. *Free Radic. Biol. Med.* 82, 22–28. doi: 10.1016/j.freeradbiomed.2015.01.028

Novo, G., Cadeddu, C., Sucato, V., Pagliaro, P., Romano, S., Tocchetti, C. G., et al. (2016b). Role of biomarkers in monitoring antiblastic cardiotoxicity. *J. Cardiovasc. Med. (Hagerstown).* 17(Suppl. 1), S27–S34. doi: 10.2459/JCM.0000000000000379

Odiete, O., Hill, M. F., and Sawyer, D. B. (2012). Neuregulin in cardiovascular development and disease. *Circ. Res.* 111, 1376–1385. doi: 10.1161/CIRCRESAHA.112.267286

Oeffinger, K. C., Mertens, A. C., Sklar, C. A., Kawashima, T., Hudson, M. M., Meadows, A. T., et al. (2006). Chronic health conditions in adult survivors of childhood cancer. *N. Engl. J. Med.* 355, 1572–1582. doi: 10.1056/NEJMsa060185

Oka, T., Akazawa, H., Naito, A. T., and Komuro, I. (2014). Angiogenesis and cardiac hypertrophy: maintenance of cardiac function and causative roles in heart failure. *Circ. Res.* 114, 565–571. doi: 10.1161/CIRCRESAHA.114.300507

Oliveira, M. S., Melo, M. B., Carvalho, J. L., Melo, I. M., Lavor, M. S., Gomes, D. A., et al. (2013). Doxorubicin cardiotoxicity and cardiac function improvement after stem cell therapy diagnosed by strain echocardiography. *J. Cancer Sci. Ther.* 5, 52–57. doi: 10.4172/1948-5956.1000184

Ozcelik, C., Erdmann, B., Pilz, B., Wettschureck, N., Britsch, S., Hübner, N., et al. (2002). Conditional mutation of the ErbB2 (HER2) receptor in cardiomyocytes leads to dilated cardiomyopathy. *Proc. Natl. Acad. Sci. U.S.A.* 99, 8880–8885. doi: 10.1073/pnas.122249299

Oztop, I., Gencer, M., Okan, T., Yaren, A., Altekin, E., Turker, S., et al. (2004). Evaluation of cardiotoxicity of a combined bolus plus infusional 5-fluorouracil/folinic acid treatment by echocardiography, plasma troponin I level, QT interval and dispersion in patients with gastrointestinal system cancers. *Jpn. J. Clin. Oncol.* 34, 262–268. doi: 10.1093/jjco/hyh047

Pagliaro, P., Moro, F., Tullio, F., Perrelli, M. G., and Penna, C. (2011). Cardioprotective pathways during reperfusion: focus on redox signaling and other modalities of cell signaling. *Antioxid. Redox Signal.* 14, 833–850. doi: 10.1089/ars.2010.3245

Pagliaro, P., and Penna, C. (2015). Redox signalling and cardioprotection: translatability and mechanism. *Br. J. Pharmacol.* 172, 1974–1995. doi: 10.1111/bph.12975

Papapetropoulos, A., Foresti, R., and Ferdinandy, P. (2015). Pharmacology of the 'gasotransmitters' NO, CO and H2S: translational opportunities. *Br. J. Pharmacol.* 172, 1395–1396. doi: 10.1111/bph.13005

Penna, C., Angotti, C., and Pagliaro, P. (2014). Protein S-nitrosylation in preconditioning and postconditioning. *Exp. Biol. Med. (Maywood)* 239, 647–662. doi: 10.1177/1535370214522935

Pereira, G. C., Pereira, S. P., Tavares, L. C., Carvalho, F. S., Magalhães-Novais, S., Barbosa, I. A., et al. (2016). Cardiac cytochrome c and cardiolipin depletion during anthracycline-induced chronic depression of mitochondrial function. *Mitochondrion* 30, 95–104. doi: 10.1016/j.mito.2016.07.005

Petrelli, F., Barni, S., Bertocchi, P., and Zaniboni, A. (2016). TAS-102, the first "cardio-gentle" fluoropyrimidine in the colorectal cancer landscape? *BMC Cancer* 16:386. doi: 10.1186/s12885-016-2409-8

Pituskin, E., Mackey, J. R., Koshman, S., Jassal, D., Pitz, M., Haykowsky, M. J., et al. (2017). Multidisciplinary approach to novel therapies in cardio-oncology research (MANTICORE 101-Breast): a randomized trial for the prevention of trastuzumab-associated cardiotoxicity. *J. Clin. Oncol.* 35, 870–877. doi: 10.1200/JCO.2016.68.7830

Pointon, A. V., Walker, T. M., Phillips, K. M., Luo, J., Riley, J., Zhang, S. D., et al. (2010). Doxorubicin *in vivo* rapidly alters expression and translation of myocardial electron transport chain genes, leads to ATP loss and caspase 3 activation. *PLoS ONE* 5:e12733. doi: 10.1371/journal.pone.0012733

Polk, A., Vaage-Nilsen, M., Vistisen, K., and Nielsen, D. L. (2013). Cardiotoxicity in cancer patients treated with 5-fluorouracil or capecitabine: a systematic review of incidence, manifestations and predisposing factors. *Cancer Treat. Rev.* 39, 974–984. doi: 10.1016/j.ctrv.2013.03.005

Polk, A., Vistisen, K., Vaage-Nilsen, M., and Nielsen, D. L. (2014). A systematic review of the pathophysiology of 5-fluorouracil-induced cardiotoxicity. *BMC Pharmacol. Toxicol.* 15:47. doi: 10.1186/2050-6511-15-47

Ponikowski, P., Voors, A. A., Anker, S. D., Bueno, H., Cleland, J. G., Coats, A. J., et al. (2016). 2016 ESC Guidelines for the diagnosis and treatment of acute and chronic heart failure: the task force for the diagnosis and treatment of acute and chronic heart failure of the European Society of Cardiology (ESC). Developed with the special contribution of the Heart Failure Association (HFA) of the ESC. *Eur. J. Heart Fail.* 18, 891–975. doi: 10.1002/ejhf.592

Rainer, P. P., Doleschal, B., Kirk, J. A., Sivakumaran, V., Saad, Z., Groschner, K., et al. (2012). Sunitinib causes dose-dependent negative functional effects on myocardium and cardiomyocytes. *BJU Int.* 110, 1455–1462. doi: 10.1111/j.1464-410X.2012.11134.x

Räsänen, M., Degerman, J., Nissinen, T. A., Miinalainen, I., Kerkelä, R., Siltanen, A., et al. (2016). VEGF-B gene therapy inhibits doxorubicin-induced cardiotoxicity by endothelial protection. *Proc. Natl. Acad. Sci. U.S.A.* 113, 13144–13149. doi: 10.1073/pnas.1616168113

Rastogi, S., Sharov, V. G., Mishra, S., Gupta, R. C., Blackburn, B., Belardinelli, L., et al. (2008). Ranolazine combined with enalapril or metoprolol prevents progressive LV dysfunction and remodeling in dogs with moderate heart failure. *Am. J. Physiol. Heart Circ. Physiol.* 295, H2149–2155. doi: 10.1152/ajpheart.00728.2008

Reck, M., Kaiser, R., Mellemgaard, A., Douillard, J. Y., Orlov, S., Krzakowski, M., et al. (2014). Docetaxel plus nintedanib versus docetaxel plus placebo in patients with previously treated non-small-cell lung cancer (LUME-Lung 1): a phase 3, double-blind, randomised controlled trial. *Lancet Oncol.* 15, 143–155. doi: 10.1016/S1470-2045(13)70586-2

Rephaeli, A., Waks-Yona, S., Nudelman, A., Tarasenko, I., Tarasenko, N., Phillips, D. R., et al. (2007). Anticancer prodrugs of butyric acid and formaldehyde protect against doxorubicin-induced cardiotoxicity. *Br. J. Cancer.* 96, 1667–1674. doi: 10.1038/sj.bjc.6603781

Riad, A., Bien, S., Westermann, D., Becher, P. M., Loya, K., Landmesser, U., et al. (2009). Pretreatment with statin attenuates the cardiotoxicity of Doxorubicin in mice. *Cancer Res.* 69, 695–699. doi: 10.1158/0008-5472.CAN-08-3076

Rohrbach, S., Yan, X., Weinberg, E. O., Hasan, F., Bartunek, J., Marchionni, M. A., et al. (1999). Neuregulin in cardiac hypertrophy in rats with aortic stenosis. Differential expression of erbB2 and erbB4 receptors. *Circulation* 100, 407–412.

Russell, E. G., and Cotter, T. G. (2015). New insight into the role of Reactive Oxygen Species (ROS) in cellular signal-transduction processes. *Int. Rev. Cell Mol. Biol.* 319, 221–254. doi: 10.1016/bs.ircmb.2015.07.004

Sabbah, H. N., Chandler, M. P., Mishima, T., Suzuki, G., Chaudhry, P., Nass, O., et al. (2002). Ranolazine, a partial fatty acid oxidation (pFOX) inhibitor, improves left ventricular function in dogs with chronic heart failure. *J. Card. Fail.* 8, 416–422. doi: 10.1054/jcaf.2002.129232

Saitoh, S., Kiyooka, T., Rocic, P., Rogers, P. A., Zhang, C., Swafford, A., et al. (2007). Redox-dependent coronary metabolic dilation. *Am. J. Physiol. Heart Circ. Physiol.* 293, H3720–H3725. doi: 10.1152/ajpheart.00436.2007

Salvatorelli, E., Menna, P., and Minotti, G. (2015). Managing anthracycline-induced cardiotoxicity: beginning with the end in mind. *Future Cardiol.* 11, 363–366. doi: 10.2217/FCA.15.35

Sandler, A., Gray, R., Perry, M. C., Brahmer, J., Schiller, J. H., Dowlati, A., et al. (2006). Paclitaxel-carboplatin alone or with bevacizumab for non-small-cell lung cancer. *N. Engl. J. Med.* 355, 2542–2550. doi: 10.1056/NEJMoa061884

Santos, D. L., Moreno, A. J., Leino, R. L., Froberg, M. K., and Wallace, K. B. (2002). Carvedilol protects against doxorubicin-induced mitochondrial cardiomyopathy. *Toxicol. Appl. Pharmacol.* 185, 218–227. doi: 10.1006/taap.2002.9532

Sawyer, D. B. (2013). Anthracyclines and heart failure. *N. Engl. J. Med.* 368, 1154–1156. doi: 10.1056/NEJMcibr1214975

Schermuly, R. T., Dony, E., Ghofrani, H. A., Pullamsetti, S., Savai, R., Roth, M., et al. (2005). Reversal of experimental pulmonary hypertension by PDGF inhibition. *J. Clin. Invest.* 115, 2811–2821. doi: 10.1172/JCI24838

Scott, J. M., Khakoo, A., Mackey, J. R., Haykowsky, M. J., Douglas, P. S., and Jones, L. W. (2011). Modulation of anthracycline-induced cardiotoxicity by aerobic exercise in breast cancer: current evidence and underlying mechanisms. *Circulation* 124, 642–650. doi: 10.1161/CIRCULATIONAHA.111.021774

Scott, J. M., Koelwyn, G. J., Hornsby, W. E., Khouri, M., Peppercorn, J., Douglas, P. S., et al. (2013). Exercise therapy as treatment for cardiovascular and oncologic disease after a diagnosis of early-stage cancer. *Semin. Oncol.* 40, 218–228. doi: 10.1053/j.seminoncol.2013.01.001

Seicean, S., Seicean, A., Alan, N., Plana, J. C., Budd, G. T., and Marwick, T. H. (2013). Cardioprotective effect of beta-adrenoceptor blockade in patients with breast cancer undergoing chemotherapy: follow-up study of heart failure. *Circ. Heart Fail.* 6, 420–426. doi: 10.1161/CIRCHEARTFAILURE.112.000055

Seicean, S., Seicean, A., Plana, J. C., Budd, G. T., and Marwick, T. H. (2012). Effect of statin therapy on the risk for incident heart failure in patients with breast cancer receiving anthracycline chemotherapy: an observational clinical cohort study. *J. Am. Coll. Cardiol.* 60, 2384–2390. doi: 10.1016/j.jacc.2012.07.067

Seymour, L., Bramwell, V., and Moran, L. A. (1999). Use of dexrazoxane as a cardioprotectant in patients receiving doxorubicin or epirubicin chemotherapy for the treatment of cancer. The Provincial Systemic Treatment Disease Site Group. *Cancer Prev. Control.* 3, 145–159.

Shinkai, A., Yoshisue, H., Koike, M., Shoji, E., Nakagawa, S., Saito, A., et al. (1999). A novel human CC chemokine, eotaxin-3, which is expressed in IL-4-stimulated vascular endothelial cells, exhibits potent activity toward eosinophils. *J. Immunol.* 163, 1602–1610.

Shoemaker, L. K., Arora, U., and Rocha Lima, C. M. (2004). 5-fluorouracil-induced coronary vasospasm. *Cancer Control.* 11, 46–49. doi: 10.1177/107327480401100107

Simunek, T., Stérba, M., Popelová, O., Adamcová, M., Hrdina, R., and Gersl, V. (2009). Anthracycline-induced cardiotoxicity: overview of studies examining the roles of oxidative stress and free cellular iron. *Pharmacol. Rep.* 61, 154–171. doi: 10.1016/S1734-1140(09)70018-0

Singh, C. K., Siddiqui, I. A., El-Abd, S., Mukhtar, H., and Ahmad, N. (2016). Combination chemoprevention with grape antioxidants. *Mol. Nutr. Food Res.* 60, 1406–1415. doi: 10.1002/mnfr.201500945

Slamon, D. J., Clark, G. M., Wong, S. G., Levin, W. J., Ullrich, A., and McGuire, W. L. (1987). Human breast cancer: correlation of relapse and survival with amplification of the HER-2/neu oncogene. *Science.* 235, 177–182. doi: 10.1126/science.3798106

Slamon, D. J., Leyland-Jones, B., Shak, S., Fuchs, H., Paton, V., Bajamonde, A., et al. (2001). Use of chemotherapy plus a monoclonal antibody against HER2 for metastatic breast cancer that overexpresses HER2. *N. Engl. J. Med.* 344, 783–792. doi: 10.1056/NEJM200103153441101

Soga, M., Kamal, F. A., Watanabe, K., Ma, M., Palaniyandi, S., Prakash, P., et al. (2006). Effects of angiotensin II receptor blocker (candesartan) in daunorubicin-induced cardiomyopathic rats. *Int. J. Cardiol.* 110, 378–385. doi: 10.1016/j.ijcard.2005.08.061

Sorrentino, M. F., Kim, J., Foderaro, A. E., and Truesdell, A. G. (2012). 5-fluorouracil induced cardiotoxicity: review of the literature. *Cardiol. J.* 19, 453–458. doi: 10.5603/CJ.2012.0084

Spallarossa, P., Garibaldi, S., Altieri, P., Fabbi, P., Manca, V., Nasti, S., et al. (2004). Carvedilol prevents doxorubicin-induced free radical release and apoptosis in cardiomyocytes *in vitro*. *J. Mol. Cell. Cardiol.* 37, 837–846. doi: 10.1016/j.yjmcc.2004.05.024

Staiano, R. I., Loffredo, S., Borriello, F., Iannotti, F. A., Piscitelli, F., Orlando, P., et al. (2016). Human lung-resident macrophages express CB1 and CB2 receptors whose activation inhibits the release of angiogenic and lymphangiogenic factors. *J. Leukoc. Biol.* 99, 531–540. doi: 10.1189/jlb.3HI1214-584R

Stefani, L., Maffulli, N., Mascherini, G., Francini, L., Petri, C., and Galanti, G. (2015). Exercise as prescription therapy: benefits in cancer and hypertensive patients. *Transl Med UniSa.* 11, 39–43.

Sterba, M., Popelová, O., Vávrová, A., Jirkovský, E., Kovaríková, P., Geršl, V., et al. (2013). Oxidative stress, redox signaling, and metal chelation in anthracycline cardiotoxicity and pharmacological cardioprotection. *Antioxid. Redox Signal.* 18, 899–929. doi: 10.1089/ars.2012.4795

Suter, T. M., and Ewer, M. S. (2013). Cancer drugs and the heart: importance and management. *Eur. Heart J.* 34, 1102–1111. doi: 10.1093/eurheartj/ehs181

Suter, T. M., Procter, M., van Veldhuisen, D. J., Muscholl, M., Bergh, J., Carlomagno, C., et al. (2007). Trastuzumab-associated cardiac adverse effects in the herceptin adjuvant trial. *J. Clin. Oncol.* 25, 3859–3865. doi: 10.1200/JCO.2006.09.1611

Swain, S. M., Ewer, M. S., Cortés, J., Amadori, D., Miles, D., Knott, A., et al. (2013). Cardiac tolerability of pertuzumab plus trastuzumab plus docetaxel in patients with HER2-positive metastatic breast cancer in CLEOPATRA: a randomized, double-blind, placebo-controlled phase III study. *Oncologist* 18, 257–264. doi: 10.1634/theoncologist.2012-0448

Swain, S. M., and Vici, P. (2004). The current and future role of dexrazoxane as a cardioprotectant in anthracycline treatment: expert panel review. *J. Cancer Res. Clin. Oncol.* 130, 1–7. doi: 10.1007/s00432-003-0498-7

Swain, S. M., Whaley, F. S., Gerber, M. C., Weisberg, S., York, M., Spicer, D., et al. (1997). Cardioprotection with dexrazoxane for doxorubicin-containing therapy in advanced breast cancer. *J. Clin. Oncol.* 15, 1318–1332. doi: 10.1200/JCO.1997.15.4.1318

Sysa-Shah, P., Tocchetti, C. G., Gupta, M., Rainer, P. P., Shen, X., Kang, B. H., et al. (2016). Bidirectional cross-regulation between ErbB2 and beta-adrenergic signalling pathways. *Cardiovasc. Res.* 109, 358–373. doi: 10.1093/cvr/cvv274

Takimoto, E., and Kass, D. A. (2007). Role of oxidative stress in cardiac hypertrophy and remodeling. *Hypertension* 49, 241–248. doi: 10.1161/01.HYP.0000254415.31362.a7

Tan, C., Tasaka, H., Yu, K. P., Murphy, M. L., and Karnofsky, D. A. (1967). Daunomycin, an antitumor antibiotic, in the treatment of neoplastic disease. Clinical evaluation with special reference to childhood leukemia. *Cancer* 20, 333–353.

Telli, M. L., Witteles, R. M., Fisher, G. A., and Srinivas, S. (2008). Cardiotoxicity associated with the cancer therapeutic agent sunitinib malate. *Ann. Oncol.* 19, 1613–1618. doi: 10.1093/annonc/mdn168

Thorn, C. F., Oshiro, C., Marsh, S., Hernandez-Boussard, T., McLeod, H., Klein, T. E., et al. (2011). Doxorubicin pathways: pharmacodynamics and adverse effects. *Pharmacogenet. Genomics.* 21, 440–446. doi: 10.1097/FPC.0b013e32833ffb56

Timolati, F., Ott, D., Pentassuglia, L., Giraud, M. N., Perriard, J. C., Suter, T. M., et al. (2006). Neuregulin-1 beta attenuates doxorubicin-induced alterations of excitation-contraction coupling and reduces oxidative stress in adult rat cardiomyocytes. *J. Mol. Cell. Cardiol.* 41, 845–854. doi: 10.1016/j.yjmcc.2006.08.002

Tocchetti, C. G., Cadeddu, C., Di Lisi, D., Femminò, S., Madonna, R., Mele, D., et al. (2017). From molecular mechanisms to clinical management of antineoplastic drug-induced cardiovascular toxicity: A translational overview. *Antioxid. Redox Signal.* doi: 10.1089/ars.2016.6930

Tocchetti, C. G., Carpi, A., Coppola, C., Quintavalle, C., Rea, D., Campesan, M., et al. (2014). Ranolazine protects from doxorubicin-induced oxidative stress and cardiac dysfunction. *Eur. J. Heart Fail.* 16, 358–366. doi: 10.1002/ejhf.50

Tocchetti, C. G., Gallucci, G., Coppola, C., Piscopo, G., Cipresso, C., Maurea, C., et al. (2013). The emerging issue of cardiac dysfunction induced by antineoplastic angiogenesis inhibitors. *Eur. J. Heart Fail.* 15, 482–489. doi: 10.1093/eurjhf/hft008

Tocchetti, C. G., Molinaro, M., Angelone, T., Lionetti, V., Madonna, R., Mangiacapra, F., et al. (2015a). nitroso-redox balance and modulation of basal myocardial function: an update from the Italian Society of Cardiovascular Research (SIRC). *Curr. Drug Targets.* 16, 895–903. doi: 10.2174/1389450116666150304103517

Tocchetti, C., Leppo, M. K., Bedja, D., Wang, Y., Weiss, R., and Paolocci, N. (2015b). Cardiac overexpression of creatine kinase improves cardiomyocytes function in heart failure and during increased redox stress. *Circ. Res.* 117:A338.

Tokarska-Schlattner, M., Zaugg, M., da Silva, R., Lucchinetti, E., Schaub, M. C., Wallimann, T., et al. (2005). Acute toxicity of doxorubicin on isolated perfused heart: response of kinases regulating energy supply. *Am. J. Physiol. Heart Circ. Physiol.* 289, H37–H47. doi: 10.1152/ajpheart.01057.2004

Van Cutsem, E., Bajetta, E., Valle, J., Köhne, C. H., Hecht, J. R., Moore, M., et al. (2011). Randomized, placebo-controlled, phase III study of oxaliplatin, fluorouracil, and leucovorin with or without PTK787/ZK 222584 in patients with previously treated metastatic colorectal adenocarcinoma. *J. Clin. Oncol.* 29, 2004–2010. doi: 10.1200/JCO.2010.29.5436

Van Cutsem, E., Hoff, P. M., Blum, J. L., Abt, M., and Osterwalder, B. (2002). Incidence of cardiotoxicity with the oral fluoropyrimidine capecitabine is typical of that reported with 5-fluorouracil. *Ann. Oncol.* 13, 484–485. doi: 10.1093/annonc/mdf108

Varga, Z. V., Kupai, K., Szucs, G., Gáspár, R., Pálóczi, J., Faragó, N., et al. (2013). MicroRNA-25-dependent up-regulation of NADPH oxidase 4 (NOX4) mediates hypercholesterolemia-induced oxidative/nitrative stress and subsequent dysfunction in the heart. *J. Mol. Cell. Cardiol.* 62, 111–121. doi: 10.1016/j.yjmcc.2013.05.009

Varricchi, G., Galdiero, M. R., Loffredo, S., Marone, G., Iannone, R., and Granata, F. (2017a). Are Mast Cells MASTers in Cancer? *Front. Immunol.* 8:424. doi: 10.3389/fimmu.2017.00424

Varricchi, G., Galdiero, M. R., Marone, G., Criscuolo, G., Triassi, M., Bonaduce, D., et al. (2017b). Cardiotoxicity of immune checkpoint inhibitors. *ESMO Open* 2:e000247. doi: 10.1136/esmoopen-2017-000247

Varricchi, G., Galdiero, M. R., Marone, G., Granata, F., and Borriello, F. (2017c). Controversial role of mast cells in skin cancers. *Exp. Dermatol.* 26, 11–17. doi: 10.1111/exd.13107

Varricchi, G., Galdiero, M. R., and Tocchetti, C. G. (2017d). Cardiac toxicity of immune checkpoint inhibitors: cardio-oncology meets immunology. *Circulation* 136, 1989–1992. doi: 10.1161/CIRCULATIONAHA.117.029626

Vincent, D. T., Ibrahim, Y. F., Espey, M. G., and Suzuki, Y. J. (2013). The role of antioxidants in the era of cardiooncology. *Cancer Chemother. Pharmacol.* 72, 1157–1168. doi: 10.1007/s00280-013-2260-4

Vlasova, I. I., Tyurin, V. A., Kapralov, A. A., Kurnikov, I. V., Osipov, A. N., Potapovich, M. V., et al. (2006). Nitric oxide inhibits peroxidase activity of cytochrome c.cardiolipin complex and blocks cardiolipin oxidation. *J. Biol. Chem.* 281, 14554–14562. doi: 10.1074/jbc.M509507200

Vorobjeva, N., Prikhodko, A., Galkin, I., Pletjushkina, O., Zinovkin, R., Sud'ina, G., et al. (2017). Mitochondrial reactive oxygen species are involved in chemoattractant-induced oxidative burst and degranulation of human neutrophils *in vitro*. *Eur. J. Cell Biol.* 96, 254–265. doi: 10.1016/j.ejcb.2017.03.003

Wang, X., Ha, T., Liu, L., Zou, J., Zhang, X., Kalbfleisch, J., et al. (2013). Increased expression of microRNA-146a decreases myocardial ischaemia/reperfusion injury. *Cardiovasc. Res.* 97, 432–442. doi: 10.1093/cvr/cvs356

Welti, J., Loges, S., Dimmeler, S., and Carmeliet, P. (2013). Recent molecular discoveries in angiogenesis and antiangiogenic therapies in cancer. *J. Clin. Invest.* 123, 3190–3200. doi: 10.1172/JCI70212

Willis, M. S., and Patterson, C. (2013). Proteotoxicity and cardiac dysfunction–Alzheimer's disease of the heart? *N. Engl. J. Med.* 368, 455–464. doi: 10.1056/NEJMra1106180

Woitek, F., Zentilin, L., Hoffman, N. E., Powers, J. C., Ottiger, I., Parikh, S., et al. (2015). Intracoronary cytoprotective gene therapy: a study of VEGF-B167 in a pre-clinical animal model of dilated cardiomyopathy. *J. Am. Coll. Cardiol.* 66, 139–153. doi: 10.1016/j.jacc.2015.04.071

Xi, L., Zhu, S. G., Das, A., Chen, Q., Durrant, D., Hobbs, D. C., et al. (2012). Dietary inorganic nitrate alleviates doxorubicin cardiotoxicity: mechanisms and implications. *Nitric Oxide.* 26, 274–284. doi: 10.1016/j.niox.2012.03.006

Yamagishi, S., and Takeuchi, M. (2005). Telmisartan is a promising cardiometabolic sartan due to its unique PPAR-gamma-inducing property. *Med. Hypotheses.* 64, 476–478. doi: 10.1016/j.mehy.2004.09.015

Yao, Y., Xu, X., Zhang, G., Zhang, Y., Qian, W., and Rui, T. (2012). Role of HMGB1 in doxorubicin-induced myocardial apoptosis and its regulation pathway. *Basic Res. Cardiol.* 107, 267. doi: 10.1007/s00395-012-0267-3

Yeh, E. T., and Bickford, C. L. (2009). Cardiovascular complications of cancer therapy: incidence, pathogenesis, diagnosis, and management. *J. Am. Coll. Cardiol.* 53, 2231–2247. doi: 10.1016/j.jacc.2009.02.050

Zamorano, J. L., Lancellotti, P., Rodriguez Muñoz, D., Aboyans, V., Asteggiano, R., Galderisi, M., et al. (2016). 2016 ESC Position Paper on cancer treatments and cardiovascular toxicity developed under the auspices of the ESC Committee for Practice Guidelines: The Task Force for cancer treatments and cardiovascular toxicity of the European Society of Cardiology (ESC). *Eur. Heart J.* 37, 2768–2801. doi: 10.1093/eurheartj/ehw211

Zanardelli, M., Micheli, L., Cinci, L., Failli, P., Ghelardini, C., and Di Cesare Mannelli, L. (2014). Oxaliplatin neurotoxicity involves peroxisome alterations. PPARgamma agonism as preventive pharmacological approach. *PLoS ONE* 9:e102758. doi: 10.1371/journal.pone.0102758

Zang, J., Wu, S., Tang, L., Xu, X., Bai, J., Ding, C., et al. (2012). Incidence and risk of QTc interval prolongation among cancer patients treated with vandetanib: a systematic review and meta-analysis. *PLoS ONE* 7:e30353. doi: 10.1371/journal.pone.0030353

Zhang, M., Perino, A., Ghigo, A., Hirsch, E., and Shah, A. M. (2013). NADPH oxidases in heart failure: poachers or gamekeepers? *Antioxid. Redox Signal.* 18, 1024–1041. doi: 10.1089/ars.2012.4550

Zhang, S., Liu, X., Bawa-Khalfe, T., Lu, L. S., Lyu, Y. L., Liu, L. F., et al. (2012). Identification of the molecular basis of doxorubicin-induced cardiotoxicity. *Nat. Med.* 18, 1639–1642. doi: 10.1038/nm.2919

Zhao, Y., McLaughlin, D., Robinson, E., Harvey, A. P., Hookham, M. B., Shah, A. M., et al. (2010). Nox2 NADPH oxidase promotes pathologic cardiac remodeling associated with Doxorubicin chemotherapy. *Cancer Res.* 70, 9287–9297. doi: 10.1158/0008-5472.CAN-10-2664

7

Redox Aspects of Chaperones in Cardiac Function

Claudia Penna[1], Matteo Sorge[2], Saveria Femminò[1], Pasquale Pagliaro[1] and Mara Brancaccio[2]**

[1] Department of Clinical and Biological Sciences, University of Torino, Torino, Italy, [2] Department of Molecular Biotechnology and Health Sciences, University of Torino, Torino, Italy

Edited by:
Antonio Colantuoni,
University of Naples Federico II, Italy

Reviewed by:
Francesco Moccia,
University of Pavia, Italy
Teresa Pasqua,
University of Calabria, Italy

***Correspondence:**
Claudia Penna
claudia.penna@unito.it
Mara Brancaccio
mara.brancaccio@unito.it

Molecular chaperones are stress proteins that allow the correct folding or unfolding as well as the assembly or disassembly of macromolecular cellular components. Changes in expression and post-translational modifications of chaperones have been linked to a number of age- and stress-related diseases including cancer, neurodegeneration, and cardiovascular diseases. Redox sensible post-translational modifications, such as S-nitrosylation, glutathionylation and phosphorylation of chaperone proteins have been reported. Redox-dependent regulation of chaperones is likely to be a phenomenon involved in metabolic processes and may represent an adaptive response to several stress conditions, especially within mitochondria, where it impacts cellular bioenergetics. These post-translational modifications might underlie the mechanisms leading to cardioprotection by conditioning maneuvers as well as to ischemia/reperfusion injury. In this review, we discuss this topic and focus on two important aspects of redox-regulated chaperones, namely redox regulation of mitochondrial chaperone function and cardiac protection against ischemia/reperfusion injury.

Keywords: cardioprotection, ischemia/reperfusion, heat shock proteins, nitrogen reactive species, reactive oxygen species, redox signaling, mitochondria

INTRODUCTION

Chaperones are proteins responsible for folding, transport, maturation, assembly, and activation of many different proteins, impacting on a wide variety of cellular processes. Chaperones act by binding to protein unfolded domains and, through different mechanisms, promoting protein re-folding and/or avoiding the formation of toxic misfolded protein aggregates. Moreover, they promote the degradation of proteins irreversibly misfolded via the ubiquitin-proteasome pathway or through autophagy. Chaperones play an important role in preserving proteins that exert their functions through considerable conformation changes, like receptors and signal transduction mediators. In these cases, protein activation and de-activation imply cyclic structural reorganization, potentially dangerous for protein stability. Moreover, chaperones play an important role in the assembly of multiprotein complexes, likely by facilitating the structural changes caused by the association of the different subunits. Chaperone proteins function in different cell compartments, including endoplasmic reticulum (ER) and mitochondria. In the ER, a specific set of chaperones is devoted to assisting the folding of proteins during their maturation, but they also take part to a quality control machinery, that induces degradation of proteins that fail to reach their active conformation and in generating signals that increase chaperone transcription and translation in case of massive protein unfolding (the Unfolded Protein Response; Groenendyk et al., 2010). In mitochondria maintaining protein folding is particularly challenging due to the specific mechanism of protein import, the presence of reactive oxygen species (ROS) and the need to assemble proteins synthesized in the cytoplasm and inside the organelle in large multiprotein complexes. Mitochondria possess specific chaperones able to face these difficult tasks and to perform a dedicated quality control (Haynes and Ron, 2010). Furthermore, chaperones are even secreted by cells and can act in the extracellular milieu by chaperoning secreted factors or by signaling through membrane receptors (Eustace and Jay, 2004; Calderwood et al., 2016).

In summary, chaperone proteins exert a number of essential functions in eukaryotic cells in physiological situations, although their action is even more crucial under stress conditions. In this review, we will focus on the role of chaperone proteins in the heart. Indeed, cardiomyocyte cytoplasm is crowded with proteins, mainly forming the specialized contractile apparatus, that interact the ones with the others building solid complexes, able to cope with relevant mechanical stress. The proper folding, assembly and turnover of this multitude of proteins depend on chaperone protein activity (Christians et al., 2014; Tarone and Brancaccio, 2014). Protein misfolding can occur due to a number of means, as genetic mutations, inaccurate post-translational modifications, excessive mechanical stretch and ROS production. Notably, the accumulation of misfolded proteins characterizes a number of cardiac diseases, like hypertrophic cardiomyopathy, idiopathic dilated cardiomyopathy, myocardial infarction and genetic cardiomyopathies. Furthermore, the induction of protein aggregates causes cardiomyopathy in animal models (Bulteau et al., 2001; Tannous et al., 2008; Tian et al., 2012; Parry et al., 2015). Accordingly, the forced expression of chaperone proteins generally protects the heart from many different stress conditions, including the production of ROS (Tarone and Brancaccio, 2014).

In this review, we consider the response of chaperones to ROS production, the redox aspects that can influence chaperone function within the heart during ischemia/reperfusion and chaperone importance in protecting the heart from deleterious consequences. We also focus on chaperone role within mitochondria, as these organelles are extremely important in cardiac activity both in physiologic and pathological conditions.

REACTIVE OXYGEN AND NITROGEN SPECIES AND REDOX SIGNALING

ROS derive from several enzymatic activities in cardiomyocytes and other cells of the cardiovascular system (e.g., endothelial and smooth muscle cells), with mitochondria representing the main source for their production. Indeed, about 2% of oxygen (O_2) consumed by cardiac mitochondria is transformed to superoxide anion ($O_2^{-\bullet}$) due to the incomplete reduction of O_2. Therefore, $O_2^{-\bullet}$ is mainly a byproduct of aerobic respiration. Following spontaneous dismutation, it is transformed to hydrogen peroxide (H_2O_2), which via the Fenton reaction can be converted in the highly reactive hydroxyl radical ($OH^\bullet$) (Turrens, 2003; Tullio et al., 2013; Henstridge et al., 2016). H_2O_2 can be inactivated by glutathione catalyzed by glutathione peroxidase or catalase (Radi et al., 1991; Arai et al., 1999).

Reactive nitrogen species (RNS) refer to the reactive molecules stemming from nitric oxide ($NO^\bullet$), the signaling gaseous molecule, which in certain conditions may act as an antioxidant. It is mainly synthesized from L-arginine by the nitric oxide synthases, NOS1 (neuronal NOS, nNOS), NOS2 (inducible NOS, iNOS) and NOS3 (endothelial NOS, eNOS). In the heart, NOS3 is mainly found in the caveolae of coronary vascular endothelium, whereas cardiomyocytes constitutively express NOS1 and NOS3 in different subcellular structures, while inducible NOS2 expression can be triggered by several stimuli, including infections, heart failure and ischemia/reperfusion (Brown and Borutaite, 2007; Tullio et al., 2013; Penna et al., 2014a). The possibility that mitochondria are important sources of $NO^\bullet$ via a mitochondrial NOS (mitoNOS) variant has been proposed. However, definitive evidence concerning the existence of mitoNOS is not yet available (Lacza et al., 2009).

Nitric oxide can be formed also by other enzymatic and non-enzymatic reactions (Penna et al., 2014a). It can also be transformed, by a redox reaction, into many reactive molecules including nitroxyl (HNO), nitrite (NO_2^-), and peroxynitrite ($ONOO^-$), each one has different functional effects (Wink et al., 2003; Brown and Borutaite, 2007; Tocchetti et al., 2011; Tullio et al., 2013; Penna et al., 2014a).

Under pathophysiological conditions, excessive, unbalanced, ROS and RNS formation may be deleterious for organelle and cell activity as they can accumulate and damage proteins, lipids, and DNA. However, it is now clear that they are also involved in many important signaling functions. Moreover, ROS and RNS can interact to shift from a form to another with more or less reactivity potential. ROS/RNS can induce discrete, reversible and site-specific modifications in proteins, controlling a redox signaling in physiological changes in channel and enzyme function, as well as regulation of transcription. On the other hand, ROS/RNS can induce alterations, diffuse and irreversible, defined as redox stress. The latter is involved in pathophysiological processes together with other pathologic conditions such as inflammation. Proteins more commonly targeted by ROS/RNS contain sensible amino acidic side chains, including cysteine, methionine and histidine, or coordinated metal centers that regulate their conformation and function (Giles et al., 2003). For instance, $NO^\bullet$ can react with $O_2^{-\bullet}$ to form $ONOO^-$, which can impair directly and irreversibly tyrosines in the proteins, yielding tyrosine nitration, a result that is frequently deleterious. $NO^\bullet$ can react also with $ONOO^-$ to form N_2O_3 which can, in turn, react with the so-called "reactive cysteines" to yield S-nitrosylation or S-nitrosylated proteins (PSNO), a result that is frequently beneficial. Indeed, S-nitrosylation sheds cysteine from further oxidation processes.

Cysteine residues of proteins display chemistry versatility, thus these residues may achieve multiple oxidation states and, therefore, are particularly suited to the task of switching from signaling to stress. Indeed, the reactive cysteines can react with ROS/RNS to produce a number of species comprising PSNO. Reactive cysteines can also react with glutathione to form mixed disulfides, such as S-glutathionylation (see below)

(Hurd et al., 2005a; Penna et al., 2014a). Intra- and intermolecular disulfide bonds (PSSP) can also occur. If ROS are excessive, protein thiol oxidation can progress to sulfinic acid (PSO_2H) and sulfonic acid (PSO_3H), leading to irreversible protein dysfunction, representing redox stress (Hurd et al., 2005b).

S-nitrosylation, which is emerging as the paradigm of redox signaling, is the incorporation of nitric oxide moiety to a sulfur atom to form the SNO bond in proteins (PSNO). S-nitrosylation being a signaling modality that acts as a reversible molecular switch resembles the phosphorylation/dephosphorylation in kinase signaling (Hess et al., 2005; Penna et al., 2014a).

An interesting process is the formation of a disulfide bond (PSSP) with a concomitant release of NO-moiety that take place by nucleophilic attack of proximal protein thiols to the site of SNO. While S-nitrosylation may occur with different reaction mechanisms, denitrosylation may be due to S-nitrosoglutathione reductase and/or the intervention of thioredoxin system (namely the cytosolic Trx1 and the mitochondrial Trx2). These are considered the two main enzymatic systems for denitrosylation, which, actually, may also occur for non-enzymatic processes (Sengupta et al., 2007; Benhar et al., 2008; Penna et al., 2014a). For instance, thioredoxins denitrosylate proteins and then thioredoxin reductase regenerates thioredoxins (Penna et al., 2014a).

As said, another modification of protein cysteine residues representing a redox signaling modality is S-glutathionylation, which refers to a covalent modification of a cysteine residue by glutathione. S-glutathionylation comprises a mixed disulfide species (PS-SG). Proteins particularly rich in cysteine are susceptible to glutathionylation especially in the presence of alkaline pH, which favors deprotonation of protein thiols and reaction with glutathione. Of course, S-glutathionylation, like other signaling processes, is reversible through a process called deglutathionylation. In this process, the main enzymes involved are glutaredoxin and thioredoxins. Also, reduction of disulfides may be responsible for deglutathionylation when the GSH pool is reduced (Beer et al., 2004).

S-nitrosylation and S-glutathionylation interact: glutathione reductase removes the NO fraction from proteins through the transnitrosation of SNO with GSH to form GSNO (S-nitrosoglutathione), which will, in turn, be converted into GSH by S-nitrosoglutathione reductase.

The dynamic S-nitrosylation/denitrosylation and glutathionylation/deglutathionylation reactions are of pivotal importance in the regulation of the cardiovascular system. For example, in transgenic models of increased or decreased activity of S-nitrosoglutathione reductase, the sepsis-induced myocardial depression is positively influenced by denitrosylation/deglutathionylation. Therefore, besides guanylyl cyclase activation and cGMP production, $NO^{\bullet}$ may affect pathophysiology via S-nitrosylation and S-glutathionylation of proteins, including chaperones (**Figure 1**; Sengupta et al., 2007; Benhar et al., 2009; Anand and Stamler, 2012; Beigi et al., 2012; Martínez-Ruiz et al., 2013).

As described above and as reported below, cells have evolved multiple fine-regulated systems to balance their redox

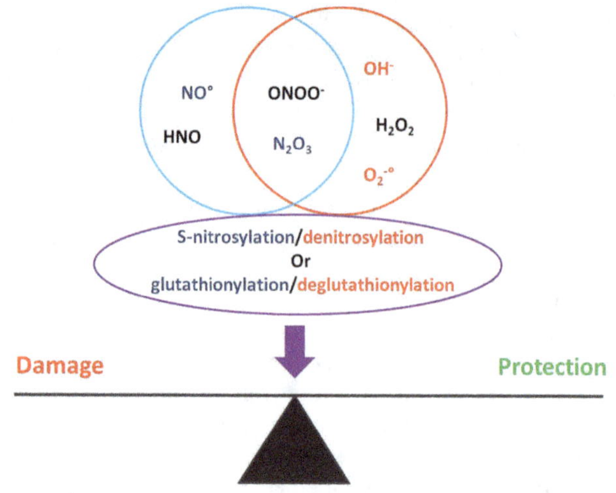

FIGURE 1 | Oxygen and nitrogen reactive species regulate S-nitrosylation and glutathionylation of proteins, impacting on cardiac pathophysiology.

homeostasis, including detoxifying enzymes and reducing proteins. The regulation of ROS levels is a critical point in cells. Indeed, ROS/RNS play important roles in different signaling pathways (Rhee, 2006; D'Autreaux and Toledano, 2007; Tullio et al., 2013). However, once ROS exceed the antioxidant capacity of the cell, it causes oxidative stress. ROS can induce important alterations in the function and structure of DNA, lipids and in particular proteins rich in cysteine, methionine, and histidine (Imlay, 2003). Interestingly, these ROS-sensible amino acidic side chains are frequently present in chaperone proteins, suggesting that ROS can regulate chaperone oxidation state and activity under oxidative stress conditions.

REDOX REGULATION OF CHAPERONE PROTEINS

Chaperones are highly conserved proteins that may play a huge protective role during cellular stress and pathologic conditions. Important redox modifications of chaperone proteins have been described in oxidative stress conditions.

HSP33 is a well-known redox-activated chaperone protein in prokaryotes that protects bacteria from oxidative stress damage, preventing protein unfolding and aggregation (Winter et al., 2008). *In vitro* experiments demonstrated that HSP33 is activated by hydrogen peroxide and heat shock through the formation of reversible disulfide bonds. A first disulfide bond in the C-terminal domain of the protein induces the unfolding of its zinc-binding domain and the linker region between the C-terminal and the N-terminal substrate-binding domain. The formation of a second disulfide bond blocks the linker region in the unfolded conformation, exposing a highly hydrophobic surface. This favors the interaction between two oxidized HSP33 in a stable chaperone-active homodimer that binds unfolded proteins under oxidizing condition (Graumann et al., 2001; Ilbert et al., 2007).

Asna1/TRC40 (transmembrane recognition complex 40), similarly to HSP33, functions as a redox-regulated chaperone during oxidative stress, in eukaryotes (Voth and Jakob, 2017). In non-stress conditions, Asna1/TRC40 is devoted to facilitating the post-translational delivery of tail-anchored proteins to the mammalian endoplasmic reticulum. However, in oxidative conditions, the formation of a disulfide bond induces a conformational change in the protein that oligomerizes and behaves as a molecular chaperone. The possibility that Asna1/TRC40 protects mammalian tissues from oxidative stress is still under investigation (Voth and Jakob, 2017). Moreover, also other proteins as the PLP-dependent aminotransferases hBCAT or the antioxidant enzymes 2-cys peroxiredoxins are known to be oxidized under severe oxidative stress condition, inducing the formation of high molecular weight oligomers or supra-molecular complexes with chaperone activity (Jang et al., 2004; El Hindy et al., 2014). In eukaryotes, redox alterations are described in various chaperone proteins, as GRP58, GRP78, HSC70, HSP90, HSP70, and HSP60 (Fratelli et al., 2002; Lind et al., 2002; Scroggins and Neckers, 2007; Wang et al., 2012). HSP90 is one of the most important molecular chaperones, involved in different signaling pathways in normal and pathological conditions. HSP90 activity is determined by its ability to hydrolyze ATP and is regulated by the binding with small co-chaperone proteins. Intriguingly, the HSP90 function is modulated also by various post-translational modifications, as phosphorylation, acetylation, ubiquitination, S-nitrosylation and oxidation (Scroggins and Neckers, 2007). In endothelial cells, $NO^{\bullet}$ binds to the thiol side chain of cysteine-597 in the C-terminal domain of HSP90, compromising its ATPase activity and thus inhibiting its chaperone function (Martínez-Ruiz et al., 2005). In human breast cancer MDA-MB-231 cells, the treatment with the cytotoxic steroid tubocapsenolide A induces an increase in oxygen reactive species and a reduction in intracellular glutathione content. In this condition, ROS determine a thiol oxidation of HSP90 causing the loss of its chaperone activity and the consequent proteasomal degradation of its client proteins (Chen et al., 2008).

TRAP1 (tumor necrosis factor receptor-associated protein 1), the mitochondrial homolog of HSP90, is subjected to S-nitrosylation in tumor cells lacking S-nitrosoglutathione reductase (GSNOR). S-nitrosylation at cysteine-501 causes an accelerated proteasomal degradation of TRAP1, inducing an increase in levels and activity of succinate dehydrogenase (SDH), normally inhibited by TRAP1, sensitizing cells to SDH-inhibitors chemotherapy. Other aspects of TRAP1 function are described below (see "Chaperones in mitochondria").

Protein Disulfide-Isomerase (PDI) is another well-known redox-dependent chaperone in humans, ubiquitously expressed and mainly localized in the endoplasmic reticulum (Hatahet and Ruddock, 2009). PDI catalyzes the folding of its substrates under oxidative conditions. PDI activity is related to its conformation, which is in turn dependent on the redox state of its active sites. In particular, the oxidation of its active sites determines the conversion of PDI from a compact to an open conformation exposing the substrates-binding surface. PDI binds to unfolded proteins and, by reducing its own disulfide bonds, induces the formation of disulfides in the substrate. The reduction of its active sites determines the return to its compact conformation, releasing the folded substrate (Wang et al., 2015).

HSP27 is a molecular chaperone active when aggregated in a high molecular weight complex. In ischemia/reperfusion (I/R) injury, HSP27 cysteine-141 forms a disulfide with a low-molecular-weight thiol, such as glutathione (S-glutathionylation), and this modification induces the disaggregation of the multimeric complex and the loss of its chaperone activity (Eaton et al., 2002).

HSP70 and HSP60 are two other chaperones susceptible to S-glutathionylation under oxidative stress conditions. The overexpression of HSP70 is protective against oxidative damage in H9C2 cells exposed to oxidative reagents or hypoxia as well as *in vivo* models subjected to ischemic injury (Marber et al., 1995; Chong et al., 1998; Okubo et al., 2001). It has been suggested that S-glutathionylation of HSP70 may potentiate its chaperone activity (Fratelli et al., 2002). A similar regulation is proposed also for HSP60, a predominantly mitochondrial chaperone known to be upregulated by the accumulation of unfolded and oxidized molecules within mitochondria. In accordance, HSP60 overexpression protects against ischemia-reperfusion injury (Fratelli et al., 2002; Lind et al., 2002).

CHAPERONES IN THE HEART

The intense, restless contractile and metabolic activities of the heart require a continuous supply of oxygen and nutrients and a tight control of synthesis, folding and turnover of macromolecules, including proteins. In the case of cardiac overload and in stress conditions, the greater myocardial energy demand may enhance the leakage of electrons from mitochondrial complexes I to III and may induce ROS formation, which may overcome the anti-oxidant cell capacity, thus damaging proteins and other target molecules. Indeed, the accurate regulation of cardiac proteostasis may be impaired by several stress conditions, including oxidative stress, causing an accumulation of damaged and misfolded proteins that exceed the cellular degradation ability. Unfolded proteins can thus aggregate in toxic oligomers and finally in bigger insoluble aggregates disrupting cardiomyocyte structure and function and leading to cardiomyopathy (Willis and Patterson, 2013; Del Monte and Agnetti, 2014; McLendon and Robbins, 2015). Nevertheless, oxidative stimuli may also induce the activation of intracellular signaling pathways to sustain the cardiac activity and prevent the onset of cardiomyopathy (Tarone and Lembo, 2003; Sorge and Brancaccio, 2016). Of note, proteins involved in signal transduction are often metastable, changing conformation during activation/deactivation processes. This feature confers to these proteins a particular propensity to denaturate in stress conditions (Conway and Lee, 2015).

The heart is rich in chaperones and co-chaperones and under stress conditions, it increases chaperone expression and activity to cope with unfolded protein accumulation and sustain the activation of protective pathways. Indeed, in the heart small heat shock proteins and bigger chaperones, as HSP90 and HSP70, work in a coordinated fashion to regulate the intracellular signaling cascade and the folding or degradation of unfolded proteins (Hartl et al., 2011; Kriegenburg et al., 2012; Tarone and Brancaccio, 2014).

HSP90 and HSP70 are considered the two most important molecular chaperones and are both rapidly induced in stressed hearts. The interaction with co-chaperones, that regulate the binding to specific targets, allow them to induce the conformational changes needed to activate/deactivate signaling molecules and their assembly in pro-survival signalosome complexes (Kupatt et al., 2004; Tarone and Brancaccio, 2014; Parry et al., 2015). This chaperone machinery also promotes the correct folding of specific "clients proteins" (http://www.picard.ch/downloads/downloads.htm) and controls the degradation of unfolded proteins and of protein aggregates, through the proteasome and the autophagosome pathways (Ficker et al., 2003; McDonough and Patterson, 2003; Carra et al., 2008; Arndt et al., 2010; Taipale et al., 2010).

Small heat shock proteins are another group of chaperones characterized by a α-crystallin domain which favors their oligomerization in supramolecular complexes with chaperone activity. Recent experimental evidence suggests an important role for these chaperones in the stressed heart. Indeed, by binding their client proteins, in some cases in association with HSP90, they are able to promote protein folding, prevent misfolded protein aggregation and support signal transduction pathways (Vos et al., 2011; Bakthisaran et al., 2015; Haslbeck and Vierling, 2015).

For example, αB-crystallin (CryAB or HSPB5) is a small chaperone fundamental for cytoskeletal proteins folding, in particular for desmin and titin. A missense mutation in its coding gene induces the formation of desmin aggregates and causes a cardiomyopathy (Vicart et al., 1998).

Other small heat shock proteins, like HSP27, HSP20, HSP22, and Melusin are induced under stress conditions favoring protein folding and pro-survival signaling activation (Sui et al., 2009; Fan and Kranias, 2011; Christians et al., 2012; Sorge and Brancaccio, 2016). The mitochondrial and protective role of these and other chaperones are described in the following paragraphs.

CHAPERONES IN CARDIAC MITOCHONDRIA

Mitochondria represent 35–40% of cardiac cell volume. Therefore the role of chaperones in these organelles is very important for cardiac function, especially in I/R and cardioprotection. Mitochondrial chaperones have been extensively studied in Saccharomyces cerevisiae elucidating a complex system that can be generalized to all the eukaryotes. In these organelles, specific chaperones assist proteins in their import and folding and protect mitochondria from different stress stimuli, like temperature and excessive ROS (**Figure 2**).

Mitochondrial HSP70 (mtHSP70), also known as Ssc1, Grp75, PBP74, mot-2 or mortalin, is considered the most important mitochondrial chaperone in higher eukaryotes. It is a member of the HSP70 family characterized by an N-terminal ATPase domain and a C-terminal peptide-binding domain. mtHSP70 is translated into the cytoplasm and transported into mitochondria where it interacts with structural mitochondrial proteins, metabolic enzymes and proteins involved in cell differentiation and survival (Wadhwa et al., 1998, 2002, 2003; Schwarzer et al., 2002). mtHSP70 is essential for pre-protein—precursors of mature proteins—import from cytosol to the mitochondrial matrix. Pre-proteins cross the double mitochondrial membrane in an extended conformation thanks to a positive charged N-terminal part, favored by the membrane electrochemical gradient (Schwartz et al., 1999). mtHSP70 forms a complex with its co-chaperone Mge1, a homolog of the bacterial Grp3 protein, that induces the release of ADP and P_i augmenting the ATPase activity of mtHSP70 (Dekker and Pfanner, 1997). Mge1 may stabilize the interaction of mtHSP70 with the inner membrane protein Tim44 to create a molecular motor that uses the energy from the ATP hydrolysis for the full translocation of the polypeptide chains inside the mitochondria (**Figure 2**; Wachter et al., 1994; Schneider et al., 1996).

Another important role of mtHSP70, not related to the translocase activity, is in protein folding and prevention of protein aggregation. Indeed mtHSP70 interacts with another cochaperone, Mdj1, a homolog of the bacterial DnaJ protein, and they associate with newly imported or neo-synthesized proteins or with misfolded aggregate proteins to mediate their folding to the native conformation (**Figure 2**; Herrmann et al., 1994; Prip-Buus et al., 1996).

Ecm10 and Ssq1 are two other HSP70 family proteins contained within mitochondria. Ecm10 is a very close homolog of mtHSP70, likely involved in different functions (Baumann et al., 2000). Ssq1 is a mtHSP70 homolog involved in the maintenance of the mitochondrial genome and in the assembly of iron/sulfur (Fe/S) containing complexes (Schilke et al., 1996, 1999). In particular, Ssq1, regulated by the co-chaperone proteins Mge1 and Jac1, is responsible for the formation of Fe/S clusters and for their assembly into functional protein complexes (**Figure 2**; Lutz et al., 2001; Schmidt et al., 2001).

HSP60 and HSP10, two chaperone proteins translated in the cytoplasm and then imported into the mitochondrial matrix play an important function in mitochondrial protein folding. HSP60 consists of a double ring system each composed of seven protein subunits (Xu et al., 1997). The co-chaperone HSP10, a homolog of the bacterial GroES, forms a cap closing the opening of the inner cavity of the HSP60 double ring, regulating substrate accessibility and ATPase activity (Martin et al., 1993; Fenton et al., 1996; David et al., 2013). Pre-folding proteins and newly imported pre-proteins enter the cavity of the complex and acquire their native conformation thanks to an ATP-dependent reaction (**Figure 2**; Ostermann et al., 1989; Brinker et al., 2001). Recent studies also indicate that HSP10 can be involved in the RasGTPase pathway, protecting myocytes from I/R damage, and that it interacts with caspase 3 and modulates Bcl-2 family factors, suggesting a potential anti-apoptotic role in cardiomyocytes (Shan et al., 2003; Lin et al., 2004).

HSP78 and Prohibitins are other significant chaperones and proteins involved in the folding process inside the mitochondria. HSP78, activated by heat stress, and Mcx1,

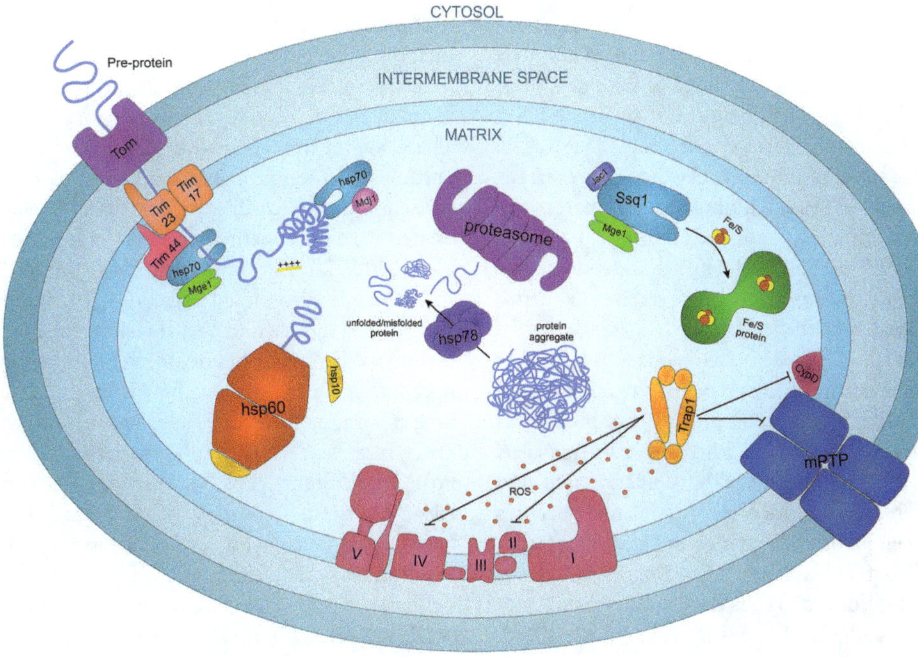

FIGURE 2 | The complex interplay of chaperone proteins in regulating the apoptotic process in cardiomyocytes.

members of the HSP100 family mediate protein folding and degradation of irreversibly damaged proteins (**Figure 2**). Prohibitins, induced after heat shock, oxidative and metabolic stress, act as foldase-unfoldase and control the AAA-proteases activity in protein degradation. Prohibitin complexes control cell proliferation, cristae morphogenesis and the functional integrity of mitochondria (van Dyck et al., 1998; Steglich et al., 1999; Krzewska et al., 2001; Nijtmans et al., 2002).

As said, mitochondria are the main sources of ROS production in the cardiomyocytes and consequently the more subjected to oxidative stress. TRAP1 is induced upon oxidative stress and characterized by an anti-oxidant and anti-apoptotic activity (Montesano Gesualdi et al., 2007). TRAP1 is strictly similar to the cytosolic HSP90, with the same domain organization. However, it has a different mechanism of folding, due to a characteristic asymmetric conformation when bound to the client in its ATP-binding state. The hydrolysis of a first ATP determines a rearrangement of the chaperone conformation and the client folding, then a second ATP hydrolysis induces the release of the client and a switch of TRAP1 conformation to its ADP-binding state (Lavery et al., 2014). TRAP1 has an important role in mitochondrial homeostasis, maintaining organelle integrity and preventing energy depletion under ROS-induced stress. In particular, TRAP1 inhibits the cytochrome oxidase (complex IV of the respiratory chain) and the succinate dehydrogenase (complex II of the respiratory chain and component of the TCA cycle), favoring the metabolic switch from oxidative phosphorylation toward aerobic glycolysis, avoiding ATP depletion and mitophagy under oxidative conditions (**Figure 2**; Sciacovelli et al., 2013; Yoshida et al., 2013). TRAP1 has also an anti-apoptotic role as it antagonizes the mitochondrial permeability transition pore (mPTP) opening by inhibiting the complex II-induced ROS release and the mPTP inducer Cyclophilin-D (**Figure 2**; Kang et al., 2007; Guzzo et al., 2014).

New chaperones have been discovered in the last years with multiple functions, as the small Tims chaperones, involved into the import and translocation of proteins and metabolites in the mitochondria, Tid1, a co-chaperone involved in mitochondrial homeostasis and cell apoptosis, and Hep1 that favors mtHSP70 folding and regulate mitochondrial proteostasis (Petrakis et al., 2009; Blamowska et al., 2012; Cheng et al., 2016). It is likely that new mitochondrial chaperones are still to be discovered.

CHAPERONES IN PHYSIOLOGICAL EXERCISE

It has been demonstrated in animals and humans that physiological stress induced by exercise modulates the activity and expression of HSPs in many tissues. Indeed, during exhaustive or very intense exercise, the temperature of the muscles can reach 45°C, which can represent a thermal shock able to induce HSPs expression. Moreover, other events, such as oxidative stress (i.e., augmented levels of $O_2^{\bullet-}$ and H_2O_2), muscle damage and inflammatory response, can occur in this type of exercise and may represent stimuli able to induce HSP expression. Nevertheless, although the production of ROS may play an important role in mediating the expression of chaperones, no definitive evidences for a redox mechanism exist in the exercise-induced chaperone expression (Dimauro et al.,

2016; Henstridge et al., 2016). Both acute and chronic exercise modulates the expression of specific HSPs in different organs in a sex-dependent and species-specific manner (Dimauro et al., 2016; Henstridge et al., 2016). Several scientific studies have described the probable relationship between induction of different HSPs and ROS generated after acute exercise in humans. Salo et al. (1991) reported that in rats, after intense and exhaustive exercise, the levels of more than 15 HSPs, including HSP70, increase in heart, liver and skeletal muscle tissues. In addition to HSP70, also αB-crystallin, HSP27, HSP60 and HSP90 were described among the chaperones induced by acute exercise in *vastus lateralis* muscle and blood cells (Fehrenbach et al., 2000; Khassaf et al., 2001; Fischer et al., 2006; Petersen et al., 2012). Other studies have suggested that also various types of chronic exercise could promote an adaptive homeostatic process that modulates the expression of different HSPs in humans. Also in this case, HSP70, αB-crystallin, HSP27, and HSP60 are upregulated and associated to a redox response. Indeed, it has been reported a good correlation between oxidative enzymes and HSP expression in skeletal muscle (Vogt et al., 2001; Morton et al., 2008; Cumming et al., 2014) and/or blood cells (i.e., leukocytes) (Simar et al., 2012; Ziemann et al., 2013; Beltran Valls et al., 2014). During repeated bouts of exercise, in the training period, the expression of stress-proteins, as the aforementioned HSPs, can occur together with the expression of antioxidants, leading to a homeostatic adaptation. This adaptation brings gradually back the HSP levels. Indeed, after weeks of training the levels of HSP70 and HSP27 return to pre-exercise levels and animals that have successfully completed a resistance training program no longer show increases in HSPs performing the training exercises. It seems that the acquired pro-reducing conditions of trained animals prevent HSP induction by ROS (Salo et al., 1991; Beltran Valls et al., 2014). Obviously, this will only be true as long as physical exercise is maintained, so that, in case of detraining, it will bring back the redox status and the new exercise bouts will be able to re-induce "stress" and the expression of HSPs (Davies, 2016).

Though the precise mechanisms linking redox aspects and HSP modulation during physiologic exercise is still not completely understood, a ROS-mediated modulation of HSP expression may be present during acute exercise and a putative homeostatic process, underpinning the involvement of several small HSPs, is described for chronic exercise (Cumming et al., 2014).

CHAPERONES IN MYOCARDIAL ISCHEMIA/REPERFUSION INJURY AND CARDIOPROTECTION

In the heart, the mismatch between oxygen supply and demand leads to myocardial ischemia, which has deleterious effects, ranging from contractile impairment to cell death. The damage due to ischemia may be exacerbated by reperfusion, inducing an I/R injury.

ROS/RNS formation and impaired antioxidant capacity are among the proposed mechanisms to explain the myocardial I/R injury. The unbalanced redox changes lead to the dysfunction of protective molecules against cellular death, including deregulation of chaperones and co-chaperones. Indeed, if chaperones do not work properly, misfolded proteins cannot be repaired and may form insoluble aggregates. These aggregates are highly dangerous for the cells and may participate in the processes leading to cardiomyocyte death and consequently to cardiovascular diseases, such as arrhythmias, dilated cardiomyopathy and heart failure (Willis and Patterson, 2010, 2013; Tarone and Brancaccio, 2014, 2015).

Although prolonged episodes of ischemia followed by reperfusion induce damage, transient episodes (a few minutes or seconds) of ischemia before or after a prolonged cardiac ischemia may induce cardioprotection with consequent reduction of infarct size, myocardial dysfunction, and arrhythmias. These procedures are referred to as ischemic preconditioning (IP) or post-conditioning (PostC), respectively (Penna et al., 2014a). Also, transient episodes of ischemia in a remote organ before (remote ischemic pre-conditioning), during (remote per-conditioning) or after (remote post-conditioning) a prolonged ischemic insult can attenuate myocardial I/R injury (Lau et al., 2017). Other physiological procedures able to induce cardioprotection are repeated short-term episodes of exercise (exercise preconditioning), that can trigger a phenotype similar to that induced by IP (Yuan et al., 2018). The same protection could be obtained with pharmacological tools (Penna et al., 2014a), given before, during or after an ischemic insult, known as pharmacological conditioning. The cardioprotective mechanisms of the various conditioning procedures (ischemic, remote or pharmacological) are strongly associated. They may induce two windows of cardioprotection: early preconditioning (first window of protection) and late preconditioning (second window of protection) (Yuan et al., 2018).

Ischemia/reperfusion as well as cardioprotective maneuvers may affect transcription factors regulating chaperones, co-chaperones, and several HSPs. In particular, a number of experimental studies report that increasing chaperones, and especially HSPs, may improve the outcome of I/R injury. Indeed, an important role for HSPs has been described in both the first and second window of protection (Dangi et al., 2015). Moreover, several drugs may be potentially cardioprotective because of their ability to affect the family of heat shock transcription factors and to promote HSP expression within the heart (Willis and Patterson, 2010, 2013; Tarone and Brancaccio, 2014).

Among transcription factors regulating chaperones, the enhancement of heat shock transcription factor 1 (HSF-1), but not the HSF-2 activity has been described after cardiac I/R in post-ischemic rat heart (Nishizawa et al., 1996). Subsequently, it has been observed that HSF-1 induction in I/R is mediated by ROS and ATP levels (Chang et al., 2001; David et al., 2013). Also, X-box binding protein 1 (XBP1), a transcription factor involved in the endoplasmic reticulum chaperone neo-formation regulates the cellular response to ischemia. Indeed, in hypoxic conditions, a dominant-negative form of XBP1 determines an increase in apoptosis in cardiomyocytes (Thuerauf et al., 2006). Moreover, activating transcription factor 6 (ATF6), a transcription factor boosting endoplasmic reticulum chaperone synthesis that is involved in the unfolded protein response, induces enhanced expression of GRP78 and GRP94 chaperones in response to I/R. ATF6 pharmacological blockade impairs heart function and augments the mortality rate after myocardial ischemia (Delisle et al., 2004; Toko et al., 2010).

HSP72/HSP70 (also known as inducible HSP70) has been the focus of many types of research in I/R and cardioprotection fields. Indeed, it has been reported that HSP70 and small HSPs, such as HSP27, induce cardioprotection against irreversible injury associated with I/R (Moghimian et al., 2014). HSP72 seems to increase at 1 week after coronary artery occlusion (Tanonaka et al., 2003). Its expression in rat hearts, induced after a single oral dose of geranylgeranyl acetone, an antiulcer agent, protects against I/R injury (Ooie et al., 2001). The expression of HSP70, instead, is rapidly induced in the ischemic-reperfused heart (Nishizawa et al., 1996). Cardioprotective effects of HSP70 have been reported in isolated adult cardiac myocytes and in transgenic mouse hearts (Knowlton et al., 1991; Heads et al., 1995; Plumier et al., 1995; Lepore et al., 2001; Okubo et al., 2001). HSP72/HSP70 participates to cardioprotection induced by exercise preconditioning, early and late protection, where HSP70 repairs unfolded proteins or may stabilize the function of the endoplasmic reticulum (Yuan et al., 2018). Although several pieces of evidence suggest that brief ischemia triggers the expression of HSP70 (Polla, 1988; Knowlton et al., 1991; Sun et al., 1995) and that HSP70 is actively associated with myocardial protection (Marber et al., 1995; Plumier et al., 1995; Chiu et al., 2003; Guisasola et al., 2006), it has been suggested that the induction of HSP72, as end effectors of protection in ischemic preconditioning, does not occur in the first, but in the second window of protection.

The overexpression of HSP70 seems also to augment the $NO^{\bullet}$ production in response to cytokine stimulation, thus protecting cultured cells from TNFα injury (Latchman, 2001). HSP70 is also present in the exosomes, small vesicles released from cells into the blood. They can transmit signals with activation of protective pathways in cardiomyocytes via toll-like receptor (TLR) 4. The cardioprotective mechanism of exosomes seems mediated by HSP70, which activates a pathway downstream of TLR4, with action on ERK1/2 and p38MAPK and phosphorylation of HSP27 (Vicencio et al., 2015).

HSP90 is essential for the integrity and correct function of numerous signaling proteins. The increased expression of HSP90 has been described in the myocardium after I/R (Nishizawa et al., 1996). Indeed, during the ischemic preconditioning, HSP90 is activated by situations of cellular stress and facilitates the mitochondrial importation of cytosolic proteins (Jiao et al., 2008). Intriguingly, HSP90 is involved in the mitochondrial importation of connexin 43, which together with the adenosine triphosphate-sensitive K^+ channels, is fundamental in cardioprotection from ischemic preconditioning (Rodriguez-Sinovas et al., 2006; Jiao et al., 2008). Furthermore, PostC improves the translocation of PKCε to mitochondria in an HSP90-dependent manner (Zhong et al., 2014). HSP90 is involved in the reduction of apoptosis and cardiomyocyte necrosis, favoring the induction of Bcl-2 anti-apoptotic protein and the inhibition of pro-apoptotic Bax in the mitochondrial fraction (Zhong et al., 2014; **Figure 3**). Yet, HSP90 binds NOS3 and stimulates its activity (Latchman, 2001) and its overexpression has been reported to reduce I/R lesions via the Akt/NOS3 pathway (Kupatt et al., 2004).

As said above, an HSP90 homolog is the TRAP1/HSP75. It is targeted to mitochondria where is fundamental for mitochondrial integrity and protection from cell death caused by oxidative stress (Montesano Gesualdi et al., 2007). Recent studies have reported the protective action of TRAP1 against I/R-induced mitochondria dysfunction and cell injury (Zhang et al., 2015). In cardiac models both I/R and hypoxia/reoxygenation protocols induced TRAP1 (Xiang et al., 2010; Kim et al., 2012). Its overexpression hinders hypoxia-induced mitochondrial injury and cell death also in isolated rat cardiomyocytes (Williamson et al., 2008).

Melusin is a chaperone protein selectively expressed in cardiac and skeletal muscles, able to act as co-chaperone in the HSP90 machinery. Melusin limits cardiomyocyte death and ameliorates adaptive hypertrophy signaling pathways in response to different stress conditions, including cardiac I/R (Penna et al., 2014b; Tarone and Brancaccio, 2015). The overexpression of Melusin confers resistance to cardiac I/R injury via activation of AKT and ERK kinases and increasing HSP90 expression (Penna et al., 2014b).

HSP60 is a chaperone considered as a good marker for monitoring myocardial damage and heart failure. Intriguingly, high anti-HSP60 antibody levels correlate with high levels of brain natriuretic peptide and with left ventricular end-diastolic dimension, and the HSP60 levels correlate with the extent of cardiac dysfunction (Novo et al., 2011). It has been reported that HSP60 increases few weeks after coronary artery occlusion in rat heart (Tanonaka et al., 2003; Toga et al., 2007; Wang et al., 2010). Also in human ischemic heart disease, HSP60 doubled its expression in comparison to control subjects (Knowlton et al.,

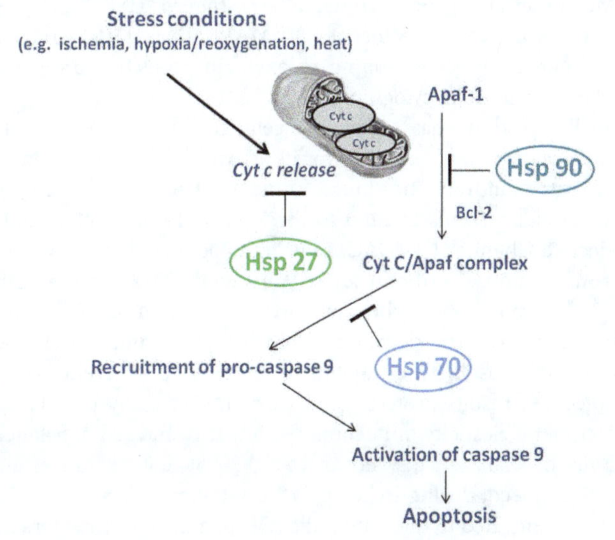

FIGURE 3 | Overview of mitochondrial chaperone proteins.

1998). HSP60 has different localizations: it is present in the exosomes and in the extra-mitochondrial cytosol of several cells. In the cardiac tissue, the cytosolic HSP60 forms complexes with Bax, Bak, and Bcl-XL, but not with Bcl-2. During hypoxia, HSP60 cellular distribution changes, leaving the cytosol and translocating to the plasma membrane (Gupta and Knowlton, 2005). In ischemic heart disease, instead, HSP60 translocates from the cytoplasm to mitochondria (Sidorik et al., 2005). Increased expression of cardiac HSP60 after 9–12 weeks of coronary artery ligation in rats has been correlated with NF-κB activation (Wang et al., 2010). However, it has been proposed that low doses of lipopolysaccharide could provide a means of reducing myocardial I/R injury by increasing HSP70 with a subsequent inhibition of NF-κB (Yao et al., 2011). This apparent discrepancy on the role of NF-κB may reflect the importance of a sequential involvement of the different chaperones in determining the protective effects in the I/R context.

HSP56/FKBP52 is part of the family of FK506-binding proteins (FKBPs) and behaves as a co-chaperone associated with HSP90 in steroid receptor complexes (Carroll et al., 2011). Recently, it has been reported that in mice the overexpression of HSP56 neither induces myocardial hypertrophy nor protects the intact heart from I/R-injury (Carroll et al., 2011). Although, HSP56 has cardiac action, it seems not protective also when induced by the cardiac-derived peptide cardiotrophin-1, which has cardioprotective properties (Brar et al., 2001).

Small HSPs involved in the response to I/R include HSP20, HSP22, HSP27 and αB-crystallin, which are often increased in response to stress. HSP27 and αB-crystallin increase in response to stress to protect against insults such as I/R (Efthymiou et al., 2004; Arrigo et al., 2007). These two proteins are vital to muscle development and assembly (Brown et al., 2007). Indeed, HSPB2/HSP27 overexpression limits I/R injury in adult cardiomyocytes (Vander Heide, 2002). Elevated levels of HSP27 may also participate to cardioprotection with anti-apoptotic effects. They preserve the integrity of actin cytoskeleton and microtubules and protect the endothelium from ischemia (Mehlen et al., 1996; Latchman, 2001). Indeed, HSP27 behaves as a downstream effector of p38 MAPK during ischemic or β-adrenergic preconditioning or oxytocin protective protocols (Marais et al., 2005; Moghimian et al., 2014).

αB-crystallin has different cellular locations and its phosphorylation is necessary for its activation and translocation to mitochondria and microfilaments (Jin et al., 2008). αB-crystallin seems to bind to the Voltage-Dependent Anion-selective Channel 1 (VDAC1) during hypoxic/redox stresses in neonatal mouse cardiomyocytes (Chis et al., 2012) and to both VDAC1 and ANT during myocardial infarction. αB-crystallin mitochondrial translocation inhibits cytochrome c release into the cytosol. αB-crystallin, by binding to different target molecules, results protective for cardiomyocytes by preserving sarcomeric elasticity, mitochondrial integrity and redox balance (Bullard et al., 2004; Maloyan et al., 2005; Rajasekaran et al., 2007). Indeed, during ischemia, αB-crystallin is phosphorylated and translocated to the contractile cell apparatus where interacts with several cytoskeletal proteins, such as desmin and actin, to maintain protein folding and to prevent aggregation (Bennardini et al., 1992; Djabali et al., 1997; Golenhofen et al., 1998; Wang et al., 2002, 2003). After I/R insult, αB-crystallin translocates to mitochondria (Martindale et al., 2005) where it may exert cardioprotective effects. Indeed, αB-crystallin KO mice show decreased contractile recovery with increased necrosis and apoptosis (Ray et al., 2001; Morrison et al., 2004; Bousette et al., 2010). Yet, cardioprotective post-conditioning induces a preservation of αB-crystallin levels in pigs and αB-crystallin-peptide administration in mice limits infarct area (Cubedo et al., 2016). Recently, it has been reported that subchronic nandrolone administration limits cardiac oxidative stress by inducing the expression of antioxidant proteins, comprising αB-crystallin, thus contributing to amelioration of post-ischemic heart performance (Pergolizzi et al., 2017).

HSP20/HSPB6 is a small HSP located in the cytoplasm that may translocate in part into the nucleus after a heart stress. Induced expression of HSP20/HSPB6 limits apoptosis and infarct size and improves cardiac contractility. HSP20 expression in I/R seems regulated, at least in part, by miR-320 (Ren et al., 2009). Inhibition of HSP20 phosphorylation may exacerbate cardiac I/R damage by suppressing autophagy and increasing other modalities of cell death (Qian et al., 2009; Edwards et al., 2011; Fan and Kranias, 2011). In ischemic conditions, HSP20 is associated to the sarcomeric structure in cardiac and skeletal muscle, as well as in cardiac myoblast cell line, H9C2 (van de Klundert and de Jong, 1999; Verschuure et al., 2002; Golenhofen et al., 2004). In cardiac cells, isoproterenol treatment induced a redistribution of HSP20 to the cytoskeleton and co-localization with actin. HSP20 can be phosphorylated in three phosphorylation sites: serine 16 by PKA/PKG; serine 59 through PKC; and serine 157 via insulin stimulation (Fan et al., 2005). Its phosphorylation at Ser16 may provide cardioprotection against β-agonist-induced apoptosis (Fan et al., 2004). Moreover, HSP20 may interact with the Bcl-2 family and the proapoptotic protein Bax. The anti-apoptotic effect of HSP20 is mediated by PKA pathway, and it prevents the translocation of Bax from the cytosol to the mitochondria, thus limiting cytochrome c release and caspase-3 activation (Fan et al., 2005).

HSPB8/HSP22 is another small HSP whose expression is swiftly induced after ischemia. It is increased also 3-fold in a pig model 1 h after reperfusion following ischemia (Depre et al., 2001) and in the hibernating myocardium in humans and swine (Depre et al., 2004). Indeed HSP22 overexpression limits apoptosis and infarct size (Depre et al., 2006; Sui et al., 2009).

Also, co-chaperones are important in determining the response to I/R stress. DnaJ-like pDJA1 increases 4-fold after reperfusion in a pig model of I/R (Depre et al., 2003). BAG-1, another co-chaperone, protects against I/R induced apoptosis (Salo et al., 1991). CHIP, a co-chaperone/ubiquitin ligase involved in protein quality control, is necessary for optimal cardioprotection after coronary occlusion in mice. Indeed, CHIP KO mouse shows a larger infarct size (Zhang et al., 2005). Ubiquitin *(UB)* is a small molecular weight protein best known for its role in the proteasomal degradation of damaged proteins. Recently, it has been reported that exogenous and prolonged treatment with UB before I/R protocol, reduces infarct size, improves heart function and decreases inflammatory response.

Whether this protection occurs with the intervention of CHIP is not clear yet (Fehrenbach et al., 2000).

CONCLUSIONS

Protein misfolding and aggregation are emerging as crucial mechanisms in inducing cardiomyopathy and ischemic damage. The ability of chaperone proteins to inhibit unfolded protein aggregation inducing their degradation and to potentiate beneficial signal transduction pathways in cardiomyocytes is responsible for chaperone-mediated cardioprotection in different pathological conditions. ROS/RNS production in the myocardium causes protein modification and unfolding, inducing mitochondrial dysfunction and cardiomyocyte loss. However, the increase in ROS/RNS levels, besides inducing chaperone expression through the activation of specific transcription factors, likely modify cardiac chaperones directly on amino acid residues and/or formation of disulfide bonds, promoting cell survival and cardiac function. This is a fascinating possibility that would contribute to explain the mechanism of conditioning in heart protection and open the way to new possible therapeutic interventions.

AUTHOR CONTRIBUTIONS

All authors listed have made a substantial, direct and intellectual contribution to the work, and approved it for publication.

ACKNOWLEDGMENTS

This work was supported by Italian Ministry of Education, University and Research (Progetto di Ricerca PRIN 2015) to MB and by Compagnia di San Paolo/University of Torino (Progetti di ricerca di Ateneo 2016) to MB and CP.

REFERENCES

Anand, P., and Stamler, J. S. (2012). Enzymatic mechanisms regulating protein S-nitrosylation: implications in health and disease. *J. Mol. Med.* 90, 233–244. doi: 10.1007/s00109-012-0878-z

Arai, M., Imai, H., Koumura, T., Yoshida, M., Emoto, K., Umeda, M., et al. (1999). Mitochondrial phospholipid hydroperoxide glutathione peroxidase plays a major role in preventing oxidative injury to cells. *J. Biol. Chem.* 274, 4924–4933. doi: 10.1074/jbc.274.8.4924

Arndt, V., Dick, N., Tawo, R., Dreiseidler, M., Wenzel, D., Hesse, M., et al. (2010). Chaperone-assisted selective autophagy is essential for muscle maintenance. *Curr. Biol.* 20, 143–148. doi: 10.1016/j.cub.2009.11.022

Arrigo, A. P., Simon, S., Gibert, B., Kretz-Remy, C., Nivon, M., Czekalla, A., et al. (2007). Hsp27 (HspB1) and alphaB-crystallin (HspB5) as therapeutic targets. *FEBS Lett.* 581, 3665–3674. doi: 10.1016/j.febslet.2007.04.033

Bakthisaran, R., Tangirala, R., and Rao Ch, M. (2015). Small heat shock proteins: role in cellular functions and pathology. *Biochim. Biophys. Acta* 1854, 291–319. doi: 10.1016/j.bbapap.2014.12.019

Baumann, F., Milisav, I., Neupert, W., and Herrmann, J. M. (2000). Ecm10, a novel hsp70 homolog in the mitochondrial matrix of the yeast Saccharomyces cerevisiae. *FEBS Lett.* 487, 307–312. doi: 10.1016/S0014-5793(00)02364-4

Beer, S. M., Taylor, E. R., Brown, S. E., Dahm, C. C., Costa, N. J., Runswick, M. J., et al. (2004). Glutaredoxin 2 catalyzes the reversible oxidation and glutathionylation of mitochondrial membrane thiol proteins: implications for mitochondrial redox regulation and antioxidant DEFENSE. *J. Biol. Chem.* 279, 47939–47951. doi: 10.1074/jbc.M408011200

Beigi, F., Gonzalez, D. R., Minhas, K. M., Sun, Q. A., Foster, M. W., Khan, S. A., et al. (2012). Dynamic denitrosylation via S-nitrosoglutathione reductase regulates cardiovascular function. *Proc. Natl. Acad. Sci. U.S.A.* 109, 4314–4319. doi: 10.1073/pnas.1113319109

Beltran Valls, M. R., Dimauro, I., Brunelli, A., Tranchita, E., Ciminelli, E., Caserotti, P., et al. (2014). Explosive type of moderate-resistance training induces functional, cardiovascular, and molecular adaptations in the elderly. *Age* 36, 759–772. doi: 10.1007/s11357-013-9584-1

Benhar, M., Forrester, M. T., and Stamler, J. S. (2009). Protein denitrosylation: enzymatic mechanisms and cellular functions. *Nat. Rev. Mol. Cell Biol.* 10, 721–732. doi: 10.1038/nrm2764

Benhar, M., Forrester, M. T., Hess, D. T., and Stamler, J. S. (2008). Regulated protein denitrosylation by cytosolic and mitochondrial thioredoxins. *Science* 320, 1050–1054. doi: 10.1126/science.1158265

Bennardini, F., Wrzosek, A., and Chiesi, M. (1992). Alpha B-crystallin in cardiac tissue. Association with actin and desmin filaments. *Circ. Res.* 71, 288–294. doi: 10.1161/01.RES.71.2.288

Blamowska, M., Neupert, W., and Hell, K. (2012). Biogenesis of the mitochondrial Hsp70 chaperone. *J. Cell Biol.* 199, 125–135. doi: 10.1083/jcb.201205012

Bousette, N., Chugh, S., Fong, V., Isserlin, R., Kim, K. H., Volchuk, A., et al. (2010). Constitutively active calcineurin induces cardiac endoplasmic reticulum stress and protects against apoptosis that is mediated by alpha-crystallin-B. *Proc. Natl. Acad. Sci. U.S.A.* 107, 18481–18486. doi: 10.1073/pnas.1013555107

Brar, B. K., Stephanou, A., Pennica, D., and Latchman, D. S. (2001). CT-1 mediated cardioprotection against ischaemic re-oxygenation injury is mediated by PI3 kinase, Akt and MEK1/2 pathways. *Cytokine* 16, 93–96. doi: 10.1006/cyto.2001.0951

Brinker, A., Pfeifer, G., Kerner, M. J., Naylor, D. J., Hartl, F. U., and Hayer-Hartl, M. (2001). Dual function of protein confinement in chaperonin-assisted protein folding. *Cell* 107, 223–233. doi: 10.1016/S0092-8674(01)00517-7

Brown, D. D., Christine, K. S., Showell, C., and Conlon, F. L. (2007). Small heat shock protein Hsp27 is required for proper heart tube formation. *Genesis* 45, 667–678. doi: 10.1002/dvg.20340

Brown, G. C., and Borutaite, V. (2007). Nitric oxide and mitochondrial respiration in the heart. *Cardiovasc. Res.* 75, 283–290. doi: 10.1016/j.cardiores.2007.03.022

Bullard, B., Ferguson, C., Minajeva, A., Leake, M. C., Gautel, M., Labeit, D., et al. (2004). Association of the chaperone alphaB-crystallin with titin in heart muscle. *J. Biol. Chem.* 279, 7917–7924. doi: 10.1074/jbc.M307473200

Bulteau, A. L., Lundberg, K. C., Humphries, K. M., Sadek, H. A., Szweda, P. A., Friguet, B., et al. (2001). Oxidative modification and inactivation of the proteasome during coronary occlusion/reperfusion. *J. Biol. Chem.* 276, 30057–30063. doi: 10.1074/jbc.M100142200

Calderwood, S. K., Gong, J., and Murshid, A. (2016). Extracellular HSPs: the complicated roles of extracellular HSPs in immunity. *Front. Immunol.* 7:159. doi: 10.3389/fimmu.2016.00159

Carra, S., Seguin, S. J., and Landry, J. (2008). HspB8 and Bag3: a new chaperone complex targeting misfolded proteins to macroautophagy. *Autophagy* 4, 237–239. doi: 10.4161/auto.5407

Carroll, C. J., Suleman, N., Davidson, S. M., Faulkes, D. J., Diss, J. K., Knight, R., et al. (2011). Transgenic overexpression of HSP56 does not result in cardiac hypertrophy nor protect from ischaemia/reperfusion injury. *Int. J. Biochem. Cell Biol.* 43, 74–79. doi: 10.1016/j.biocel.2010.09.020

Chang, J., Knowlton, A. A., Xu, F., and Wasser, J. S. (2001). Activation of the heat shock response: relationship to energy metabolites. A ^{31}P NMR study in rat hearts. *Am. J. Physiol. Heart Circ. Physiol.* 280, H426–H433. doi: 10.1152/ajpheart.2001.280.1.H426

Chen, W. Y., Chang, F. R., Huang, Z. Y., Chen, J. H., Wu, Y. C., and Wu, C. C. (2008). Tubocapsenolide A, a novel withanolide, inhibits proliferation and induces apoptosis in MDA-MB-231 cells by thiol oxidation of heat shock proteins. *J. Biol. Chem.* 283, 17184–17193. doi: 10.1074/jbc.M709447200

Cheng, L. H., Hung, K. F., Lee, T. C., Huang, C. Y., Chiu, W. T., Lo, J. F., et al. (2016). Mitochondrial co-chaperone protein Tid1 is required for energy homeostasis during skeletal myogenesis. *Stem Cell Res. Ther.* 7:185. doi: 10.1186/s13287-016-0443-8

Chis, R., Sharma, P., Bousette, N., Miyake, T., Wilson, A., Backx, P. H., et al. (2012). alpha-Crystallin B prevents apoptosis after H_2O_2 exposure in mouse neonatal cardiomyocytes. *Am. J. Physiol. Heart Circ. Physiol.* 303, H967–H978. doi: 10.1152/ajpheart.00040.2012

Chiu, J. H., Tsou, M. T., Tung, H. H., Tai, C. H., Tsai, S. K., Chih, C. L., et al. (2003). Preconditioned somatothermal stimulation on median nerve territory increases myocardial heat shock protein 70 and protects rat hearts against ischemia-reperfusion injury. *J. Thorac. Cardiovasc. Surg.* 125, 678–685. doi: 10.1067/mtc.2003.29

Chong, K. Y., Lai, C. C., Lille, S., Chang, C., and Su, C. Y. (1998). Stable overexpression of the constitutive form of heat shock protein 70 confers oxidative protection. *J. Mol. Cell. Cardiol.* 30, 599–608. doi: 10.1006/jmcc.1997.0623

Christians, E. S., Ishiwata, T., and Benjamin, I. J. (2012). Small heat shock proteins in redox metabolism: implications for cardiovascular diseases. *Int. J. Biochem. Cell Biol.* 44, 1632–1645. doi: 10.1016/j.biocel.2012.06.006

Christians, E. S., Mustafi, S. B., and Benjamin, I. J. (2014). Chaperones and cardiac misfolding protein diseases. *Curr. Protein Pept. Sci.* 15, 189–204. doi: 10.2174/1389203715666140331111518

Conway, M. E., and Lee, C. (2015). The redox switch that regulates molecular chaperones. *Biomol. Concepts* 6, 269–284. doi: 10.1515/bmc-2015-0015

Cubedo, J., Vilahur, G., Casaní, L., Mendieta, G., Gómez-Jabalera, E., Juan-Babot, O., et al. (2016). Targeting the molecular mechanisms of ischemic damage: protective effects of alpha-crystallin-B. *Int. J. Cardiol.* 215, 406–416. doi: 10.1016/j.ijcard.2016.04.072

Cumming, K. T., Raastad, T., Holden, G., Bastani, N. E., Schneeberger, D., Paronetto, M. P., et al. (2014). Effects of vitamin C and E supplementation on endogenous antioxidant systems and heat shock proteins in response to endurance training. *Physiol. Rep.* 2:e12142. doi: 10.14814/phy2.12142

Dangi, S. S., Gupta, M., Dangi, S. K., Chouhan, V. S., Maurya, V. P., Kumar, P., et al. (2015). Expression of HSPs: an adaptive mechanism during long-term heat stress in goats (Capra hircus). *Int. J. Biometeorol.* 59, 1095–1106. doi: 10.1007/s00484-014-0922-5

D'Autréaux, B., and Toledano, M. B. (2007). ROS as signalling molecules: mechanisms that generate specificity in ROS homeostasis. *Nat. Rev. Mol. Cell Biol.* 8, 813–824. doi: 10.1038/nrm2256

David, S., Bucchieri, F., Corrao, S., Czarnecka, A. M., Campanella, C., Farina, F., et al. (2013). Hsp10: anatomic distribution, functions, and involvement in human disease. *Front. Biosci.* 5, 768–778. doi: 10.2741/E657

Davies, K. J. (2016). Adaptive homeostasis. *Mol. Aspects Med.* 49, 1–7. doi: 10.1016/j.mam.2016.04.007

Dekker, P. J., and Pfanner, N. (1997). Role of mitochondrial GrpE and phosphate in the ATPase cycle of matrix Hsp70. *J. Mol. Biol.* 270, 321–327. doi: 10.1006/jmbi.1997.1131

Del Monte, F., and Agnetti, G. (2014). Protein post-translational modifications and misfolding: new concepts in heart failure. *Proteomics Clin. Appl.* 8, 534–542. doi: 10.1002/prca.201400037

Delisle, B. P., Anson, B. D., Rajamani, S., and January, C. T. (2004). Biology of cardiac arrhythmias: ion channel protein trafficking. *Circ. Res.* 94, 1418–1428. doi: 10.1161/01.RES.0000128561.28701.ea

Depre, C., Kim, S. J., John, A. S., Huang, Y., Rimoldi, O. E., Pepper, J. R., et al. (2004). Program of cell survival underlying human and experimental hibernating myocardium. *Circ. Res.* 95, 433–440. doi: 10.1161/01.RES.0000138301.42713.18

Depre, C., Tomlinson, J. E., Kudej, R. K., Gaussin, V., Thompson, E., Kim, S. J., et al. (2001). Gene program for cardiac cell survival induced by transient ischemia in conscious pigs. *Proc. Natl. Acad. Sci. U.S.A.* 98, 9336–9341. doi: 10.1073/pnas.171297498

Depre, C., Wang, L., Sui, X., Qiu, H., Hong, C., Hedhli, N., et al. (2006). H11 kinase prevents myocardial infarction by preemptive preconditioning of the heart. *Circ. Res.* 98, 280–288. doi: 10.1161/01.RES.0000201284.45482.e8

Depre, C., Wang, L., Tomlinson, J. E., Gaussin, V., Abdellatif, M., Topper, J. N., et al. (2003). Characterization of pDJA1, a cardiac-specific chaperone found by genomic profiling of the post-ischemic swine heart. *Cardiovasc. Res.* 58, 126–135. doi: 10.1016/S0008-6363(02)00845-3

Dimauro, I., Mercatelli, N., and Caporossi, D. (2016). Exercise-induced ROS in heat shock proteins response. *Free Radic. Biol. Med.* 98, 46–55. doi: 10.1016/j.freeradbiomed.2016.03.028

Djabali, K., de Nechaud, B., Landon, F., and Portier, M. M. (1997). AlphaB-crystallin interacts with intermediate filaments in response to stress. *J. Cell Sci.* 110(Pt 21), 2759–2769.

Eaton, P., Fuller, W., and Shattock, M. J. (2002). S-thiolation of HSP27 regulates its multimeric aggregate size independently of phosphorylation. *J. Biol. Chem.* 277, 21189–21196. doi: 10.1074/jbc.M200591200

Edwards, H. V., Cameron, R. T., and Baillie, G. S. (2011). The emerging role of HSP20 as a multifunctional protective agent. *Cell. Signal.* 23, 1447–1454. doi: 10.1016/j.cellsig.2011.05.009

Efthymiou, C. A., Mocanu, M. M., de Belleroche, J., Wells, D. J., Latchmann, D. S., and Yellon, D. M. (2004). Heat shock protein 27 protects the heart against myocardial infarction. *Basic Res. Cardiol.* 99, 392–394. doi: 10.1007/s00395-004-0483-6

El Hindy, M., Hezwani, M., Corry, D., Hull, J., El Amraoui, F., Harris, M., et al. (2014). The branched-chain aminotransferase proteins: novel redox chaperones for protein disulfide isomerase–implications in Alzheimer's disease. *Antioxid. Redox Signal.* 20, 2497–2513. doi: 10.1089/ars.2012.4869

Eustace, B. K., and Jay, D. G. (2004). Extracellular roles for the molecular chaperone, hsp90. *Cell Cycle* 3, 1098–1100. doi: 10.4161/cc.3.9.1088

Fan, G. C., and Kranias, E. G. (2011). Small heat shock protein 20 (HspB6) in cardiac hypertrophy and failure. *J. Mol. Cell. Cardiol.* 51, 574–577. doi: 10.1016/j.yjmcc.2010.09.013

Fan, G. C., Chu, G., and Kranias, E. G. (2005). Hsp20 and its cardioprotection. *Trends Cardiovasc. Med.* 15, 138–141. doi: 10.1016/j.tcm.2005.05.004

Fan, G. C., Chu, G., Mitton, B., Song, Q., Yuan, Q., and Kranias, E. G. (2004). Small heat-shock protein Hsp20 phosphorylation inhibits beta-agonist-induced cardiac apoptosis. *Circ. Res.* 94, 1474–1482. doi: 10.1161/01.RES.0000129179.66631.00

Fehrenbach, E., Niess, A. M., Schlotz, E., Passek, F., Dickhuth, H. H., and Northoff, H. (2000). Transcriptional and translational regulation of heat shock proteins in leukocytes of endurance runners. *J. Appl. Physiol.* 89, 704–710. doi: 10.1152/jappl.2000.89.2.704

Fenton, W. A., Weissman, J. S., and Horwich, A. L. (1996). Putting a lid on protein folding: structure and function of the co-chaperonin, GroES. *Chem. Biol.* 3, 157–161. doi: 10.1016/S1074-5521(96)90257-4

Ficker, E., Dennis, A. T., Wang, L., and Brown, A. M. (2003). Role of the cytosolic chaperones Hsp70 and Hsp90 in maturation of the cardiac potassium channel HERG. *Circ. Res.* 92, e87–e100. doi: 10.1161/01.RES.0000079028.31393.15

Fischer, C. P., Hiscock, N. J., Basu, S., Vessby, B., Kallner, A., Sjöberg, L. B., et al. (2006). Vitamin E isoform-specific inhibition of the exercise-induced heat shock protein 72 expression in humans. *J. Appl. Physiol.* 100, 1679–1687. doi: 10.1152/japplphysiol.00421.2005

Fratelli, M., Demol, H., Puype, M., Casagrande, S., Eberini, I., Salmona, M., et al. (2002). Identification by redox proteomics of glutathionylated proteins in oxidatively stressed human T lymphocytes. *Proc. Natl. Acad. Sci. U.S.A.* 99, 3505–3510. doi: 10.1073/pnas.052592699

Giles, N. M., Watts, A. B., Giles, G. I., Fry, F. H., Littlechild, J. A., and Jacob, C. (2003). Metal and redox modulation of cysteine protein function. *Chem. Biol.* 10, 677–693. doi: 10.1016/S1074-5521(03)00174-1

Golenhofen, N., Ness, W., Koob, R., Htun, P., Schaper, W., and Drenckhahn, D. (1998). Ischemia-induced phosphorylation and translocation of stress protein alpha B-crystallin to Z lines of myocardium. *Am. J. Physiol.* 274(5 Pt 2), H1457–H1464.

Golenhofen, N., Perng, M. D., Quinlan, R. A., and Drenckhahn, D. (2004). Comparison of the small heat shock proteins alphaB-crystallin, MKBP, HSP25, HSP20, and cvHSP in heart and skeletal muscle. *Histochem. Cell Biol.* 122, 415–425. doi: 10.1007/s00418-004-0711-z

Graumann, J., Lilie, H., Tang, X., Tucker, K. A., Hoffmann, J. H., Vijayalakshmi, J., et al. (2001). Activation of the redox-regulated molecular chaperone Hsp33–a two-step mechanism. *Structure* 9, 377–387. doi: 10.1016/S0969-2126(01)00599-8

Groenendyk, J., Sreenivasaiah, P. K., Kim, D. H., Agellon, L. B., and Michalak, M. (2010). Biology of endoplasmic reticulum stress in the heart. *Circ. Res.* 107, 1185–1197. doi: 10.1161/CIRCRESAHA.110.227033

Guisasola, M. C., Desco Mdel, M., Gonzalez, F. S., Asensio, F., Dulin, E., Suarez, A., et al. (2006). Heat shock proteins, end effectors of myocardium ischemic preconditioning? *Cell Stress Chaperones* 11, 250–258. doi: 10.1379/CSC-181R1.1

Gupta, S., and Knowlton, A. A. (2005). HSP60, Bax, apoptosis and the heart. *J. Cell. Mol. Med.* 9, 51–58. doi: 10.1111/j.1582-4934.2005.tb00336.x

Guzzo, G., Sciacovelli, M., Bernardi, P., and Rasola, A. (2014). Inhibition of succinate dehydrogenase by the mitochondrial chaperone TRAP1 has anti-oxidant and anti-apoptotic effects on tumor cells. *Oncotarget* 5, 11897–11908. doi: 10.18632/oncotarget.2472

Hartl, F. U., Bracher, A., and Hayer-Hartl, M. (2011). Molecular chaperones in protein folding and proteostasis. *Nature* 475, 324–332. doi: 10.1038/nature10317

Haslbeck, M., and Vierling, E. (2015). A first line of stress defense: small heat shock proteins and their function in protein homeostasis. *J. Mol. Biol.* 427, 1537–1548. doi: 10.1016/j.jmb.2015.02.002

Hatahet, F., and Ruddock, L. W. (2009). Protein disulfide isomerase: a critical evaluation of its function in disulfide bond formation. *Antioxid. Redox Signal.* 11, 2807–2850. doi: 10.1089/ars.2009.2466

Haynes, C. M., and Ron, D. (2010). The mitochondrial UPR - protecting organelle protein homeostasis. *J. Cell Sci.* 123(Pt 22), 3849–3855. doi: 10.1242/jcs.075119

Heads, R. J., Latchman, D. S., and Yellon, D. M. (1995). Differential stress protein mRNA expression during early ischaemic preconditioning in the rabbit heart and its relationship to adenosine receptor function. *J. Mol. Cell. Cardiol.* 27, 2133–2148. doi: 10.1016/S0022-2828(95)91299-1

Henstridge, D. C., Febbraio, M. A., and Hargreaves, M. (2016). Heat shock proteins and exercise adaptations. Our knowledge thus far and the road still ahead. *J. Appl. Physiol.* 120, 683–691. doi: 10.1152/japplphysiol.00811.2015

Herrmann, J. M., Stuart, R. A., Craig, E. A., and Neupert, W. (1994). Mitochondrial heat shock protein 70, a molecular chaperone for proteins encoded by mitochondrial DNA. *J. Cell Biol.* 127, 893–902. doi: 10.1083/jcb.127.4.893

Hess, D. T., Matsumoto, A., Kim, S. O., Marshall, H. E., and Stamler, J. S. (2005). Protein S-nitrosylation: purview and parameters. *Nat. Rev. Mol. Cell Biol.* 6, 150–166. doi: 10.1038/nrm1569

Hurd, T. R., Costa, N. J., Dahm, C. C., Beer, S. M., Brown, S. E., Filipovska, A., et al. (2005a). Glutathionylation of mitochondrial proteins. *Antioxid. Redox Signal.* 7, 999–1010. doi: 10.1089/ars.2005.7.999

Hurd, T. R., Filipovska, A., Costa, N. J., Dahm, C. C., and Murphy, M. P. (2005b). Disulphide formation on mitochondrial protein thiols. *Biochem. Soc. Trans.* 33(Pt 6), 1390–1393. doi: 10.1042/BST0331390

Ilbert, M., Horst, J., Ahrens, S., Winter, J., Graf, P. C., Lilie, H., et al. (2007). The redox-switch domain of Hsp33 functions as dual stress sensor. *Nat. Struct. Mol. Biol.* 14, 556–563. doi: 10.1038/nsmb1244

Imlay, J. A. (2003). Pathways of oxidative damage. *Annu. Rev. Microbiol.* 57, 395–418. doi: 10.1146/annurev.micro.57.030502.090938

Jang, H. H., Lee, K. O., Chi, Y. H., Jung, B. G., Park, S. K., Park, J. H., et al. (2004). Two enzymes in one; two yeast peroxiredoxins display oxidative stress-dependent switching from a peroxidase to a molecular chaperone function. *Cell* 117, 625–635. doi: 10.1016/j.cell.2004.05.002

Jiao, J. D., Garg, V., Yang, B., and Hu, K. (2008). Novel functional role of heat shock protein 90 in ATP-sensitive K+ channel-mediated hypoxic preconditioning. *Cardiovasc. Res.* 77, 126–133. doi: 10.1093/cvr/cvm028

Jin, J. K., Whittaker, R., Glassy, M. S., Barlow, S. B., Gottlieb, R. A., and Glembotski, C. C. (2008). Localization of phosphorylated alphaB-crystallin to heart mitochondria during ischemia-reperfusion. *Am. J. Physiol. Heart Circ. Physiol.* 294, H337–H344. doi: 10.1152/ajpheart.00881.2007

Kang, B. H., Plescia, J., Dohi, T., Rosa, J., Doxsey, S. J., and Altieri, D. C. (2007). Regulation of tumor cell mitochondrial homeostasis by an organelle-specific Hsp90 chaperone network. *Cell* 131, 257–270. doi: 10.1016/j.cell.2007.08.028

Khassaf, M., Child, R. B., McArdle, A., Brodie, D. A., Esanu, C., and Jackson, M. J. (2001). Time course of responses of human skeletal muscle to oxidative stress induced by nondamaging exercise. *J. Appl. Physiol.* 90, 1031–1035. doi: 10.1152/jappl.2001.90.3.1031

Kim, H. K., Kang, S. W., Jeong, S. H., Kim, N., Ko, J. H., Bang, H., et al. (2012). Identification of potential target genes of cardioprotection against ischemia-reperfusion injury by express sequence tags analysis in rat hearts. *J. Cardiol.* 60, 98–110. doi: 10.1016/j.jjcc.2012.02.004

Knowlton, A. A., Brecher, P., and Apstein, C. S. (1991). Rapid expression of heat shock protein in the rabbit after brief cardiac ischemia. *J. Clin. Invest.* 87, 139–147. doi: 10.1172/JCI114963

Knowlton, A. A., Kapadia, S., Torre-Amione, G., Durand, J. B., Bies, R., Young, J., et al. (1998). Differential expression of heat shock proteins in normal and failing human hearts. *J. Mol. Cell. Cardiol.* 30, 811–818. doi: 10.1006/jmcc.1998.0646

Kriegenburg, F., Ellgaard, L., and Hartmann-Petersen, R. (2012). Molecular chaperones in targeting misfolded proteins for ubiquitin-dependent degradation. *FEBS J.* 279, 532–542. doi: 10.1111/j.1742-4658.2011.08456.x

Krzewska, J., Langer, T., and Liberek, K. (2001). Mitochondrial Hsp78, a member of the Clp/Hsp100 family in Saccharomyces cerevisiae, cooperates with Hsp70 in protein refolding. *FEBS Lett.* 489, 92–96. doi: 10.1016/S0014-5793(00)02423-6

Kupatt, C., Dessy, C., Hinkel, R., Raake, P., Daneau, G., Bouzin, C., et al. (2004). Heat shock protein 90 transfection reduces ischemia-reperfusion-induced myocardial dysfunction via reciprocal endothelial NO synthase serine 1177 phosphorylation and threonine 495 dephosphorylation. *Arterioscler. Thromb. Vasc. Biol.* 24, 1435–1441. doi: 10.1161/01.ATV.0000134300.87476.d1

Lacza, Z., Pankotai, E., and Busija, D. W. (2009). Mitochondrial nitric oxide synthase: current concepts and controversies. *Front. Biosci.* 14, 4436–4443. doi: 10.2741/3539

Latchman, D. S. (2001). Heat shock proteins and cardiac protection. *Cardiovasc. Res.* 51, 637–646. doi: 10.1016/S0008-6363(01)00354-6

Lau, J. K., Pennings, G. J., Yong, A., and Kritharides, L. (2017). Cardiac remote ischaemic preconditioning: mechanistic and clinical considerations. *Heart Lung Circ.* 26, 545–553. doi: 10.1016/j.hlc.2016.11.006

Lavery, L. A., Partridge, J. R., Ramelot, T. A., Elnatan, D., Kennedy, M. A., and Agard, D. A. (2014). Structural asymmetry in the closed state of mitochondrial Hsp90 (TRAP1) supports a two-step ATP hydrolysis mechanism. *Mol. Cell* 53, 330–343. doi: 10.1016/j.molcel.2013.12.023

Lepore, D. A., Knight, K. R., Anderson, R. L., and Morrison, W. A. (2001). Role of priming stresses and Hsp70 in protection from ischemia-reperfusion injury in cardiac and skeletal muscle. *Cell Stress Chaperones* 6, 93–96. doi: 10.1379/1466-1268(2001)006<0093:ROPSAH>2.0.CO;2

Lin, K. M., Hollander, J. M., Kao, V. Y., Lin, B., Macpherson, L., and Dillmann, W. H. (2004). Myocyte protection by 10 kD heat shock protein (Hsp10) involves the mobile loop and attenuation of the Ras GTP-ase pathway. *FASEB J.* 18, 1004–1006. doi: 10.1096/fj.03-0348fje

Lind, C., Gerdes, R., Hamnell, Y., Schuppe-Koistinen, I., von Löwenhielm, H. B., Holmgren, A., et al. (2002). Identification of S-glutathionylated cellular proteins during oxidative stress and constitutive metabolism by affinity purification and proteomic analysis. *Arch. Biochem. Biophys.* 406, 229–240. doi: 10.1016/S0003-9861(02)00468-X

Lutz, T., Westermann, B., Neupert, W., and Herrmann, J. M. (2001). The mitochondrial proteins Ssq1 and Jac1 are required for the assembly of iron sulfur clusters in mitochondria. *J. Mol. Biol.* 307, 815–825. doi: 10.1006/jmbi.2001.4527

Maloyan, A., Sanbe, A., Osinska, H., Westfall, M., Robinson, D., Imahashi, K., et al. (2005). Mitochondrial dysfunction and apoptosis underlie the pathogenic process in alpha-B-crystallin desmin-related cardiomyopathy. *Circulation* 112, 3451–3461. doi: 10.1161/CIRCULATIONAHA.105.572552

Marais, E., Genade, S., Salie, R., Huisamen, B., Maritz, S., Moolman, J. A., et al. (2005). The temporal relationship between p38 MAPK and HSP27 activation in ischaemic and pharmacological preconditioning. *Basic Res. Cardiol.* 100, 35–47. doi: 10.1007/s00395-004-0495-7

Marber, M. S., Mestril, R., Chi, S. H., Sayen, M. R., Yellon, D. M., and Dillmann, W. H. (1995). Overexpression of the rat inducible 70-kD heat stress protein in a transgenic mouse increases the resistance of the heart to ischemic injury. *J. Clin. Invest.* 95, 1446–1456. doi: 10.1172/JCI117815

Martin, J., Mayhew, M., Langer, T., and Hartl, F. U. (1993). The reaction cycle of GroEL and GroES in chaperonin-assisted protein folding. *Nature* 366, 228–233. doi: 10.1038/366228a0

Martindale, J. J., Wall, J. A., Martinez-Longoria, D. M., Aryal, P., Rockman, H. A., Guo, Y., et al. (2005). Overexpression of mitogen-activated protein kinase kinase 6 in the heart improves functional recovery from ischemia *in vitro* and protects against myocardial infarction *in vivo*. *J. Biol. Chem.* 280, 669–676. doi: 10.1074/jbc.M406690200

Martínez-Ruiz, A., Araújo, I. M., Izquierdo-Álvarez, A., Hernansanz-Agustín, P., Lamas, S., and Serrador, J. M. (2013). Specificity in S-nitrosylation: a short-range mechanism for NO signaling? *Antioxid. Redox Signal.* 19, 1220–1235. doi: 10.1089/ars.2012.5066

Martínez-Ruiz, A., Villanueva, L., González de Orduña, C., López-Ferrer, D., Higueras, M. A., Tarín, C., et al. (2005). S-nitrosylation of Hsp90 promotes the inhibition of its ATPase and endothelial nitric oxide synthase regulatory activities. *Proc. Natl. Acad. Sci. U.S.A.* 102, 8525–8530. doi: 10.1073/pnas.0407294102

McDonough, H., and Patterson, C. (2003). CHIP: a link between the chaperone and proteasome systems. *Cell Stress Chaperones* 8, 303–308. doi: 10.1379/1466-1268(2003)008<0303:CALBTC>2.0.CO;2

McLendon, P. M., and Robbins, J. (2015). Proteotoxicity and cardiac dysfunction. *Circ. Res.* 116, 1863–1882. doi: 10.1161/CIRCRESAHA.116.305372

Mehlen, P., Schulze-Osthoff, K., and Arrigo, A. P. (1996). Small stress proteins as novel regulators of apoptosis. Heat shock protein 27 blocks Fas/APO-1- and staurosporine-induced cell death. *J. Biol. Chem.* 271, 16510–16514. doi: 10.1074/jbc.271.28.16510

Moghimian, M., Faghihi, M., Karimian, S. M., Imani, A., and Mobasheri, M. B. (2014). Upregulated Hsp27 expression in the cardioprotection induced by acute stress and oxytocin in ischemic reperfused hearts of the rat. *Chin. J. Physiol.* 57, 329–334. doi: 10.4077/CJP.2014.BAC257

Montesano Gesualdi, N., Chirico, G., Pirozzi, G., Costantino, E., Landriscina, M., and Esposito, F. (2007). Tumor necrosis factor-associated protein 1 (TRAP-1) protects cells from oxidative stress and apoptosis. *Stress* 10, 342–350. doi: 10.1080/10253890701314863

Morrison, L. E., Whittaker, R. J., Klepper, R. E., Wawrousek, E. F., and Glembotski, C. C. (2004). Roles for alphaB-crystallin and HSPB2 in protecting the myocardium from ischemia-reperfusion-induced damage in a KO mouse model. *Am. J. Physiol. Heart Circ. Physiol.* 286, H847–H855. doi: 10.1152/ajpheart.00715.2003

Morton, J. P., Maclaren, D. P., Cable, N. T., Campbell, I. T., Evans, L., Kayani, A. C., et al. (2008). Trained men display increased basal heat shock protein content of skeletal muscle. *Med. Sci. Sports Exerc.* 40, 1255–1262. doi: 10.1249/MSS.0b013e31816a7171

Nijtmans, L. G., Artal, S. M., Grivell, L. A., and Coates, P. J. (2002). The mitochondrial PHB complex: roles in mitochondrial respiratory complex assembly, ageing and degenerative disease. *Cell. Mol. Life Sci.* 59, 143–155. doi: 10.1007/s00018-002-8411-0

Nishizawa, J., Nakai, A., Higashi, T., Tanabe, M., Nomoto, S., Matsuda, K., et al. (1996). Reperfusion causes significant activation of heat shock transcription factor 1 in ischemic rat heart. *Circulation* 94, 2185–2192. doi: 10.1161/01.CIR.94.9.2185

Novo, G., Cappello, F., Rizzo, M., Fazio, G., Zambuto, S., Tortorici, E., et al. (2011). Hsp60 and heme oxygenase-1 (Hsp32) in acute myocardial infarction. *Transl. Res.* 157, 285–292. doi: 10.1016/j.trsl.2011.01.003

Okubo, S., Wildner, O., Shah, M. R., Chelliah, J. C., Hess, M. L., and Kukreja, R. C. (2001). Gene transfer of heat-shock protein 70 reduces infarct size *in vivo* after ischemia/reperfusion in the rabbit heart. *Circulation* 103, 877–881. doi: 10.1161/01.CIR.103.6.877

Ooie, T., Takahashi, N., Saikawa, T., Nawata, T., Arikawa, M., Yamanaka, K., et al. (2001). Single oral dose of geranylgeranylacetone induces heat-shock protein 72 and renders protection against ischemia/reperfusion injury in rat heart. *Circulation* 104, 1837–1843. doi: 10.1161/hc3901.095771

Ostermann, J., Horwich, A. L., Neupert, W., and Hartl, F. U. (1989). Protein folding in mitochondria requires complex formation with hsp60 and ATP hydrolysis. *Nature* 341, 125–130. doi: 10.1038/341125a0

Parry, T. L., Melehani, J. H., Ranek, M. J., and Willis, M. S. (2015). Functional amyloid signaling via the inflammasome, necrosome, and signalosome: new therapeutic targets in heart failure. *Front. Cardiovasc. Med.* 2:25. doi: 10.3389/fcvm.2015.00025

Penna, C., Angotti, C., and Pagliaro, P. (2014a). Protein S-nitrosylation in preconditioning and postconditioning. *Exp. Biol. Med.* 239, 647–662. doi: 10.1177/1535370214522935

Penna, C., Brancaccio, M., Tullio, F., Rubinetto, C., Perrelli, M. G., Angotti, C., et al. (2014b). Overexpression of the muscle-specific protein, melusin, protects from cardiac ischemia/reperfusion injury. *Basic Res. Cardiol.* 109:418. doi: 10.1007/s00395-014-0418-9

Pergolizzi, B., Carriero, V., Abbadessa, G., Penna, C., Berchialla, P., De Francia, S., et al. (2017). Subchronic nandrolone administration reduces cardiac oxidative markers during restraint stress by modulating protein expression patterns. *Mol. Cell. Biochem.* 434, 51–60. doi: 10.1007/s11010-017-3036-7

Petersen, A. C., McKenna, M. J., Medved, I., Murphy, K. T., Brown, M. J., Della Gatta, P., et al. (2012). Infusion with the antioxidant N-acetylcysteine attenuates early adaptive responses to exercise in human skeletal muscle. *Acta Physiol.* 204, 382–392. doi: 10.1111/j.1748-1716.2011.02344.x

Petrakis, N., Alcock, F., and Tokatlidis, K. (2009). Mitochondrial ATP-independent chaperones. *IUBMB Life* 61, 909–914. doi: 10.1002/iub.235

Plumier, J. C., Ross, B. M., Currie, R. W., Angelidis, C. E., Kazlaris, H., Kollias, G., et al. (1995). Transgenic mice expressing the human heat shock protein 70 have improved post-ischemic myocardial recovery. *J. Clin. Invest.* 95, 1854–1860. doi: 10.1172/JCI117865

Polla, B. S. (1988). A role for heat shock proteins in inflammation? *Immunol. Today* 9, 134–137. doi: 10.1016/0167-5699(88)91199-1

Prip-Buus, C., Westerman, B., Schmitt, M., Langer, T., Neupert, W., and Schwarz, E. (1996). Role of the mitochondrial DnaJ homologue, Mdj1p, in the prevention of heat-induced protein aggregation. *FEBS Lett.* 380, 142–146. doi: 10.1016/0014-5793(96)00049-X

Qian, J., Ren, X., Wang, X., Zhang, P., Jones, W. K., Molkentin, J. D., et al. (2009). Blockade of Hsp20 phosphorylation exacerbates cardiac ischemia/reperfusion injury by suppressed autophagy and increased cell death. *Circ. Res.* 105, 1223–1231. doi: 10.1161/CIRCRESAHA.109.200378

Radi, R., Turrens, J. F., Chang, L. Y., Bush, K. M., Crapo, J. D., and Freeman, B. A. (1991). Detection of catalase in rat heart mitochondria. *J. Biol. Chem.* 266, 22028–22034.

Rajasekaran, N. S., Connell, P., Christians, E. S., Yan, L. J., Taylor, R. P., Orosz, A., et al. (2007). Human alpha B-crystallin mutation causes oxido-reductive stress and protein aggregation cardiomyopathy in mice. *Cell* 130, 427–439. doi: 10.1016/j.cell.2007.06.044

Ray, P. S., Martin, J. L., Swanson, E. A., Otani, H., Dillmann, W. H., and Das, D. K. (2001). Transgene overexpression of alphaB crystallin confers simultaneous protection against cardiomyocyte apoptosis and necrosis during myocardial ischemia and reperfusion. *FASEB J.* 15, 393–402. doi: 10.1096/fj.00-0199com

Ren, X. P., Wu, J., Wang, X., Sartor, M. A., Jones, K., Qian, J., et al. (2009). MicroRNA-320 is involved in the regulation of cardiac ischemia/reperfusion injury by targeting heat-shock protein 20. *Circulation* 119, 2357–2366. doi: 10.1161/CIRCULATIONAHA.108.814145

Rhee, S. G. (2006). Cell signaling. H_2O_2, a necessary evil for cell signaling. *Science* 312, 1882–1883. doi: 10.1126/science.1130481

Rodriguez-Sinovas, A., Boengler, K., Cabestrero, A., Gres, P., Morente, M., Ruiz-Meana, M., et al. (2006). Translocation of connexin 43 to the inner mitochondrial membrane of cardiomyocytes through the heat shock protein 90-dependent TOM pathway and its importance for cardioprotection. *Circ. Res.* 99, 93–101. doi: 10.1161/01.RES.0000230315.56904.de

Salo, D. C., Donovan, C. M., and Davies, K. J. (1991). HSP70 and other possible heat shock or oxidative stress proteins are induced in skeletal muscle, heart, and liver during exercise. *Free Radic. Biol. Med.* 11, 239–246. doi: 10.1016/0891-5849(91)90119-N

Schilke, B., Forster, J., Davis, J., James, P., Walter, W., Laloraya, S., et al. (1996). The cold sensitivity of a mutant of Saccharomyces cerevisiae lacking a mitochondrial heat shock protein 70 is suppressed by loss of mitochondrial DNA. *J. Cell Biol.* 134, 603–613. doi: 10.1083/jcb.134.3.603

Schilke, B., Voisine, C., Beinert, H., and Craig, E. (1999). Evidence for a conserved system for iron metabolism in the mitochondria of *Saccharomyces cerevisiae*. *Proc. Natl. Acad. Sci. U.S.A.* 96, 10206–10211. doi: 10.1073/pnas.96.18.10206

Schmidt, S., Strub, A., Röttgers, K., Zufall, N., and Voos, W. (2001). The two mitochondrial heat shock proteins 70, Ssc1 and Ssq1, compete for the cochaperone Mge1. *J. Mol. Biol.* 313, 13–26. doi: 10.1006/jmbi.2001.5013

Schneider, H. C., Westermann, B., Neupert, W., and Brunner, M. (1996). The nucleotide exchange factor MGE exerts a key function in the ATP-dependent cycle of mt-Hsp70-Tim44 interaction driving mitochondrial protein import. *EMBO J.* 15, 5796–5803.

Schwartz, M. P., Huang, S., and Matouschek, A. (1999). The structure of precursor proteins during import into mitochondria. *J. Biol. Chem.* 274, 12759–12764. doi: 10.1074/jbc.274.18.12759

Schwarzer, C., Barnikol-Watanabe, S., Thinnes, F. P., and Hilschmann, N. (2002). Voltage-dependent anion-selective channel (VDAC) interacts with the dynein light chain Tctex1 and the heat-shock protein PBP74. *Int. J. Biochem. Cell Biol.* 34, 1059–1070. doi: 10.1016/S1357-2725(02)00026-2

Sciacovelli, M., Guzzo, G., Morello, V., Frezza, C., Zheng, L., Nannini, N., et al. (2013). The mitochondrial chaperone TRAP1 promotes neoplastic growth by inhibiting succinate dehydrogenase. *Cell Metab.* 17, 988–999. doi: 10.1016/j.cmet.2013.04.019

Scroggins, B. T., and Neckers, L. (2007). Post-translational modification of heat-shock protein 90: impact on chaperone function. *Expert Opin. Drug Discov.* 2, 1403–1414. doi: 10.1517/17460441.2.10.1403

Sengupta, R., Ryter, S. W., Zuckerbraun, B. S., Tzeng, E., Billiar, T. R., and Stoyanovsky, D. A. (2007). Thioredoxin catalyzes the denitrosation of low-molecular mass and protein S-nitrosothiols. *Biochemistry* 46, 8472–8483. doi: 10.1021/bi700449x

Shan, Y. X., Liu, T. J., Su, H. F., Samsamshariat, A., Mestril, R., and Wang, P. H. (2003). Hsp10 and Hsp60 modulate Bcl-2 family and mitochondria apoptosis signaling induced by doxorubicin in cardiac muscle cells. *J. Mol. Cell. Cardiol.* 35, 1135–1143. doi: 10.1016/S0022-2828(03)00229-3

Sidorik, L., Kyyamova, R., Bobyk, V., Kapustian, L., Rozhko, O., Vigontina, O., et al. (2005). Molecular chaperone, HSP60, and cytochrome P450 2E1 co-expression in dilated cardiomyopathy. *Cell Biol. Int.* 29, 51–55. doi: 10.1016/j.cellbi.2004.11.011

Simar, D., Malatesta, D., Mas, E., Delage, M., and Caillaud, C. (2012). Effect of an 8-weeks aerobic training program in elderly on oxidative stress and HSP72 expression in leukocytes during antioxidant supplementation. *J. Nutr. Health Aging* 16, 155–161. doi: 10.1007/s12603-011-0106-5

Sorge, M., and Brancaccio, M. (2016). Melusin promotes a protective signal transduction cascade in stressed hearts. *Front. Mol. Biosci.* 3:53. doi: 10.3389/fmolb.2016.00053

Steglich, G., Neupert, W., and Langer, T. (1999). Prohibitins regulate membrane protein degradation by the m-AAA protease in mitochondria. *Mol. Cell. Biol.* 19, 3435–3442. doi: 10.1128/MCB.19.5.3435

Sui, X., Li, D., Qiu, H., Gaussin, V., and Depre, C. (2009). Activation of the bone morphogenetic protein receptor by H11kinase/Hsp22 promotes cardiac cell growth and survival. *Circ. Res.* 104, 887–895. doi: 10.1161/CIRCRESAHA.108.192328

Sun, J. Z., Tang, X. L., Knowlton, A. A., Park, S. W., Qiu, Y., and Bolli, R. (1995). Late preconditioning against myocardial stunning. An endogenous protective mechanism that confers resistance to postischemic dysfunction 24 h after brief ischemia in conscious pigs. *J. Clin. Invest.* 95, 388–403. doi: 10.1172/JCI1 17667

Taipale, M., Jarosz, D. F., and Lindquist, S. (2010). HSP90 at the hub of protein homeostasis: emerging mechanistic insights. *Nat. Rev. Mol. Cell Biol.* 11, 515–528. doi: 10.1038/nrm2918

Tannous, P., Zhu, H., Nemchenko, A., Berry, J. M., Johnstone, J. L., Shelton, J. M., et al. (2008). Intracellular protein aggregation is a proximal trigger of cardiomyocyte autophagy. *Circulation* 117, 3070–3078. doi: 10.1161/CIRCULATIONAHA.107.763870

Tanonaka, K., Toga, W., Yoshida, H., and Takeo, S. (2003). Myocardial heat shock protein changes in the failing heart following coronary artery ligation. *Heart Lung Circ.* 12, 60–65. doi: 10.1046/j.1444-2892.2003.00139.x

Tarone, G., and Brancaccio, M. (2014). Keep your heart in shape: molecular chaperone networks for treating heart disease. *Cardiovasc. Res.* 102, 346–361. doi: 10.1093/cvr/cvu049

Tarone, G., and Brancaccio, M. (2015). The muscle-specific chaperone protein melusin is a potent cardioprotective agent. *Basic Res. Cardiol.* 110:10. doi: 10.1007/s00395-015-0466-9

Tarone, G., and Lembo, G. (2003). Molecular interplay between mechanical and humoral signalling in cardiac hypertrophy. *Trends Mol. Med.* 9, 376–382. doi: 10.1016/S1471-4914(03)00164-3

Thuerauf, D. J., Marcinko, M., Gude, N., Rubio, M., Sussman, M. A., and Glembotski, C. C. (2006). Activation of the unfolded protein response in infarcted mouse heart and hypoxic cultured cardiac myocytes. *Circ. Res.* 99, 275–282. doi: 10.1161/01.RES.0000233317.70421.03

Tian, Z., Zheng, H., Li, J., Li, Y., Su, H., and Wang, X. (2012). Genetically induced moderate inhibition of the proteasome in cardiomyocytes exacerbates myocardial ischemia-reperfusion injury in mice. *Circ. Res.* 111, 532–542. doi: 10.1161/CIRCRESAHA.112.270983

Tocchetti, C. G., Stanley, B. A., Murray, C. I., Sivakumaran, V., Donzelli, S., Mancardi, D., et al. (2011). Playing with cardiac "redox switches": the "HNO way" to modulate cardiac function. *Antioxid. Redox Signal.* 14, 1687–1698. doi: 10.1089/ars.2010.3859

Toga, W., Tanonaka, K., and Takeo, S. (2007). Changes in Hsp60 level of the failing heart following acute myocardial infarction and the effect of long-term treatment with trandolapril. *Biol. Pharm. Bull.* 30, 105–110. doi: 10.1248/bpb.30.105

Toko, H., Takahashi, H., Kayama, Y., Okada, S., Minamino, T., Terasaki, F., et al. (2010). ATF6 is important under both pathological and physiological states in the heart. *J. Mol. Cell. Cardiol.* 49, 113–120. doi: 10.1016/j.yjmcc.2010.03.020

Tullio, F., Angotti, C., Perrelli, M. G., Penna, C., and Pagliaro, P. (2013). Redox balance and cardioprotection. *Basic Res. Cardiol.* 108:392. doi: 10.1007/s00395-013-0392-7

Turrens, J. F. (2003). Mitochondrial formation of reactive oxygen species. *J. Physiol.* 552(Pt 2), 335–344. doi: 10.1113/jphysiol.2003.049478

van de Klundert, F. A., and de Jong, W. W. (1999). The small heat shock proteins Hsp20 and alphaB-crystallin in cultured cardiac myocytes: differences in cellular localization and solubilization after heat stress. *Eur. J. Cell Biol.* 78, 567–572. doi: 10.1016/S0171-9335(99)80022-3

van Dyck, L., Dembowski, M., Neupert, W., and Langer, T. (1998). Mcx1p, a ClpX homologue in mitochondria of *Saccharomyces cerevisiae*. *FEBS Lett.* 438, 250–254. doi: 10.1016/S0014-5793(98)01310-6

Vander Heide, R. S. (2002). Increased expression of HSP27 protects canine myocytes from simulated ischemia-reperfusion injury. *Am. J. Physiol. Heart Circ. Physiol.* 282, H935–H941. doi: 10.1152/ajpheart.00660.2001

Verschuure, P., Croes, Y., van den IJssel, P. R., Quinlan, R. A., de Jong, W. W., and Boelens, W. C. (2002). Translocation of small heat shock proteins to the actin cytoskeleton upon proteasomal inhibition. *J. Mol. Cell. Cardiol.* 34, 117–128. doi: 10.1006/jmcc.2001.1493

Vicart, P., Caron, A., Guicheney, P., Li, Z., Prévost, M. C., Faure, A., et al. (1998). A missense mutation in the alphaB-crystallin chaperone gene causes a desmin-related myopathy. *Nat. Genet.* 20, 92–95. doi: 10.1038/1765

Vicencio, J. M., Yellon, D. M., Sivaraman, V., Das, D., Boi-Doku, C., Arjun, S., et al. (2015). Plasma exosomes protect the myocardium from ischemia-reperfusion injury. *J. Am. Coll. Cardiol.* 65, 1525–1536. doi: 10.1016/j.jacc.2015.02.026

Vogt, M., Puntschart, A., Geiser, J., Zuleger, C., Billeter, R., and Hoppeler, H. (2001). Molecular adaptations in human skeletal muscle to endurance training under simulated hypoxic conditions. *J. Appl. Physiol.* 91, 173–182. doi: 10.1152/jappl.2001.91.1.173

Vos, M. J., Zijlstra, M. P., Carra, S., Sibon, O. C., and Kampinga, H. H. (2011). Small heat shock proteins, protein degradation and protein aggregation diseases. *Autophagy* 7, 101–103. doi: 10.4161/auto.7.1.13935

Voth, W., and Jakob, U. (2017). Stress-activated chaperones: a first line of defense. *Trends Biochem. Sci.* 42, 899–913. doi: 10.1016/j.tibs.2017.08.006

Wachter, C., Schatz, G., and Glick, B. S. (1994). Protein import into mitochondria: the requirement for external ATP is precursor-specific whereas intramitochondrial ATP is universally needed for translocation into the matrix. *Mol. Biol. Cell* 5, 465–474. doi: 10.1091/mbc.5.4.465

Wadhwa, R., Taira, K., and Kaul, S. C. (2002). An Hsp70 family chaperone, mortalin/mthsp70/PBP74/Grp75: what, when, and where? *Cell Stress Chaperones* 7, 309–316. doi: 10.1379/1466-1268(2002)007<0309:AHFCMM>2.0.CO;2

Wadhwa, R., Takano, S., Robert, M., Yoshida, A., Nomura, H., Reddel, R. R., et al. (1998). Inactivation of tumor suppressor p53 by mot-2, a hsp70 family member. *J. Biol. Chem.* 273, 29586–29591. doi: 10.1074/jbc.273.45.29586

Wadhwa, R., Yaguchi, T., Hasan, M. K., Taira, K., and Kaul, S. C. (2003). Mortalin-MPD (mevalonate pyrophosphate decarboxylase) interactions and their role in control of cellular proliferation. *Biochem. Biophys. Res. Commun.* 302, 735–742. doi: 10.1016/S0006-291X(03)00226-2

Wang, C., Yu, J., Huo, L., Wang, L., Feng, W., and Wang, C. C. (2012). Human protein-disulfide isomerase is a redox-regulated chaperone activated by oxidation of domain a'. *J. Biol. Chem.* 287, 1139–1149. doi: 10.1074/jbc.M111.303149

Wang, L., Wang, X., and Wang, C. C. (2015). Protein disulfide-isomerase, a folding catalyst and a redox-regulated chaperone. *Free Radic. Biol. Med.* 83, 305–313. doi: 10.1016/j.freeradbiomed.2015.02.007

Wang, X., Klevitsky, R., Huang, W., Glasford, J., Li, F., and Robbins, J. (2003). AlphaB-crystallin modulates protein aggregation of abnormal desmin. *Circ. Res.* 93, 998–1005. doi: 10.1161/01.RES.0000102401.77712.ED

Wang, X., Osinska, H., Gerdes, A. M., and Robbins, J. (2002). Desmin filaments and cardiac disease: establishing causality. *J. Card. Fail.* 8, S287–S292. doi: 10.1054/jcaf.2002.129279

Wang, Y., Chen, L., Hagiwara, N., and Knowlton, A. A. (2010). Regulation of heat shock protein 60 and 72 expression in the failing heart. *J. Mol. Cell. Cardiol.* 48, 360–366. doi: 10.1016/j.yjmcc.2009.11.009

Williamson, C. L., Dabkowski, E. R., Dillmann, W. H., and Hollander, J. M. (2008). Mitochondria protection from hypoxia/reoxygenation injury with mitochondria heat shock protein 70 overexpression. *Am. J. Physiol. Heart Circ. Physiol.* 294, H249–H256. doi: 10.1152/ajpheart.00775.2007

Willis, M. S., and Patterson, C. (2010). Hold me tight: role of the heat shock protein family of chaperones in cardiac disease. *Circulation* 122, 1740–1751. doi: 10.1161/CIRCULATIONAHA.110.942250

Willis, M. S., and Patterson, C. (2013). Proteotoxicity and cardiac dysfunction–Alzheimer's disease of the heart? *N. Engl. J. Med.* 368, 455–464. doi: 10.1056/NEJMra1106180

Wink, D. A., Miranda, K. M., Katori, T., Mancardi, D., Thomas, D. D., Ridnour, L., et al. (2003). Orthogonal properties of the redox siblings nitroxyl and nitric oxide in the cardiovascular system: a novel redox paradigm. *Am. J. Physiol. Heart Circ. Physiol.* 285, H2264–H2276. doi: 10.1152/ajpheart.00531.2003

Winter, J., Ilbert, M., Graf, P. C., Ozcelik, D., and Jakob, U. (2008). Bleach activates a redox-regulated chaperone by oxidative protein unfolding. *Cell* 135, 691–701. doi: 10.1016/j.cell.2008.09.024

Xiang, F., Huang, Y. S., Shi, X. H., and Zhang, Q. (2010). Mitochondrial chaperone tumour necrosis factor receptor-associated protein 1 protects cardiomyocytes from hypoxic injury by regulating mitochondrial permeability transition pore opening. *FEBS J.* 277, 1929–1938. doi: 10.1111/j.1742-4658.2010.07615.x

Xu, Z., Horwich, A. L., and Sigler, P. B. (1997). The crystal structure of the asymmetric GroEL-GroES-(ADP)7 chaperonin complex. *Nature* 388, 741–750. doi: 10.1038/41944

Yao, Y. W., Zhang, G. H., Zhang, Y. Y., Li, W. D., Wang, C. H., Yin, C. Y., et al. (2011). Lipopolysaccharide pretreatment protects against ischemia/reperfusion injury via increase of HSP70 and inhibition of NF-kappaB. *Cell Stress Chaperones* 16, 287–296. doi: 10.1007/s12192-010-0242-6

Yoshida, S., Tsutsumi, S., Muhlebach, G., Sourbier, C., Lee, M. J., Lee, S., et al. (2013). Molecular chaperone TRAP1 regulates a metabolic switch between mitochondrial respiration and aerobic glycolysis. *Proc. Natl. Acad. Sci. U.S.A.* 110, E1604–E1612. doi: 10.1073/pnas.1220659110

Yuan, Y., Pan, S. S., and Shen, Y. J. (2018). Cardioprotection of exercise preconditioning involving heat shock protein 70 and concurrent autophagy: a potential chaperone-assisted selective macroautophagy effect. *J. Physiol. Sci.* 68, 55–67. doi: 10.1007/s12576-016-0507-7

Zhang, C., Xu, Z., He, X. R., Michael, L. H., and Patterson, C. (2005). CHIP, a cochaperone/ubiquitin ligase that regulates protein quality control, is required for maximal cardioprotection after myocardial infarction in mice. *Am. J. Physiol. Heart Circ. Physiol.* 288, H2836–H2842. doi: 10.1152/ajpheart.01122.2004

Zhang, P., Lu, Y., Yu, D., Zhang, D., and Hu, W. (2015). TRAP1 Provides protection against myocardial ischemia-reperfusion injury by ameliorating mitochondrial dysfunction. *Cell. Physiol. Biochem.* 36, 2072–2082. doi: 10.1159/000430174

Zhong, G. Q., Tu, R. H., Zeng, Z. Y., Li, Q. J., He, Y., Li, S., et al. (2014). Novel functional role of heat shock protein 90 in protein kinase C-mediated ischemic postconditioning. *J. Surg. Res.* 189, 198–206. doi: 10.1016/j.jss.2014.01.038

Ziemann, E., Zembroñ-Lacny, A., Kasperska, A., Antosiewicz, J., Grzywacz, T., Garsztka, T., et al. (2013). Exercise training-induced changes in inflammatory mediators and heat shock proteins in young tennis players. *J. Sports Sci. Med.* 12, 282–289.

8

Ticagrelor Improves Endothelial Function by Decreasing Circulating Epidermal Growth Factor (EGF)

Francesco Vieceli Dalla Sega[1,2,3], *Francesca Fortini*[1,2,3], *Giorgio Aquila*[1,2], *Rita Pavasini*[4], *Simone Biscaglia*[4], *Davide Bernucci*[4], *Annamaria Del Franco*[4], *Elisabetta Tonet*[4], *Paola Rizzo*[3,5], *Roberto Ferrari*[2,3,4] *and Gianluca Campo*[3,4*]

[1] Department of Medical Sciences, University of Ferrara, Ferrara, Italy, [2] Maria Cecilia Hospital, GVM Care & Research, E.S. Health Science Foundation, Cotignola, Italy, [3] Department of Morphology, Surgery and Experimental Medicine, University of Ferrara, Ferrara, Italy, [4] Cardiovascular Institute, Azienda Ospedaliero-Universitaria di Ferrara, Cona, Italy, [5] Laboratory for Technologies of Advanced Therapies, University of Ferrara, Ferrara, Italy

Edited by:
Pasquale Pagliaro,
Università degli Studi di Torino, Italy

Reviewed by:
Marco Moscarelli,
Imperial College London,
United Kingdom
Rossella Rota,
Bambino Gesù Ospedale Pediatrico
(IRCCS), Italy

***Correspondence:**
Gianluca Campo
cmpglc@unife.it

Ticagrelor is one of the most powerful $P2Y_{12}$ inhibitor. We have recently reported that, in patients with concomitant Stable Coronary Artery Disease (SCAD) and Chronic Obstructive Pulmonary Disease (COPD) undergoing percutaneous coronary intervention (PCI), treatment with ticagrelor, as compared to clopidogrel, is associated with an improvement of the endothelial function (Clinical Trial NCT02519608). In the present study, we showed that, in the same population, after 1 month treatment with ticagrelor, but not with clopidogrel, there is a decrease of the circulating levels of epidermal growth factor (EGF) and that these changes in circulating levels of EGF correlate with on-treatment platelet reactivity. Furthermore, in human umbilical vein endothelial cells (HUVEC) incubated with sera of the patients treated with ticagrelor, but not with clopidogrel there is an increase of p-eNOS levels. Finally, analyzing the changes in EGF and p-eNOS levels after treatment, we observed an inverse correlation between p-eNOS and EGF changes only in the ticagrelor group. Causality between EGF and eNOS activation was assessed *in vitro* in HUVEC where we showed that EGF decreases eNOS activity in a dose dependent manner. Taken together our data indicate that ticagrelor improves endothelial function by lowering circulating EGF that results in the activation of eNOS in the vascular endothelium.

Keywords: epidermal growth factor (EGF), eNOS, ticagrelor, endothelial function, stable coronary artery disease (SCAD), chronic obstructive pulmonary disease (COPD), EGF

INTRODUCTION

Ticagrelor is one of the most powerful $P2Y_{12}$ inhibitor (Motovska et al., 2018). Unlike other $P2Y_{12}$ inhibitors, ticagrelor exerts some pleiotropic effects acting mainly on endothelial function in several settings (Schnorbus et al., 2014; Li et al., 2016; Campo et al., 2017; Kim et al., 2017). In a recent randomized clinical trial, in patients with concomitant stable coronary artery disease (SCAD) and chronic obstructive pulmonary disease (COPD) undergoing percutaneous coronary intervention (PCI), we demonstrated that 1 month treatment with ticagrelor, as compared to clopidogrel, is associated with an improvement in markers of endothelial function, such as a reduction of endothelial apoptosis and endothelial nitric oxide (NO) production, a reduction in ROS levels in PBMC as well as a more effective reduction of platelet reactivity (Campo et al., 2017).

At the state of the art the reason of the effect of ticagrelor on endothelial function is not completely characterized. One of the possible mechanism behind its pleiotropic effects could be related to the ability of ticagrelor to increase adenosine plasma concentration by inhibiting the adenosine type-1 equilibrative nucleoside transporter (ENT1) (Sumaya and Storey, 2017). Nonetheless, this view has been argued by some studies showing that ticagrelor is not always able to increase adenosine plasma concentration (van den Berg et al., 2015). This implies that increased plasma adenosine, at least in some circumstances, may not represent the only mechanism by which ticagrelor improves endothelial function and that other molecular targets may be involved.

It is well-established that circulating cytokines, such as TNF-α, cause increased endothelial apoptosis and inhibit eNOS activity in endothelial cells (Agnoletti et al., 1999; Valgimigli et al., 2003). Hence, this is a sub-analysis of The comparisoN between ticAgrelor and clopidogrel effect on endoTHelial platelet ANd iNflammation parameters in patiEnts with SCAD and COPD study, aiming to investigate the underlying mechanism of ticagrelor- mediated improvement of endothelial function, comparing the effect on cytokines level of 1 month treatment of ticagrelor vs. clopidogrel, and then assessing p-eNOS levels in endothelial cells treated with patient's sera and investigating possible correlations between cytokines changes and this marker of endothelial function.

MATERIALS AND METHODS

Study Design/Population/Randomization and Interventions

This is a sub-study of the clinical trial "The comparisoN between ticAgrelor and clopidogrel effect on endoTHelial platelet ANd iNflammation parameters in patiEnts with SCAD and COPD" undergoing PCI (NATHAN-NEVER). The clinical trial was registered at www.clinicaltrials.gov with the identifier NCT02519608. The protocol was approved by "Comitato Etico Unico della Provincia di Ferrara." All subjects gave written informed consent in accordance with the Declaration of Helsinki. Details of the design of the study and the outcomes of the clinical trial are reported in Campo et al. (2017). Briefly, population inclusion criteria were: (1) age >18 years; (2) ability to provide informed written consent; (3) SCAD diagnosis with coronary artery angiography (CAA) and PCI; (4) COPD diagnosis confirmed by spirometry. Main exclusion criteria were: (1) prior administration of $P2Y_{12}$ inhibitor (clopidogrel, ticlopidine, prasugrel, ticagrelor) or of anticoagulant drugs; (2) known intolerance to clopidogrel or ticagrelor; (3) prior intracranial hemorrhage; (4) cerebrovascular accident and/or active major bleeding and/or major surgery within the last 30 days and (5) other known inflammatory chronic disorders. Randomization /interventions: 46 patients were enrolled and randomly assigned to receive, on top of aspirin, clopidogrel, or ticagrelor. To minimize potential confounding effects, randomization was stratified according to the presence of diabetes and COPD severity.

Inflammation Parameters (Cytokines/Chemokines) Analysis

Sera ($n = 20$ per group) were kept at −80°C and thawed only once before performing the MILLIPLEX MAP Human Cytokine/Chemokine Panel assay (Merck Millipore, Billerica, MA), a multiplex immunoassay, which allows the simultaneous detection and quantification of the following 29 human cytokines/chemokines: epidermal growth factor (EGF), Eotaxin, granulocyte colony-stimulating factor (G-CSF), granulocyte monocyte colony-stimulating factor (GM-CSF), interferon (IFN) -α2, IFN-γ, interleukin (IL)-10, IL-12(p40), IL-12(p70), IL-13, IL-15, 1L-17α, IL-1 receptor antagonist (ra), IL-1α, IL-1β, IL-2, IL-3, IL-4, IL-5, IL-6, IL-7, IL-8, inducible protein (IP)-10 (CXCL10), monocyte chemoattractant protein (MCP)-1, macrophage inflammatory protein (MIP)-1α, MIP-1β, tumor necrosis factor (TNF) -α, TNF-β, and vascular endothelial growth factor (VEGF). Samples were processed following the manufacturer's instructions and data were analyzed by MAGPIX instrument provided with the MILLIPLEX-Analyst Software.

Platelet Function Analysis

On-treatment platelet reactivity (PR) was assessed by the VerifyNow^{TM} system (Accumetrics, San Diego, CA, USA), using a specific assay to evaluate $P2Y_{12}$ inhibitors (VerifyNow $P2Y_{12}{}^{TM}$). The results were expressed as $P2Y_{12}$ reaction unit (PRU).

Cell Culture

HUVECs pools, purchased from Life Technologies, were plated on 1.5% gelatin-coated tissue culture dishes and maintained in basal medium M200 (Life Technologies, Carlsbad, CA, USA) containing 2% FBS and growth factors (EGM-2, Life Technologies, Carlsbad, CA, USA) at 37°C with 5% CO_2. Cells from passages 2 to 4 were actively proliferating (70–90% confluent) when samples were harvested and analyzed. EGM-2 contains EGF among other growth factors, in the experiments where HUVECs were treated with different concentrations of EGF cells were seeded and grown in EGM-2 without EGF and different concentrations of recombinant human EGF (rhEGF) were added 48 h prior to cell lysis.

ELISA

Activation of eNOS in HUVEC was assessed by ELISA (Cell Signaling Technology, Danvers, USA) with antibody specific for the phosphorylated form of eNOS (p-eNOS Ser1177) following manufacturer instructions. Briefly, HUVECs were treated for 48 h with patient's sera ($n = 18$ per group) or were grown in M200 supplemented with EGM2 without EGF. Analysis of eNOS activation were performed after 48 h incubation with patient's sera or different concentrations of rhEGF. Protein concentration of each lysate was quantified by using Pierce BCA Protein Assay Kit (Thermo Scientific, Wilmington, USA) and 10 μg of total protein extract was used for each well. Data were expressed as p-eNOS levels as absorbance at 488 nm.

Western Blot

Western blot analysis was carried out to detect expression of total eNOS and β-actin as previously described (Fortini et al., 2017). Briefly, cells were lysed in RIPA buffer and protein concentration of each lysate was quantified by Pierce BCA Protein Assay Kit (Thermo Scientific, Wilmington, USA). The same amount of total protein (10 μg) was loaded in each lane, then proteins were separated on 7% NuPAGE gels (Life Technologies, Carlsbad, CA. USA). Proteins were transferred to PVDF membranes and were incubated overnight at 4°C with primary antibodies, washed three times in TBS/Tween 0.1%, and then incubated for 1 h at room temperature with secondary peroxidase-conjugated antibodies. Membranes were washed three times in TBS/Tween 0.1% and developed using Western Lightning ECL Pro (PerkinElmer, Waltham, MA). Images were obtained by exposing membranes to Chemidoc. Immunoreactive bands were analyzed with ImageLab analysis software (Bio Rad, Hercules, CA). Mouse antibody against eNOS was from BD Biosciences (Franklin Lakes, New Jersey, USA), mouse monoclonal against β-actin and secondary anti-mouse antibody were from Sigma-Aldrich (St. Louis, MS, USA). β-actin was used for normalization in the quantitative evaluation of western blots after verifying that β-actin levels were not affected by any treatment in comparison to total protein evaluated by staining with Ponceau (Sigma-Aldrich, Saint Louis, MO).

Statistical Analysis

Normal distribution of the variables was explored with the Kolmogorov–Smirnov test and with the Shapiro test (alpha = 0.05). Variables were presented with mean ± standard deviation or median ± interquartile range. Normally distributed variables were compared by *t*-test and one-way ANOVA; otherwise the Mann-Whitney U and Kruskal-Wallis tests were used. For comparisons between two groups two-tailed unpaired Student's *t*-tests were used except for the comparisons in the before and after analysis in which two-tailed paired Student's *t*-tests were used. When more than two groups were compared, one-way ANOVA with Student-Newman-Keuls method for multiple comparisons was used. Correlations between EGF and p-eNOS or, EGF and PR were assessed using Spearman correlation test (alpha = 0.05). In cells experiments with exogenous EGF results are expressed as mean ± *SD* of at least three independent experiments. Statistical analysis was perfomed with Graphpad Prism 6.0 (Graphpad Software, La Jolla, CA).

RESULTS

Cytokines/Chemokines

As previously reported, after 1 month treatment of ticagrelor or clopidogrel, serum levels of inflammation-related cytokines/chemokines, in patients with concomitant SCAD and COPD undergoing PCI, did not statistically differ (Campo et al., 2017). In this study, the effect of each treatment on cytokine level was further investigated with a before and after statistical analysis. We found that there is a significant decrease in the serum levels of EGF in patients treated with ticagrelor, but not in the clopidogrel group. EGF serum concentration was log- normally distributed, as tested with the Kolmogorov–Smirnov test. Accordingly, EGF levels in the different groups were expressed as log[EGF] (**Figures 1A,B**) and further analyses were performed using log-transformed EGF values. Difference between log[EGF] means before and after treatment with ticagrelor was 0.21 ($p < 0.01$; 95% CI difference of means = 0.09–0.33).

Correlation Between EGF Changes and Platelet Reactivity

As previously reported, ticagrelor is more powerful in inhibiting PR compared with clopidogrel (Lemesle et al., 2015; Campo et al., 2017). After 1-month treatment, changes in EGF levels correlated with on-treatment platelet reactivity ($R = 0.355$; $p = 0.020$) (**Figure 2**).

Changes in p-eNOS Levels Changes and Correlation With EGF

In HUVECs treated with patient's sera we found an increase of p-eNOS only in those of patients treated with ticagrelor at 1 month compared to the baseline (OD 2.0 at baseline vs. 2.7 after 1 month; $p < 0.01$). Furthermore, we observed a significant difference in p-eNOS levels between HUVEC treated with the sera of the two treatment groups (OD 2.1 vs. 2.7, clopidogrel, and ticagrelor, respectively; $p < 0.01$) (**Figure 3**).

We then analyzed the changes in EGF and p-eNOS levels after 1 month treatment with the two different antiplatelet drugs. The efficacy in modulating EGF or p-eNOS of clopidogrel or ticagrelor was expressed as ratio of EGF or p-eNOS levels after 1 month over the respective EGF or p-eNOS at baseline. Fold-times changes of EGF ($EGF_{1month}/EGF_{baseline}$) and of p-eNOS ($p\text{-}eNOS_{1month}/p\text{-}eNOS_{baseline}$) are shown in **Figures 4A,B**. Ticagrelor was shown to be more powerful in decreasing EGF compared to clopidogrel ($p = 0.042$) and also more efficient in increasing p-eNOS ($p = 0.020$). In addition, correlation analyses between changes in EGF and in p-eNOS levels (**Figures 5A,B**) showed a correlation between EGF and p-eNOS ratio in the ticagrelor ($R = -0.571$; $p = 0.002$) but not in the clopidogrel group ($R = 0.100$; $p = 0.714$).

Effect of Exogenous EGF on eNOS in HUVECs

To assess a possible causal relationship between EGF levels and eNOS activation we treated HUVEC with different concentrations of EGF and we evaluated p-eNOS levels. We found that p-eNOS levels quantified by ELISA were decreased by EGF in a dose-dependent manner (**Figure 6A**). In addition, we analyzed by western blotting the total eNOS content in HUVEC treated with different concentration of EGF and we found that also total eNOS protein was diminished by EGF in a dose-dependent manner (**Figure 6B**).

DISCUSSION

In this study we report that, in patients with SCAD and COPD undergoing PCI, 1 month treatment with ticagrelor, but not with

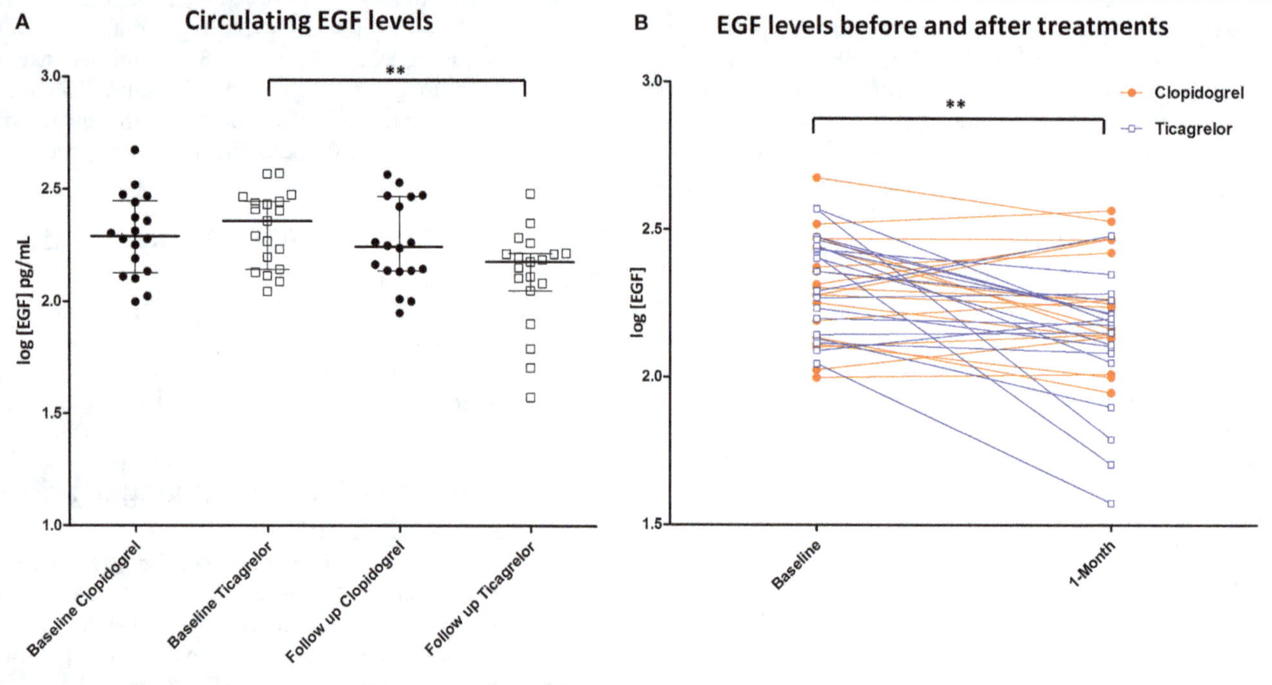

FIGURE 1 | (A) EGF levels in the serum of patients at baseline and after 1 month of treatment. Black circle: patient randomized to clopidogrel. White square: patient randomized to ticagrelor. $^{**}P < 0.01$; **(B)** EGF levels of patients representation before and after treatments. Orange circle: patient randomized to clopidogrel. Blue squares: patient randomized to ticagrelor. $^{**}P < 0.01$.

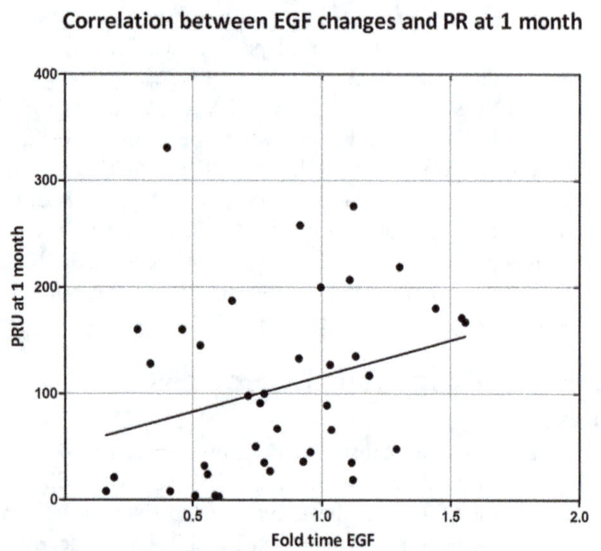

FIGURE 2 | Correlation between on-treatment platelet reactivity at 1 month and EGF changes. On treatment platelet reactivity was measured by VerifyNow after and expressed as $P2Y_{12}$ reaction unit (PRU). EGF changes were expressed as ratio between serum EGF concentration at 1 month over serum EGF concentration at baseline. Correlation was assessed by Spearman correlation test: $R = 0.350$; $p = 0.020$.

clopidogrel, results in a decrease of serum EGF concentration (**Figures 1A,B**). EGF can be secreted in the blood stream by different cellular sources such as submandibular gland (Tsutsumi et al., 1986), kidney (Staruschenko et al., 2013), and platelets (Ben-Ezra et al., 1990; Feng et al., 2012). However, the individual contribution of the different sources of circulating EGF as well as how the EGF levels are physiologically determined are not known.

EGF is a small protein constituted by 53 amino acids and three intramolecular disulfide bridges, and it is the founding member of the EGF-family of proteins. EGF acts by specifically binding to epidermal growth factor receptor (EGFR) on the cell membrane (Carpenter and Cohen, 1990). EGFR is a transmembrane receptor that controls signal transduction pathways that ultimately lead to survival, differentiation, and/or cell proliferation (Zeng and Harris, 2014). Activation of EGFR is known to be involved in many pathological processes such as endothelial dysfunction (Mehta et al., 2008), hypertension (Zhou et al., 2009), restenosis (Chan et al., 2003; Shafi et al., 2009), atherogenesis (Dreux et al., 2006), and cardiac remodeling (Iwamoto et al., 2003). More recently, it has been also shown that EGFR inhibition in T cells reduces atherosclerosis development (Zeboudj et al., 2018). The precise contribution of specific EGFR ligands is still poorly understood in the cardiovascular context but different lines of evidence have revealed that EGF can negatively affect endothelial function (Belmadani et al., 2008; Kassan et al., 2015), vascular tone regulation (Lundstam et al., 2007; Sumaya and Storey, 2017) and that it provokes proliferation of vascular smooth muscle cells (Berk et al., 1985).

We found a correlation, even if not particularly strong ($R = 0.350$), between changes in serum EGF concentrations and on-treatment platelet reactivity after pharmacological treatment

(**Figure 2**). Certainly, other factors could be involved in the level of PR and this will be the object of our future studies. EGF is present in platelets α-granules from where it can be secreted in the blood stream following degranulation (Lev-Ran et al., 1990; Blair and Flaumenhaft, 2009; Bertrand-Duchesne et al., 2010; Durante et al., 2013). Notably, it is known that inhibiting $P2Y_{12}$ receptors not only blocks platelet aggregation but also reduces release of mediators from α-granules (Zhao et al., 2001; Storey et al., 2002). In this study, we did not investigate the mechanism by which EGF is decreased by ticagrelor, but based on the current knowledge, it appears likely that the observed decrease in the serum EGF could be due to a decrease in the EGF released by platelets.

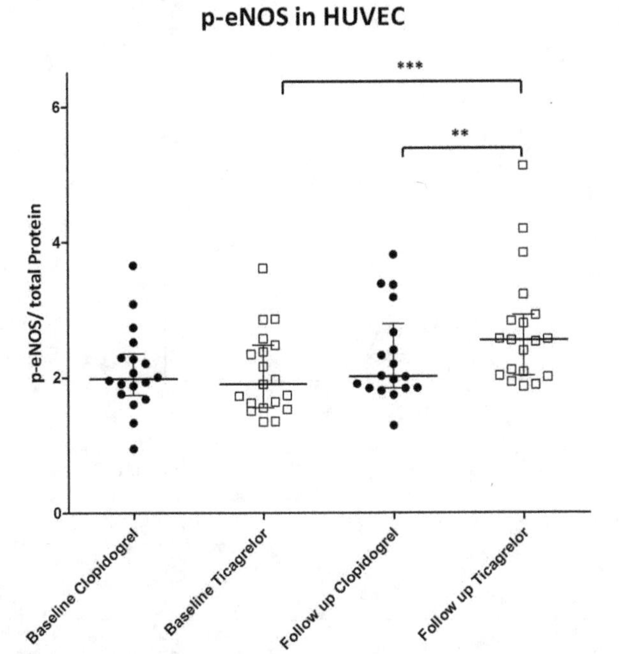

FIGURE 3 | p-eNOS in HUVEC treated with patient's sera at baseline and after 1 month of treatment. Black circle: patient randomized to clopidogrel. p-eNOS levels are expressed as OD at 450 nm. White square: patient randomized to ticagrelor. $^{**}P < 0.01$; $^{***}P < 0.001$.

Moreover, we showed that in HUVEC treated with sera of patients of the ticagrelor group at 1 month there is a higher activation of eNOS, in comparison to clopidogrel at the same time point (**Figure 3**). Interestingly, we found a negative correlation between changes in levels of circulating EGF and in eNOS activation in the ticagrelor arm (**Figure 5B**), but not in the clopidogrel group (**Figure 5A**). Taken together our data suggest that EGF interferes with eNOS activation. The role of EGF in decreasing eNOS activity has already been reported in animal models: in diabetic mice EGFR activation, resulting in eNOS activity impairment, is implicated in mesenteric resistance artery (MRA) dysfunction (Belmadani et al., 2008); in the same model, endogenous EGF decreased p-eNOS levels (Kassan et al., 2015). Here we showed *in vitro* that EGF is able to decrease both eNOS phosphorylation (**Figure 6A**) and total eNOS protein (**Figures 6B,C**) in a dose-dependent manner in HUVECs. Taken together our data indicate that ticagrelor is able to reduce circulating EGF levels and that, in turn, lower serum EGF positively affects the endothelial function by facilitating eNOS activity.

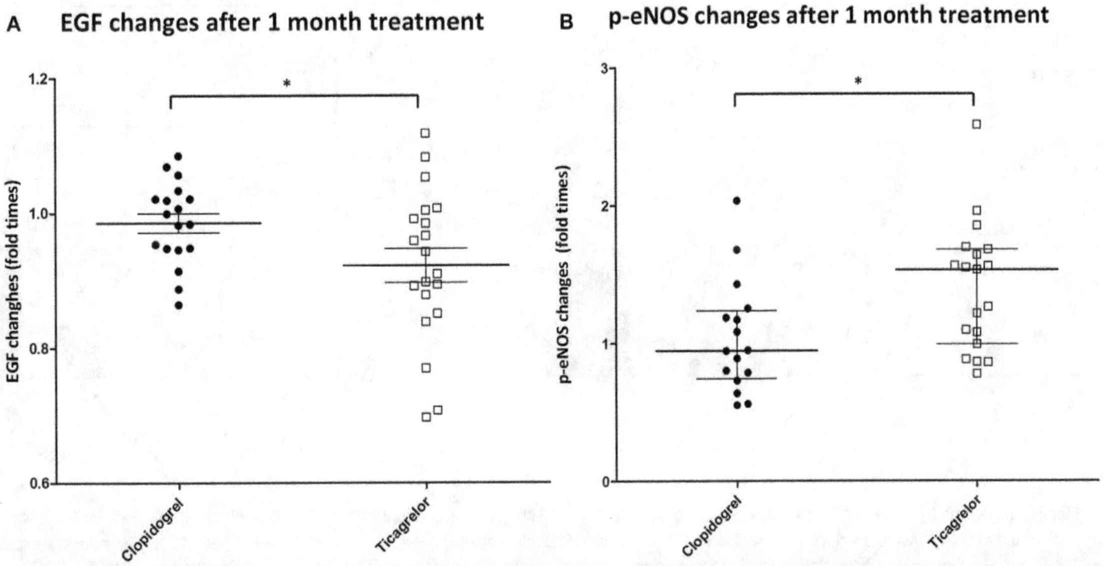

FIGURE 4 | (A) Changes in EGF levels in the serum of patients (on the y-axis is shown the ratio between EGF levels after 1 month of treatment and at baseline). Black circle: patient randomized to clopidogrel. White square: patient randomized to ticagrelor. $^{*}P < 0.05$. **(B)** Changes in p-eNOS levels in HUVEC treated with patient's sera (on the y-axis is shown the ratio between p-eNOS levels in HUVEC treated with patient's sera after 1 month of treatment and at baseline). Black circle: patient randomized to clopidogrel. White square: patient randomized to ticagrelor. $^{*}P < 0.05$.

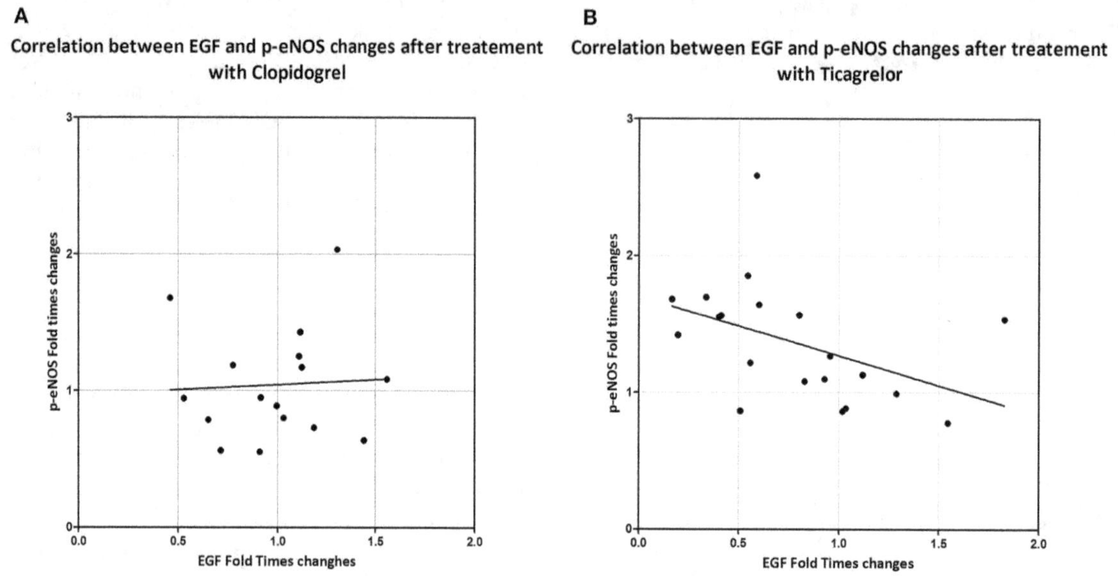

FIGURE 5 | Correlation between changes in levels of circulating EGF (ratio between EGF levels after 1 month of treatment and at baseline) and of p-eNOS in serum treated HUVEC (ratio between p-eNOS levels in HUVEC treated with patient's sera after 1 month of treatment and at baseline) in patients treated with clopidogrel **(A)** or with ticagrelor **(B)**. Correlation was assessed by Spearman correlation test. Clopidogrel: $R = 0.100$; $p = 0.714$. Ticagrelor: $R = -0.571$; $p = 0.002$.

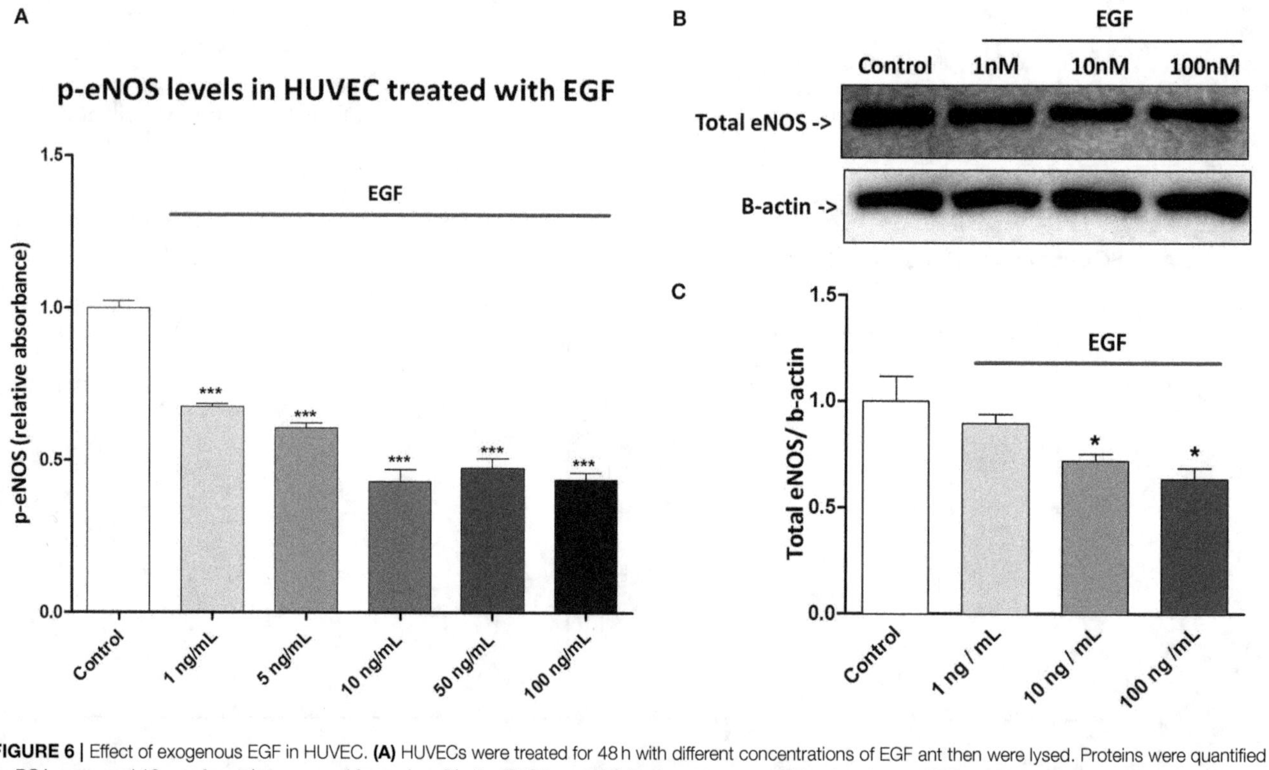

FIGURE 6 | Effect of exogenous EGF in HUVEC. **(A)** HUVECs were treated for 48 h with different concentrations of EGF ant then were lysed. Proteins were quantified by BCA assay and 10 μg of protein were used for each well in the ELISA. p-eNOS levels were expressed as absorbance (OD) at 450 nm. Results are expressed as mean ± SD of three independent experiments. ***$P < 0.001$ (comparison between control and treatment). **(B)** HUVECs were treated for 48 h with EGF. Lysates were electrophoresed and immunoblotted with total eNOS antibody, β-actin antibody was used to ensure equal loading. Images are representative of one of three independent experiments. **(C)** Densitometric analysis of western blot. *$P < 0.05$ (comparison between control and treatments).

In conclusion, we showed that the positive effect of ticagrelor on endothelial function is, at least in part, mediated by its capacity to lower EGF that in turn results in a better eNOS activation. Our data suggest that lower platelet reactivity could result in lower EGF release by platelets through a $P2Y_{12}$-mediated mechanism. This would imply that ticagrelor improvement of endothelial function is not only due to mechanisms linked to increased adenosine availability but could also be directly connected to its higher efficacy in diminishing platelet reactivity.

AUTHOR CONTRIBUTIONS

FVDS and FF: Performed *in vitro* experiments; FVDS and PR: Analyzed the data and wrote the paper; GC and RF: Designed and supervised the clinical trial and provided critical revision of data; GA, RP, SB, DB, and ADF: Participated to clinical assessments, collection of samples, and laboratory analyses. All authors reviewed data and results, and approved the final version of the manuscript.

FUNDING

This study was partially supported by a research grant [ESR-14-10659] by AstraZeneca, which had no role in collecting, analyzing, and interpreting data; manuscript writing; and the decision to submit the paper for publication.

ACKNOWLEDGMENTS

We thank Antonio Pannuti for his valuable advice in the statistical data analysis and interpretation.

REFERENCES

Agnoletti, L., Curello, S., Bachetti, T., Malacarne, F., Gaia, G., Comini, L., et al. (1999). Serum from patients with severe heart failure downregulates eNOS and is proapoptotic: role of tumor necrosis factor. *Circulation* 100, 1983–1991.

Belmadani, S., Palen, D. I., Gonzalez-Villalobos, R. A., Boulares, H. A., and Matrougui, K. (2008). Elevated epidermal growth factor receptor phosphorylation induces resistance artery dysfunction in diabetic db/db mice. *Diabetes* 57, 1629–1637. doi: 10.2337/db07-0739

Ben-Ezra, J., Sheibani, K., Hwang, D. L., and Lev-Ran, A. (1990). Megakaryocyte synthesis is the source of epidermal growth factor in human platelets. *Am. J. Pathol.* 137, 755–759.

Berk, B. C., Brock, T. A., Webb, R. C., Taubman, M. B., Atkinson, W. J., Gimbrone, M. A., et al. (1985). Epidermal growth factor, a vascular smooth muscle mitogen, induces rat aortic contraction. *J. Clin. Invest.* 75, 1083–1086. doi: 10.1172/JCI111772

Bertrand-Duchesne, M. P., Grenier, D., and Gagnon, G. (2010). Epidermal growth factor released from platelet-rich plasma promotes endothelial cell proliferationin *in vitro*. *J. Periodont. Res.* 45, 87–93. doi: 10.1111/j.1600-0765.2009.01205.x

Blair, P., and Flaumenhaft, R. (2009). Platelet α-granules: basic biology and clinical correlates. *Blood Rev.* 23, 177–189. doi: 10.1016/j.blre.2009.04.001

Campo, G., Vieceli Dalla Sega, F., Pavasini, R., Aquila, G., Gallo, F., Fortini, F., et al. (2017). Biological effects of ticagrelor over clopidogrel in patients with stable coronary artery disease and chronic obstructive pulmonary disease. *Thromb. Haemost.* 117, 1208–1216. doi: 10.1160/TH16-12-0973

Carpenter, G., and Cohen, S. (1990). Epidermal growth factor. *J. Biol. Chem.* 265, 7709–7712.

Chan, A. K., Kalmes, A., Hawkins, S., Daum, G., and Clowes, A. W. (2003). Blockade of the epidermal growth factor receptor decreases intimal hyperplasia in balloon-injured rat carotid artery. *J. Vasc. Surg.* 37, 644–649. doi: 10.1067/mva.2003.92

Dreux, A. C., Lamb, D. J., Modjtahedi, H., and Ferns, G. A. (2006). The epidermal growth factor receptors and their family of ligands: their putative role in atherogenesis. *Atherosclerosis* 186, 38–53. doi: 10.1016/j.atherosclerosis.2005.06.038

Durante, C., Agostini, F., Abbruzzese, L., Toffola, R. T., Zanolin, S., Suine, C., et al. (2013). Growth factor release from platelet concentrates: analytic quantification and characterization for clinical applications. *Vox Sang.* 105, 129–136. doi: 10.1111/vox.12039

Feng, X., Scheinberg, P., Samsel, L., Rios, O., Chen, J., McCoy, J. P., et al. (2012). Decreased plasma cytokines are associated with low platelet counts in aplastic anemia and immune thrombocytopenic purpura. *J. Thromb. Haemost.* 10, 1616–1623. doi: 10.1111/j.1538-7836.2012.04757.x

Fortini, F., Vieceli Dalla Sega, F., Caliceti, C., Aquila, G., Pannella, M., Pannuti, A., et al. (2017). Estrogen receptor β-dependent Notch1 activation protects vascular endothelium against tumor necrosis factor α (TNFα)-induced apoptosis. *J. Biol. Chem.* 292, 18178–18191. doi: 10.1074/jbc.M117.790121

Iwamoto, R., Yamazaki, S., Asakura, M., Takashima, S., Hasuwa, H., Miyado, K., et al. (2003). Heparin-binding EGF-like growth factor and ErbB signaling is essential for heart function. *Proc. Natl. Acad. Sci. U.S.A.* 100, 3221–3226. doi: 10.1073/pnas.0537588100

Kassan, M., Ait-Aissa, K., Ali, M., Trebak, M., and Matrougui, K. (2015). Augmented EGF receptor tyrosine kinase activity impairs vascular function by NADPH oxidase-dependent mechanism in type 2 diabetic mouse. *Biochim. Biophys. Acta Mol. Cell Res.* 1853, 2404–2410. doi: 10.1016/j.bbamcr.2015.05.032

Kim, H. K., Jeong, M. H., Lim, K. S., Kim, J. H., Lim, H. C., Kim, M. C., et al. (2017). Effects of ticagrelor on neointimal hyperplasia and endothelial function, compared with clopidogrel and prasugrel, in a porcine coronary stent restenosis model. *Int. J. Cardiol.* 240, 326–331. doi: 10.1016/j.ijcard.2017.04.108

Lemesle, G., Schurtz, G., Bauters, C., and Hamon, M. (2015). High on-treatment platelet reactivity with ticagrelor versus prasugrel: a systematic review and meta-analysis. *J. Thromb. Haemost.* 13, 931–942. doi: 10.1111/jth.12907

Lev-Ran, A., Hwang, D. L., and Snyder, D. S. (1990). Human serum and plasma have different sources of epidermal growth factor. *Am. J. Physiol. Regul. Integr. Comp. Physiol.* 259, R545–R548. doi: 10.1152/ajpregu.1990.259.3.R545

Li, Z., Li, Y., Zhang, T., Miao, W., and Su, G. (2016). Comparison of the influence of ticagrelor and clopidogrel on inflammatory biomarkers and vascular endothelial function for patients with ST-segment elevation myocardial infarction receiving emergency percutaneous coronary intervention: study protocol for a randomized controlled trial. *Trials* 17:75. doi: 10.1186/s13063-016-1168-9

Lundstam, U., Hägg, U., Bergmann Sverrisdottir, Y., Svensson, L. E., and Gan, L.-M. (2007). Epidermal growth factor levels are related to diastolic blood pressure and carotid artery stiffness. *Scand. Cardiov. J.* 41, 308–312. doi: 10.1080/14017430701439508

Mehta, V. B., Zhou, Y., Radulescu, A., and Besner, G. E. (2008). HB-EGF stimulates eNOS expression and nitric oxide production and promotes eNOS dependent angiogenesis. *Growth Factors* 26, 301–315. doi: 10.1080/08977190802393596

Motovska, Z., Hlinomaz, O., Kala, P., Hromadka, M., Knot, J., Varvarovsky, I., et al. (2018). 1-year outcomes of patients undergoing primary angioplasty for myocardial infarction treated with prasugrel versus ticagrelor. *J. Am. Coll. Cardiol.* 71, 371–381. doi: 10.1016/j.jacc.2017.11.008

Schnorbus, B., Daiber, A., Jurk, K., Warnke, S., König, J., Krahn, U., et al. (2014). Effects of clopidogrel, prasugrel and ticagrelor on endothelial function, inflammatory and oxidative stress parameters and platelet function in patients undergoing coronary artery stenting for an acute coronary syndrome. A randomised, prospective, controlled study. *BMJ Open* 4:e005268. doi: 10.1136/bmjopen-2014-005268

Shafi, S., Lamb, D., Modjtahedi, H., and Ferns, G. (2009). Periadventitial delivery of anti-EGF receptor antibody inhibits neointimal macrophage accumulation after angioplasty in a hypercholesterolaemic rabbit. *Int. J. Exp. Pathol.* 91, 224–234. doi: 10.1111/j.1365-2613.2009.00700.x

Staruschenko, A., Palygin, O., Ilatovskaya, D. V., and Pavlov, T. S. (2013). Epidermal growth factors in the kidney and relationship to hypertension. *Am. J. Physiol. Renal Physiol.* 305, F12–F20. doi: 10.1152/ajprenal.00112.2013

Storey, R. F., Judge, H. M., Wilcox, R. G., and Heptinstall, S. (2002). Inhibition of ADP-induced P-selectin expression and platelet-leukocyte conjugate formation by clopidogrel and the P2Y12 receptor antagonist AR-C69931MX but not aspirin. *Thromb. Haemost.* 88, 488–494. doi: 10.1055/s-0037-1613242

Sumaya, W., and Storey, R. F. (2017). Ticagrelor. *Int. Cardiol. Clin.* 6, 49–55. doi: 10.1016/j.iccl.2016.08.004

Tsutsumi, O., Kurachi, H., and Oka, T. (1986). A physiological role of epidermal growth factor in male reproductive function. *Science* 233, 975–977. doi: 10.1126/science.3090686

Valgimigli, M., Merli, E., Malagutti, P., Soukhomovskaia, O., Cicchitelli, G., Macri, G., et al. (2003). Endothelial dysfunction in acute and chronic coronary syndromes: evidence for a pathogenetic role of oxidative stress. *Arch. Biochem. Biophys.* 420, 255–261. doi: 10.1016/j.abb.2003.07.006

van den Berg, T. N., El Messaoudi, S., Rongen, G. A., van den Broek, P. H., Bilos, A., Donders, A. R., et al. (2015). Ticagrelor does not inhibit adenosine transport at relevant concentrations: a Randomized Cross-Over Study in healthy subjects *in vivo*. *PLoS ONE* 10:e0137560. doi: 10.1371/journal.pone.0137560

Zeboudj, L., Maitre, M., Guyonnet, L., Laurans, L., Joffre, J., Lemarie, J., et al. (2018). Selective EGF-receptor inhibition in CD4(+) T cells induces anergy and limits atherosclerosis. *J. Am. Coll. Cardiol.* 71, 160–172. doi: 10.1016/j.jacc.2017.10.084

Zeng, F., and Harris, R. C. (2014). Epidermal growth factor, from gene organization to bedside. *Semin. Cell Dev. Biol.* 28, 2–11. doi: 10.1016/j.semcdb.2014.01.011

Zhao, L., Bath, P., and Heptinstall, S. (2001). Effects of combining three different antiplatelet agents on platelets and leukocytes in whole blood *in vitro*. *Br. J. Pharmacol.* 134, 353–358. doi: 10.1038/sj.bjp.0704248

Zhou, Y., Brigstock, D., and Besner, G. E. (2009). Heparin-binding EGF-like growth factor is a potent dilator of terminal mesenteric arterioles. *Microvasc. Res.* 78, 78–85. doi: 10.1016/j.mvr.2009.04.006

9

Potentially Common Therapeutic Targets for Multiple Sclerosis and Ischemic Stroke

Roberto Paternò[1] and Jean-Marc Chillon[2,3]*

[1] *Dipartimento di Medicina Clinica e Chirurgia, Università degli Studi di Napoli Federico II, Naples, Italy,* [2] *Mécanismes Physiopathologiques et Conséquences des Calcifications Cardiovasculaires (EA 7517), Faculty of Pharmacy, University of Picardie Jules Verne, Amiens, France,* [3] *Direction de la Recherche Clinique et de l'Innovation, CHU Amiens Picardie, Amiens, France*

Edited by:
Pasquale Pagliaro,
Università degli Studi di Torino, Italy

Reviewed by:
Thorsten Rudroff,
Colorado State University,
United States
Rosa Iodice,
Università degli Studi di Napoli
Federico II, Italy

***Correspondence:**
Roberto Paternò
rpaterno@unina.it

Ischemic stroke (IS) and multiple sclerosis (MS) are two pathologies of the central nervous system (CNS). At the first look, this appears to be the only similarity between the two diseases, as they seem quite different. Indeed IS has an acute onset compared to MS which develops chronically; IS is consecutive to blood clot migrating to cerebral blood vessels or decrease in cerebral blood flow following atherosclerosis or decreases in cardiac output, whereas MS is an immune disease associated with neurodegeneration. However, both pathologies share similar pathologic pathways and treatments used in MS have been the object of studies in IS. In this mini-review we will discuss similarities between IS and MS on astrocytes and neuroinflammation hallmarks emphasizing the potential for treatments.

Keywords: multiple sclerosis, ischemic stroke, common pathway, common therapy, neuroinflammation

INTRODUCTION

Ischemic stroke (IS) and multiple sclerosis (MS) are two pathologies of the central nervous system (CNS). It has been proposed that the two pathologies may share similar pathological pathways involving particularly glutamate release, oxidative stress, and reactive oxygen species (ROS). During IS, activation of glutamate receptors following the release of this excitatory neurotransmitter leads to an increase in intracellular calcium and activation of nitric oxide synthase and NADPH oxidase pathways. The resulting increases in ROS contribute to neuronal death, increases in blood–brain barrier (BBB) permeability and ischemic lesion development (for review see Forrester et al., 2018). Similarly, glutamate may be involved in MS development. Oligodendrocytes, the myelin-producing cells of the CNS, are vulnerable to glutamate excitotoxicity via glutamate receptors activation. ROS generated following glutamate receptors activation may contribute to demyelination and neuronal degradation in MS (for review, see Gilgun-Sherki et al., 2004; Iodice et al., 2017).

ASTROCYTES

Astrocytes and Stroke

For a long time, glia cells were believed to be only structural cells. It is now well known that glia cells such as astrocytes or microglia play a role in the CNS functions in physiological and pathological conditions. Indeed, astrocytes regulate ion and neurotransmitters homeostasis, metabolically support neurons, and monitor synaptic activity (for review, see Parpura et al., 2012). Astrocytes glutamate transporters play a major role in glutamate clearance and excitotoxicity by removing glutamate from the extracellular space and maintaining it below neurotoxic levels (Rothstein et al., 1996). It has been reported that glial glutamate transporter (GLT-1) may have a dual effect in stroke by taking up glutamate and thus protecting neurons in the early stages of ischemia and by releasing glutamate and triggering neurons death with prolonged ischemia (Mitani and Tanaka, 2003). Furthermore, astrocytes form a functional syncytium thanks to gap junctions composed of the channel protein connexin43 (Giaume et al., 1991). Such syncytium may protect the CNS during IS by dispersing potassium or glutamate released from neuron in the extracellular space and accumulated by astrocytes. Indeed, infarct volumes were significantly increased in connexin43 heterozygous null mice compared to wild type mice (Siushansian et al., 2001). Reactive astrogliosis also occurs following CNS injury with beneficial and deleterious effects. Astrogliosis involves morphological and functional changes and contribute to glial scar that may protect preserved healthy tissues from inflammation but also may decrease ischemic tissue recovery by reducing axons regeneration. Actually, glial scar may be beneficial in the early stages of stroke allowing to limit lesion size but deleterious if not resolved by decreasing neuroplasticity and CNS regeneration (Pekny et al., 2014). Several factors such as p53 (Ahn et al., 2015), p38 mitogen-activated protein kinase (Roy Choudhury et al., 2014), macrophage-derived osteopontin (Gliem et al., 2015), acute-phase protein pentraxin-3 (Rodriguez-Grande et al., 2014), and CD36 (Bao et al., 2012) are involved in astrocytes activation (see Sofroniew, 2009 for more information).

Astrocytes and MS

In MS, microglia activation has been shown in all clinical subtypes of the disease (Prineas et al., 2001), astrocytes produce a glial scar when inflammation decreases. In recent studies, the astrocytes are recognized as early and highly active players during MS lesion formation and as having beneficial and detrimental roles during MS lesion evolution. Studies indicate that astroglial myelin phagocytosis is an early event that takes place before the damaged myelin is removed by macrophages. Thus modulation of early astroglia responses can be a possible target for MS treatment (Ponath et al., 2017).

In MS, all aspects of glutamate homeostasis are impaired, indicating that glutamate excitotoxicity is an essential mechanism in the pathogenesis of the disease. Many studies have shown that glutamate levels are increased in the cerebrospinal fluid (CSF) (Sarchielli et al., 2003) and in acute lesions of MS patients (Srinivasan et al., 2005). There is an increase of glutaminase expression in macrophages and microglia in close proximity to dystrophic axons. In addition, in experimental autoimmune encephalomyelitis (EAE), an animal model of MS (Werner et al., 2001), there is a correlation between glutaminase expression and axonal damage.

Today, several mechanisms have been taken into account that may link astrocytic glutamate release with the glutamate excitotoxicity present in MS, and all these mechanisms involve microglia activation; in fact, after activation, these cells release adenosine triphosphate (ATP), which activates the P2Y1 receptor on astrocytes, leading to glutamate release (Pascual et al., 2012). Considering that in MS immunoinflammatory and neurodegenerative processes coexist, the glutamate excitotoxicity could be the missing link between them. This concept has practical value in developing innovative therapy that should take into account the immunosuppression as well as the neuroprotection.

Astrocyte-Targeted Strategies

Astrocyte-Targeted Strategies in Stroke (Table 1)

Astrocyte-targeted-strategies may be an option for stroke therapy. Increasing astrocyte survival during ischemic stress is associated with an increased neuronal survival. Indeed, astrocyte targeted overexpression of heat shock protein 72 and superoxide dismutase 2 increases astrocyte resistance to ischemic stress and preserves CA1 neurons following forebrain ischemia (Xu et al., 2010). Similarly, pyruvate increases the synthesis of glutathione, an antioxydant protecting cells from toxins such as free radicals. Pyruvate administration protects against glutamate-induced toxicity in mixed culture of cortex cells but not in pure neuronal cultures (Miao et al., 2011). Furthermore, addition of astroglia to the pure neuronal cultures restores pyruvate-associated neuronal protection (Miao et al., 2011). Other experiments indicate that upregulation of GLT-1 expression in astrocytes with ceftriaxone (Ouyang et al., 2007; Verma et al., 2010) or viral-mediated gene delivery (Weller et al., 2008) protects neurons from ischemia. Another potential target for stroke therapy is p53 as it has been shown that inhibition of p53 activity prevents astrocyte activation and astrocyte impaired glutamate intake (Ahn et al., 2015). Another potential targets for astrocytes and ischemic protection are microRNAs. MicroRNAs, some of them expressed in astrocytes, appear to be involved in the regulation of cerebral ischemia and may be targets to improve stroke outcome (Ouyang et al., 2014). Indeed increasing levels of microRNA-29a, a microRNA strongly expressed in astrocytes, protects neurons during forebrain ischemia (Ouyang et al., 2013). Finally, some experiments also suggest that astrocytes may be implicated in the induction of brain ischemic tolerance by preconditioning. This was linked to an upregulation of P2X7 receptors by astrocytes following preconditioning (Hirayama et al., 2015).

Astrocyte-Targeted Strategies in MS (Table 1)

The P2X7 receptor has also been implicated in the pathogenesis of MS. P2X7R immunoreactivity is increased in activated microglia/macrophages in spinal cord during MS (Yiangou et al., 2006). In addition, pharmacological inhibition of the receptor diminishes astrogliosis in rat EAE and reduces neurological symptoms (Grygorowicz et al., 2016). However, conflicting results have been obtained in this animal model of MS. In fact P2X7 receptor knockout mice are more resistant to EAE than wild-type mice (Sharp et al., 2008). On the other hand, in another study, the P2X7 receptor knockdown mice have a more severe EAE (Chen and Brosnan, 2006). Conflicting

TABLE 1 | Common therapeutic targets for multiple sclerosis and ischemic stroke.

Targets	Molecular patterns	Consequences
Astrocytes	- Overexpression of heat shock protein 72	↑ astrocytes resistance to ischemic stress (Xu et al., 2010)
	- Overexpression of superoxide dismutase 2	↑ astrocytes resistance to ischemic stress (Xu et al., 2010)
	- Pyruvate	↑ glutathione (antioxidant) synthesis (Miao et al., 2011)
	- Ceftriaxone	↑ glial glutamate transporter (Ouyang et al., 2007; Verma et al., 2010)
	- Inhibition of p53	↓ astrocytes activation (Ahn et al., 2015)
	- microRNA-29a	↑ neurons survival during ischemia (Ouyang et al., 2013)
	- P2X7 receptors	↑ brain ischemic tolerance by preconditioning (Hirayama et al., 2015)
Blood–Brain Barrier	- Insulin growth factor 1	↑ BBB integrity (Bake et al., 2014)
	- Overexpression of heat Shock protein 27	↑ BBB integrity (Shi et al., 2017)
	- Preservation of tight junction by Sac-1004	↑ BBB integrity (Zhang H. et al., 2017)
	- Blockade of α4 integrin	↓ peripheral immune cells infiltration Becker et al., 2001; Investigators, 2001; Relton et al., 2001; Liesz et al., 2011b; Langhauser et al., 2014; Llovera et al., 2015; Elkins et al., 2017)
Neuroinflammation	- Fumarate	Immunomodulatory and antioxidant properties (Lin et al., 2016)
	- Fingolimod	↓ lymphocytes influx and thrombo-inflammation (Liesz et al., 2011a; Kraft et al., 2013; Fu et al., 2014)
	- Nrf2 activation	↓ microglia activation and CNS peripheral cells infiltration (Kuo et al., 2017)
	- IL1 inhibitor	↓ inflammatory cytokines expression (Zhang D.D. et al., 2017)
	- IL33	↑ anti-inflammatory Th2 responses (Luo et al., 2014; Korhonen et al., 2015)
	- IL4	Modulation of microglia activation (Korhonen et al., 2015; Xia et al., 2015; Zhao et al., 2015)
	- Protein kinases inhibitors	↑ M2-polarized microglia (Lee and Suk, 2017)
	- microRNA	↑ M2-polarized microglia (Ni et al., 2015; Hamzei Taj et al., 2016)
	- TNF-α	↓ inflammation (mixed results) (Sumbria et al., 2012; Clausen et al., 2014; Pires et al., 2014; Probert, 2015; Palle et al., 2017; Wu et al., 2017)
	- IL6	↓inflammation (Maimone et al., 1997; Beauchemin and Carruthers, 2016; Kleiter et al., 2016; Wang et al., 2016)

results were also observed regarding P2X7 receptors and IS. On one side, activation of P2X7 receptors appears necessary for inducing ischemic tolerance by preconditioning (Bindra et al., 2014; Hirayama et al., 2015) and attenuate brain edema after IS (Kaiser et al., 2016). On the other side, P2X7 receptors are involved in microglial cell (Eyo et al., 2013) and neuronal death (Arbeloa et al., 2012) during oxygen-glucose deprivation.

NEUROINFLAMMATION

Immune Cells Infiltration/Blood–Brain Barrier Dysfunction and Stroke

The brain initial innate response to stroke is essentially mediated by microglia, the resident macrophage of the CNS. This initial step is then followed by infiltration of immune cells such as neutrophils, macrophage/monocytes, T cells (Ma et al., 2017). In ischemic conditions, neurons release damage associated molecular patterns (DAMPs) leading to glial (microglia and astrocytes) activation and chemokines liberation. This will lead to endothelial cells activation, with expression of adhesion molecules allowing interaction between peripheral immune cells and endothelial cells followed by diapedesis (Strecker et al., 2017). Furthermore, microglia activation induces the production of ROS through the activation of NADPH oxidase associated with BBB disruption (Sumi et al., 2010). Other pro-inflammatory cytokines, such as tumor necrosis factor (TNF-α) and interleukin (IL)1β are also secreted by activated microglia and contribute to BBB dysfunction (Da Fonseca et al., 2014). Microglia can also express matrix metalloproteinase (MMP) following activation (Del Zoppo et al., 2007). MMP also play a role in BBB dysfunction during IS following degradation of tight junction proteins (Liu et al., 2012; Li et al., 2013). This may contribute to the deleterious role of MMP-9 in the development of brain injury after focal cerebral ischemia (Asahi et al., 2000). Finally, it has been reported that all microglia in the penumbra are associated to endothelial cells within 24 h post reperfusion and destroy endothelial cells by phagocytosis contributing to BBB disruption (Jolivel et al., 2015). It has also been reported that other cells than microglia, such as mast cells, are potentially initiators of BBB dysfunction and neuroinflammation (McKittrick et al., 2015). Peripheral immune cells infiltration following BBB disruption release anti-microbial enzymes, reactive oxygen/nitrogen species and chemokines responsible for further inflammation and BBB dysfunction (Strecker et al., 2017).

M1 Phenotype Versus M2 Phenotype and Stroke

When activated, immune cells can acquire 2 phenotypes, M1 activated phenotype and M2 activated phenotype (Olah et al., 2011; Easton, 2013; Patel et al., 2013). The M1 phenotype is characterized by high expression of destructive pro-inflammatory mediators and contributes to ischemic lesions extension. In contrast, the M2 phenotype presents neuroprotective properties. Furthermore, M2 phenotype facilitates phagocytosis, thus reducing secondary inflammatory reaction and making space for newborn neurons. It has been observed that microglia and macrophages respond dynamically to ischemic injury with, first, an increase in the protective M2 phenotype followed by a transition to the pro-inflammatory M1 phenotype (Hu et al., 2012). Several factors may contribute to immune cells polarization. Ischemic neurons may contribute to M1 microglial activation by releasing soluble FAS ligand (Meng et al., 2016). In contrast, neurons in the penumbra produce IL4, a cytokine with the ability to polarize macrophages to the M2 phenotype (Zhao et al., 2015).

M1 Phenotype Versus M2 Phenotype and MS

In both MS and experimental animal models of MS, intracerebral M1 phenotype cells (Broholm et al., 2004) as well as M2 phenotype (Boven et al., 2006) have been detected. Reactive microglia/macrophages exert both neurodestructive and neuroprotective effects in MS contributing to the most common clinical presentation of MS, the relapsing-remitting form. It has been observed that both M1 and M2 activation states can occur at the same time in EAE, and that the M1 to M2 ratio is a key factor in relapse of EAE (Miron et al., 2013). The M1 state is associated with progressive EAE whereas the M2 state may suppress the clinical symptoms of EAE (Ransohoff and Perry, 2009). It has also been observed that both MS and EAE are characterized by predominance of M1 microglia in the acute or early phase of the disease (Mikita et al., 2011). M1 markers appear in normal-appearing white matter and in active and inactive white matter lesions, whereas M2 markers are mainly expressed in the perivascular space (Zhang et al., 2011). For both stroke and MS, considering M1 and M2 polarization, the therapy must be developed to prevent excessive microglial activities but also to preserve their protective functions.

Cytokines and Chemokines Involved in Stroke

In a recent review, Iadecola and Anrather listed mediators of post-ischemic inflammation. They separated mediators involved in the initiation, the amplification and the resolution of IS (Iadecola and Anrather, 2011). Considering cytokines, IL1α and IL1β and TNF-α are involved in the initiation of post-ischemic inflammation. Then, IL1, 6, 10, 17, 20, and TNF-α contributes to the amplification of the neuroinflammation whereas TGF-β, IL10, 17, and 23 contribute to its resolution (Iadecola and Anrather, 2011). Numerous chemokines such as CCL5, CXCL4, CXCL7, CX3CL1, (initiation) and CCL2, CCL3, CCL5, CXCL2/3, and CXCL8 (amplification) also contributes to post-stroke inflammation (Iadecola and Anrather, 2011). Other mediators include adhesion molecules, proteases, and small molecules such as prostanoids and leukotriens for initiation and iNOS, C0X-2 and NADPH oxidase for amplification (Iadecola and Anrather, 2011).

Neuroinflammation-Targeted Strategies

Neuroinflammation-Targeted Strategies and Stroke (Table 1)

Considering the importance of neuroinflammation in ischemic stroke, immunomodulation appears like an interesting therapeutic option. Immunomodulation is currently used for MS treatment and several drugs used in MS have been evaluated in ischemic stroke. Fumarate, because of its immunomodulatory and antioxidant properties, suppresses pro-inflammatory cytokines in *in vitro* and *in vivo* stroke models. This is associated with a decrease in infarct size and an improvement in behavioral outcome (Lin et al., 2016). In animal models of ischemic stroke, treatment with fingolimod is associated with mixed results. In one study, fingolimod reduced post-stroke lymphocytes influx but had no favorable impact on infarct volume and behavioral dysfunction (Liesz et al., 2011a). In another study it has been shown that fingolimod has stroke-protective action by reduction of thrombo-inflammation but not by a direct neuroprotective effect (Kraft et al., 2013). Furthermore, in a small clinical trial, oral fingolimod within 72h of stroke onset was associated with decreased microvascular permeability, attenuated neurological deficits and improved recovery (Fu et al., 2014). Few papers on the impact of glatiramer in IS are available. The results are somewhat contradictory with either no reduction of infarct volume or improvement in neurological deficit in mice (Poittevin et al., 2013; Kraft et al., 2014) or an improvement of neurological deficit and an increase in neurogenesis and decrease in infarct volume in rats (Ibarra et al., 2007; Cruz et al., 2015).

Other treatments modulating directly or indirectly neuroinflammation may present an interest for stroke therapy. Indeed, it has been reported that activation of Nrf2 is associated with a decrease in microglia activation and CNS peripheral cell infiltration as well as a protection against IS in mice (Kuo et al., 2017). It has also been shown that a fusion protein, which fused the natural inhibitor of IL1, the IL1 receptor antagonist, with a cell penetrating peptide, alleviates brain infarction, cerebral edema, neurological deficit score, motor performance and inflammatory cytokines expression (Zhang D.D. et al., 2017). Several IL may also present an interest. For example, IL33 is protective against ischemic insult by promoting the anti-inflammatory Th2 responses (Luo et al., 2014; Korhonen et al., 2015). This protective effect seems also related to the induction of IL4 secretion (Korhonen et al., 2015). It has been previously reported that IL4 is secreted by ischemic neurons as an endogenous defense mechanism by modulating microglia activation (Zhao et al., 2015). Indeed, M2-polarized microglia with its anti-inflammatory profile is a promising therapeutic option for stroke therapy (Xia et al., 2015). Other potential targets to decrease microglia-mediated neuroinflammation by increasing M2-polarized microglia are protein kinases inhibitors (Lee and Suk, 2017) or microRNA such as let-7c-5p (Ni et al., 2015) or microRNA-124 (Hamzei Taj et al., 2016). As, as previously mentioned, neuroinflammation involves infiltration by peripheral immune cells of the CNS, other potential therapies for stroke prevention may be to decrease such infiltration. Decreasing BBB disruption may do this. Indeed, preservation of the BBB integrity by insulin growth factor 1 (Bake et al., 2014), overexpression of heat shock protein 27 (Shi et al., 2017), or preservation of tight junction by Sac-1004 (Zhang H. et al., 2017) is associated with an improved post-stroke neurological outcome. Another possibility to decrease peripheral immune cells infiltration is to modulate adhesion molecule. Blockade of α4 integrin can protect the brain against ischemic injuries in experimental models of IS (Becker et al., 2001; Relton et al., 2001; Liesz et al., 2011b). In contrast, blockade of α4 integrin was ineffective to protect from acute IS (Langhauser et al., 2014). This apparent discrepancy may be explained by the results of a preclinical multicenter trial on anti CD49d treatment for acute brain ischemia (Llovera et al., 2015). Indeed, treatment with CD49d-specific antibodies reduced leukocytes invasion and infarct volume in stroke model associated with small cortical infarction but not in stroke model associated with large ischemic lesion suggesting that treatment efficacy may depend on infarct severity or localization (Llovera et al., 2015). In humans, anti ICAM-1 therapy worsened stroke outcome in a clinical trial (Investigators, 2001) whereas treatment with natalizumab, an α4 integrin blocker, did not reduce infarct growth but had a beneficial effect on functional outcome (Elkins et al., 2017). Noteworthy, natalizumab is currently used as MS treatments and its use in experimental models of IS once again emphasizes the similarities between the 2 pathologies.

Few data are available on the impact of TNF-α blocking on IS lesions. It has been observed that patients with psoriasis and treated with TNF-α inhibitors had a lower cardiovascular event risk compared to patients treated with phototherapy (Wu et al., 2018) or methotrexate (Wu et al., 2017). Furthermore, anti TNF-α therapy ameliorates functional outcomes after stroke by altering the peripheral immune response but without any impact on infarct volume (Clausen et al., 2014). One of the

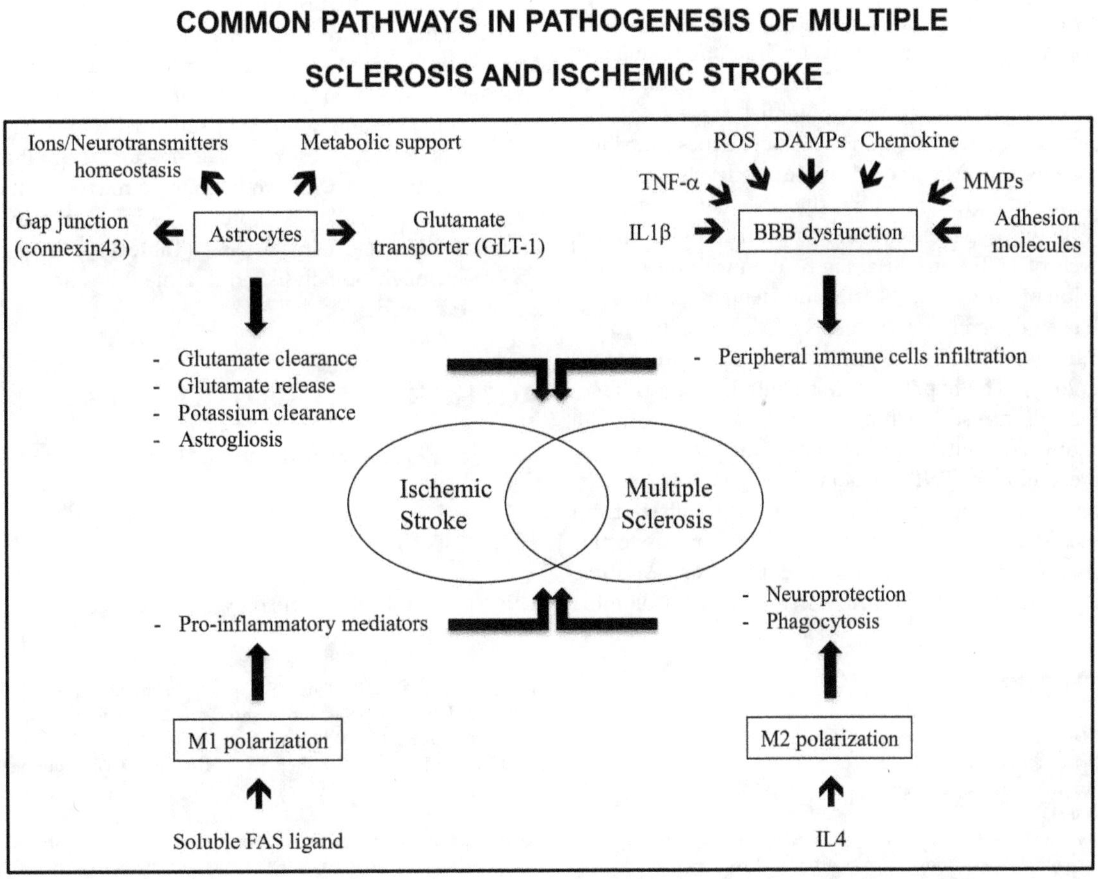

FIGURE 1 | Common pathways in pathogenesis of multiple sclerosis and ischemic stroke include astrocytes, BBB dysfunction and M1/M2 polarization. Astrocytes are involved in ions and neurotransmitters homeostasis and metabolic support. Gap junctions as well as glutamate transporters allow for glutamate uptake and clearance. Similarly, gap junctions allow for potassium clearance. Stored glutamate may be released by astrocytes and may be responsible for delayed lesions. In the same way astrogliosis has deleterious and protective effects. It protects preserved tissue from inflammation but decreased neurogenesis in ischemic tissue. Inflammatory markers such as TNF-α or IL1-β, reactive oxygen species, danger associated molecular patterns (DAMPs, molecules released from necrotic cells), chemokines, matrix metalloproteinases (MMPs), and adhesion molecules expression contribute to BBB disruption and peripheral immune cells infiltration. M1 polarization of immune cells is associated with an increase in pro-inflammatory mediators and deleterious effects on neuronal lesions. In contrast, M2 polarization is associated with neuroprotection and dead cells phagocytosis allowing for a decrease in inflammation.

potential problems for IS treatments with anti TNF-α therapy may be BBB crossing. Indeed engineering of a BBB crossing TNF-α inhibitor allowed to decrease infarct volume and to improve neurological outcome in a stroke experimental model (Sumbria et al., 2012). However, we have to remain cautious and more data are necessary on the impact of TNF-α inhibitors on IS as it has been observed that TNF-α inhibition was associated with increased ischemic damage following a decrease in innate immune response from the brain (Pires et al., 2014). Considering IL6, it has been reported that pre-treatment with tocilizumab, a monoclonal antibody against IL6 in a rat model of ischemic stroke, prevents neuronal cell apoptosis (Wang et al., 2016).

In conclusion, targeting of neuroinflammation appears a promising option in IS treatment. Several clinical trials have been performed or are underway to evaluate clinical outcome in patients (for review see (Veltkamp and Gill, 2016)).

Neuroinflammation-Targeted Strategies and MS (Table 1)

It is well known that MS is an immume disease and the scope of this review is not to describe inflammatory pathways involved in MS. Most if not all of MS treatments are immunomodulatory or immunosuppressive drugs. In this field, several inflammatory factors may be identified as new potential targets for MS treatment. Indeed, several studies show that cytokines contribute to the pathogenesis of MS. Indeed, increased levels of TNF-α can be found in active lesions within the CNS as well as in the serum and CSF of MS patients (Wen et al., 2012). Furthermore, increased levels of TNF-α in CSF are in relation with the severity and progression of the disease (Sharief and Hentges, 1991). Thus studies have been done in mouse models of MS to test treatment strategy aiming to block TNF-α with very encouraging results (Palle et al., 2017). The hypothesis that neutralization of TNF-α may reduce or arrest MS progression was evaluated in a phase II randomized, multicenter, placebo-controlled study using lenercept, a recombinant TNFR1 fusion protein. However results were discouraging as patients treated with lenercept suffered from increased disease activity. These results suggest that non-selective blockade of TNF-α is detrimental (The Lenercept Multiple Sclerosis Study Group and The University of British Columbia Ms/Mri Analysis Group, 1999). One possible explanation could be that TNF-α may exert both proinflammatory effects and protective functions, for example, mediating remyelination in the CNS under pathological conditions (Probert, 2015). Other cytokines could be involved in the pathogenesis of MS as increased levels of IL6 have been found in active plaques of individuals suffering from MS (Maimone et al., 1997). It has also been reported that IL6-deficient animals were fully resistant to EAE (Kleiter et al., 2016). However, we have to remain cautious as a report described a patient with rheumatoid arthritis who developed MS during anti-IL6 therapy (Beauchemin and Carruthers, 2016). Furthermore, it has been reported that patients treated with anti-TNF-α therapies are at risk to develop clinical signs of MS. Putting all these data together we can speculate that IL6 may have beneficial effect in patients with MS.

CONCLUSION AND PERSPECTIVES

IS and MS share common pathological pathways such as astrocytes activation, BBB disruption and microglia/macrophages polarization (**Figure 1**). This allows emphasizing similar treatments. Already, drugs commonly delivered for MS treatment have been the object of clinical trials for IS care using their immunomodulation potential. Potential innovative treatments targeting astrocytes activation, BBB integrity and neuroinflammation with modulation of microglia/macrophages polarization or cytokines expression have been the subjects of animal studies and clinical trials (**Table 1**). This is of interest as, except for thrombolysis, no treatment has been identified to decrease IS burden.

AUTHOR CONTRIBUTIONS

RP conceived and wrote the article. J-MC wrote the article.

FUNDING

This work was partly granted by Prindex s.r.l.

REFERENCES

Ahn, K. C., Mackenzie, E. M., Learman, C. R., Hall, T. C., Weaver, C. L., Dunbar, G. L., et al. (2015). Inhibition of p53 attenuates ischemic stress-induced activation of astrocytes. *Neuroreport* 26, 862–869. doi: 10.1097/WNR.0000000000000439

Arbeloa, J., Perez-Samartin, A., Gottlieb, M., and Matute, C. (2012). P2X7 receptor blockade prevents ATP excitotoxicity in neurons and reduces brain damage after ischemia. *Neurobiol. Dis.* 45, 954–961. doi: 10.1016/j.nbd.2011.12.014

Asahi, M., Asahi, K., Jung, J. C., Del Zoppo, G. J., Fini, M. E., and Lo, E. H. (2000). Role for matrix metalloproteinase 9 after focal cerebral ischemia: effects of gene knockout and enzyme inhibition with BB-94. *J. Cereb. Blood Flow Metab.* 20, 1681–1689. doi: 10.1097/00004647-200012000-00007

Bake, S., Selvamani, A., Cherry, J., and Sohrabji, F. (2014). Blood brain barrier and neuroinflammation are critical targets of IGF-1-mediated neuroprotection in stroke for middle-aged female rats. *PLoS One* 9:e91427. doi: 10.1371/journal.pone.0091427

Bao, Y., Qin, L., Kim, E., Bhosle, S., Guo, H., Febbraio, M., et al. (2012). CD36 is involved in astrocyte activation and astroglial scar formation. *J. Cereb. Blood Flow Metab.* 32, 1567–1577. doi: 10.1038/jcbfm.2012.52

Beauchemin, P., and Carruthers, R. (2016). MS arising during Tocilizumab therapy for rheumatoid arthritis. *Mult. Scler.* 22, 254–256. doi: 10.1177/1352458515623862

Becker, K., Kindrick, D., Relton, J., Harlan, J., and Winn, R. (2001). Antibody to the alpha4 integrin decreases infarct size in transient focal cerebral ischemia in rats. *Stroke* 32, 206–211. doi: 10.1161/01.STR.32.1.206

Bindra, C. S., Jaggi, A. S., and Singh, N. (2014). Role of P2X7 purinoceptors in neuroprotective mechanism of ischemic postconditioning in mice. *Mol. Cell. Biochem.* 390, 161–173. doi: 10.1007/s11010-014-1967-9

Boven, L. A., Van Meurs, M., Van Zwam, M., Wierenga-Wolf, A., Hintzen, R. Q., Boot, R. G., et al. (2006). Myelin-laden macrophages are anti-inflammatory, consistent with foam cells in multiple sclerosis. *Brain* 129, 517–526. doi: 10.1093/brain/awh707

Broholm, H., Andersen, B., Wanscher, B., Frederiksen, J. L., Rubin, I., Pakkenberg, B., et al. (2004). Nitric oxide synthase expression and enzymatic activity in multiple sclerosis. *Acta Neurol. Scand.* 109, 261–269. doi: 10.1111/j.1600-0404.2004.00207.x

Chen, L., and Brosnan, C. F. (2006). Exacerbation of experimental autoimmune encephalomyelitis in P2X7R-/- mice: evidence for loss of apoptotic activity in lymphocytes. *J. Immunol.* 176, 3115–3126. doi: 10.4049/jimmunol.176.5.3115

Clausen, B. H., Degn, M., Martin, N. A., Couch, Y., Karimi, L., Ormhoj, M., et al. (2014). Systemically administered anti-TNF therapy ameliorates functional outcomes after focal cerebral ischemia. *J. Neuroinflammation* 11:203. doi: 10.1186/s12974-014-0203-6

Cruz, Y., Lorea, J., Mestre, H., Kim-Lee, J. H., Herrera, J., Mellado, R., et al. (2015). Copolymer-1 promotes neurogenesis and improves functional recovery after acute ischemic stroke in rats. *PLoS One* 10:e0121854. doi: 10.1371/journal.pone.0121854

Da Fonseca, A. C., Matias, D., Garcia, C., Amaral, R., Geraldo, L. H., Freitas, C., et al. (2014). The impact of microglial activation on blood-brain barrier in brain diseases. *Front. Cell Neurosci.* 8:362. doi: 10.3389/fncel.2014.00362

Del Zoppo, G. J., Milner, R., Mabuchi, T., Hung, S., Wang, X., Berg, G. I., et al. (2007). Microglial activation and matrix protease generation during focal cerebral ischemia. *Stroke* 38, 646–651. doi: 10.1161/01.STR.0000254477.34231.cb

Easton, A. S. (2013). Neutrophils and stroke - can neutrophils mitigate disease in the central nervous system? *Int. Immunopharmacol.* 17, 1218–1225. doi: 10.1016/j.intimp.2013.06.015

Elkins, J., Veltkamp, R., Montaner, J., Johnston, S. C., Singhal, A. B., Becker, K., et al. (2017). Safety and efficacy of natalizumab in patients with acute ischaemic stroke (ACTION): a randomised, placebo-controlled, double-blind phase 2 trial. *Lancet Neurol.* 16, 217–226. doi: 10.1016/S1474-4422(16)30357-X

Eyo, U. B., Miner, S. A., Ahlers, K. E., Wu, L. J., and Dailey, M. E. (2013). P2X7 receptor activation regulates microglial cell death during oxygen-glucose deprivation. *Neuropharmacology* 73, 311–319. doi: 10.1016/j.neuropharm.2013.05.032

Forrester, S. J., Kikuchi, D. S., Hernandes, M. S., Xu, Q., and Griendling, K. K. (2018). Reactive oxygen species in metabolic and inflammatory signaling. *Cir. Res.* 122, 877–902. doi: 10.1161/CIRCRESAHA.117.311401

Fu, Y., Zhang, N., Ren, L., Yan, Y., Sun, N., Li, Y. J., et al. (2014). Impact of an immune modulator fingolimod on acute ischemic stroke. *Proc. Natl. Acad. Sci. U.S.A.* 111, 18315–18320. doi: 10.1073/pnas.1416166111

Giaume, C., Fromaget, C., El Aoumari, A., Cordier, J., Glowinski, J., and Gros, D. (1991). Gap junctions in cultured astrocytes: single-channel currents and characterization of channel-forming protein. *Neuron* 6, 133–143. doi: 10.1016/0896-6273(91)90128-M

Gilgun-Sherki, Y., Melamed, E., and Offen, D. (2004). The role of oxidative stress in the pathogenesis of multiple sclerosis: the need for effective antioxidant therapy. *J. Neurol.* 251, 261–268. doi: 10.1007/s00415-004-0348-9

Gliem, M., Krammes, K., Liaw, L., Van Rooijen, N., Hartung, H. P., and Jander, S. (2015). Macrophage-derived osteopontin induces reactive astrocyte polarization and promotes re-establishment of the blood brain barrier after ischemic stroke. *Glia* 63, 2198–2207. doi: 10.1002/glia.22885

Grygorowicz, T., Welniak-Kaminska, M., and Struzynska, L. (2016). Early P2X7R-related astrogliosis in autoimmune encephalomyelitis. *Mol. Cell. Neurosci.* 74, 1–9. doi: 10.1016/j.mcn.2016.02.003

Hamzei Taj, S., Kho, W., Riou, A., Wiedermann, D., and Hoehn, M. (2016). MiRNA-124 induces neuroprotection and functional improvement after focal cerebral ischemia. *Biomaterials* 91, 151–165. doi: 10.1016/j.biomaterials.2016.03.025

Hirayama, Y., Ikeda-Matsuo, Y., Notomi, S., Enaida, H., Kinouchi, H., and Koizumi, S. (2015). Astrocyte-mediated ischemic tolerance. *J. Neurosci.* 35, 3794–3805. doi: 10.1523/JNEUROSCI.4218-14.2015

Hu, X., Li, P., Guo, Y., Wang, H., Leak, R. K., Chen, S., et al. (2012). Microglia/macrophage polarization dynamics reveal novel mechanism of injury expansion after focal cerebral ischemia. *Stroke* 43, 3063–3070. doi: 10.1161/STROKEAHA.112.659656

Iadecola, C., and Anrather, J. (2011). The immunology of stroke: from mechanisms to translation. *Nat. Med.* 17, 796–808. doi: 10.1038/nm.2399

Ibarra, A., Avendano, H., and Cruz, Y. (2007). Copolymer-1 (Cop-1) improves neurological recovery after middle cerebral artery occlusion in rats. *Neurosci. Lett.* 425, 110–113. doi: 10.1016/j.neulet.2007.08.038

Investigators, E. A. S. T. (2001). Use of anti-ICAM-1 therapy in ischemic stroke: results of the Enlimomab Acute Stroke Trial. *Neurology* 57, 1428–1434. doi: 10.1212/WNL.57.8.1428

Iodice, R., Manganelli, F., and Dubbioso, R. (2017). The therapeutic use of non-ivasive brain stimulation in multiple sclerosis - a review. *Restor. Nurol. Neurosci.* 35, 497–509. doi: 10.3233/RNN-170735

Jolivel, V., Bicker, F., Biname, F., Ploen, R., Keller, S., Gollan, R., et al. (2015). Perivascular microglia promote blood vessel disintegration in the ischemic penumbra. *Acta Neuropathol.* 129, 279–295. doi: 10.1007/s00401-014-1372-1

Kaiser, M., Penk, A., Franke, H., Krugel, U., Norenberg, W., Huster, D., et al. (2016). Erratum to: lack of functional P2X7 receptor aggravates brain edema development after middle cerebral artery occlusion. *Purinergic Signal.* 12, 735–736. doi: 10.1007/s11302-016-9523-6

Kleiter, I., Ayzenberg, I., Araki, M., Yamamura, T., and Gold, R. (2016). Tocilizumab, MS, and NMOSD. *Mult. Scler.* 22, 1891–1892. doi: 10.1177/1352458516643395

Korhonen, P., Kanninen, K. M., Lehtonen, S., Lemarchant, S., Puttonen, K. A., Oksanen, M., et al. (2015). Immunomodulation by interleukin-33 is protective in stroke through modulation of inflammation. *Brain Behav. Immun.* 49, 322–336. doi: 10.1016/j.bbi.2015.06.013

Kraft, P., Gob, E., Schuhmann, M. K., Gobel, K., Deppermann, C., Thielmann, I., et al. (2013). FTY720 ameliorates acute ischemic stroke in mice by reducing thrombo-inflammation but not by direct neuroprotection. *Stroke* 44, 3202–3210. doi: 10.1161/STROKEAHA.113.002880

Kraft, P., Gobel, K., Meuth, S. G., and Kleinschnitz, C. (2014). Glatiramer acetate does not protect from acute ischemic stroke in mice. *Exp. Transl. Stroke Med.* 6:4. doi: 10.1186/2040-7378-6-4

Kuo, P. C., Yu, I. C., Scofield, B. A., Brown, D. A., Curfman, E. T., Paraiso, H. C., et al. (2017). 3H-1,2-Dithiole-3-thione as a novel therapeutic agent for the treatment of ischemic stroke through Nrf2 defense pathway. *Brain Behav. Immun.* 62, 180–192. doi: 10.1016/j.bbi.2017.01.018

Langhauser, F., Kraft, P., Gob, E., Leinweber, J., Schuhmann, M. K., Lorenz, K., et al. (2014). Blocking of alpha4 integrin does not protect from acute ischemic stroke in mice. *Stroke* 45, 1799–1806. doi: 10.1161/STROKEAHA.114.005000

Lee, S. H., and Suk, K. (2017). Emerging roles of protein kinases in microglia-mediated neuroinflammation. *Biochem. Pharmacol.* 146, 1–9. doi: 10.1016/j.bcp.2017.06.137

Li, D. D., Song, J. N., Huang, H., Guo, X. Y., An, J. Y., Zhang, M., et al. (2013). The roles of MMP-9/TIMP-1 in cerebral edema following experimental acute cerebral infarction in rats. *Neurosci. Lett.* 550, 168–172. doi: 10.1016/j.neulet.2013.06.034

Liesz, A., Sun, L., Zhou, W., Schwarting, S., Mracsko, E., Zorn, M., et al. (2011a). FTY720 reduces post-ischemic brain lymphocyte influx but does not improve outcome in permanent murine cerebral ischemia. *PLoS One* 6:e21312. doi: 10.1371/journal.pone.0021312

Liesz, A., Zhou, W., Mracsko, E., Karcher, S., Bauer, H., Schwarting, S., et al. (2011b). Inhibition of lymphocyte trafficking shields the brain against deleterious neuroinflammation after stroke. *Brain* 134, 704–720. doi: 10.1093/brain/awr008

Lin, R., Cai, J., Kostuk, E. W., Rosenwasser, R., and Iacovitti, L. (2016). Fumarate modulates the immune/inflammatory response and rescues nerve cells and neurological function after stroke in rats. *J Neuroinflammation* 13:269. doi: 10.1186/s12974-016-0733-1

Liu, J., Jin, X., Liu, K. J., and Liu, W. (2012). Matrix metalloproteinase-2-mediated occludin degradation and caveolin-1-mediated claudin-5 redistribution contribute to blood-brain barrier damage in early ischemic stroke stage. *J. Neurosci.* 32, 3044–3057. doi: 10.1523/JNEUROSCI.6409-11.2012

Llovera, G., Hofmann, K., Roth, S., Salas-Perdomo, A., Ferrer-Ferrer, M., Perego, C., et al. (2015). Results of a preclinical randomized controlled multicenter trial (pRCT): Anti-CD49d treatment for acute brain ischemia. *Sci. Transl. Med.* 7:299ra121. doi: 10.1126/scitranslmed.aaa9853

Luo, Y., Zhou, Y., Xiao, W., Liang, Z., Dai, J., Weng, X., et al. (2014). Interleukin-33 ameliorates ischemic brain injury in experimental stroke through promoting

Th2 response and suppressing Th17 response. *Brain Res.* 1597, 86–94. doi: 10.1016/j.brainres.2014.12.005

Ma, Y., Wang, J., Wang, Y., and Yang, G. Y. (2017). The biphasic function of microglia in ischemic stroke. *Prog. Neurobiol.* 157, 247–272. doi: 10.1016/j.pneurobio.2016.01.005

Maimone, D., Guazzi, G. C., and Annunziata, P. (1997). IL-6 detection in multiple sclerosis brain. *J. Neurol. Sci.* 146, 59–65. doi: 10.1016/S0022-510X(96)00283-3

McKittrick, C. M., Lawrence, C. E., and Carswell, H. V. (2015). Mast cells promote blood brain barrier breakdown and neutrophil infiltration in a mouse model of focal cerebral ischemia. *J. Cereb. Blood Flow Metab.* 35, 638–647. doi: 10.1038/jcbfm.2014.239

Meng, H. L., Li, X. X., Chen, Y. T., Yu, L. J., Zhang, H., Lao, J. M., et al. (2016). Neuronal soluble fas ligand drives M1-microglia polarization after cerebral ischemia. *CNS Neurosci. Ther.* 22, 771–781. doi: 10.1111/cns.12575

Miao, Y., Qiu, Y., Lin, Y., Miao, Z., Zhang, J., and Lu, X. (2011). Protection by pyruvate against glutamate neurotoxicity is mediated by astrocytes through a glutathione-dependent mechanism. *Mol. Biol. Rep.* 38, 3235–3242. doi: 10.1007/s11033-010-9998-0

Mikita, J., Dubourdieu-Cassagno, N., Deloire, M. S., Vekris, A., Biran, M., Raffard, G., et al. (2011). Altered M1/M2 activation patterns of monocytes in severe relapsing experimental rat model of multiple sclerosis. Amelioration of clinical status by M2 activated monocyte administration. *Mult. Scler.* 17, 2–15. doi: 10.1177/1352458510379243

Miron, V. E., Boyd, A., Zhao, J. W., Yuen, T. J., Ruckh, J. M., Shadrach, J. L., et al. (2013). M2 microglia and macrophages drive oligodendrocyte differentiation during CNS remyelination. *Nat. Neurosci.* 16, 1211–1218. doi: 10.1038/nn.3469

Mitani, A., and Tanaka, K. (2003). Functional changes of glial glutamate transporter GLT-1 during ischemia: an in vivo study in the hippocampal CA1 of normal mice and mutant mice lacking GLT-1. *J. Neurosci.* 23, 7176–7182. doi: 10.1523/JNEUROSCI.23-18-07176.2003

Ni, J., Wang, X., Chen, S., Liu, H., Wang, Y., Xu, X., et al. (2015). MicroRNA let-7c-5p protects against cerebral ischemia injury via mechanisms involving the inhibition of microglia activation. *Brain Behav. Immun.* 49, 75–85. doi: 10.1016/j.bbi.2015.04.014

Olah, M., Biber, K., Vinet, J., and Boddeke, H. W. (2011). Microglia phenotype diversity. *CNS Neurol. Disord. Drug Targets* 10, 108–118. doi: 10.2174/187152711794488575

Ouyang, Y. B., Voloboueva, L. A., Xu, L. J., and Giffard, R. G. (2007). Selective dysfunction of hippocampal CA1 astrocytes contributes to delayed neuronal damage after transient forebrain ischemia. *J. Neurosci.* 27, 4253–4260. doi: 10.1523/JNEUROSCI.0211-07.2007

Ouyang, Y. B., Xu, L., Lu, Y., Sun, X., Yue, S., Xiong, X. X., et al. (2013). Astrocyte-enriched miR-29a targets PUMA and reduces neuronal vulnerability to forebrain ischemia. *Glia* 61, 1784–1794. doi: 10.1002/glia.22556

Ouyang, Y. B., Xu, L., Yue, S., Liu, S., and Giffard, R. G. (2014). Neuroprotection by astrocytes in brain ischemia: importance of microRNAs. *Neurosci. Lett.* 565, 53–58. doi: 10.1016/j.neulet.2013.11.015

Palle, P., Monaghan, K. L., Milne, S. M., and Wan, E. C. K. (2017). Cytokine signaling in multiple sclerosis and its therapeutic applications. *Med. Sci.* 5:E0023. doi: 10.3390/medsci5040023

Parpura, V., Heneka, M. T., Montana, V., Oliet, S. H., Schousboe, A., Haydon, P. G., et al. (2012). Glial cells in (patho)physiology. *J. Neurochem.* 121, 4–27. doi: 10.1111/j.1471-4159.2012.07664.x

Pascual, O., Ben Achour, S., Rostaing, P., Triller, A., and Bessis, A. (2012). Microglia activation triggers astrocyte-mediated modulation of excitatory neurotransmission. *Proc. Natl. Acad. Sci. U.S.A.* 109, E197–E205. doi: 10.1073/pnas.1111098109

Patel, A. R., Ritzel, R., Mccullough, L. D., and Liu, F. (2013). Microglia and ischemic stroke: a double-edged sword. *Int. J. Physiol. Pathophysiol. Pharmacol.* 5, 73–90.

Pekny, M., Wilhelmsson, U., and Pekna, M. (2014). The dual role of astrocyte activation and reactive gliosis. *Neurosci. Lett.* 565, 30–38. doi: 10.1016/j.neulet.2013.12.071

Pires, P. W., Girgla, S. S., Moreno, G., Mcclain, J. L., and Dorrance, A. M. (2014). Tumor necrosis factor-alpha inhibition attenuates middle cerebral artery remodeling but increases cerebral ischemic damage in hypertensive rats. *Am. J. Physiol. Heart Circ. Physiol.* 307, H658–H669. doi: 10.1152/ajpheart.00018.2014

Poittevin, M., Deroide, N., Azibani, F., Delcayre, C., Giannesini, C., Levy, B. I., et al. (2013). Glatiramer Acetate administration does not reduce damage after cerebral ischemia in mice. *J. Neuroimmunol.* 254, 55–62. doi: 10.1016/j.jneuroim.2012.09.009

Ponath, G., Ramanan, S., Mubarak, M., Housley, W., Lee, S., Sahinkaya, F. R., et al. (2017). Myelin phagocytosis by astrocytes after myelin damage promotes lesion pathology. *Brain* 140, 399–413. doi: 10.1093/brain/aww298

Prineas, J. W., Kwon, E. E., Cho, E. S., Sharer, L. R., Barnett, M. H., Oleszak, E. L., et al. (2001). Immunopathology of secondary-progressive multiple sclerosis. *Ann. Neurol.* 50, 646–657. doi: 10.1002/ana.1255

Probert, L. (2015). TNF and its receptors in the CNS: the essential, the desirable and the deleterious effects. *Neuroscience* 302, 2–22. doi: 10.1016/j.neuroscience.2015.06.038

Ransohoff, R. M., and Perry, V. H. (2009). Microglial physiology: unique stimuli, specialized responses. *Annu. Rev. Immunol.* 27, 119–145. doi: 10.1146/annurev.immunol.021908.132528

Relton, J. K., Sloan, K. E., Frew, E. M., Whalley, E. T., Adams, S. P., and Lobb, R. R. (2001). Inhibition of alpha4 integrin protects against transient focal cerebral ischemia in normotensive and hypertensive rats. *Stroke* 32, 199–205. doi: 10.1161/01.STR.32.1.199

Rodriguez-Grande, B., Swana, M., Nguyen, L., Englezou, P., Maysami, S., Allan, S. M., et al. (2014). The acute-phase protein PTX3 is an essential mediator of glial scar formation and resolution of brain edema after ischemic injury. *J. Cereb. Blood Flow Metab.* 34, 480–488. doi: 10.1038/jcbfm.2013.224

Rothstein, J. D., Dykes-Hoberg, M., Pardo, C. A., Bristol, L. A., Jin, L., Kuncl, R. W., et al. (1996). Knockout of glutamate transporters reveals a major role for astroglial transport in excitotoxicity and clearance of glutamate. *Neuron* 16, 675–686. doi: 10.1016/S0896-6273(00)80086-0

Roy Choudhury, G., Ryou, M. G., Poteet, E., Wen, Y., He, R., Sun, F., et al. (2014). Involvement of p38 MAPK in reactive astrogliosis induced by ischemic stroke. *Brain Res.* 1551, 45–58. doi: 10.1016/j.brainres.2014.01.013

Sarchielli, P., Greco, L., Floridi, A., Floridi, A., and Gallai, V. (2003). Excitatory amino acids and multiple sclerosis: evidence from cerebrospinal fluid. *Arch. Neurol.* 60, 1082–1088. doi: 10.1001/archneur.60.8.1082

Sharief, M. K., and Hentges, R. (1991). Association between tumor necrosis factor-alpha and disease progression in patients with multiple sclerosis. *N. Engl. J. Med.* 325, 467–472. doi: 10.1056/NEJM199108153250704

Sharp, A. J., Polak, P. E., Simonini, V., Lin, S. X., Richardson, J. C., Bongarzone, E. R., et al. (2008). P2x7 deficiency suppresses development of experimental autoimmune encephalomyelitis. *J. Neuroinflammation* 5, 33. doi: 10.1186/1742-2094-5-33

Shi, Y., Jiang, X., Zhang, L., Pu, H., Hu, X., Zhang, W., et al. (2017). Endothelium-targeted overexpression of heat shock protein 27 ameliorates blood-brain barrier disruption after ischemic brain injury. *Proc. Natl. Acad. Sci. U.S.A.* 114, E1243–E1252. doi: 10.1073/pnas.1621174114

Siushansian, R., Bechberger, J. F., Cechetto, D. F., Hachinski, V. C., and Naus, C. C. (2001). Connexin43 null mutation increases infarct size after stroke. *J. Comp. Neurol.* 440, 387–394. doi: 10.1002/cne.1392

Sofroniew, M. V. (2009). Molecular dissection of reactive astrogliosis and glial scar formation. *Trends Neurosci.* 32, 638–647. doi: 10.1016/j.tins.2009.08.002

Srinivasan, R., Sailasuta, N., Hurd, R., Nelson, S., and Pelletier, D. (2005). Evidence of elevated glutamate in multiple sclerosis using magnetic resonance spectroscopy at 3 T. *Brain* 128, 1016–1025. doi: 10.1093/brain/awh467

Strecker, J. K., Schmidt, A., Schabitz, W. R., and Minnerup, J. (2017). Neutrophil granulocytes in cerebral ischemia - Evolution from killers to key players. *Neurochem. Int.* 107, 117–126. doi: 10.1016/j.neuint.2016.11.006

Sumbria, R. K., Boado, R. J., and Pardridge, W. M. (2012). Brain protection from stroke with intravenous TNFalpha decoy receptor-Trojan horse fusion protein. *J. Cereb. Blood Flow Metab.* 32, 1933–1938. doi: 10.1038/jcbfm.2012.97

Sumi, N., Nishioku, T., Takata, F., Matsumoto, J., Watanabe, T., Shuto, H., et al. (2010). Lipopolysaccharide-activated microglia induce dysfunction of the blood-brain barrier in rat microvascular endothelial cells co-cultured with microglia. *Cell Mol. Neurobiol.* 30, 247–253. doi: 10.1007/s10571-009-9446-7

The Lenercept Multiple Sclerosis Study Group and The University of British Columbia Ms/Mri Analysis Group (1999). TNF neutralization in MS: results of a randomized, placebo-controlled multicenter study. *Neurology* 53, 457–465.

Veltkamp, R., and Gill, D. (2016). Clinical Trials of Immunomodulation in Ischemic Stroke. *Neurotherapeutics* 13, 791–800. doi: 10.1007/s13311-016-0458-y

Verma, R., Mishra, V., Sasmal, D., and Raghubir, R. (2010). Pharmacological evaluation of glutamate transporter 1 (GLT-1) mediated neuroprotection following cerebral ischemia/reperfusion injury. *Eur. J. Pharmacol.* 638, 65–71. doi: 10.1016/j.ejphar.2010.04.021

Wang, S., Zhou, J., Kang, W., Dong, Z., and Wang, H. (2016). Tocilizumab inhibits neuronal cell apoptosis and activates STAT3 in cerebral infarction rat model. *Bosn. J. Basic Med. Sci.* 16, 145–150. doi: 10.17305/bjbms.2016.853

Weller, M. L., Stone, I. M., Goss, A., Rau, T., Rova, C., and Poulsen, D. J. (2008). Selective overexpression of excitatory amino acid transporter 2 (EAAT2) in astrocytes enhances neuroprotection from moderate but not severe hypoxia-ischemia. *Neuroscience* 155, 1204–1211. doi: 10.1016/j.neuroscience.2008.05.059

Wen, S. R., Liu, G. J., Feng, R. N., Gong, F. C., Zhong, H., Duan, S. R., et al. (2012). Increased levels of IL-23 and osteopontin in serum and cerebrospinal fluid of multiple sclerosis patients. *J. Neuroimmunol.* 244, 94–96. doi: 10.1016/j.jneuroim.2011.12.004

Werner, P., Pitt, D., and Raine, C. S. (2001). Multiple sclerosis: altered glutamate homeostasis in lesions correlates with oligodendrocyte and axonal damage. *Ann. Neurol.* 50, 169–180. doi: 10.1002/ana.1077

Wu, J. J., Guerin, A., Sundaram, M., Dea, K., Cloutier, M., and Mulani, P. (2017). Cardiovascular event risk assessment in psoriasis patients treated with tumor necrosis factor-alpha inhibitors versus methotrexate. *J. Am. Acad. Dermatol.* 76, 81–90. doi: 10.1016/j.jaad.2016.07.042

Wu, J. J., Sundaram, M., Cloutier, M., Gauthier-Loiselle, M., Guerin, A., Singh, R., et al. (2018). The risk of cardiovascular events in psoriasis patients treated with tumor necrosis factor-alpha inhibitors versus phototherapy: an observational cohort study. *J. Am. Acad. Dermatol.* 79, 60–68. doi: 10.1016/j.jaad.2018.02.050

Xia, C. Y., Zhang, S., Gao, Y., Wang, Z. Z., and Chen, N. H. (2015). Selective modulation of microglia polarization to M2 phenotype for stroke treatment. *Int. Immunopharmacol.* 25, 377–382. doi: 10.1016/j.intimp.2015.02.019

Xu, L., Emery, J. F., Ouyang, Y. B., Voloboueva, L. A., and Giffard, R. G. (2010). Astrocyte targeted overexpression of Hsp72 or SOD2 reduces neuronal vulnerability to forebrain ischemia. *Glia* 58, 1042–1049. doi: 10.1002/glia.20985

Yiangou, Y., Facer, P., Durrenberger, P., Chessell, I. P., Naylor, A., Bountra, C., et al. (2006). COX-2, CB2 and P2X7-immunoreactivities are increased in activated microglial cells/macrophages of multiple sclerosis and amyotrophic lateral sclerosis spinal cord. *BMC Neurol.* 6:12. doi: 10.1186/1471-2377-6-12

Zhang, D. D., Zou, M. J., Zhang, Y. T., Fu, W. L., Xu, T., Wang, J. X., et al. (2017). A novel IL-1RA-PEP fusion protein with enhanced brain penetration ameliorates cerebral ischemia-reperfusion injury by inhibition of oxidative stress and neuroinflammation. *Exp. Neurol.* 297, 1–13. doi: 10.1016/j.expneurol.2017.06.012

Zhang, H., Park, J. H., Maharjan, S., Park, J. A., Choi, K. S., Park, H., et al. (2017). Sac-1004, a vascular leakage blocker, reduces cerebral ischemia-reperfusion injury by suppressing blood-brain barrier disruption and inflammation. *J. Neuroinflammation* 14, 122. doi: 10.1186/s12974-017-0897-3

Zhang, Z., Zhang, Z. Y., Schittenhelm, J., Wu, Y., Meyermann, R., and Schluesener, H. J. (2011). Parenchymal accumulation of CD163+ macrophages/microglia in multiple sclerosis brains. *J. Neuroimmunol.* 237, 73–79. doi: 10.1016/j.jneuroim.2011.06.006

Zhao, X., Wang, H., Sun, G., Zhang, J., Edwards, N. J., and Aronowski, J. (2015). Neuronal Interleukin-4 as a modulator of microglial pathways and ischemic brain damage. *J. Neurosci.* 35, 11281–11291. doi: 10.1523/JNEUROSCI.1685-15.2015

10

Cardiovascular Adaptive Homeostasis in Exercise

Kelvin J. A. Davies[1,2,3*]

[1] Leonard Davis School of Gerontology of the Ethel Percy Andrus Gerontology Center, University of Southern California, Los Angeles, CA, United States, [2] Molecular and Computational Biology Program, Department of Biological Sciences, Dornsife College of Letters, Arts, and Sciences, University of Southern California, Los Angeles, CA, United States, [3] Department of Biochemistry and Molecular Medicine, USC Keck School of Medicine, University of Southern California, Los Angeles, CA, United States

Edited by:
Pasquale Pagliaro,
Università degli Studi di Torino, Italy

Reviewed by:
Antonio Crisafulli,
Università degli Studi di Cagliari, Italy
Tommaso Angelone,
University of Calabria, Italy

***Correspondence:**
Kelvin J. A. Davies
kelvin@usc.edu

Adaptive Homeostasis has been defined as, "The transient expansion or contraction of the homeostatic range in response to exposure to sub-toxic, non-damaging, signaling molecules or events, or the removal or cessation of such molecules or events." (Davies, 2016). I propose that one of the most significant examples of adaptive homeostasis may be the adaptation of the cardiovascular system to exercise training. In particular, endurance type training involves the generation of increased levels of free radicals such as ubisemiquinone, superoxide, nitric oxide, and other (non-radical) reactive oxygen species such as hydrogen peroxide (H_2O_2), in a repetitive manner, typically several times per week. As long as the training intensity and duration are sub-maximal and not exhaustive these reactive species do not cause damage, but rather activate signal transduction pathways to induce mitochondrial biogenesis—the foundation of increased exercise endurance. Particularly important are the NFκB and Nrf2 signal transduction pathways which respond to reactive oxygen and nitrogen species generated during exercise. As with other examples of adaptive homeostasis the effects are transient, lasting only as long as the training is maintained. Unfortunately, the ability to adapt to exercise training declines with age, perhaps as a result of impaired Nrf2 and NFκB signaling, as does adaptive homeostasis capacity in general. Since this is an Hypothesis/Theory Paper and not a review, I have not tried to provide a comprehensive discussion of all the literature relating to exercise adaptation and the cardiovascular system. Rather, I have attempted to develop the Hypothesis or Theory that adaptive homeostasis is the foundation for adaptation of the cardiovascular system to exercise training, largely based on work from my own laboratory, that of close collaborators, and that of key contributors over a period of almost 40 years.

Keywords: adaptive homeostasis, exercise, cardiovascular system, redox regulation, signal transduction, Nrf2, mitochondria, free radicals

INTRODUCTION

Adaptive Homeostasis has been defined as, "The transient expansion or contraction of the homeostatic range in response to exposure to sub-toxic, non-damaging, signaling molecules or events, or the removal or cessation of such molecules or events." (Davies, 2016). Adaptive Homeostasis applies to the expansion or contraction of the homeostatic range, for any given physiological parameter, including heart rate, blood pressure, cardiac stroke volume or output, respiratory rate and volume, etc. Although Adaptive Homeostasis pertains to any signaling event that can regulate multiple physiological functions, such as heat, cold, osmotic stress, acid/base changes, nutrients, etc. the concept was actually first described (Davies, 2016) and subsequently further developed (Davies et al., 2017; Lomeli et al., 2017; Pomatto and Davies, 2017; Pomatto et al., 2017a,b,c, 2018a; 2018b; Walker et al., 2018; Zhou et al., 2018) as a function of oxidation/reduction ("Redox") signaling. Furthermore, the "seeds" for the whole concept of adaptive homeostasis originate with studies of cardiovascular adaptation to exercise (e.g., Davies et al., 1981, 1982a,b,c, 1984). Thus, Adaptive Homeostasis would appear to be an especially good fit for this Special Research Topic on "Redox and Nitrosative Signaling in Cardiovascular System: from Physiological Response to Disease."

Recently, we published more generalized treatises on the contribution of diminished adaptive homeostasis to multiple age-related diseases, including cardiovascular disorders (Davies et al., 2017; Lomeli et al., 2017; Pomatto and Davies, 2017), but here I will attempt to target the cardiovascular system, and its responses to exercise training, specifically. Please note that this is an Hypothesis/Theory Paper and not a review. Therefore, I have not tried to provide a comprehensive discussion of all the literature relating to exercise adaptation and the cardiovascular system, and I apologize to all those whose important work has been omitted. Rather, I have attempted to develop the Hypothesis or Theory, largely based on work from my laboratory and that of close collaborators over a period of almost 40 years, that adaptive homeostasis is the basis for adaptation of the cardiovascular system to exercise training.

DIFFERENTIATING ENDURANCE AND SPRINT TRAINING ADAPTATIONS

One of the first studied cardiovascular signaling responses is the exercise training effect. Exercise training also represents one of the most widely experienced cardiovascular adaptations affecting humans. In early studies, Holloszy et al. (Holloszy, 1967, 2008; Terjung et al., 1973) had demonstrated significant cardiovascular and skeletal muscle adaptations to endurance exercise training. In a series of studies in the late 1970's and early 1980's we set about trying to differentiate the very different adaptive responses to physical exercise training of an endurance type, vs. sprint or strength training (Davies et al., 1981, 1982b). We also sought to determine the mechanism(s) underlying exercise training adaptations although, at that time, little was known about biological signal transduction pathways. We used young male Sprague-Dawley laboratory rats to study adaptation to endurance training [10 weeks of daily treadmill running, for 5 days per week at a speed of 26.8 m/min (1.0 mph), and a slope of 8.5° (15% grade)]. Initially the rats ran for only 20 min but this was gradually increased each day such that, by week 5 (and for the next 5 weeks) the rats each ran for 120 min per day. This training protocol caused only a small (14%) increase in VO_{2max} (maximum amount of oxygen that an animal can utilize during intense, or maximal exercise) but increased endurance capacity (run time to exhaustion in a treadmill run at a constant, sub-VO_{2max} work load) four-fold and greatly increased (actually doubled) the mitochondrial content of skeletal muscles (Davies et al., 1981).

Unlike the program of endurance training described above, a regimen of sprint training (lasting 4 weeks) did not result in any significant increases in muscle mitochondrial oxidase capacity, or in total muscle mitochondrial mass, and only increased VO_{2max} by a modest 15% (Davies et al., 1982b). The sprint training program did, however, increase the capacity for high intensity workload, also called VO_{2max} work load (maximal treadmill speed at 15% grade) by 25%. The protocol used for sprint training, over a 4 week period, involved starting each session with a 2-min "warm-up" at a treadmill speed of 26.8 m/min, and then gradually increasing treadmill speed during the third minute to 97 m/min. The rats were then required to complete two 1-min periods of sprinting at 97 m/min each day (with a 10 s rest in between). To ensure that they were acclimatized to running on the treadmill (but not actually trained) control rats ran for 5 min at 26.8 m/min, twice per week. Despite the increases in VO_{2max} work load resulting from sprint training, there was no increase in endurance capacity and (as already noted above) muscle mitochondrial oxidase capacity and muscle mitochondrial mass also did not change. These results were taken as evidence that muscle mitochondrial total mass and oxidase capacity are closely coupled with exercise endurance capacity, but that VO_{2max} must be determined by other factors (Davies et al., 1982b).

In fact, the above studies (Davies et al., 1981, 1982b) also suggested that VO_{2max} might be largely determined by the oxygen carrying capacity of blood and not a function limited by mitochondrial respiration. To further test these relationships, we next used three experimental interventions with the same strain of laboratory rats described above: (1) Dietary Iron deficiency and dietary repletion (Davies et al., 1982a; Maguire et al., 1982), (2) Dietary iron deficiency and blood transfusion (Davies et al., 1984), and (3) Dietary Vitamin E (α tocopherol) deficiency (Quintanilha and Davies, 1982; Quintanilha et al., 1982).

Abbreviations: Nrf2, nuclear factor erythroid-derived 2-related factor 2; NFκB, nuclear factor kappa-light-chain-enhancer of activated B cells; VO_{2max}, maximum amount of oxygen that an individual can utilize during intense, or maximal exercise; Hb, hemoglobin; $O_2^{\bullet-}$, superoxide anion radical; H_2O_2, hydrogen peroxide; $NO^{\bullet}$, nitric oxide radical; H_2O_2, hydrogen peroxide; EDL, extensor digitorum longus muscle; RCAN1-4, regulator of calcineurin protein 1-4; HSP70, heat shock protein 70; OGG1, DNA damage repair enzyme 8-oxoguanine-DNA glycosylase; MnSOD, manganese superoxide dismutase (mitochondrial); GSH, reduced glutathione; GSSG, oxidized glutathione; TFAM, mitochondrial transcription factor A; PGC-1α, peroxisome proliferator-activated receptor-gamma coactivator 1-alpha PGC-1α; NRF-1, nuclear respiratory factor 1; NRF-2, nuclear respiratory factor 2; P38MAPK, mitogen-activated protein kinase A; AMPK, AMP-activated protein kinase; SIRT1, Sirtuin1; Keap1, Kelch-like ECH-associated protein 1; Cul3, Cullin3; Akt, the RAC-alpha serine/threonine-protein kinase encoded by the *AKT* gene (also known as protein kinase B, or PKB); PKC γ, protein kinase C gamma; EPRE or ARE, electrophile response element or antioxidant response element; NFE2L1 or Nrf1, Nuclear factor erythroid-derived 2-related factor 1 (sometimes written as Nrf1, but which has an official symbol of NFE2L1); Bach1, transcription regulator protein Bach1; cMyc, Myelocytomatosis oncogene cellular homolog; MPP+, 1-methyl-4-phenylpyridine.

The effects of dietary iron deficiency and dietary iron repletion on exercise performance were investigated in young male Sprague-Dawley rats (Davies et al., 1982a; Maguire et al., 1982). Iron deficiency was established in young, male rats by feeding them a low-iron diet with only 2 mg iron/kg, whereas the diet fed to control animals contained 50 mg iron/kg. After 42 days, rats fed the low-iron diet had blood hemoglobin (Hb) levels of only 3.6 ± 0.5 g/dl, whereas the control rats exhibited blood Hb of 13.7 ± 0.6 g/dl. In the iron-deficient animals, we observed 60–85% lower muscle mitochondrial oxidative capacities in comparison with controls; presumably this resulted from 30% lower mitochondrial content of muscles and significantly lower mitochondrial enzyme specific activities. In the iron-deficient rats, both VO_2 max and VO_2 max work load were 50% lower than seen in control animals, and exercise endurance capacity was 90% lower. To reverse deficiency, the low-iron rats were next switched to the control (iron-sufficient) diet and we carefully mapped out the time course of iron repletion and the recovery of muscle mitochondrial and exercise parameters. Blood Hb was markedly in only 3 days and was accompanied by significant improvements in both VO_{2max} and VO_{2max} work load. Importantly, however, neither mitochondrial bioenergetic functions, nor the mitochondrial content of muscle, nor muscle mitochondrial oxidative capacity, exhibited significant increases before day 5 of iron repletion, and exercise endurance capacity also did not increase before day 5. From these studies of iron-deficiency and repletion we were persuaded that muscle mitochondrial oxidase capacity probably does not normally impose a limit on VO_{2max} or VO_{2max} work load. Similarly, we concluded that the oxidative capacity of muscle (i.e., functional mitochondria) probably does limit exercise endurance capacity. Parallel studies, on the same animals, revealed that the iron deficiency protocol severely depleted mitochondrial iron sulfur proteins and cytochromes, which then caused severe limitations of up to 70–80% in the electron transport capacity, and ATP production, of mitochondria (Davies et al., 1982a; Maguire et al., 1982).

Although the above studies of iron deficiency and repletion provided temporal evidence for a dissociation between muscle mitochondrial oxidative capacity and VO_{2max}/VO_{2max} workload and, conversely, provided temporal evidence for a strong association between muscle mitochondrial oxidative capacity and endurance capacity and between the oxygen carrying capacity of blood and VO_{2max} workload, no causal relationships could be concluded. To attempt to delineate cause and effect we utilized dietary iron deficiency and blood transfusions using young male weanling Sprague-Dawley rats (Davies et al., 1984). Using the same iron-deficient and control diets described above, we found that only 21 days of dietary iron deficiency caused significant anemia (Hb, 3.9 vs. 14.2 g/dl in controls) and major loss of function of muscle mitochondria, such that skeletal muscle mitochondrial total oxidative capacity was as much as 90% lower than see in control rats. VO_{2max} apparently declined by 50% as a result of iron deficiency and the maximal endurance capacity (time to exhaustion in a separate treadmill run at a constant, sub-VO_{2max} work load) of iron-deficient rats was only 10% of that seen in control animals. We next took the iron deficient rats and artificially increased their blood Hb by transfusion with packed erythrocytes. Conversely, we decreased the Hb levels of control rats by withdrawing blood and transfusing them with plasma. These procedures enabled us to match the Hb of both iron-deficient and control rats at a common value of approximately 9.5 g/dl. Raising the Hb of iron-deficient animals immediately corrected their exercise VO_{2max} such that it was only 15% below control values but, importantly, we observed no improvement whatsoever in exercise endurance capacity. These interventional experiments yielded a direct demonstration that VO_{2max} and endurance capacity depend on rather different physiological functions. Based on these results, it was posited that oxygen delivery to tissues is a major determinant of VO_{2max} but, in contrast, muscle mitochondrial capacity is a major determinant of exercise endurance capacity (Davies et al., 1984). It should also be mentioned, however, that what determines VO_{2max} is still the subject of some debate, with some investigators favoring a "cardiocentric" viewpoint whereas others consider skeletal muscles as the limiting factor.

There are also some neural reflexes that regulate the cardiovascular apparatus. One of these is the so called muscle metaboreflex, which adjusts the cardiovascular response on the basis of the metabolic conditions of working muscles. It has been speculated that in some cardiovascular diseases, and in the sedentary state, detraining affects this reflex by increasing matabolite accumulation and decreasing muscle oxidative capacity. For instance, this is the so called "muscle hypothesis" of heart failure. The interaction of intrinsic muscle factors and neural signaling may, thus, represent a potential link between fatigue, cardiovascular disregulation, and the effect of training in these pathologies.

Taken together, the above studies of endurance training; sprint training; iron deficiency, dietary repletion, and blood transfusion; and vitamin E deficiency all point to the conclusion that the mitochondrial content of muscle and, of course, mitochondrial competence have a major role in determining exercise endurance capacity. Furthermore, increased mitochondrial biogenesis during endurance exercise training would seem to be a key factor in exercise adaptive homeostasis.

UBISEMIQUINONE, SUPEROXIDE, AND HYDROGEN PEROXIDE IN EXERCISE

Our exercise studies also demonstrated, for the first time, unequivocally that free radical generation in skeletal muscles and liver increases during exercise, and is especially evident during exhaustive exercise (Davies and Hochstein, 1982; Davies et al., 1982c). Previous work by Tappel et al. (Dillard et al., 1978) had suggested that exercise caused increased free radical generation that could be measured as expired pentane but this indirect methodology was criticized as being subject to large errors due to variable pentane production by gut flora and fauna, and various other investigators produced equivocal results with other measures of lipid peroxidation. Our work used the direct approach of actually measuring free radical signals by electron spin resonance spectroscopy, and demonstrated increased concentrations of mitochondrial ubisemiquinone radicals in both muscle and liver, following exercise (Davies et al., 1982c). We were actually able to identify two discrete "pools" of semi-stabilized ubisemiquinone with stability constants high enough to support the physiological significance of Peter Mitchell's "Q Cycle Hypothesis" (Davies and Hochstein, 1982). Of greater importance for the current discussion, however, is the observation that reduction of molecular oxygen to the superoxide anion radical ($O_2^{\bullet-}$) by ubisemiquinone is a major source of intracellular $O_2^{\bullet-}$ generation, and much if not most of the $O_2^{\bullet-}$ so generated rapidly dismutates to form hydrogen peroxide (H_2O_2) (Cadenas and Davies, 2000).

Following heavy exercise, we found increases of 100–200% in observable concentrations of free radicals in rat muscles and liver (Davies et al., 1982c). The free radical signals we could observe and measure via electron spin resonance spectroscopy were largely attributable to mitochondrial ubisemiquinone radicals (Davies and Hochstein, 1982). Exhaustive exercise (but not exercise at a training level) caused significant damage, including lipid peroxidation, diminished sarcoplasmic reticulum and endoplasmic reticulum integrity, and diminished respiratory control of mitochondria. In a parallel study, we found that Vitamin E deficiency, which sensitizes animals to increased free radical oxidative damage, caused a similar damage profile (in membranes, sarcoplasmic/endoplasmic reticulum, and mitochondria) even without making the animals exercise (Davies et al., 1982c; Quintanilha and Davies, 1982; Quintanilha et al., 1982). Our earlier studies indicated that endurance capacity in exercise is principally governed by the functional muscle mitochondrial mass (Davies et al., 1981, 1982a,b, 1984), and when we exercise tested the vitamin E deficient animals (with their impaired muscle mitochondria), we found that their endurance was indeed 40% lower than that of controls (Davies et al., 1982c). These findings further strengthened our interpretation that exercise training of a serious but sub-maximal nature slightly increases free radical (ubisemiquinone and $O_2^{\bullet-}$) and H_2O_2 generation, and that this is an important component of exercise adaptation. In contrast, maximal exercise to exhaustion increases free radical and H_2O_2 generation to dangerously high levels that can cause significant cellular damage.

Interestingly, our studies showed that the generation of $O_2^{\bullet-}$ by purified mitochondria studied *in vitro*, increased as a function of temperature (Salo et al., 1991). When we exposed mitochondria to temperatures seen in exercising human beings (Brooks et al., 1971a,b) we found that temperature-induced partial uncoupling of oxygen consumption and ATP production accounted for the increased $O_2^{\bullet-}$ generation (Salo et al., 1991). Thus, it is possible that temperature-induced fluctuations in the fidelity with which ubisemiquinone, and other electron carriers, such as complexes I and III, can direct electrons along the mitochondrial respiratory chain, resulting in a "leakage" of electrons directly to oxygen, may account for both significant $O_2^{\bullet-}$ generation in exercise and a limit to exercise capacity.

Of course, today everyone recognizes both $O_2^{\bullet-}$ and H_2O_2 as major intracellular signaling molecules. In 1983, however, when we first demonstrated ubisemiquinone radicals in exercise, such relationships were not understood. Despite this lack of mechanistic understanding, we wrote, "It is tempting to propose that exercise induced free radicals .... may be the initiating stimulus to mitochondrial biogenesis." (Davies et al., 1982c). Viewed with the hindsight of current knowledge, the results suggest that increased concentrations of ubisemiquinone radicals, and the $O_2^{\bullet-}$ and H_2O_2 generated by interaction of ubisemiquinone (and/or complexes I and III) with molecular oxygen may provide a stimulus to the adaptive homeostasis, including the mitochondrial biogenesis, which results from endurance training.

EXERCISE-INDUCED GENERATION OF REACTIVE OXYGEN/NITROGEN SPECIES BY XANTHINE OXIDASE AND BY NEUTROPHILS AND OTHER PHAGOCYTIC CELLS

Since our original publications, several groups have verified increased generation of free radicals, and other reactive oxygen/nitrogen species in exercise (e.g., see Packer et al., 2008; Sachdev and Davies, 2008). In addition to the $O_2^{\bullet-}$ and H_2O_2 generated by ubisemiquinone, as described above, other investigators have also described additional mitochondrial and extra-mitochondrial sources of reactive oxygen/nitrogen species in exercise (reviewed in Sachdev and Davies, 2008).

Xanthine oxidase is one such source of exercise-induced $O_2^{\bullet-}$ and H_2O_2 generation, as described by Viña et al. (Heunks et al., 1999; Viña et al., 2000). These investigators noted that xanthine dehydrogenase could be converted to xanthine oxidase during intensive exercise, perhaps due to transient hypoxia. The xanthine oxidase so produced may then generate $O_2^{\bullet-}$ and H_2O_2 rather than the NADH generated by its parent xanthine dehydrogenase. Importantly, the xanthine oxidase inhibitor allopurinol blocked much of the oxidation seen in tissues from intensively exercised animals.

McArdle et al. (1999) proposed that that exhaustive, eccentric, or prolonged exercise may increase generation of reactive oxygen/nitrogen species as a result of neutrophils, as well as other phagocytic type cells, overwhelming antioxidant defenses as part of an intensified immune response to cellular injury. For example, McArdle et al. (1999) reported increased concentrations of oxidized glutathione in extensor digitorum longus (EDL) muscles 3 days after an extensive program of injury-inducing contractions, although no significant glutathione oxidation was actually evident a few hours following exercise. Other investigators have also reported neutrophil/phagocyte activation and reactive oxygen/nitrogen species generation with very long duration, extreme intensity, or exhaustive exercise (Singh et al., 1994; Wareski et al., 2000; Quindry et al., 2003; Morozov et al., 2006).

Part of the problem with whole animal (or human) studies of reactive oxygen/nitrogen species, especially in exercise, is the sheer difficulty of making accurate measurements of species that are, by their very nature, short lived in biological systems. After reviewing the literature on generation of such species by mitochondrial ubisemiquinone (and/or mitochondrial complexes I and III), xanthine oxidase, neutrophils and other phagocytes, and various ill-defined sources, I think there are some valuable conclusions we may draw. First, it seems clear that there can be multiple sources of $O_2^{\bullet -}$, H_2O_2, and other reactive oxygen/nitrogen species in exercise. Second, there is clearly a major difference between endurance exercise and sprint or strength training. Third, both the intensity and the duration of an exercise session affect the generation of reactive oxygen/nitrogen species. Fourth, generation of reactive oxygen/nitrogen species at low levels during non-exhaustive exercise (e.g., daily training sessions) appears to be involved in mitochondrial biogenesis whereas very high levels of reactive oxygen/nitrogen species generation during exhaustive exercise appear to contribute to tissue injury.

SHOCK AND STRESS PROTEINS IN EXERCISE ADAPTATION

Very heavy or exhaustive exercise induces heat-shock (in humans involving muscle temperatures that can reach 45°C, and human core body temperatures as high as 44°C), oxidative stress (as evidenced by increased levels of $O_2^{\bullet -}$ and H_2O_2), and tissue damage, whereas daily exercise training at much lower intensity and duration promotes mitochondrial biogenesis (100–200% increases muscle mitochondrial mass). Following such intense and exhaustive exercise in rats, the levels of more than 15 heat shock or oxidative stress proteins, including HSP70, were elevated in skeletal muscle, heart, and liver tissues (Salo et al., 1991). Different patterns of protein transcriptional responses (incorporation of [^{3}H]leucine into newly-synthesized proteins) were observed in soleus, plantaris, and EDL muscles, probably reflecting differential involvement in the exercise session and/or differential responses to heat shock and oxidative stress. Heart, liver, and skeletal muscles also exhibited diverse patterns of responses to heat shock *in vitro*, nevertheless increased levels of some five proteins, in particular HSP70 and an unidentified 106 kDa protein, were common findings.

Focusing more on HSP70, we found that mRNA levels (as measured by Northern blot with a [^{32}P]-labeled *HSP70* cDNA probe), were significantly elevated in both skeletal muscle and cardiac muscle following exercise, and following either both heat-shock or oxidative stress of *ex vivo* tissues exposed to oxidative stress or heat-shock *in vitro* (Salo et al., 1991). In exhaustive exercise studies the levels of *HSP70* mRNA in skeletal muscles crested some 30–60 min after the end of the exercise session, and gradually decreased thereafter such that control levels were re-established in another 5 h. HSP70 transcription and translation may thus be seen as an appropriate physiological response to both the elevated temperatures and increased oxidation typical of heavy exercise. Extreme hyperthermia in very heavy and exhaustive exercise might actually be the proximal source for increased oxidation, because we also discovered, in this same study, a temperature-dependent uncoupling of muscle mitochondria (studied *in vitro*), with concomitant increases in $O_2^{\bullet -}$ production: the higher the temperature applied, the more $O_2^{\bullet -}$ generation was increased (Salo et al., 1991). Both HSP70 and HSP90 play major roles in the transport of nuclear encoded polypeptides into mitochondria, since the bulk of essential mitochondrial proteins are actually encoded in the cell nucleus and transcribed on cytoplasmic ribosomes. Thus, HSP70 and HSP90 may be vital links in the molecular mechanism of exercise-induced mitochondrial biogenesis (Salo et al., 1991). As noted above, however, there are major differences between a program of daily exercise endurance training at sub-maximal intensity and duration, and a single bout of maximal and exhaustive exercise. Thus, although it is much easier to measure the greatly increased production/generation of heat-shock or oxidative-stress proteins and free radicals or related oxidants following intense exercise to exhaustion, I propose that the much smaller elevations in these same species that occur in sub-maximal exercise, as a person trains to increase endurance, are important factors in signaling for mitochondrial biogenesis.

Importantly, rats that have actually completed a successful endurance exercise training program no longer exhibit increases in any shock or stress proteins (including no change in HSP70) at exercise levels or durations that produce significant shock/stress protein expression in untrained rats (Salo et al., 1991). This result can now be seen as an early demonstration of a key aspect of adaptive homeostasis: that the normal physiological range can be temporarily expanded in response to signaling molecules or events, but will return to its basal range if signaling is stopped for a sufficient period. In this case, exercise training is the "event" which (mediated by signaling molecules such as of $O_2^{\bullet -}$ and H_2O_2) temporarily expands the physiological range for exercise tolerance such that (after weeks of training) the daily exercise workout level is no longer a stress; of course, as predicted by the adaptive homeostasis theory (Davies, 2016), this will only be true for as long as exercise training is kept up, so that a return to sedentary lifestyle will cause the expanded physiological range to gradually contract back to pre-training dimensions.

Working with close collaborators at the University of Rennes in France, we have described how exhaustive exercise increases transcription/translation of the calcineurin inhibitor RCAN1-4 (Regulator of Calcineurin 1-4) in rat skeletal muscles (Emrani et al., 2015). We had previously shown that RCAN1-4 (originally called Adapt78, DSCR1, or calcipressin) is part of a repertoire of immediate oxidative stress proteins that actually helps to improve adaptation to oxidants by inhibiting calcineurin, which dephosphorylates and inactivates many other proteins required for adaptation (Crawford et al., 1997; Ermak et al., 2002; Harris et al., 2005; Davies et al., 2007).

The levels of RCAN1-4 were elevated in both EDL and gastrocnemius muscles of rats, but not in their soleus muscles, following exercise to exhaustion (Emrani et al., 2015). Importantly, as something of an internal control, calcineurin enzymatic activity declined in EDL and gastrocnemius as levels of its inhibitor RCAN1 rose, but was unchanged in soleus muscles where RCAN1 also did not increase. Unexpectedly, the expression of calcineurin protein actually decreased in EDL, gastrocnemius, and soleus for (thus far) unexplained reasons. Another indicator of oxidative stress, protein oxidation, was also elevated in EDL and gastrocnemius muscles, but not in soleus muscles. It was concluded that oxidative "signals" generated during exercise, doubtless reactive oxygen/nitrogen species, increased the expression of RCAN1-4 protein in EDL and gastrocnemius muscles. We, therefore, proposed that up-regulation of RCAN1-4 transcription/translation and thus, induction of the signal transduction pathways that it regulates, is a significant element involved in physiological adaptative homeostasis stimulated by reactive oxygen/nitrogen species generated during exercise (Emrani et al., 2015).

Exercise also modifies the level/activity of the of mitochondrial outer-membrane-associated DNA damage repair enzyme 8-oxoguanine DNA glycosylase (OGG1) in skeletal muscle (Radak et al., 2009). Following 8 weeks of a swimming endurance training program, mitochondrial levels of carbonylated proteins were decreased (compared with control animals) and nuclear OGG1 activity was increased. These effects were reversed during de-training. Interestingly, OGG1 levels in muscle were increased following exercise endurance training, and this increase was reversed to control levels by de-training. It seems possible that endurance training may actually increase the transport of OGG1 across the mitochondrial membranes and into the matrix, thus potentially increasing the capacity for OGG1-mediated repair of oxidized DNA. In contrast, the decline in muscle OGG1 levels seen with physical inactivity could actually diminish the effective transport of OGG1 into mitochondria and decrease DNA repair (Radak et al., 2009). Finally, the mitochondrial Lon protease which protects the mitochondrial matrix against accumulation of oxidatively damaged proteins by selectively degrading them (Bota and Davies, 2002; Bota et al., 2002; Pomatto et al., 2016) is significantly induced by exercise (Koltai et al., 2012).

SIGNAL TRANSDUCTION PATHWAYS REGULATING CARDIOVASCULAR ADAPTATIVE HOMEOSTASIS IN EXERCISE

From the work of many laboratories it has become abundantly clear that many forms of transient adaptation are mediated by discrete signal transduction pathways. Thus, for example, the shock, stress, or adaptive proteins discussed in the section above do not just increase (or decrease) expression on their own. Instead, dedicated signal transduction pathways exist within all cells to initiate, regulate, and terminate adaptive gene expression responses. Such adaptive homeostasis related signal transduction pathways involve sensor proteins in the cytoplasm which undergo a series of complex protein–protein interactions, transport proteins for nuclear translocation, and binding to specific regulator regions of target proteins to initiate increased transcription. Similarly, inhibitory sensor proteins can regulate the systematic down-regulation of gene expression once the need for an adaptive response has passed. Several such signal transduction pathways that operate during exercise adaptation are discussed in the sub-sections below.

The NFκB Signal Transduction Pathway in Exercise Adaptation

The nuclear factor kappa-light-chain-enhancer of activated B cells, or NFκB, signal transduction pathway contributes to adaptation and protection from oxidative stress. Under non-stressful conditions, the NFκB transcription factor resides in the cytosol, where it is bound to its specific inhibitor protein, IκB (Baeuerle and Baltimore, 1988a). Following exposure to H_2O_2 (or some other reactive oxygen species), NFκB is translocated to the cell nucleus, where it can bind to the upstream promoter regions of multiple target genes through its DNA binding subunits, p50 and p65. Binding of p50 and p65 to target gene promoters then elicits transcriptional activation of those target genes (Baeuerle and Baltimore, 1988b; Meyer et al., 1994). The gene encoding the mitochondrial (manganese containing) form of superoxide dismutase, or Mn-SOD, contains one such upstream promoter region, and its expression is upregulated by NFκB. Binding of NFκB to the Mn-SOD gene promoter region was originally reported by Wan et al. (1994), but the finding by Hollander et al. that an exhaustive exercise session significantly increased expression of Mn-SOD did not come for several years (Hollander et al., 2001). These results, subsequently confirmed by Ji et al. (2004), provided an example that exercise can induce adaptation and increased protection through superoxide dismutase.

Gomez-Cabrera et al. (2005) examined the effect of xanthine oxidase, via the inhibitory activity of allopurinol on NFκB activation in rats, following intensive exercise to exhaustion. The investigators found that that if, the rats received a dose of allopurionol prior to exercise, they exhibited far less oxidation of glutathione (GSH oxidized to GSSG) than did rats that were exercised with no allopurionol pre-treatment. The results were interpreted to mean that normally during intense exercise to exhaustion glutathione is oxidized by H_2O_2 generated by xanthine oxidase but that this can be prevented by inhibiting xanthine oxidase with allopurinol. Importantly, the allopurionol-treated rats also exhibited significantly less adaptation through the NFκB pathway. For example, the activity of Mn-SOD, among that of other inducible enzymes, increased significantly in the control animals after exhaustive exercise but was induced to a far lesser extent in rats that had received the allopurinol pre-treatment. These results provided additional evidence that NFκB plays a significant role in adaptation to oxidative stress via triggering by H_2O_2. Indeed, it has been found that NFκB can remain bound to target genes for many hours, or even for days, after exercise (Hollander et al., 2001) presumably causing continued elevated transcription of multiple adaptive enzymes (Gomez-Cabrera et al., 2005), thereby and playing a very important role in adapting to exercise-induced oxidative damage. Because of these observations, Gomez-Cabrera et al. (2005) also suggested that if reactive oxygen species play such major roles in initiating adaptive responses (for example via NFκB) then the practice of supplementing the diets of athletes with antioxidants should probably be reconsidered, or even discarded.

Mitochondrial Biogenesis Signal Transduction Pathways—Mitochondrial Transcription Factor a (TFAM) and Peroxisome Proliferator-Activated Receptor-Gamma Coactivator 1-Alpha (PGC-1α)—In Exercise Adaptation

Mitochondrial transcription factor A (TFAM) peroxisome proliferator-activated receptor-gamma coactivator 1-alpha (PGC-1α) are major regulators of the mitochondrial genome (Gleyzer et al., 2005; Kaasik, 2009). In contrast nuclear respiratory factors1 and 2 (abbreviated NRF-1 and NRF-2 respectively), can control expression of many nuclear genes that actually encode mitochondrial proteins. TFAM, NRF-1, and NRF-2 are, in turn, controlled by peroxisome proliferator-activated receptor-gamma coactivator 1-alpha (PGC-1α) (Olesen et al., 2010). PGC-1α induces mitochondrial biogenesis, following activation (phosphorylation) by the mitogen-activated protein kinase (p38 MAPK) or AMP-activated protein kinase (AMPK) (Holloszy, 2008; Viña et al., 2009; Olsen, 2010). Additionally it has been shown that Sirtuin1 (SIRT1), also known as NAD-dependent deacetylase sirtuin-1, catalyzes PGC-1α deacetylation, which also activates the coactivator (Wareski et al., 2000; Nemoto et al., 2005).

Researchers have found that PGC-1α is readily induced by both acute and regular exercise and plays a significant role in muscle mitochondrial biogenesis (Terada et al., 2002; Pilegaard et al., 2003; Ikeda et al., 2006; Hart et al., 2014; Marton et al., 2015). In most of these studies, SIRT1, AMPK, NRF-1, and TFAM also accompanies (or preceded) mitochondrial biogenesis (Koltai et al., 2017). Of particular significance is the finding that aging is associated with a significant decline in mitochondrial biogenesis, but that exercise training can partially reverse this trend (Koltai et al., 2012). Importantly, PGC-1α levels decline with age but are at least partially restored with exercise training (Koltai et al., 2012). Also at least partially restored to "youthful" levels by exercise training in this study were SIRT1, AMPK, NRF-1, and TFAM, as well as actual markers of increased mitochondrial biogenesis.

The Nuclear Factor Erythroid-Derived 2-Related Factor 2 (Nrf2) Signal Transduction Pathway in Exercise Adaptation

The Keap1-Nrf2 signal transduction pathway is vitally important in regulating cellular and organismal adaptation to reactive oxygen and nitrogen species. This relationship is a widely observed biological phenomenon that has been verified (with Nrf2 orthologs) in numerous eukaryotic systems, including yeast, various mammalian/human cells, *Caenorhabditis elegans* nematode worms, *Drosophila melanogaster* flies, mice, rats, and human beings (Pickering et al., 2012; Zhang et al., 2015; Davies et al., 2017; Pomatto and Davies, 2017; Pomatto et al., 2017c, 2018a,b; Raynes et al., 2017). In mammals, Nrf2 is found in the cytoplasm where it forms part of a complex with Keap1 and several other proteins. The Cullin3 (Cul3) component of the Keap1-Nrf2 complex is actually an E3-ubiquitin ligase enzyme that rapidly polyubiquitinylates Nrf2 thus causing its degradation by the 26S proteasome. Since Nrf2 is synthesized at high levels, this process ensures that cytoplasmic Nrf2 undergoes constant and rapid turnover.

Upon exposure to oxidants or electrophiles, Nrf2 detaches from the Keap1 (Kelch-like ECH-associated protein 1 complex, avoids polyubiquitinylation, and instead undergoes phosphorylation by the serine/threonine kinase Akt (the RAC-alpha serine/threonine-protein kinase encoded by the *AKT* gene, also known as protein kinase B, or PKB) and protein kinase C gamma (PKC γ). Phosphorylated Nrf2 is then transported into the cell nucleus where it can bind to the upstream electrophile response elements or EPRE's (also called antioxidant response elements, or ARE's) of hundreds of target genes involved in cellular protection and adaptive homeostasis. Binding of Nrf2 to a target gene's EPRE/ARE causes increased transcription and translation, and elevated levels of the protective/adaptive protein encoded by that gene. Activation of the Nrf2 signal transduction pathway is a key, required, element for many forms of effective adaptive homeostasis, and inhibiting or blocking activation also forstalls adaptation. Nuclear factor erythroid-derived 2-related factor 1 (sometimes written as Nrf1, but which has an official symbol of NFE2L1) often binds to EPRE/ARE sites where it only poorly induces transcription and is, thus often seen as an inhibitor of Nrf2 responses (although NFE2L1 has its own target genes as well). In addition, both the transcription regulator protein Bach1 and the oncogene cMyc (Myelocytomatosis oncogene cellular homolog) appear to act as true physiological inhibitors of Nrf2 signaling (by different mechanisms) and both increase with age (Zhang et al., 2015; Zhou et al., 2018); this finding may go some way to explaining the loss of Nrf2 signaling responsiveness with aging.

If any tissue might be expected to undergo adaptive homeostasis in response to exercise training it would be skeletal muscle, and careful studies indicate that this is actually the case (Davies et al., 1981, 1982a,b, 1984). A strong link between Nrf2 signaling and mitochondrial biogenesis in exercise was reported by Merry and Ristow (2016). These authors reported that reactive oxygen and nitrogen species activate Nrf2 signaling in exercise, and work through induction of NRF-1 and TFAM to induce mitochondrial biogenesis and production of antioxidant enzymes in skeletal muscles. The authors further reported that mice with impaired Nrf2 signaling were unable to increase mitochondrial mass, endurance capacity, or whole body energy expenditure to the same extent as wild-type mice, following a 5 week program of treadmill endurance training. The duration and intensity of exercise also clearly affects Nrf2 signaling responses, with longer and more intense bouts of exercise being more effective (Li et al., 2015).

Even though the myocardium is constantly at work throughout life, Muthusamy et al. (2012) found that a session of acute endurance exercise resulted in Nrf2 signaling, with resultant enhancement of several antioxidant protective systems and defense pathways in the heart muscle of wild-type mice. Importantly, this protective example of adaptive homeostasis was not seen in Nrf2 double mutant mice. In a study published in

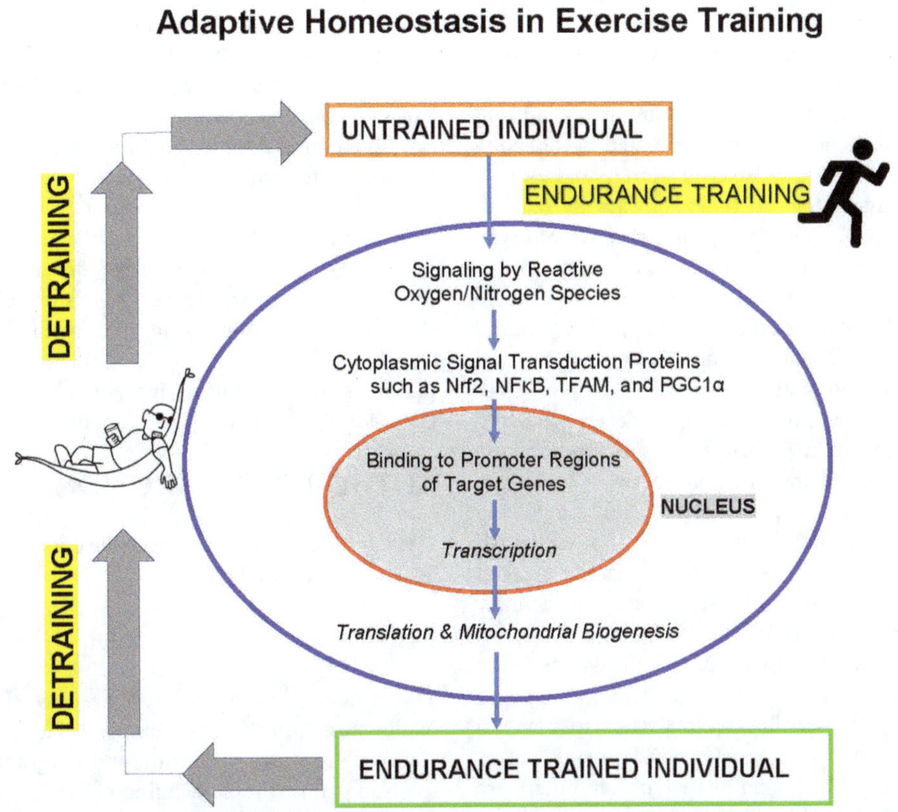

FIGURE 1 | Adaptive homeostasis in exercise training. Reactive oxygen and nitrogen species such as $O_2^{\bullet-}$, H_2O_2, and $NO^{\bullet}$ activate cytoplasmic signaling proteins such as Nrf2, NFκB, TFAM, and PGC1α to translocate to the cell nucleus where they bind to upstream promoter regions of hundreds of target genes to initiate transcription and (ultimately) translation. The protein products of these target genes include mitochondrial proteins encoded in the nucleus, leading to mitochondria biogenesis, and numerous other adaptive and protective proteins. These changes in gene expression and increased mitochondrial biogenesis (in addition to other metabolic alterations) lead to increased exercise endurance capacity. The training effect is a transient process of expanding the range of adaptive homeostasis and it only lasts as long as the training stimulus is maintained. If training is discontinued then detraining results in adaptive homeostasis returning the range of endurance capacity to pre-training levels.

the same year, Gounder et al. (2012) reported that Nrf2 signaling is normally impaired in the hearts of aged mice (and humans). They found that aged mice (>23 months) exhibited multiple signs of significant cardiac oxidative stress following a single bout of high-intensity endurance-type exercise, in comparison with young mice (∼2 months). Furthermore, the aged mice failed to elicit a significant Nrf2 response to the endurance test. In a study of human males, Done et al. (2016) found that a single bout of cycling exercise elicited substantial Nrf2-dependent gene expression in peripheral blood mononuclear cells collected from young (23 ± 1 years) men, whereas the Nrf2 responses of aged (63 ± 1 years) men were significantly blunted. Providing more hope for the future, however, Gounder et al. (2012) found that a 6 week program of daily exercise training at more moderate levels was successful in eliciting an Nrf2-dependent adaptive response. This result raises the hope that older individuals may still be able to reap the benefits of Nrf2-dependent adaptive homeostasis, as long as the exercise stimulus is not too intense or exhaustive.

Another tissue/organ that might not have been expected to exhibit exercise adaptations is the brain. Nevertheless, Tsou et al. (2015) reported that 4 weeks of treadmill exercise training effectively diminished several of the negative neuronal effects of 1-methyl-4-phenylpyridine (MPP+) in a rodent model of Parkinson disease. The authors implicated Nrf2 signaling in their positive results, and further found that Nrf2 knock-down, using a lentivirus-carried shNrf2 delivery system, blocked the protective effects of exercise training. These results, and those above, indicate that Nrf2 has a widespread systemic role in exercise adaptation, including mitochondrial biogenesis. More in-depth reviews of the role(s) of Nrf2 in exercise adaptive homeostasis have recently been published (Done and Traustadóttir, 2016; Madhusudhanan and Rajasekaran, 2016).

CONCLUSIONS

The studies discussed above show that endurance exercise training involves significant adaptive homeostasis of the cardiovascular system, including extensive biogenesis of mitochondria. In fact, muscle mitochondrial oxidative capacity can now be seen as a major determinant of endurance exercise capability, and types of training that do not increase mitochondrial biogenesis (e.g., sprint training) also do not increase endurance capacity. Furthermore, impairment of mitochondrial functionality and capacity (e.g., by iron deficiency or vitamin E deficiency) imposes major limitations to exercise endurance capacity (**Figure 1**).

Adaptive homeostasis during exercise training is mediated by discrete signal transduction pathways operated by signaling proteins such as NFκB, TFAM, PGC-1α, Nrf2, and others. Redox regulation of signal transduction pathways by reactive oxygen species such as $O_2^{\bullet -}$ and H_2O_2, and reactive nitrogen species such as $NO^{\bullet}$ (the nitric oxide radical), is a key factor in inducing mitochondrial biogenesis and increased cellular damage protection. Importantly, effective redox signaling, mitochondrial biogenesis, and increasing endurance capacity come as a result of sub-maximal intensity/duration exercise bouts. In other words, low levels of reactive oxygen/nitrogen species generated during serious but sub-maximal exercise training sessions are effective in recruiting signal transduction pathways to induce mitochondrial biogenesis. In contrast, exercise sessions involving maximal intensity or maximal endurance (e.g., exercise to exhaustion) generate much higher levels of reactive oxygen and nitrogen species that cause cellular damage and actually diminish effective adaptation. Thus, damage is not a necessary, or desirable, component of exercise adaptive homeostasis in the cardiovascular system.

Finally, the ability of the cardiovascular system to adapt to exercise training diminishes with age. Obviously, many factors are involved in producing the "aging phenotype," and there are clearly many components that contribute to age-related declines, but one important factor appears to be progressively ineffective redox signal transduction and mitochondrial biogenesis with advancing age. In this regard, increasing levels of the Nrf2 inhibitors Bach1 and cMyc, that are observed with advancing age, may contribute to an age-dependent compromise of exercise adaptive homeostasis in the cardiovascular system. On a more positive note, with which to end, Kwak (2013) found that although aging is typically associated with a gradual decline in cardiac function, "*.....exercise training not only improves cardiac function but also decreases the risk of heart disease.*" Specifically, Kwak found that chronic exercise training effectively diminished the age-associated mitochondrial-mediated apoptosis in the aging heart (reviewed in Kwak, 2013), giving hope that alternative pathways or mechanisms may exist to mediate the beneficial effects of exercise in older individuals.

AUTHOR CONTRIBUTIONS

The author confirms being the sole contributor of this work and approved it for publication.

FUNDING

The author was funded by grant # ES003598 from the National Institute of Environmental Health Sciences of the US National Institutes of Health, and by grant # AG052374 from the National Institute on Aging of the US National Institutes of Health.

REFERENCES

Baeuerle, P. A., and Baltimore, D. (1988a). Activation of DNA-binding activity in an apparently cytoplasmic precursor of the NF-kappa B transcription factor. *Cell* 53, 211–217. doi: 10.1016/0092-8674(88)90382-0

Baeuerle, P. A., and Baltimore, D. (1988b). I kappa B: a specific inhibitor of the NF-kappa B transcription factor. *Science* 242, 540–546.

Bota, D. A., van Remmen, H., and Davies, K. J. A. (2002). Modulation of Lon protease activity and aconitase turnover with aging and oxidative stress. *FEBS Lett.* 532, 103–106 doi: 10.1016/S0014-5793(02)03638-4

Bota, D., and Davies, K. J. A. (2002). Lon protease preferentially degrades oxidized mitochondrial aconitase by an ATP-stimulated mechanism. *Nat. Cell Biol.* 4, 674–680. doi: 10.1038/ncb836

Brooks, G. A., Hittelman, K. J., Faulkner, J. A., and Beyer, R. E. (1971a). Temperature, skeletal muscle mitochondrial functions, and oxygen debt. *Am. J. Physiol.* 220, 1053–1059.

Brooks, G. A., Hittelman, K. J., Faulkner, J. A., and Beyer, R. E. (1971b). Tissue temperatures and whole-animal oxygen consumption after exercise. *Am. J. Physiol.* 221, 427–431.

Cadenas, E., and Davies, K. J. A. (2000). Mitochondrial free radical production, oxidative stress, and aging. *Free Radic. Biol. Med.* 29, 222–2230.

Crawford, D. R., Leahy, K. P., Abramova, N., Lan, L., Wang, Y., and Davies, K. J. A. (1997). Hamster adapt78, mRNA is a down syndrome critical region homologue that is inducible by oxidative stress. *Arch. Biochem. Biophys.* 342, 6–12.

Davies, K. J. A. (2016). Adaptive homeostasis. *Mol. Aspects Med.* 49, 1–7. doi: 10.1016/j.mam.2016.04.007

Davies, J. M. S., Cillard, J., Friguet, B., Cadenas, E., Cadet, J., Cayce, R., et al. (2017). The oxygen paradox, the French Paradox, and age-related diseases. *GeroScience* 39, 499–550. doi: 10.1007/s11357-017-0002-y

Davies, K. J. A., Donovan, C. M., Refino, C. J., Brooks, G. A., Packer, L., and Dallman, P. R. (1984). Distinguishing the effects of anemia and muscle iron deficiency on exercise bioenergetics in the rat. *Am. J. Physiol.: Endocrinol. Metab.* 246, E535–E543. doi: 10.1152/ajpendo.1984.246.6.E535

Davies, K. J. A., Ermak, G., Rothermel, B. A., Pritchard, M., Heitman, J., Ahnn, J., et al. (2007). Renaming the DSCR1/Adapt78 gene family as RCAN: regulators of calcineurin. *FASEB J.* 21, 3023–3028. doi: 10.1096/fj.06-7246com

Davies, K. J. A., and Hochstein, P. (1982). Ubisemiquinone radicals in liver: implications for a mitochondrial Q cycle *in vivo*. *Biochem. Biophys. Res. Commun.* 107, 1292-1299.

Davies, K. J. A., Maguire, J. J., Brooks, G. A., Dallman, P. R., and Packer, L. (1982a). Muscle mitochondrial bioenergetics, oxygen supply, and work capacity during dietary iron deficiency and repletion. *Am. J. Physiol. Endocrinol. Metab.* 242, E418-E427.

Davies, K. J. A., Packer, L., and Brooks, G. A. (1981). Biochemical adaptation of mitochondria, muscle, and whole animal respiration to endurance training. *Arch. Biochem. Biophys.* 209, 539–554.

Davies, K. J. A., Packer, L., and Brooks, G. A. (1982b). Exercise bioenergetics following sprint training. *Arch. Biochem. Biophys.* 215, 260-265.

Davies, K. J. A., Quintanilha, A. T., Brooks, G. A., and Packer, L. (1982c). Free radicals and tissue damage produced by exercise. *Biochem. Biophys. Res. Commun.* 107, 1198-1205.

Dillard, C. J., Litov, R. E., Savin, W. M., Dumelin, E. E., and Tappel, A. L. (1978). Effects of exercise, Vitamin, E., and ozone on pulmonary function and lipid peroxidation. *J. Appl. Physiol.* 45, 927–932.

Done, A. J., and Traustadóttir, T. (2016). Nrf2 mediates redox adaptations to exercise. *Redox Biol.* 10, 191–199. doi: 10.1016/j.redox.2016.10.003

Done, A. J., Gage, M. J., Nieto, N. C., and Traustadóttir, T. (2016). Exercise-induced Nrf2 signaling is impaired in aging. *Free Radic. Biol. Med.* 96, 130–138. doi: 10.1016/j.freeradbiomed.2016.04

Emrani, B. R., Rébillard, A., Lefeuvre, L., Gratas-Delamarche, A., Ermak, G., Davies, K. J. A., et al. (2015). The calcineurin antagonist, RCAN1-4 is induced by exhaustive exercise in skeletal muscle. *Free Radic. Biol. Med.* 87, 290–299. doi: 10.1016/j.freeradbiomed.2015.06.023

Ermak, G., Harris, C., and Davies, K. J. A. (2002). The DSCR1 (Adapt78) Isoform 1 protein, "Calcipressin 1" inhibits calcineurin and protects against acute calcium-mediated stress damage, including transient oxidative stress. *FASEB J.* 16, 814–824. doi: 10.1096/fj.01-0846com

Gleyzer, N., Vercauteren, K., and Scarpulla, R. C. (2005). Control of mitochondrial transcription specificity factors (TFB1M and TFB2M) by nuclear respiratory factors (NRF-1 and NRF-2) and PGC-1 family coactivators. *Mol. Cell Biol.* 25, 1354–1366. doi: 10.1128/MCB.25.4.1354-1366.2005

Gomez-Cabrera, M. C., Borras, C., Pallardo, F. V., Sastre, J., Ji, L. L., and Viña, J. (2005). Decreasing xanthine oxidase-mediated oxidative stress prevents useful cellular adaptations to exercise in rats. *J. Physiol.* 567, 113–120. doi: 10.1113/jphysiol.2004.080564

Gounder, S., Kannan, S., Devadoss, D., Miller, C. J., Whitehead, K. S., Odelberg, S. J., et al. (2012). Impaired transcriptional activity of Nrf2 in age-related myocardial oxidative stress is reversible by moderate exercise training. *PLOS ONE* 7:e45697. doi: 10.1371/journal.pone.0045697

Harris, C. D., Ermak, G., and Davies, K. J. A. (2005). Multiple roles of the DSCR1 (Adapt78 or RCAN1) gene and its protein product calcipressin 1 (or RCAN1) in disease. *Cell Mol. Life Sci.* 62, 2477–2486. doi: 10.1007/s00018-005-5085-4

Hart, N., Sarga, L., Koch, L. G., Britton, S. L., Ngo, J. K., Davies, K. J. A., et al. (2014). Resveratrol enhances exercise-induced adaptive responses in rats selectively bred for low running performance. *Dose Response* 12, 57–71.

Heunks, L. M., Viña, J., van Herwaarden, C. L., Folgering, H. T., Gimeno, A., and Dekhuijzen, P. N. (1999). Xanthine oxidase is involved in exercise-induced oxidative stress in chronic obstructive pulmonary disease. *Am. J. Physiol.* 277, R1697–R1704. doi: 10.1152/ajpregu.1999.277.6.R1697

Hollander, J., Fiebig, R., Gore, M., Ookawara, T., Ohno, H., and Ji, L. L. (2001). Superoxide dismutase gene expression is activated by a single bout of exercise in rat skeletal muscle. *Pflügers Arch. Eur. J. Physiol.* 442, 426–434.

Holloszy, J. O. (1967). Biochemical adaptations in muscle. effects of exercise on mitochondrial oxygen uptake and respiratory enzyme activity in skeletal muscle. *J. Biol. Chem.* 242, 2278–2282.

Holloszy, J. O. (2008). Regulation by exercise of skeletal muscle content of mitochondria and GLUT4. *J. Physiol. Pharmacol.* 59(Suppl. 7), 5–18.

Ikeda, S., Kawamoto, H., Kasaoka, K., Hitomi, Y., Kizaki, T., Sankai, Y., et al. (2006). Muscle type-specific response of PGC-1alpha and oxidative enzymes during voluntary wheel running in mouse skeletal muscle. *Acta Physiol.* 188, 217–223. doi: 10.1111/j.1748-1716.2006.01623.x

Ji, L. L., Gomez-Cabrera, M. C., Steinhafel, N., and Viña, J. (2004). Acute exercise activates nuclear factor (NF)-kappaB signaling pathway in rat skeletal muscle. *FASEB J.* 18, 1499–1506. doi: 10.1096/fj.04-1846com

Kaasik, A. (2009). PGC-1α and PGC-1β regulate mitochondrial density in neurons. *J. Biol. Chem.* 284, 21379–21385. doi: 10.1074/jbc.M109.018911

Koltai, E., Bori, Z., Chabert, C., Dubouchaud, H., Naito, H., Machida, S., et al. (2017). SIRT1 may play a crucial role in overload induced hypertrophy of skeletal muscle: an hypothesis. *J. Physiol.* 595, 3361–3376. doi: 10.1113/JP273774

Koltai, E., Hart, N., Bori, Z., Taylor, A. W., Goto, S., Ngo, J. K., et al. (2012). Age-associated declines in mitochondrial biogenesis and protein quality control factors are minimized by exercise training. *Am. J. Physiol. Regul. Integr. Comp. Physiol.* 303, R127–R134. doi: 10.1152/ajpregu.00337.2011

Kwak, H.-B. (2013). Effects of aging and exercise training on apoptosis in the heart. *J. Exerc. Rehabil.* 9, 212–219. doi: 10.12965/jer.130002

Li, T., He, S., Liu, S., Kong, Z., Wang, J., and Zhang, Y. (2015). Effects of different exercise durations on Keap1-Nrf2-ARE pathway activation in mouse skeletal muscle. *Free Radic. Res.* 49, 1269–1274. doi: 10.3109/10715762.2015.1066784

Lomeli, N., Bota, D., and Davies, K. J. A. (2017). The role of diminished stress resistance, and defective adaptive homeostasis in age related diseases. *Clin. Sci.* 131, 2573–2599. doi: 10.1042/CS20160982

Madhusudhanan, N., and Rajasekaran, N. S. (2016). Exercise, Nrf2 and antioxidant signaling in cardiac aging. *Front. Physiol.* 7:241. doi: 10.3389/fphys.2016.00241

Maguire, J. J., Davies, K. J. A., Dallman, P. R., and Packer, L. (1982). Effects of dietary iron deficiency on iron-sulfur proteins and bioenergetic functions of skeletal muscle mitochondria. *Biochim. Biophys. Acta* 679, 210-220.

Marton, O. L., Koltai, E., Takeda, M., Koch, L. G., Britton, S. L., Davies, K. J. A., et al. (2015). Mitochondrial biogenesis-associated factors underlie the magnitude of response to aerobic endurance training in rats. *Pflügers Arch. Eur. J. Physiol.* 467, 779–788. doi: 10.1007/s00424-014-1554-7

McArdle, A., van der Meulen, J. H., Catapano, M., Symons, M. C., Faulkner, J. A., and Jackson, M. J. (1999). Free radical activity following contraction-induced injury to the extensor digitorum longus muscles of rats. *Free Radic. Biol. Med.* 26, 1085–1091.

Merry, T. L., and Ristow, M. (2016). Nuclear factor erythroid-derived 2-like 2 (NFE2L2, Nrf2) mediates exercise-induced mitochondrial biogenesis and the anti-oxidant response in mice. *J. Physiol.* 594, 5195–5207. doi: 10.1113/JP271957

Meyer, M., Pahl, H. L., and Baeuerle, P. A. (1994). Regulation of the transcription factors NF-kappa B and AP-1 by redox changes. *Chem. Biol. Interact.* 91, 91–100. doi: 10.1016/0009-2797(94)90029-9

Morozov, V. I., Tsyplenkov, P. V., GoGolberg, N. D., and Kalinski, M. I. (2006). The effects of high-intensity exercise on skeletal muscle neutrophil myeloperoxidase in untrained and trained rats. *Eur. J. Appl. Physiol.* 97, 716–722.

Muthusamy, V. R., Kannan, S., Sadhaasivam, K., Gounder, S. S., Davidson, C. J., Boeheme, C., et al. (2012). Acute exercise stress activates Nrf2/ARE signaling and promotes antioxidant mechanisms in the myocardium. *Free Radic. Biol. Med.* 52, 366–376. doi: 10.1016/j.freeradbiomed.2011.10.440

Nemoto, S., Fergusson, M. M., and Finkel, T. (2005). SIRT1 functionally interacts with the metabolic regulator and transcriptional coactivator PGC-1α. *J. Biol. Chem.* 280, 16456–16460. doi: 10.1074/jbc.M501485200

Olesen, J., Kiilerich, K., and Pilegaard, H. (2010). PGC-1α-mediated adaptations in skeletal muscle. *Pflügers Arch.* 460, 153–162. doi: 10.1007/s00424-010-0834-0

Packer, L., Cadenas, E., and Davies, K. J. A. (2008). Free radicals and exercise: an introduction. *Free Radic. Biol. Med.* 44, 123–125. doi: 10.1016/j.freeradbiomed.2007.05.031

Pickering, A. M., Linder, R. A., Zhang, H., Forman, H. J., and Davies, K. J. A. (2012). Nrf2-dependent induction of proteasome and Pa28αβ regulator are required for adaptation to oxidative stress. *J. Biol. Chem.* 287, 10021–10031. doi: 10.1074/jbc.M111.277145

Pilegaard, H., Saltin, B., and Neufer, P.D. (2003). Exercise induces transient transcriptional activation of the PGC-1α gene in human skeletal muscle. *J. Physiol.* 546, 851–858. doi: 10.1113/jphysiol.2002.034850

Pomatto, L. C. D., Cline, M., Woodward, N., Morgan, T., Finch, C. E., Forman, H. J., et al. (2018b). Nano-particulate exposure impacts proteasome response in young and middle-aged female mice. *Free Radic. Biol. Med.* [Epub ahead of print].

Pomatto, L. C. D., Tower, J., and Davies, K. J. A. (2018a). Sexual dimorphism and aging differentially regulate adaptive homeostasis in *Drosophila melanogaster*. *J. Gerontol. Ser. A.* 73, 141–149. doi: 10.1093/gerona/glx083

Pomatto, L. C. D., Wong, S., Tower, J., and Davies, K. J. A. (2017a). Sex-specific differences in adaptation in *D. melanogaster* wild-type strains. *Arch. Biochem. Biophys.* 636, 57–70.

Pomatto, L. C.-D., and Davies, K. J. A. (2017). The decline of adaptive homeostasis in ageing. *J. Physiol.* 595, 7275–7309. doi: 10.1113/JP275072

Pomatto, L. C.-D., Davies, K. J. A., and Tower, J. G. (2016). The mitochondrial Lon protease is required for age-specific and sex-specific adaptation to oxidative stress. *Curr. Biol. Cell Press* 27, 1–15. doi: 10.1016/j.cub.2016.10.044

Pomatto, L. C.-D., Wong, S., Carney, C., Shen, B., Tower, J., and Davies, K. J. A. (2017b). Age- and sex-specific function of the 20s proteasome and the Nrf2/CncC signal transduction pathway in oxidative stress adaptation and resistance in *Drosophila melanogaster*. *Aging* 9, 1153–1178. doi: 10.18632/aging.101218

Pomatto, L. C. D., Wong, S., Tower, J., and Davies, K. J. A. (2017c). Sex-specific adaptive homeostasis in *D. melanogaster* depends on increased proteolysis by the 20S Proteasome: data-in-Brief. *Data Brief.* 17, 653–661. doi: 10.1016/j.dib.2018.01.044

Quindry, J. C., Stone, W. L., King, J., and Broeder, C. E. (2003). The effects of acute exercise on neutrophils and plasma oxidative stress. *Med. Sci. Sports Exerc.* 35, 1139–1145 doi: 10.1249/01.MSS.0000074568.82597.0B

Quintanilha, A. T., and Davies, K. J. A. (1982). Vitamin E deficiency and photosensitization of electron transport carriers in microsomes. *FEBS Lett.* 139, 241-244.

Quintanilha, A. T., Packer, L., Davies, J. M. S., Racanelli, T. L., and Davies, K. J. A. (1982). Membrane effects of vitamin E deficiency: bioenergetic and surface charge density studies of skeletal muscle and liver mitochondria. *Ann. N. Y. Acad. Sci.* 393, 32-47.

Radak, Z., Atalay, M., Jakus, J., Boldogh, I., Davies, K. J. A., and Goto, S. (2009). Exercise improves import of 8-oxoguanine DNA glycosylase into the mitochondrial matrix of skeletal muscle and enhances the relative activity. *Free Radic. Biol. Med.* 46, 238–243. doi: 10.1016/j.freeradbiomed.2008.10.022

Raynes, R., Juarez, C., Pomatto, L. C., Sieburth, D., and Davies, K. J. A. (2017). Aging and SKN-1-dependent loss of 20S proteasome adaptation to oxidative stress in *C. elegans*. *J. Gerontol. A. Biol. Sci. Med. Sci.* 72, 143–151. doi: 10.1093/gerona/glw093

Sachdev, S., and Davies, K. J. A. (2008). Production, detection, and adaptive responses to free radicals in exercise. *Free Radic. Biol. Med.* 44, 215–223. doi: 10.1016/j.freeradbiomed.2007.07.019

Salo, D. C., Donovan, C. M., and Davies, K. J. A. (1991). HSP70 and other possible heat shock or oxidative stress proteins are induced in skeletal muscle, heart, and liver during exercise. *Free Radical Biol. Med.* 11, 239–246. doi: 10.1016/0891-5849(91)90119-N

Singh, A., Failla, M. L., and Deuster, P. A. (1994). Exercise-induced changes in immune function: effects of zinc supplementation. *J. Appl. Physiol.* 76, 2298–2303. doi: 10.1152/jappl.1994.76.6.2298

Terada, S., Goto, M., Kato, M., Kawanaka, K., Shimokawa, T., and Tabata, I. (2002). Effects of low-intensity prolonged exercise on PGC-1 mRNA expression in rat epitrochlearis muscle. *Biochem. Biophys. Res. Commun.* 296, 350–354. doi: 10.1016/S0006-291X(02)00881-1

Terjung, R. L., Klinkerfuss, G. H., Baldwin, K. M., Winder, W. W., and Holloszy, J. O. (1973). Effect of exhausting exercise on rat heart mitochondria. *Am. J. Physiol.* 225, 300–305. doi: 10.1152/ajplegacy.1973.225.2.300

Tsou, Y.-H., Shi, C.-T., Ching, C.-H., Huang, J.-Y., Jen, C.J., Kuo, Y.-M., et al. (2015). Treadmill exercise activates Nrf2 antioxidant system to protect the nigrostriatal dopaminergic neurons from MPP+ toxicity. *Exp. Neurol.* 263, 50–62. doi: 10.1016/j.expneurol.2014.09.021

Viña, J., Gimeno, A., Sastre, J., Desco, C., Aseni, M., Pallardo, F. V., et al. (2000). Mechanisms of free radical production in exhaustive exercise in humans and rats; role of xanthine oxidase and protection by allopurinol. *IUBMB Life* 49, 539–544. doi: 10.1080/15216540050167098

Viña, J., Gomez-Cabrera, M. C., Borras, C., Froio, T., Sanchis-Gomar, F., Martinez-Bello, V. E., et al. (2009). Mitochondrial biogenesis in exercise and in ageing. *Adv. Drug Deliv. Rev.* 61, 1369–1374. doi: 10.1016/j.addr.2009.06.006

Walker, C. L., Pomatto, L. C.-D., Tripathi, D., and Davies, K. J. A. (2018). Redox regulation of homeostasis and proteostasis in peroxisomes. *Physiol. Rev.* 98, 89–115. doi: 10.1152/physrev.00033.2016

Wan, X. S., Devalaraja, M. N., and St Clair, D. K. (1994). Molecular structure and organization of the human manganese superoxide dismutase gene. *DNA Cell Biol.* 13, 1127–1136. doi: 10.1089/dna.1994.13.1127

Wareski, P., Vaarmann, A., Choubey, V., Safiulina, D., Liiv, J., Kuum, M., et al. (2000). Effect of exhaustive exercise on human neutrophils in athletes. *Luminescence* 15, 15–20. doi: 10.1002/(SICI)1522-7243(200001/02)15:1<15::AID-BIO570>3.0.CO;2-O

Zhang, H., Davies, K. J. A., and Forman, H. J. (2015). Oxidative stress response and Nrf2 signaling in aging. *Free Radic. Biol. Med.* 88, 314–336. doi: 10.1016/j.freeradbiomed.2015.05.036

Zhou, L., Zhang, H., Davies, K. J. A., and Forman, H. J. (2018). Aging-related decline in the induction of Nrf2-regulated antioxidant genes in human bronchial epithelial cells. *Redox Biol.* 14, 35–40. doi: 10.1016/j.redox.2017.08.014

11

Alternative Splicing of NOX4 in the Failing Human Heart

Zoltán V. Varga[1,2†], *Márton Pipicz*[3†], *Júlia A. Baán*[3], *Tamás Baranyai*[2], *Gábor Koncsos*[1], *Przemyslaw Leszek*[4], *Mariusz Kuśmierczyk*[5], *Fátima Sánchez-Cabo*[6], *Pablo García-Pavía*[7], *Gábor J. Brenner*[1], *Zoltán Giricz*[1,8], *Tamás Csont*[3], *Luca Mendler*[3,9], *Enrique Lara-Pezzi*[10], *Pál Pacher*[2*] and *Péter Ferdinandy*[1,3,8*]

[1] *Cardiometabolic Research Group, Department of Pharmacology and Pharmacotherapy, Semmelweis University, Budapest, Hungary,* [2] *Laboratory of Cardiovascular Physiology and Tissue Injury, National Institute on Alcohol Abuse and Alcoholism, National Institutes of Health, Bethesda, MD, United States,* [3] *Department of Biochemistry, Faculty of Medicine, University of Szeged, Szeged, Hungary,* [4] *Department of Heart Failure and Transplantology, Cardinal Stefan Wyszyński Institute of Cardiology, Warszawa, Poland,* [5] *Department of Cardiac Surgery and Transplantology, Cardinal Stefan Wyszyński Institute of Cardiology, Warszawa, Poland,* [6] *Bioinformatics Unit, Centro Nacional de Investigaciones Cardioavsculares Carlos III, Madrid, Spain,* [7] *Heart Failure and Inherited Cardiac Diseases Unit, Department of Cardiology, Hospital Universitario Puerta de Hierro Majadahonda, Madrid, Spain,* [8] *Pharmahungary Group, Szeged, Hungary,* [9] *Faculty of Medicine, Institute of Biochemistry II, Goethe University, Frankfurt, Germany,* [10] *Centro de Investigaciones Cardiovasculares Carlos III, Madrid, Spain*

Edited by:
Pasquale Pagliaro, Università degli Studi di Torino, Italy

Reviewed by:
Giulio Agnetti, Johns Hopkins University, United States
Nina Kaludercic, National Research Council of Italy (CNR), Italy

***Correspondence:**
Pál Pacher
pacher@mail.nih.gov
Péter Ferdinandy
peter.ferdinandy@pharmahungary.com

† *These authors have contributed equally to this work.*

Increased oxidative stress is a major contributor to the development and progression of heart failure, however, our knowledge on the role of the distinct NADPH oxidase (NOX) isoenzymes, especially on NOX4 is controversial. Therefore, we aimed to characterize NOX4 expression in human samples from healthy and failing hearts. Explanted human heart samples (left and right ventricular, and septal regions) were obtained from patients suffering from heart failure of ischemic or dilated origin. Control samples were obtained from donor hearts that were not used for transplantation. Deep RNA sequencing of the cardiac transcriptome indicated extensive alternative splicing of the NOX4 gene in heart failure as compared to samples from healthy donor hearts. Long distance PCR analysis with a universal 5′-3′ end primer pair, allowing amplification of different splice variants, confirmed the presence of the splice variants. To assess translation of the alternatively spliced transcripts we determined protein expression of NOX4 by using a specific antibody recognizing a conserved region in all variants. Western blot analysis showed up-regulation of the full-length NOX4 in ischemic cardiomyopathy samples and confirmed presence of shorter isoforms both in control and failing samples with disease-associated expression pattern. We describe here for the first time that NOX4 undergoes extensive alternative splicing in human hearts which gives rise to the expression of different enzyme isoforms. The full length NOX4 is significantly upregulated in ischemic cardiomyopathy suggesting a role for NOX4 in ROS production during heart failure.

Keywords: cardiomyopathy, oxidative stress, cardiac dysfunction, myocardium, aging

INTRODUCTION

In spite of an overall decrease in coronary artery disease-related mortality, the number of patients suffering from heart failure is increasing steeply in aging societies (Rich, 2001; Bui et al., 2011). Aging has a considerable impact on the heart and the vasculature, partially by promoting a prooxidative milieu (Csiszar et al., 2002; Donato et al., 2007; Dai et al., 2012; Martin-Fernandez and Gredilla, 2016). In accordance, increased oxidative stress and subsequent redox imbalance has been implicated in the development and progression of heart failure (Keith et al., 1998; Ungvari et al., 2005). Reactive oxygen species (ROS) production at a basal level may induce profound adaptive changes in intracellular pathways, however, higher concentrations of ROS induces tissue damage. ROS are derived from several intracellular sources, including mitochondrial respiratory complexes, NADPH oxidases (NOX), xanthine oxidase, mono-amino oxidases, and uncoupled nitric oxide synthase, among others. Although, the majority of these enzymes generates ROS as a by-product of dysfunctional activity, the only known role of the NOX family is ROS production. This fact makes NOXs intriguing targets for pharmacotherapy, allowing selective targeting of disease-specific ROS production (Altenhofer et al., 2012, 2015). To our present knowledge, the NOX family is composed of five different enzymes (NOX1, NOX2, NOX3, NOX4, and NOX5) and five subunits, known as phox proteins (Leto et al., 2009; Sirokmany et al., 2016). NOX enzymes have been proven to be involved both in experimental models (Li et al., 2002; Byrne et al., 2003) and in humans suffering from advanced heart failure (Heymes et al., 2003). In a landmark paper, Heymes et al. described an overall increase in NOX activity in human failing hearts, however, surprisingly, they found no change in the overall level of expression of oxidase subunits in failing hearts (Heymes et al., 2003), suggesting a novel NOX as a potential source of ROS production.

The NADPH oxidase 4 (NOX4) isoenzyme has been discovered in 2000, in the renal cortex (Geiszt et al., 2000). However, it has been proven later that many other cell types (including cardiomyocytes) also express NOX4 (Byrne et al., 2003; Varga et al., 2013). According to a recent study, mitochondrial NOX4 activity is a critical regulator of fatty acid β-oxidation in macrophages (Moon et al., 2016), an effect that has been also described in cardiomyocytes (Nabeebaccus et al., 2015).

Interestingly, in contrast to the inducible NOX2, NOX4 displays constitutive mRNA expression, which is fine-tuned by delicate epigenetic mechanisms, involving microRNA-dependent posttranscriptional repression (Varga et al., 2013). In addition, NOX4 might have alternative mRNA splice variants (Goyal et al., 2005) that might further complicate understanding the role of NOX4 in normal physiology and in pathological conditions. Accordingly, in the last decade, several conflicting results have been published, giving rise to many controversy on the NOX4 field. So far, both superoxide and hydrogen peroxide have been proposed as a product of NOX4 activity (Shiose et al., 2001; Takac et al., 2011; Nisimoto et al., 2014). Mitochondrial localization of NOX4 is still a question of debate (Hirschhauser et al., 2015), while a recent paper suggest nuclear/perinuclear localization of NOX4 (Matsushima et al., 2013). In addition, NOX4 has been described both as detrimental and protective in mouse models of heart failure (Kuroda et al., 2010; Zhang et al., 2010; Nabeebaccus et al., 2015; Zhao et al., 2015; Matsushima et al., 2016).

Therefore, here we aimed to characterize and assess the expression of NOX4 in the failing human hearts with unbiased transcriptomics methods followed by validations at the protein level. In addition, we put special emphasis to characterize alternative splicing of NOX4 in healthy and failing human hearts.

MATERIALS AND METHODS

Study Design

All experimental procedures were done in accordance with the ethical standards of the responsible institutional and national committee on human experimentation, adhering to the Helsinki Declaration (1975). Written informed consent was obtained from all patients involved in the study according to the protocol approved by the Local Ethics Committees of the Institute of Cardiology, Warszawa, Poland and Hospital Universitario Puerta de Hierro Majadahonda, Madrid, Spain (IK-NP-0021-24/1426/14, 272-19/12/11). Healthy human hearts were obtained from organ donor patients (CONT, $n = 5$) whose hearts were not used for transplantation due to technical reasons (e.g., donor/recipient incompatibility). The donors did not have any relevant previous cardiological history or any abnormalities in ECG and echocardiography (LV dimensions/contractility within normal ranges). Explanted failing hearts were obtained from patients suffering from end-stage, advanced heart failure of non-ischemic (i.e., dilated cardiomyopathy, DCM, $n = 5$) or ischemic (ICM, $n = 5$) etiology.

Preparation of Tissue Samples

Human tissue samples were taken at the time of heart explanation (avoiding scarred, fibrotic, or adipose tissue, endocardium, epicardium, or coronary vessels). The samples were rinsed immediately in saline, blotted dry, frozen in liquid nitrogen and kept at −80°C until further processing.

Rat heart and kidney tissues were harvested from male Wistar rats (250–300 g). The samples were snap frozen and crushed to small pieces in a mortar with pestle in liquid nitrogen.

RNA Sequencing

Whole transcriptome sequencing was performed, and data regarding NOX4 transcript were used and evaluated in the present project. Total RNA was isolated after homogenization of frozen myocardial samples using RNAeasy columns (Qiagen) as previously described (Lopez-Olaneta et al., 2014). RNA integrity was assessed using an Agilent Bioanalyzer and reverse-transcribed. Amplified cDNA (1 μg) was sonicated to an average size of 100–300 bp and used with the TruSeq DNA Sample Preparation v2 Kit (Illumina) to generate index-tagged sequencing libraries. Libraries were applied to Genome Analyzer IIx (Illumina) followed by standard RNA sequencing protocol to generate 80–120 M of paired end 75 bp-long reads. Reads were further processed using the CASAVA package (Illumina) and cutadapt software (Extended Experimental Procedure). Resulting reads were mapped to the ensemble human genome v75 and quantified on the transcriptome using RSEM (Li and Dewey, 2011). From RSEM we used the IsoPct information (percentage of the gene expression accounted by each transcript) in each sample to identify isoforms potentially undergoing alternative splicing.

Long-Distance PCR Analysis of Alternatively Spliced mRNA Transcripts

Total RNA was isolated from homogenized left ventricle (LV) of the CONT, DCM, or ICM patients with the guanidinium thiocyanate-phenol-chloroform extraction method, as described earlier (Baan et al., 2015). RNA was reverse transcribed with MMLV-Reverse Transcriptase (Invitrogen, USA). For the detection of the alternatively spliced transcript levels of NOX4, long-distance PCR was carried out with a high fidelity Pfu polymerase (G-Biosciences, USA) with cycling conditions set as an initial denaturation step for 5 min at 95°C, followed by 40 cycles of 30 s at 95°C for template denaturation, 30 s for annealing phase at 55°C, and 3.5 min at 72°C for extension. Length of the specific PCR products was verified on 1.5% agarose gels stained with GelRed (Biotium, USA). Primer pairs for the long distance amplification of NOX4 were designed to amplify from a conserved region from all splice variants. The primer sequences were the following: forward primer 5′-TGCTGTATAACCAAGGGCCA-3′, reverse primer 5′-GGTCCACAACAGAAAACACCA-3′. The primers were designed by Primer 3 Input (version 0.4.0) software and tested to avoid primer dimer formation, unspecific amplification and self-priming formation.

Western Blot Analysis of NOX4

In order to investigate whether NOX4 expression is altered at the protein level in the failing human heart, western blot analysis was performed. Frozen tissue samples from left ventricle (LV) and right ventricle (RV) as well as from inter-ventricular septum (IVS) were homogenized in NP-40 lysis buffer (150 mM NaCl, 50 mM Tris, 1% NP-40) for NOX4 or with RIPA buffer for ERK with a tissue to homogenization buffer ratio of 1:4 containing protease and phosphatase inhibitors (AEBSF, Aprotinin, Bestatin, E-64, Leupeptin, Pepstatin A, sodium orthovanadate and sodium fluoride) (Sigma-Aldrich, St. Louis, MO, USA). Protein concentrations were assessed by the bicinchoninic acid method using the provided bovine serum albumin as standard (Pierce Biotechnologies, USA). Equal amounts of protein were loaded from each sample onto 10% SDS-polyacrylamide gels. For optimal results, in case of NOX4 blots, samples were mixed with Laemmli sample buffer without using reducing agents or sample boiling. After separation by electrophoresis, proteins were transferred (wet transfer, 2.5 h) onto nitrocellulose membrane (Amersham Biosciences, Piscataway, USA). Transfer was controlled by Ponceau S staining. The membrane was blocked with 5% non-fat dry milk in 0.1% TBS-T overnight at 4°C. After the blocking step, the membrane was incubated with a rabbit polyclonal primary antibody (dissolved in 1% non-fat dry milk in 0.1% TBS-T, 1:1,000 dilution) against NOX4 (NB110-58851, Novus Biologicals, United Kingdom)—reported to specifically recognize NOX4 protein (Basuroy et al., 2009; Maalouf et al., 2012; Siuda et al., 2012)—, or by a mouse monoclonal antibody recognizing pERK1/2 or total ERK (9106 and 9107 Cell Signaling technology, Danvers, MA, USA) for 2 h at room temperature (NOX4) or overnight at 4°C (ERK), followed by washing with 0.1% TBS-T (3 times for 10 min). After washing, the membrane was incubated with a secondary antibody (horseradish peroxidase-conjugated affinity purified goat anti-rabbit, 1:5,000 dilution, Dako, Denmark; horseradish peroxidase-conjugated affinity purified horse anti-mouse, 1:5,000 dilution, Cell Signaling Technology, USA) in 1% non-fat dry milk in 0.1% TBS-T for 1 h at room temperature. Then the membrane was washed again 3 times for 10 min. For detection of the bands, the membrane was incubated with ECL-Plus reagent (Amersham Biosciences, USA) for 5 min and then visualized. Band densities were evaluated by using Quantity One software (Bio-Rad Imaging System, USA). Equal loading was assessed by determining and normalizing to GAPDH content of each sample. Briefly, stripped membranes were probed with a primary antibody that recognizes GAPDH (1:10,000 dilution, Cell Signaling Technology, Danvers, MA, USA) for 2 h at room temperature, followed by washing with TBS-T. Then the membrane was incubated with horseradish peroxidase-conjugated affinity purified goat anti-rabbit antibody (1:20,000 dilution) for 1 h at room temperature. The membrane was washed again and band visualization and evaluation of band densities were done as describe above. There was no significant difference in GAPDH between groups.

TABLE 1 | Clinical characteristics of study population.

	CON	DCM	ICM
Number of samples	5	5	5
Gender (female/male)	3/2	2/3	4/1
Age (year)	29 ± 9	39 ± 10	57 ± 11
NYHA functional class III/IV, *n*	n.a.	0/5	3/2
LVED, mm	n.a.	68 ± 4	71 ± 4
LVSD, mm	n.a.	63 ± 5	61 ± 8
PW, mm	n.a.	9.5 ± 0.5	10 ± 1.5
IVS, mm	n.a.	10 ± 0.7	11 ± 1.5
LVEF, %	n.a.	16 ± 3	23 ± 3

Values are given in mean ± S.E.M. CON, healthy control individuals; DCM, dilated cardiomyopathy; ICM, ischemic cardiomyopathy; NYHA, New York Heart Association; LVED, left ventricular end-diastolic diameter; LVSD, left ventricular end-systolic diameter; PW, posterior wall thickness; IVS, interventricular septum thickness; LVEF, left ventricular ejection fraction; n.a., not applicable.

Statistical Analysis

Statistical analysis was performed by one-way ANOVA using Prism software (GraphPad Software, Inc., San Diego, USA), as appropriate. All data were expressed as means ± S.E.M. For all analyses, a $p < 0.05$ was considered statistically significant.

RESULTS

Study Patients

A detailed summary of clinical characteristics and medication of study subjects are shown in **Table 1**. Patients of both genders were enrolled in all groups. The age of patients suffering from ischemic cardiomyopathy differed significantly from both control and dilated cardiomyopathy patients as expected, since ischemic cardiomyopathy leads to end-stage heart failure later and in older population than dilated cardiomyopathy. DCM and ICM patients were in either New York Heart Association (NYHA) class III or IV with no difference in major cardiac functional parameters. All patients were treated with angiotensin-converting enzyme inhibitors, beta-blockers and diuretics, however, aspirin and statins were only used in the treatment regime of ICM. Control subjects received intravenous treatment composed of very low catecholamine infusion (norepinephrine: 0.1–0.2 μg/kg/min, dopamine: 1–2 μg/kg/min). Adequate fluid balance was maintained before heart explanation with intravenous fluids (e.g., hydroxyethyl starch) and desmopressin.

NOX4 Transcript Variants Are Detected in Human Hearts

The full length NOX4 A consist of 18 different exons, giving rise to the transcription of a 1,733 bp mRNA (**Figure 1A**). The majority of isoforms lack one or more exons as a result of alternative splicing. With an unbiased RNA sequencing approach, we aimed to characterize the abundance of NOX4 splicing events. (**Figure 1B**) shows the detection of splice variants (based on the Ensembl database) as detected by RNA sequencing in control and failing human hearts. Currently there are 17 NOX4-related entries, out of them 16 were detected in control and failing human samples. Two sequences are only retained introns (ENST0000524473 and ENST0000525278), and ENST529343 has a premature stop codon potentially leading to non-sense-mediated mRNA decay. However, the retained intron sequence, ENST0000524473 was detectable in almost all samples.

It is also noteworthy that more alternative splicing events were detected in the failing hearts (control average four events, failing average 5.6 events). This was further confirmed by a long distance PCR analysis that is shown on (**Figure 1C**). By using a universal 5′-3′ end primer pair and a high fidelity enzyme and longer amplification time, we were able the detect several NOX4 related transcripts, showing on one hand that the detected bands are corresponding to the predicted and expected splice variants, while on the other hand, it is also detectable on the agarose gel picture that there is extensive splicing in the failing hearts when compared to the healthy control left ventricular tissue.

NOX4 Protein Variants Are Present in Failing Human Hearts with a Spatial and Disease-Specific Distribution

To detect NOX4 variants at protein level, we used a polyclonal antibody recognizing a conserved region of the protein (C-terminal region) present in all transcript variants. During our pilot experiments, we recognized that even in rodent samples (rat kidney and heart) there is some extent of alternative splicing, with a predominant expression of the 67-kDa band in both tissues (**Figure 2A**).

However, in human hearts and using non-reducing loading conditions this observation became more obvious (**Figure 2B, Supplementary Figure 1**). Both in healthy control and failing human hearts significant amounts of alternatively spliced forms were detected. In ICM samples, the robust upregulation of the 26-kDa form and downregulation of the 28-kDa form was observed in all regions of the heart. Since the electrophoretic mobility difference between the two forms is small, it is also possible that we detected a posttranslational modification (e.g., deglycosylation—Goyal et al., 2005) of the same isoform. The 58-kDa form showed a significant upregulation in the IVS of the ischemic failing hearts. In addition, we detected a significant increase of the full length NOX4 (in non-reducing conditions the major band is detected at the level of 90 kDa possibly as a complex of a 67-kDa NOX4 with the p22 phox) in the IVS of ischemic failing hearts that was associated with a tendency of upregulation in the left ventricle as well (**Figure 2C, Supplementary Figure 1**).

In DCM samples, a significant upregulation of the 58-kDa variant was seen, together with a tendency of increased full length 90-kDa complex, similarly to the ICM samples (**Figure 2D, Supplementary Figure 2**).

To study the link between the observed difference in the expression of the 28-kDa isoform and ERK1/2 phosphorylation (Anilkumar et al., 2013), we performed pERK/ERK Western blots from left ventricular samples. We found significantly increased phosphorylation of ERK1/2 in the ICM samples as compared to CON samples, whereas there was an increase both in phosphor-ERK and total-ERK levels when normalized to GAPDH in DCM samples. These suggest activation of hypertrophic ERK signaling independently from changes in NOX4D expression in these samples (**Supplementary Figure 3**).

DISCUSSION

We described here for the first time that the NOX4 gene undergoes alternative splicing in the human heart resulting in at least three different protein isoforms. The full length NOX4 is significantly upregulated in heart failure, while a smaller 28-kDa isoform shows downregulation in ischemic failing hearts.

Alternative splicing is a critical process in RNA maturation ensuring expression of functionally diverse proteins from individual genes. Frequency of splicing events is estimated to be really high, according to Pan and colleagues more than 85% of the multi-exon genes contain at least one alternative splicing event (Pan et al., 2008). Since alternative splicing is usually tissue specific, and in many cases changes in alternative splicing occur in a disease-specific manner during progression of the disease, detection of splicing events could serve as a disease-specific or disease stage-specific biomarker. In addition, regulation of alternative splicing might affect disease outcome, pointing to the theranostic potential of splicing events (Le et al., 2015). Although, gene expression patterns in cardiac diseases have been extensively studied over the last years, our overall knowledge in terms of splicing events and the resulting protein isoforms and their association with disease states is still very limited. The variability in splicing may alter protein structure, thereby influencing subcellular protein localization, and the overall function of the particular protein. In the myocardium, alternative splicing of sarcomeric genes, cardiac ion channels, and cell signaling proteins have been reported so far, leading to the development of cardiomyopathies and arrhythmias (Gao et al., 2011; Guo et al., 2012; Lara-Pezzi et al., 2013; Maatz et al., 2014). Among NOX family members, it is known that both NOX1 (Arakawa et al., 2006) and NOX2 (Kuhns et al., 2010; Harrison et al., 2012) enzymes undergo alternative splicing. Interestingly, in lymphocytes of patients suffering from chronic granulomatosus disease due to mutations in the CYBB gene (i.e., gp91 phox)

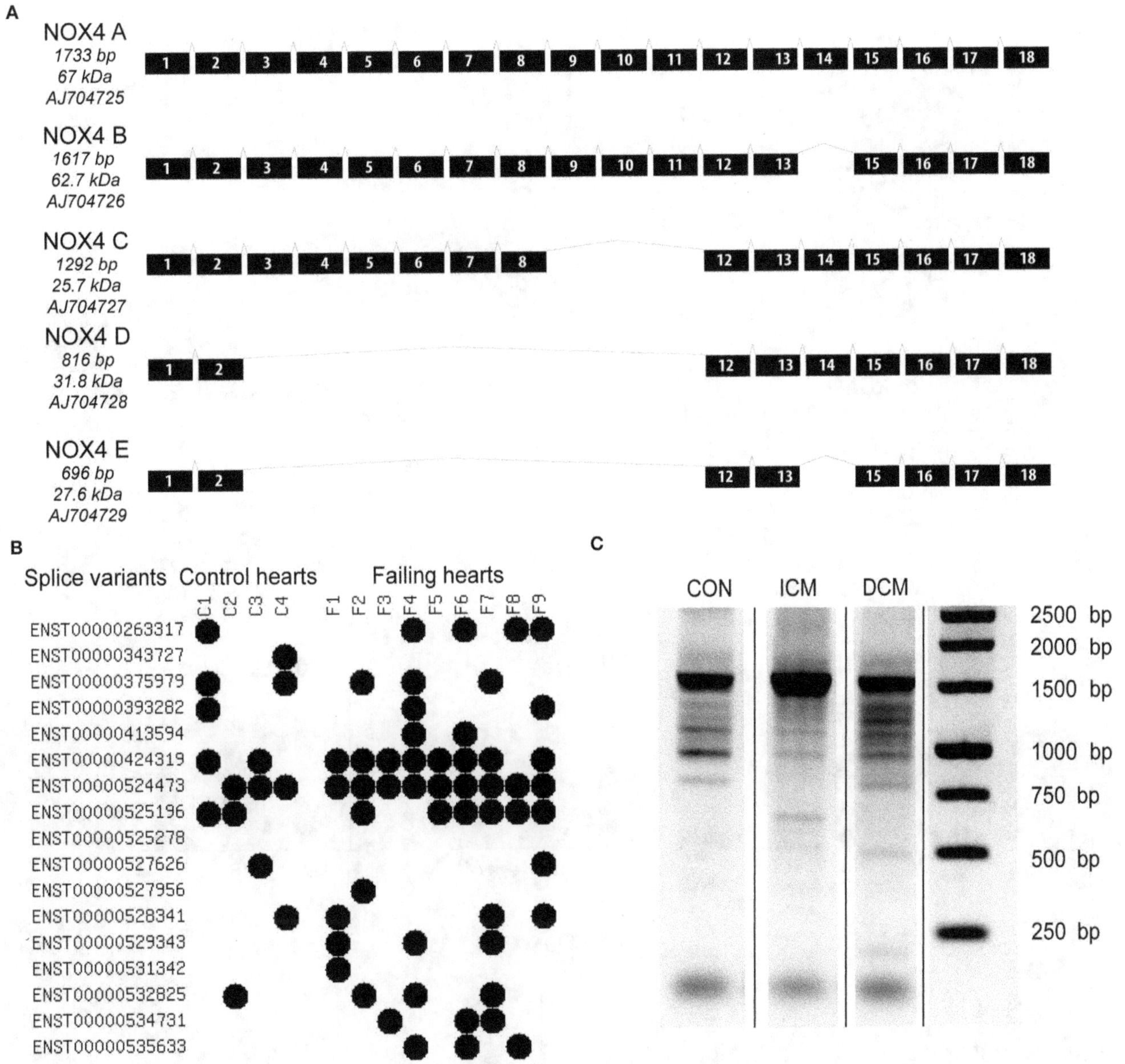

FIGURE 1 | Known transcript variants of the NOX4 messenger RNA as original described in a human endothelial cell line by Goyal et al. (2005) **(A)**. Splice variants detected in control and failing human hearts by RNA sequencing **(B)**. Each variant is annotated to an individual code in the Ensembl database. Black dots represent the presence of the variant in the sample. Long distance PCR analysis to detect NOX4 transcripts **(C)**. CON, control; ICM, ischemic cardiomyopathy; DCM, dilated cardiomyopathy.

IFN-γ is capable of partially correcting mRNA processing defects and improves splicing efficiency (Condino-Neto and Newburger, 2000). To date NOX4 transcripts variants have been reported only in cell lines, including alveolar epithelial cells (Goyal et al., 2005), vascular smooth muscle cells, endothelial cells, fibroblasts, and cardiomyocytes (Anilkumar et al., 2013). Nevertheless, the functional role of the transcripts is still largely unknown. Anilkumar et al. have reported that the 28-kDa splice variant (aka. NOX4D) is predominantly expressed in the nucleus, and produces ROS that can activate kinase signaling cascades, such as MAPK, and ROS-dependent extracellular-signal-regulated kinases (ERK1/2) (Anilkumar et al., 2013), that may potentially contribute to nuclear redox homeostasis (Hansen et al., 2006). These observations are interesting in light of our present results, since we observed a marked switch in the expression/posttranslational modification of the 28-kDa isoform, showing lower expression levels in the hearts of ischemic cardiomyopathy patients. In our samples, however, we found increased ERK phosphorylation both in ICM and DCM samples, suggesting a potentially NOX4D-independent activation of hypertrophic signaling during heart failure (Rose et al., 2010; Yeh et al., 2010).

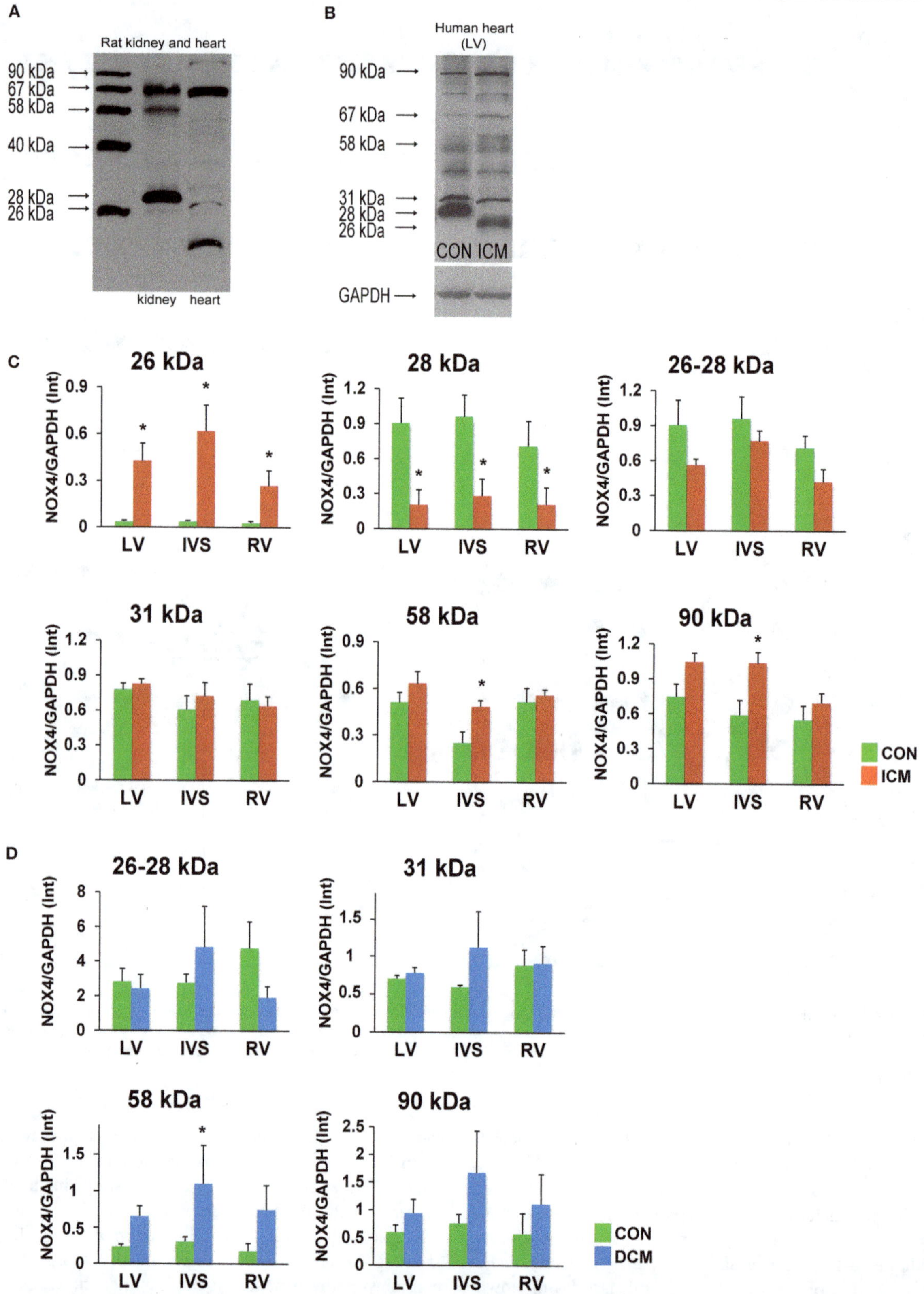

FIGURE 2 | Alternative splicing of NOX4 in rat kidney and heart **(A)**. Alternative splicing of NOX4 in human hearts **(B)**. Quantitative evaluation of spliced NOX4 isoforms in ICM samples **(C)**. Quantitative evaluation of spliced NOX4 isoforms in DCM samples **(D)**. Data are mean ± S.E.M. $n = 5$/group. $^*p < 0.05$. LV, left ventricle; IVS, interventricular septum; RV, right ventricle; ICM, ischemic cardiomyopathy; DCM, dilated cardiomyopathy.

Given the controversies in the NOX4 field, differences in splicing events might also contribute to the different phenotypes seen in the NOX4 knockout animals. So far four different knock-out models have been published with deletions of different exons (exons 1/2, exon 4, exon 9, or exons 14/15; for review please see: Altenhofer et al., 2012). Therefore, it is possible that, in a tissue specific manner, deletion of exon 4 or exon 9 may result in the expression of NOX4 variants (NOX4D and E) leading to residual NOX4 activity that complicates the interpretation of the results seen in knock-out mice studies.

From a drug developmental point of view, alternative splicing might be an important factor to consider as drug candidates may have different effects on the spliced variants (e.g., a splice event might underlie drug resistance de Necochea-Campion et al., 2016). Therefore, NOX4 inhibitors currently under clinical testing (e.g., GKT137831 from GenKyoTex S.A., VAS2870 from Vasopharm GmbH, GLX351322 from Glucox Biotech AB—see for review: Altenhofer et al., 2015) may also affect the activity of splice variants differently that may in turn influence efficacy and safety.

LIMITATIONS

A limitation of the present observational study is that our conclusions are based on descriptive data from a limited set of human samples. Due to the significant differences in the age of the ICM patients and the healthy controls, we cannot rule out the effect of age and the presence of different cardiovascular comorbidities (Ferdinandy et al., 2007, 2014) on the observed differences. Although mRNA and protein data clearly implicate the presence of the alternative splice variants of NOX4, we have not provided direct evidence by sequencing the proteins after immunoprecipitation with the antibody used in the present study.

CONCLUSIONS

In summary, our present study provides the first description that the NOX4 mRNA undergoes alternative splicing in the human heart, resulting in at least three different protein isoforms. The full length NOX4 is significantly upregulated due to heart failure that might contribute to ROS production in the failing hearts, while a smaller 28-kDa isoform shows downregulation in ischemic failing hearts possibly having important roles in redox signaling of subcellular compartments. Disease specific expression pattern of NOX4 isoforms may provide new diagnostic and therapeutic targets in heart failure, and disease-specific splicing events might represent a new factor to consider when developing NOX4-modulator drugs.

AUTHOR CONTRIBUTIONS

ZVV, MP, JAB, TB, GK, GJB, ZG, and LM performed *in vitro* experiments. ZVV analyzed data, drafted figures, and the manuscript. PL, MK, and PG-P provided patient materials and clinical data. FS-C performed bioinformatic analysis. ZVV, LM, TC, EL-P, PP, and PF conceptualized the project, provided necessary materials, and wrote the manuscript.

ACKNOWLEDGMENTS

The study was supported by the grants from the Hungarian Scientific Research Fund (OTKA ANN107803, OTKA K109737 to PF) by the National Research, Development and Innovation Fund of Hungary (Project no. NVKP_16-1-2016-0017 has been implemented with the support provided from the National Research, Development and Innovation Fund of Hungary, financed under the NVKP_16 funding scheme). ZVV was supported by the National Program of Excellence (TAMOP 4.2.4.A/1-11-1-2012-0001) and by the Rosztoczy Foundation. PF was a Szentagothai Fellow of the National Program of Excellence (TAMOP 4.2.4.A/2-11-1-2012-0001). ZG held a "János Bolyai Fellowship" from the Hungarian Academy of Sciences (awarded in 2013 and 2017). TB is supported by the UNKP-16-3 New National Excellence Program of The Ministry of Human Capacities. PP is supported by the Intramural Research Program of NIAAA. PF is a vice chair, PL and ZG are management committee members of the EU-Cardioprotection COST Action CA16225.

SUPPLEMENTARY MATERIAL

Supplementary Figure 1 | Original Western blots for NOX4 **(A)**, GAPDH **(B)**, and total protein staining by Ponceau S stain **(C)** in left ventricular (LV), right ventricular (RV), and interventricular septal regions (IVS) of ischemic cardiomyopathy patients (ICM).

Supplementary Figure 2 | Original Western blots for NOX4 **(A)**, GAPDH **(B)**, and total protein staining by Ponceau S stain **(C)** in left ventricular (LV), right ventricular (RV), and interventricular septal regions (IVS) of dilated cardiomyopathy patients (DCM).

Supplementary Figure 3 | Original Western blots for phosphorylated ERK1/2, total ERK1/2, GAPDH and total protein staining by Ponceau S stain in left ventricular (LV) samples of ischemic (ICM—**A**) or dilated cardiomyopathy patients (DCM—**B**), respectively. Data are mean ± S.E.M. $n = 5$/group. *$p < 0.05$.

REFERENCES

Altenhofer, S., Kleikers, P. W., Radermacher, K. A., Scheurer, P., Rob Hermans, J. J., Schiffers, P., et al. (2012). The NOX toolbox: validating the role of NADPH oxidases in physiology and disease. *Cell. Mol. Life Sci.* 69, 2327–2343. doi: 10.1007/s00018-012-1010-9

Altenhofer, S., Radermacher, K. A., Kleikers, P. W., Wingler, K., and Schmidt, H. H. (2015). Evolution of NADPH oxidase inhibitors: selectivity and mechanisms for target engagement. *Antioxid. Redox Signal.* 23, 406–427. doi: 10.1089/ars.2013.5814

Anilkumar, N., San Jose, G., Sawyer, I., Santos, C. X., Sand, C., Brewer, A. C., et al. (2013). A 28-kDa splice variant of NADPH oxidase-4 is nuclear-localized and involved in redox signaling in vascular cells. *Arterioscler. Thromb. Vasc. Biol.* 33, e104–e112. doi: 10.1161/ATVBAHA.112.300956

Arakawa, N., Katsuyama, M., Matsuno, K., Urao, N., Tabuchi, Y., Okigaki, M., et al. (2006). Novel transcripts of Nox1 are regulated by alternative promoters and expressed under phenotypic modulation of vascular smooth muscle cells. *Biochem. J.* 398, 303–310. doi: 10.1042/BJ20060300

Baan, J. A., Varga, Z. V., Leszek, P., Kusmierczyk, M., Baranyai, T., Dux, L., et al. (2015). Myostatin and IGF-I signaling in end-stage human heart failure: a qRT-PCR study. *J. Transl. Med.* 13:1. doi: 10.1186/s12967-014-0365-0

Basuroy, S., Bhattacharya, S., Leffler, C. W., and Parfenova, H. (2009). Nox4 NADPH oxidase mediates oxidative stress and apoptosis caused by TNF-alpha in cerebral vascular endothelial cells. *Am. J. Physiol. Cell Physiol.* 296, C422–C432. doi: 10.1152/ajpcell.00381.2008

Bui, A. L., Horwich, T. B., and Fonarow, G. C. (2011). Epidemiology and risk profile of heart failure. *Nat. Rev. Cardiol.* 8, 30–41. doi: 10.1038/nrcardio.2010.165

Byrne, J. A., Grieve, D. J., Bendall, J. K., Li, J. M., Gove, C., Lambeth, J. D., et al. (2003). Contrasting roles of NADPH oxidase isoforms in pressure-overload versus angiotensin II-induced cardiac hypertrophy. *Circ. Res.* 93, 802–805. doi: 10.1161/01.RES.0000099504.30207.F5

Condino-Neto, A., and Newburger, P. E. (2000). Interferon-gamma improves splicing efficiency of CYBB gene transcripts in an interferon-responsive variant of chronic granulomatous disease due to a splice site consensus region mutation. *Blood* 95, 3548–3554.

Csiszar, A., Ungvari, Z., Edwards, J. G., Kaminski, P., Wolin, M. S., Koller, A., et al. (2002). Aging-induced phenotypic changes and oxidative stress impair coronary arteriolar function. *Circ. Res.* 90, 1159–1166. doi: 10.1161/01.RES.0000020401.61826.EA

Dai, D. F., Chen, T., Johnson, S. C., Szeto, H., and Rabinovitch, P. S. (2012). Cardiac aging: from molecular mechanisms to significance in human health and disease. *Antioxid. Redox Signal.* 16, 1492–1526. doi: 10.1089/ars.2011.4179

de Necochea-Campion, G. P Shouse, Q., Zhou, S., Mirshahidi, S., and Chen, C. S. (2016). Aberrant splicing and drug resistance in AML. *J. Hematol. Oncol.* 9:85. doi: 10.1186/s13045-016-0315-9

Donato, A. J., Eskurza, I., Silver, A. E., Levy, A. S., Pierce, G. L., Gates, P. E., et al. (2007). Direct evidence of endothelial oxidative stress with aging in humans: relation to impaired endothelium-dependent dilation and upregulation of nuclear factor-kappaB. *Circ. Res.* 100, 1659–1666. doi: 10.1161/01.RES.0000269183.13937.e8

Ferdinandy, P., Hausenloy, D. J., Heusch, G., Baxter, G. F., and Schulz, R. (2014). Interaction of risk factors, comorbidities, and comedications with ischemia/reperfusion injury and cardioprotection by preconditioning, postconditioning, and remote conditioning. *Pharmacol. Rev.* 66, 1142–1174. doi: 10.1124/pr.113.008300

Ferdinandy, P., Schulz, R., and Baxter, G. F. (2007). Interaction of cardiovascular risk factors with myocardial ischemia/reperfusion injury, preconditioning, and postconditioning. *Pharmacol. Rev.* 59, 418–458. doi: 10.1124/pr.107.06002

Gao, G., Xie, A., Huang, S. C., Zhou, A., Zhang, J., Herman, A. M., et al. (2011). Role of RBM25/LUC7L3 in abnormal cardiac sodium channel splicing regulation in human heart failure. *Circulation* 124, 1124–1131. doi: 10.1161/CIRCULATIONAHA.111.044495

Geiszt, M., Kopp, J. B., Varnai, P., and Leto, T. L. (2000). Identification of renox, an NAD(P)H oxidase in kidney. *Proc. Natl. Acad. Sci. U.S.A.* 97, 8010–8014. doi: 10.1073/pnas.130135897

Goyal, P., Weissmann, N., Rose, F., Grimminger, F., Schafers, H. J., Seeger, W., et al. (2005). Identification of novel Nox4 splice variants with impact on ROS levels in A549 cells. *Biochem. Biophys. Res. Commun.* 329, 32–39. doi: 10.1016/j.bbrc.2005.01.089

Guo, W., Schafer, S., Greaser, M. L., Radke, M. H., Liss, M., Govindarajan, T., et al. (2012). RBM20, a gene for hereditary cardiomyopathy, regulates titin splicing. *Nat. Med.* 18, 766–773. doi: 10.1038/nm.2693

Hansen, J. M., Go, Y. M., and Jones, D. P. (2006). Nuclear and mitochondrial compartmentation of oxidative stress and redox signaling. *Annu. Rev. Pharmacol. Toxicol.* 46, 215–234. doi: 10.1146/annurev.pharmtox.46.120604.141122

Harrison, C. B., Selemidis, S., Guida, E., King, P. T., Sobey, C. G., and Drummond, G. R. (2012). NOX2beta: a novel splice variant of NOX2 that regulates NADPH oxidase activity in macrophages. *PLoS ONE* 7:e48326. doi: 10.1371/journal.pone.0048326

Heymes, C., Bendall, J. K., Ratajczak, P., Cave, A. C., Samuel, J. L., Hasenfuss, G., et al. (2003). Increased myocardial NADPH oxidase activity in human heart failure. *J. Am. Coll. Cardiol.* 41, 2164–2171. doi: 10.1016/S0735-1097(03)00471-6

Hirschhauser, C., Bornbaum, J., Reis, A., Bohme, S., Kaludercic, N., Menabo, R., et al. (2015). NOX4 in mitochondria: yeast two-hybrid-based interaction with complex I without relevance for basal reactive oxygen species? *Antioxid. Redox Signal.* 23, 1106–1112. doi: 10.1089/ars.2014.6238

Keith, M., Geranmayegan, A., Sole, M. J., Kurian, R., Robinson, A., Omran, A. S., et al. (1998). Increased oxidative stress in patients with congestive heart failure. *J. Am. Coll. Cardiol.* 31, 1352–1356. doi: 10.1016/S0735-1097(98)00101-6

Kuhns, D. B., Alvord, W. G., Heller, T., Feld, J. J., Pike, K. M., Marciano, B. E., et al. (2010). Residual NADPH oxidase and survival in chronic granulomatous disease. *N. Engl. J. Med.* 363, 2600–2610. doi: 10.1056/NEJMoa1007097

Kuroda, J., Ago, T., Matsushima, S., Zhai, P., Schneider, M. D., and Sadoshima, J. (2010). NADPH oxidase 4 (Nox4) is a major source of oxidative stress in the failing heart. *Proc. Natl. Acad. Sci. U.S.A.* 107, 15565–15570. doi: 10.1073/pnas.1002178107

Lara-Pezzi, E., Gomez-Salinero, J., Gatto, A., and Garcia-Pavia, P. (2013). The alternative heart: impact of alternative splicing in heart disease. *J. Cardiovasc. Transl. Res.* 6, 945–955. doi: 10.1007/s12265-013-9482-z

Le, K. Q., Prabhakar, B. S., Hong, W. J., and Li, L. C. (2015). Alternative splicing as a biomarker and potential target for drug discovery. *Acta Pharmacol. Sin.* 36, 1212–1218. doi: 10.1038/aps.2015.43

Leto, T. L., Morand, S., Hurt, D., and Ueyama, T. (2009). Targeting and regulation of reactive oxygen species generation by Nox family NADPH oxidases. *Antioxid. Redox Signal.* 11, 2607–2619. doi: 10.1089/ars.2009.2637

Li, B., and Dewey, C. N. (2011). RSEM: accurate transcript quantification from RNA-Seq data with or without a reference genome. *BMC Bioinformatics* 12:323. doi: 10.1186/1471-2105-12-323

Li, J. M., Gall, N. P., Grieve, D. J., Chen, M., and Shah, A. M. (2002). Activation of NADPH oxidase during progression of cardiac hypertrophy to failure. *Hypertension* 40, 477–484. doi: 10.1161/01.HYP.0000032031.30374.32

Lopez-Olaneta, M. M., Villalba, M., Gomez-Salinero, J. M., Jimenez-Borreguero, L. J., Breckenridge, R., Ortiz-Sanchez, P., et al. (2014). Induction of the calcineurin variant CnAbeta1 after myocardial infarction reduces post-infarction ventricular remodelling by promoting infarct vascularization. *Cardiovasc. Res.* 102, 396–406. doi: 10.1093/cvr/cvu068

Maalouf, R. M., Eid, A. A., Gorin, Y. C., Block, K., Escobar, G. P., Bailey, S., et al. (2012). Nox4-derived reactive oxygen species mediate cardiomyocyte injury in early type 1 diabetes. *Am. J. Physiol. Cell Physiol.* 302, C597–C604. doi: 10.1152/ajpcell.00331.2011

Maatz, H., Jens, M., Liss, M., Schafer, S., Heinig, M., Kirchner, M., et al. (2014). RNA-binding protein RBM20 represses splicing to orchestrate cardiac pre-mRNA processing. *J. Clin. Invest.* 124, 3419–3430. doi: 10.1172/JCI74523

Martin-Fernandez, B., and Gredilla, R. (2016). Mitochondria and oxidative stress in heart aging. *Age* 38, 225–238. doi: 10.1007/s11357-016-9933-y

Matsushima, S., Kuroda, J., Ago, T., Zhai, P., Park, J. Y., Xie, L. H., et al. (2013). Increased oxidative stress in the nucleus caused by Nox4 mediates oxidation of HDAC4 and cardiac hypertrophy. *Circ. Res.* 112, 651–663. doi: 10.1161/CIRCRESAHA.112.279760

Matsushima, S., Kuroda, J., Zhai, P., Liu, T., Ikeda, S., Nagarajan, N., et al. (2016). Tyrosine kinase FYN negatively regulates NOX4 in cardiac remodeling. *J. Clin. Invest.* 126, 3403–3416. doi: 10.1172/JCI85624

Moon, J. S., Nakahira, K., Chung, K. P., DeNicola, G. M., Koo, M. J., Pabon, M. A., et al. (2016). NOX4-dependent fatty acid oxidation promotes NLRP3 inflammasome activation in macrophages. *Nat. Med.* 22, 1002–1012. doi: 10.1038/nm.4153

Nabeebaccus, A., Hafstad, A., Eykyn, T., Yin, X., Brewer, A., Zhang, M., et al. (2015). Cardiac-targeted NADPH oxidase 4 in the adaptive cardiac remodelling of the murine heart. *Lancet* 385(Suppl. 1), S73. doi: 10.1016/S0140-6736(15)60388-9

Nisimoto, Y., Diebold, B. A., Cosentino-Gomes, D., and Lambeth, J. D. (2014). Nox4: a hydrogen peroxide-generating oxygen sensor. *Biochemistry* 53, 5111–5120. doi: 10.1021/bi500331y

Pan, Q., Shai, O., Lee, L. J., Frey, B. J., and Blencowe, B. J. (2008). Deep surveying of alternative splicing complexity in the human transcriptome by high-throughput sequencing. *Nat. Genet.* 40, 1413–1415. doi: 10.1038/ng.259

Rich, M. W. (2001). Heart failure in the 21st century: a cardiogeriatric syndrome. *J. Gerontol.* 56, M88–M96. doi: 10.1093/gerona/56.2.M88

Rose, B. A., Force, T., and Wang, Y. (2010). Mitogen-activated protein kinase signaling in the heart: angels versus demons in a heart-breaking tale. *Physiol. Rev.* 90, 1507–1546. doi: 10.1152/physrev.00054.2009

Shiose, A., Kuroda, J., Tsuruya, K., Hirai, M., Hirakata, H., Naito, S., et al. (2001). A novel superoxide-producing NAD(P)H oxidase in kidney. *J. Biol. Chem.* 276, 1417–1423. doi: 10.1074/jbc.M007597200

Sirokmany, G., Donko, A., and Geiszt, M. (2016). Nox/Duox family of NADPH oxidases: lessons from knockout mouse models. *Trends Pharmacol. Sci.* 37, 318–327. doi: 10.1016/j.tips.2016.01.006

Siuda, D., Zechner, U., El Hajj, N., Prawitt, D., Langer, D., Xia, N., et al. (2012). Transcriptional regulation of Nox4 by histone deacetylases in human endothelial cells. *Basic Res. Cardiol.* 107:283. doi: 10.1007/s00395-012-0283-3

Takac, I., Schroder, K., Zhang, L., Lardy, B., Anilkumar, N., Lambeth, J. D., et al. (2011). The E-loop is involved in hydrogen peroxide formation by the NADPH oxidase NOX4. *J. Biol. Chem.* 286, 13304–13313. doi: 10.1074/jbc.M110.192138

Ungvari, Z., Gupte, S. A., Recchia, F. A., Batkai, S., and Pacher, P. (2005). Role of oxidative-nitrosative stress and downstream pathways in various forms of cardiomyopathy and heart failure. *Curr. Vasc. Pharmacol.* 3, 221–229. doi: 10.2174/1570161054368607

Varga, Z. V., Kupai, K., Szucs, G., Gaspar, R., Paloczi, J., Farago, N., et al. (2013). MicroRNA-25-dependent up-regulation of NADPH oxidase 4 (NOX4) mediates hypercholesterolemia-induced oxidative/nitrative stress and subsequent dysfunction in the heart. *J. Mol. Cell. Cardiol.* 62, 111–121. doi: 10.1016/j.yjmcc.2013.05.009

Yeh, C. C., Li, H., Malhotra, D., Turcato, S., Nicholas, S., Tu, R., et al. (2010). Distinctive ERK and p38 signaling in remote and infarcted myocardium during post-MI remodeling in the mouse. *J. Cell. Biochem.* 109, 1185–1191. doi: 10.1002/jcb.22498

Zhang, M., Brewer, A. C., Schroder, K., Santos, C. X., Grieve, D. J., Wang, M., et al. (2010). NADPH oxidase-4 mediates protection against chronic load-induced stress in mouse hearts by enhancing angiogenesis. *Proc. Natl. Acad. Sci. U.S.A.* 107, 18121–18126. doi: 10.1073/pnas.1009700107

Zhao, Q. D., Viswanadhapalli, S., Williams, P., Shi, Q., Tan, C., Yi, X., et al. (2015). NADPH oxidase 4 induces cardiac fibrosis and hypertrophy through activating Akt/mTOR and NFkappaB signaling pathways. *Circulation* 131, 643–655. doi: 10.1161/CIRCULATIONAHA.114.011079

12

Ranolazine Attenuates Trastuzumab-Induced Heart Dysfunction by Modulating ROS Production

Gennaro Riccio [1], Salvatore Antonucci [2], Carmela Coppola [3], Chiara D'Avino [4,5], Giovanna Piscopo [3], Danilo Fiore [4], Carlo Maurea [3], Michele Russo [6], Domenica Rea [7], Claudio Arra [7], Gerolama Condorelli [4], Fabio Di Lisa [2], Carlo G. Tocchetti [6], Claudia De Lorenzo [4,5]* and Nicola Maurea [3]**

[1] Department of Pharmacy, Federico II University, Naples, Italy, [2] Department of Biomedical Sciences and CNR Institute of Neuroscience, University of Padova, Padova, Italy, [3] Division of Cardiology, National Cancer Institute, G. Pascale Foundation, Naples, Italy, [4] Department of Molecular Medicine and Medical Biotechnology, Federico II University, Naples, Italy, [5] CEINGE Biotecnologie Avanzate, Naples, Italy, [6] Department of Translational Medical Sciences, Federico II University, Naples, Italy, [7] Department of Animal Experimental Research, National Cancer Institute, G. Pascale Foundation, Naples, Italy

Edited by:
Pasquale Pagliaro,
Università degli Studi di Torino, Italy

Reviewed by:
Lucio Barile,
Cardiocentro Ticino, Switzerland
Sartiani Laura,
University of Florence, Italy

***Correspondence:**
Carlo G. Tocchetti
carlogabriele.tocchetti@unina.it
Claudia De Lorenzo
cladelor@unina.it
Nicola Maurea
n.maurea@istitutotumori.na.it

The ErbB2 blocker trastuzumab improves survival in oncologic patients, but can cause cardiotoxicity. The late Na+ current inhibitor ranolazine has been shown to counter experimental HF, including doxorubicin cardiotoxicity (a condition characterized by derangements in redox balance), by lowering the levels of reactive oxygen species (ROS). Since ErbB2 can modulate ROS signaling, we tested whether trastuzumab cardiotoxicity could be blunted by ranolazine via redox-mediated mechanisms. Trastuzumab decreased fractional shortening and ejection fraction in mice, but ranolazine prevented heart dysfunction when co-administered with trastuzumab. Trastuzumab cardiotoxicity was accompanied by elevations in natriuretic peptides and matrix metalloproteinase 2 (MMP2) mRNAs, which were not elevated with co-treatment with ranolazine. Trastuzumab also increased cleavage of caspase-3, indicating activation of the proapoptotic machinery. Again, ranolazine prevented this activation. Interestingly, Neonatal Rat Ventricular Myocytes (NRVMs), labeled with MitoTracker Red and treated with trastuzumab, showed only a small increase in ROS compared to baseline conditions. We then stressed trastuzumab-treated cells with the beta-agonist isoproterenol to increase workload, and we observed a significant increase of probe fluorescence, compared with cells treated with isoproterenol alone, reflecting induction of oxidative stress. These effects were blunted by ranolazine, supporting a role for *I*Na inhibition in the regulation of redox balance also in trastuzumab cardiotoxicity.

Keywords: trastuzumab cardiotoxicity, ranolazine, heart function, heart failure, oxidative stress

INTRODUCTION

ErbB2 (also called HER2) is tyrosine kinase receptor, member of the human epidermal growth factor receptor family, and is overexpressed in 25–30% of breast cancers (Slamon et al., 1987). Trastuzumab is the prototypical anti-ErbB2 drug, and the first developed and most widely used biologic anticancer agent. Since its introduction in 1998, trastuzumab has dramatically improved the clinical history of breast cancer patients, but unfortunately it has been shown to cause cardiac dysfunction (Bloom et al., 2016; Moslehi, 2016; Zamorano et al., 2016; Armenian et al., 2017), since ErbB2 has been proven to be an important modulator of myocardial function (Force et al., 2007; Eschenhagen et al., 2011). Indeed, in the heart, ErbB2 seems to mediate cell survival and functionality (De Keulenaer et al., 2010; Ky et al., 2013; Lim et al., 2015), and also cardiac regeneration (D'Uva et al., 2015), and it seems to be stimulated upon cardiac adverse hemodynamics or other stress, such as doxorubicin (De Keulenaer et al., 2010; Tocchetti et al., 2017). It has been hypothesized that ErbB2 blockers can hamper cardiomyocytes, especially when exposed to other stressors, such as pressure or volume overload or anthracyclines, eventually leading to cardiac dysfunction (de Korte et al., 2007; Gabrielson et al., 2007; Ewer and Ewer, 2010). Hence, this co-administration is now possibly avoided in clinics (Slamon et al., 2001; Suter et al., 2007), since trastuzumab can exacerbate or induce anthracycline toxicity: once trastuzumab blocks the protective mechanisms of ErbB2, the oxidative damage from anthracyclines can increase (Ewer and Ewer, 2010). Importantly, ErbB2 has been shown to modulate doxorubicin-induced redox damage (Timolati et al., 2006), while its blockade is able to induce myocytes death through redox-dependent pathways (Gordon et al., 2009). In addition, ErbB2 overexpressor mice showed upregulation of antioxidant enzymes and protection from anthracyclines cardiotoxicity (Belmonte et al., 2015).

The late Na+ current inhibitor ranolazine has emerged as a potential therapeutic to treat experimental heart failure (Sabbah et al., 2002; Rastogi et al., 2008), and has also been recently indicated as a promising cardio-oncological drug (Minotti, 2013). We and others (Tocchetti et al., 2014; Cappetta et al., 2017) have demonstrated that ranolazine is also able to blunt experimental doxorubicin cardiotoxicity. Also, we had previously shown that trastuzumab can cause experimental heart dysfunction (Riccio et al., 2009; Fedele et al., 2012). Hence, here we hypothesize that ranolazine is also able to blunt heart dysfunction induced by trastuzumab in animal and cellular models.

MATERIALS AND METHODS

Trastuzumab Treatment Protocol *in Vivo*

C57Bl/6 mice (2–4 months old, Harlan Italy, San Piero al Natisone, Udine, Italy) were injected with a cumulative dose of 2 nM trastuzumab (Genentech, South San Francisco, CA, USA) via seven daily intraperitoneal injections (2.25 mg/kg i.p., TRA group), as for our well-established protocol (Fedele et al., 2012). No mortality was associated with this dosing regimen. Another group of mice was treated orally with ranolazine (Ranexa, Menarini, 305 mg/kg/day, doses comparable Reagan-Shaw et al., 2008 with those used clinically in humans of 750 mg twice daily, below the human maximal dosing of 1 g twice daily) for 10 days (RAN group; Tocchetti et al., 2014), and another group, after 3 days of ranolazine, started receiving trastuzumab concomitantly with ranolazine for 7 days (RAN+TRA group). Sham animals were used as controls. For *ex vivo* analyses, animals were sacrificed by cervical dislocation after anesthesia with tilotamine (0.09 mg/g), zolazepam (0.09 mg/g), and 0.01% atropine (0.0 4 ml/g); hearts were then excised and processed for further studies. Eight to ten animals per group were studied for all protocols.

Transthoracic Echocardiography

In vivo cardiac function was assessed by transthoracic echocardiography in sedated 2- to 4-month-old WT C57BL6 mice (Harlan Italy, San Piero al Natisone, UD, Italy) using a Vevo 2100 high-resolution imaging system (40-MHz transducer, VisualSonics, Toronto, ON, Canada). Mice were anesthetized with Tilotamine (0.09 mg/g), Zolazepam (0.09 mg/g), and 0.01% atropine (0.04 ml/g). Cardiac function was evaluated by non-invasive echocardiography in basal conditions, after 7 days of treatment with trastuzumab, or after 3 days of pre-treatment with ranolazine followed by co-administration of ranolazine and trastuzumab for 7 days. Studies and analysis were performed blinded to heart condition. Data are presented as mean ± standard error of the mean (SEM) unless otherwise noted. Between-group differences were assessed by Student's *t*-test or one-way analysis if variance (ANOVA) as appropriate. Statistical significance was defined as $P < 0.05$.

The animal experiments described herein were carried out in accordance with the recommendations of Italian regulations for experimentation on animals. The protocol was approved by the ethical committee and met the standards required by Directive 2010/63/EU of the European Parliament.

RNA Extraction and Real-Time PCR

Fresh frozen tissue was mechanically homogenized and total RNA was extracted by using Trizol (Invitrogen, Milan, Italy) according to the manufacturer's protocol. Reverse transcription of total RNA was performed starting from equal amounts of total RNA/sample (500 ng) using SuperScript® III Reverse Transcriptase (Invitrogen, Milan, Italy). RT-PCR was used to assess the mRNAs of ANP, MMP2, and GAPDH (the latter as an internal reference), as previously described (Tocchetti et al., 2014). Experiments were carried out in triplicate for each data point, and data analysis was performed with Applied Biosystems'StepOnePlus™ Real-Time PCR System.

Western Blotting Analysis of the Apoptotic Pathway

Murine hearts were processed as previously described (Tocchetti et al., 2014). Anti-caspase 3, anti-cleaved caspase 3, anti-GAPDH (Cell Signaling Technology), or anti-Actin antibody (Sigma), followed by anti-rabbit, HRP-conjugated IgGs from goat antiserum (Thermo Scientific) were used to detect proteins involved in the apoptotic pathway. The signal from secondary antibodies was visualized by enhanced chemiluminescence detection (ECL western blotting detection kit, Thermo Scientific). The signal intensity of reactive bands was quantitatively measured with a phosphorimager (GS-710, Biorad) or by the open source software ImageJ (NIH, USA).

Isolation and Culture of Neonatal Rat Ventricular Myocytes (NRVMs)

NRVMs were isolated from 1 to 3 days old Wistar rats. Hearts were excised, fragmented and dissociated at 4°C overnight with an enzyme solution containing trypsin (Invitrogen), under continuous stirring. The day after, fragments were further dissociated with an enzymatic solution containing Collagenase type I (Gibco). Cells were purified and resuspended in growth medium consisting of MEM (Invitrogen) supplemented with 10% fetal bovine serum (Gibco) and antibiotics (100 U/ml penicillin and 100 μg/ml streptomycin).

Cells were pre-plated for 90 min in order to separate NRVMs from fibroblasts. NRVMs were counted and opportunely diluted with MEM supplemented with 10% FBS, antibiotics, non-essential amino acids (NEAA) and 0.1 mM BrdU, necessary to inhibit cell proliferation, and the plated onto slides pre-treated with gelatin 0.1%.

Measurement of Formation of Reactive Oxygen Species

NRVMs were seeded in 6-well plates at a density of 3×10^5/well and ranolazine (10 μM) and trastuzumab (2 μM), alone or in combination, were added.

After 24 h, cells were incubated for 15 min at 37°C with 10 nM MitoTracker Red CM-H2XRos (MTR, Molecular Probes, λec = 579 nm, λem = 599 nm) in HBSS. Following the incubation, cells were washed twice with HBSS and slides were analyzed using the fluorescence microscope Zeiss Axlovert 100 M and a 63x oil immersion objective.

In the kinetic experiment, NRVMs were treated with ranolazine (10 μM) and trastuzumab (2 μM), alone or in combination. After 24 h, cells were incubated with 10 nM MitoTracker Red CM-H_2XRos as shown before. Three baseline images were taken at frame rate 1/5 min, and then 4 μM Isoproterenol (ISO) was added for 1 h.

Statistical Analyses

For most studies, between-group differences were assessed by Student's *t*-test or one-way ANOVA as appropriate. Statistical analysis was performed with OriginPro 8 SR0 v8.0724. Differences among the groups in parameters assessed by reverse transcription–PCR (RT–PCR) or western blotting were evaluated using the non-parametric Kruskal–Wallis test and adjusted for multiple comparisons with the Bonferroni method Statistical analysis were performed with SPSS statistical package (14.0 version).

Statistical significance was defined as $P < 0.05$.

RESULTS

Ranolazine Attenuates Trastuzumab-Induced Heart Dysfunction in Mice

First, we tested the beneficial role of ranolazine on trastuzumab induced cardiotoxicity *in vivo* in a mouse model. To this aim, groups of 8–10 mice were treated with trastuzumab and ranolazine as described in the Methods section. Echocardiography was performed before and after the treatments.

After 7 days, in trastuzumab-treated mice, fractional shortening (FS) decreased to 54 ± 3.86%, $p < 0.0005$ vs. 60.29 ± 2.47% (sham), ejection fraction (EF) to 84.33 ±3.08%, $p < 0.0005$ vs. 91.26 ± 2.03% (sham). However, in mice treated with ranolazine plus trastuzumab, FS and EF were not significantly reduced (FS 59.40 ± 3.13%; EF 89.80 ± 2.28%; **Figure 1**).

Ranolazine Prevents Cardiac Fetal Gene Reprograming and Extracellular Matrix Remodeling in Trastuzumab Treated Hearts

At the end of the *in vivo* treatment, mice were euthanized, and hearts were removed and processed for mRNA expression analyses and detection of myocardial stress and apoptosis. All analyses were performed in parallel experiments on sham animals. In accordance with the alterations of contractile function, trastuzumab enhanced ANP and MMP2 mRNAs compared with sham. However, when mice were pre-treated with ranolazine, ANP, and MMP2 mRNA levels were lower compared to TRA (**Figure 2**).

Ranolazine Reduces Trastuzumab-Induced Apoptosis

We then investigated the impact of ranolazine on trastuzumab-induced cell death. Excised murine hearts of treated mice were handled as described above, then lysed and analyzed by Western blotting with an anti-Caspase antibody. Trastuzumab activated apoptosis significantly, as shown by the enhanced cleavage of caspase-3. Caspase-3 fragmentation did not occur when mice were co-administered with RAN+TRA (**Figure 3**).

Ranolazine Limits the Production of Reactive Oxygen Species Induced by Trastuzumab in NRVMs

To test whether ranolazine protective effects are achieved by a reduction of ROS generated upon trastuzumab administration, ROS formation was monitored in NRVMs. NRVMs labeled with MitoTracker Red and treated for 24 h with Trastuzumab showed a modest increase of probe fluorescence, compared with untreated cells, reflecting induction of oxidative stress, which was not blunted by ranolazine.

Considering that trastuzumab exerts its cardiotoxic effects especially in presence of cardiac stressors (de Korte et al., 2007; De Keulenaer et al., 2010; Ewer and Ewer, 2010; Tocchetti et al., 2017), and that the beating heart is normally subject to preload and afterload, we then incubated NRVM with the beta stimulator isoproterenol (ISO; Tocchetti et al., 2012) to simulate workload conditions. Interestingly, the concomitant administration of TRA and ISO produced a significant increase in ROS compared to ISO alone, and such increase could be blunted by RAN (**Figure 4**).

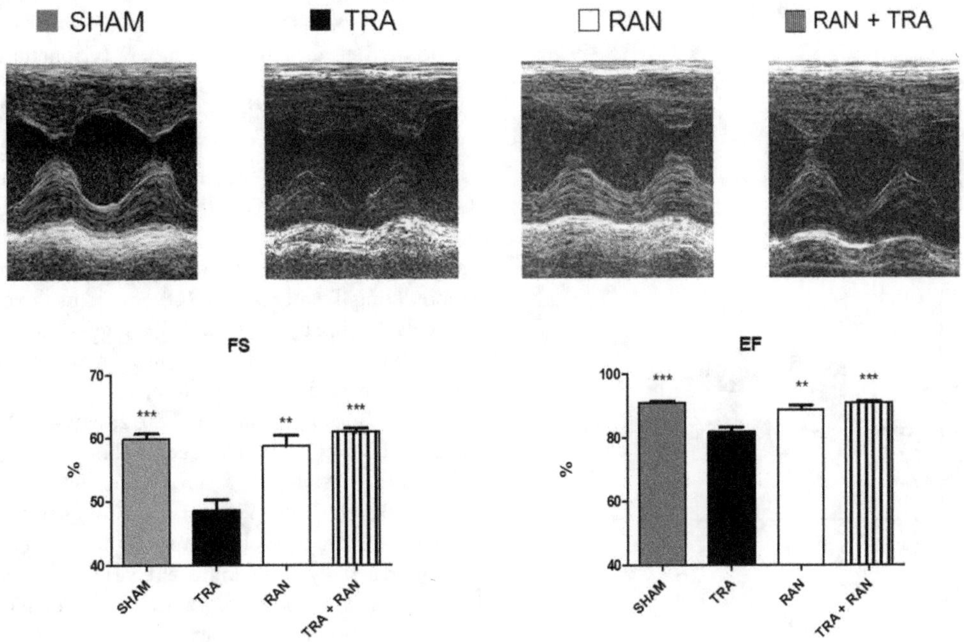

FIGURE 1 | Ranolazine protects from trastuzumab-related cardiac dysfunction. Ranolazine blunts reductions in fractional shortening (FS) and ejection fraction (EF) induced by trastuzumab (**$p < 0.01$ vs TRA; ***$p < 0.001$ vs TRA).

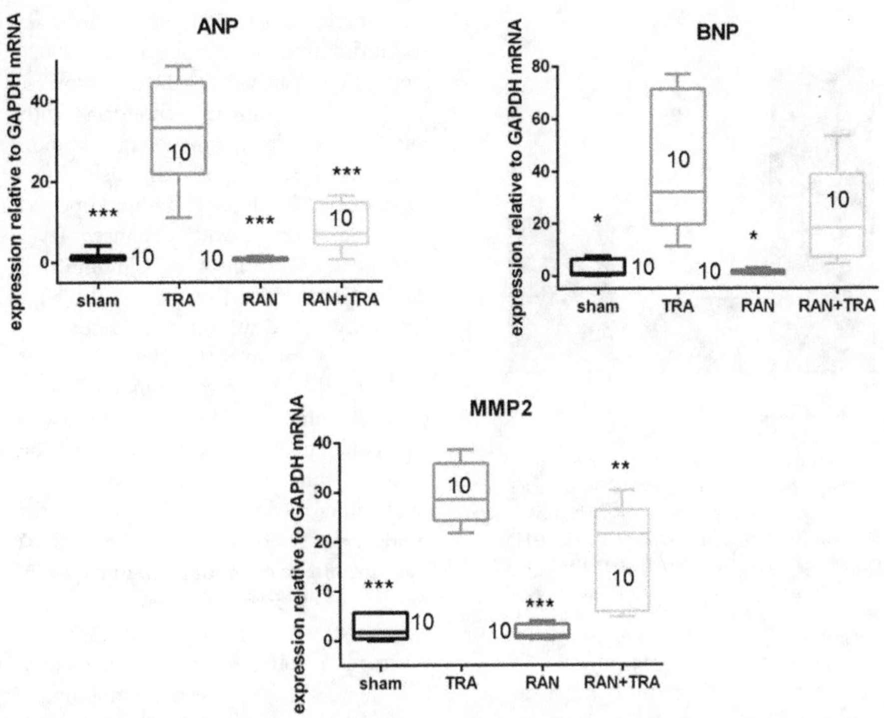

FIGURE 2 | Effects of ranolazine on cardiac fetal gene reprogramming. ANP, BNP, and MMP2 mRNA expressions induced by trastuzumab were reduced in mice pretreated with ranolazine (*$p < 0.05$ vs. TRA; **$p < 0.005$; ***$p < 0.0005$).

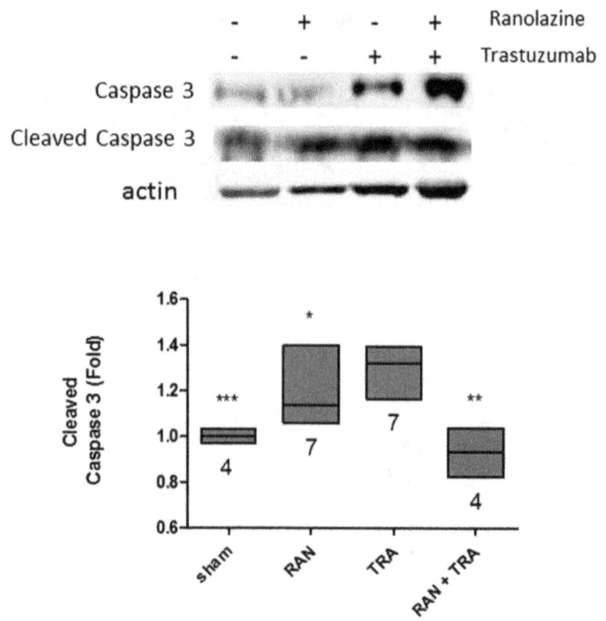

FIGURE 3 | Apoptotic pathway analysis in hearts of treated mice. Caspase 3 activation triggered by trastuzumab, was reduced by ranolazine treatment (*$p < 0.05$ vs. TRA; **$p < 0.005$ vs. TRA; ***$p < 0.0005$ vs. TRA).

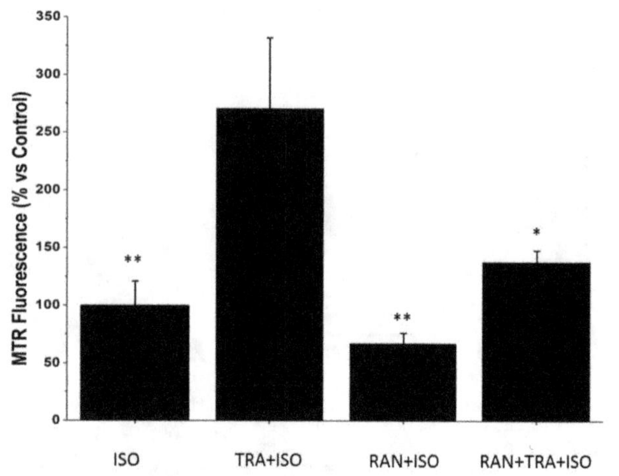

FIGURE 4 | Ranolazine (RAN) reduces Reactive Oxygen Species (ROS) formation induced by Trastuzumab (TRA) and isoproterenol (ISO). Neonatal Rat Ventricular Myocytes (NRVMs) untreated or treated for 24 h with 2 μM TRA, with 10 μM Ran or with 2 μM TRA and 10 μM Ran, were incubated for 1 h with 4 μM Iso. Microscopy analysis of cells labeled with the fluorescent probe Mitotracker Red CM-H2XRos was performed to detect the degree of mitochondrial oxidative stress. Data are normalized to the control after 24 h + 1 h of treatment with isoproterenol. n ISO: 24; n TRA+ISO: 22; n RAN+ISO: 19; n RAN+TRA+ISO: 20. *$p < 0.05$ vs. TRA; **$p < 0.01$ vs. TRA.

DISCUSSION

The introduction of trastuzumab in therapeutic protocols for ErbB2+ breast cancer has revolutionized the prognosis of patients affected by this disease, but unfortunately this therapy is characterized with a relevant incidence of cardiac dysfunction and HF, especially when associated with anthracyclines. We (Tocchetti et al., 2014) and others (Cappetta et al., 2017) have shown that the late *I*Na inhibitor ranolazine is able to blunt cardiac dysfunction induced by anthracyclines by decreasing ROS production. The data presented here suggest that ranolazine is also able to blunt trastuzumab cardiotoxicity, and this effect seems to involve a reduction in oxidative stress. Indeed, redox mechanisms have also been proposed for the neuregulin/ErbB2 pathway. This pathway has been shown to play a role in modulating the increase in ROS caused by doxorubicin in animal models (Timolati et al., 2006), suggesting that cardiotoxicity from ErbB2 blockade can also involve a dysregulation of redox homeostasis (Mercurio et al., 2016). Importantly, beside anthracyclines (Menna et al., 2012; Sawyer, 2013; Stěrba et al., 2013; Ghigo et al., 2016), redox abnormalities are involved in the pathophysiology of cardiotoxic effects caused by several antineoplastic drugs (Ferroni et al., 2011), including new biologic anti-cancer drugs, such as intracellular signaling inhibitors, that are increasingly used in recent years (Tocchetti et al., 2017). Such drugs may be cardiotoxic, since they block pathways that are major modulators of myocardial function, especially under conditions of cardiac stress, such as hypertension or hypertrophy (Suter and Ewer, 2013), with mechanisms of action that often involve redox dysregulation as well.

The importance of ErbB2 in the heart has been particularly emphasized by seminal studies that demonstrated that ErbB2 cardiac KO mice were affected by dilated cardiomyopathy, with increased susceptibility to anthracycline-induced damage to cardiomyocytes (Crone et al., 2002; Ozcelik et al., 2002). Conversely, cardiac ErbB2 overexpressor mice showed lower levels of ROS in mitochondria, with reduced ROS levels and less cell death in neonatal cardiomyocytes isolated from ErbB2(tg) hearts upon administration of anthracyclines, due to increased levels of glutathione peroxidase 1 (GPx1) protein and GPx activity, with enhanced levels of two known GPx activators, c-Abl, and Arg (Belmonte et al., 2015; Tocchetti et al., 2017). Furthermore, block of ErbB2 has been correlated with cardiomyocyte death through reactive oxygen species-dependent pathways (Gordon et al., 2009).

Along this line, our results in NRVM show that attenuation of trastuzumab toxicity with ranolazine is indeed obtained by reducing ROS production, and our *in vivo* data show better LV function with ranolazine+trastuzumab compared with trastuzumab alone. The fact that trastuzumab elicited only a modest rise in ROS in non-stressed NRVM is compatible with the cardiotoxic effect of ErbB2 blockers that might be negligible *per se*, but exacerbated when administered under conditions of cardiac stress or in previously diseased hearts (e.g., increased pressure or volume overload) or in presence of cardiovascular risk factors (age, obesity, smoking, hypertension, previous exposure to anthracyclines; Denegri et al., 2016; Tocchetti et al., 2017).

The inhibition of late INa with ranolazine has been proposed as a therapeutic strategy in many *in vivo* and *in vitro* models of heart dysfunction (Sabbah et al., 2002; Rastogi et al., 2008; Coppini et al., 2013, 2017) and in particular, ranolazine has been shown to be able to blunt LV dysfunction in experimental models of doxorubicin cardiotoxcicity by lowering oxidative stress (Tocchetti et al., 2014; Cappetta et al., 2017). By reducing elevated [Na+]i levels that, are commonly elevated in conditions of cardiac dysfunction (Bers, 2001; Pieske and Houser, 2003), ranolazine could prevent calcium overload and the occurrence of oxidative damage by reducing ROS production, with an advantage over ordinary antioxidant treatments that counteract ROS after their generation (Zeitz et al., 2002; Maack et al., 2006; Song et al., 2006; Wagner et al., 2006; Erickson et al., 2008; Kohlhaas et al., 2010; Tocchetti et al., 2014).

In the setting of heart disease, ROS play a role in pathophysiological remodeling, cellular death, and LV dysfunction (Sawyer et al., 2002; Giordano, 2005; Takimoto and Kass, 2007; Nediani et al., 2011). The molecular signaling pathways that link ROS to LV hypertrophy, remodeling, and failure include alpha- and beta-adrenergic and angiotensin II (AT1) receptor stimulation, as well as modifications of a wide number of proteins that include stress kinases, nuclear transcription factors, collagen and metalloproteinases, calcium channels, myofilaments and proteins involved in the excitation–contraction coupling machinery. A key role is played by a rise in cytosolic Ca2+ levels that lead to expression changes of several genes involved in cardiac pathophysiological hypertrophy and remodeling of the heart (Arcaro et al., 2016) with increases in interstitial fibrosis and expression of profibrotic genes (Zhao et al., 2010). Abnormalities of the extracellular matrix and adverse remodeling are also exacerbated by ROS (Kandasamy et al., 2010). Importantly, our data show that ranolazine is able to blunt the effects produced by trastuzumab on important components of LV remodeling such as myocyte death and fibrosis, and to reverse the expression changes of important genes such as NPs and MMPs, eventually mitigating the occurrence of cardiac dysfunction measured by echocardiography.

LIMITATIONS OF THE STUDY

In human pathology trastuzumab is administered to cancer patients, while here we studied experimental trastuzumab cardiotoxicity in C57BL6 mice without cancer. Of course, further studies in mice with cancer will have to be performed. Nevertheless, C57BL6 mice, that are commonly used in models of experimental heart failure, also have a compromised immune system that in part may mimic cancer.

CONCLUSIONS

Our data support previous findings on the efficacy of ranolazine in experimental heart dysfunction (Sabbah et al., 2002; Rastogi et al., 2008; Coppini et al., 2013, 2017; Tocchetti et al., 2014; Cappetta et al., 2017). We acknowledge that further experiments may be necessary to conclude that the mechanism of action involves the levels of ROS, also considering that ranolazine has been recently shown to be able to antagonize β-adrenergic stimulation and decrease myofilaments Ca2+ sensitivity (Flenner et al., 2016), with little therapeutic efficacy in a HCM murine model *in vivo*. Nevertheless, we show that in the cardio-oncologic setting, beside doxorubicin cardiotoxicity (Tocchetti et al., 2014; Cappetta et al., 2017), RAN could also be a promising cardioprotective drug in the setting of trastuzumab toxicity. More efforts involving both experimental and clinical studies will be needed in order to establish whether ranolazine might be introduced clinically in the therapeutic strategies that aim at addressing cardiotoxicity induced by trastuzumab or anthracyclines.

AUTHOR CONTRIBUTIONS

GR, SA, CDA, DF, and CM: performed *in vitro* experiments; CC and DR: performed *in vivo* experiments; GR, SA, CC, GP, DF, MR, DR, and CGT: analyzed data, drafted figures, and the manuscript; CA, GC, FDL, CDL, and NM: provided necessary materials; FDL, CGT, CDL, and NM: conceptualized the project; CGT and CDL: wrote the manuscript.

ACKNOWLEDGMENTS

The authors are grateful for kind support from Giorgia Sorrentino of National Cancer Institute Pascale, Naples, Italy. This work was supported by a grant from the Italian Ministry of Health, and by AIRC (IG, Rif. 18473) to GC.

REFERENCES

Arcaro, A., Pirozzi, F., Angelini, A., Chimenti, C., Crotti, L., Giordano, C., et al. (2016). Novel perspectives in redox biology and pathophysiology of failing myocytes: modulation of the intramyocardial redox milieu for therapeutic interventions-a review article from the working group of cardiac cell biology, Italian society of cardiology. *Oxid. Med. Cell. Longev.* 2016:6353469. doi: 10.1155/2016/6353469

Armenian, S. H., Lacchetti, C., Barac, A., Carver, J., Constine, L. S., Denduluri, N., et al. (2017). Prevention and monitoring of cardiac dysfunction in survivors of adult cancers: American Society of Clinical Oncology Clinical Practice Guideline. *J. Clin. Oncol.* 35, 893–911. doi: 10.1200/JCO.2016.70.5400

Belmonte, F., Das, S., Sysa-Shah, P., Sivakumaran, V., Stanley, B., Guo, X., et al. (2015). ErbB2 overexpression upregulates antioxidant enzymes, reduces basal levels of reactive oxygen species, and protects against doxorubicin cardiotoxicity. *Am. J. Physiol. Heart Circ. Physiol.* 309, H1271–H1280. doi: 10.1152/ajpheart.00517.2014

Bers, D. M. (2001). *Excitation–Contraction Coupling and Cardiac Contractile Force, 2nd Edn.* Dordrecht: Kluwer Academic Publishers.

Bloom, M. W., Hamo, C. E., Cardinale, D., Ky, B., Nohria, A., Baer, L., et al. (2016). Cancer therapy-related cardiac dysfunction and heart failure: part 1: definitions, pathophysiology, risk factors, and imaging. *Circ. Heart Fail.* 9:e002661. doi: 10.1161/CIRCHEARTFAILURE.115.002661

Cappetta, D., Esposito, G., Coppini, R., Piegari, E., Russo, R., Ciuffreda, L. P., et al. (2017). Effects of ranolazine in a model of doxorubicin-induced left ventricle diastolic dysfunction. *Br. J. Pharmacol.* 174, 3696–3712. doi: 10.1111/bph.13791

Coppini, R., Ferrantini, C., Yao, L., Fan, P., Del Lungo, M., Stillitano, F., et al. (2013). Late sodium current inhibition reverses electromechanical dysfunction in human hypertrophic cardiomyopathy. *Circulation* 127, 575–584. doi: 10.1161/CIRCULATIONAHA.112.134932

Coppini, R., Mazzoni, L., Ferrantini, C., Gentile, F., Pioner, J. M., Laurino, A., et al. (2017). Ranolazine prevents phenotype development in a mouse model of hypertrophic cardiomyopathy. *Circ. Heart Fail.* 10:e003565. doi: 10.1161/CIRCHEARTFAILURE.116.003565

Crone, S. A., Zhao, Y. Y., Fan, L., Gu, Y., Minamisawa, S., Liu, Y., et al. (2002). ErbB2 is essential in the prevention of dilated cardiomyopathy. *Nat. Med.* 8, 459–465. doi: 10.1038/nm0502-459

De Keulenaer, G. W., Doggen, K., and Lemmens, K. (2010). The vulnerability of the heart as a pluricellular paracrine organ: lessons from unexpected triggers of heart failure in targeted ErbB2 anticancer therapy. *Circ. Res.* 106, 35–46. doi: 10.1161/CIRCRESAHA.109.205906

de Korte, M. A., de Vries, E. G., Lub-de Hooge, M. N., Jager, P. L., Gietema, J. A., van der Graaf, W. T., et al. (2007). 111Indium-trastuzumab visualises myocardial human epidermal growth factor receptor 2 expression shortly after anthracycline treatment but not during heart failure: a clue to uncover the mechanisms of trastuzumab-related cardiotoxicity. *Eur. J. Cancer* 43, 2046–2051. doi: 10.1016/j.ejca.2007.06.024

Denegri, A., Moccetti, T., Moccetti, M., Spallarossa, P., Brunelli, C., and Ameri, P. (2016). Cardiac toxicity of trastuzumab in elderly patients with breast cancer. *J. Geriatr. Cardiol.* 13, 355–363. doi: 10.11909/j.issn.1671-5411.2016.04.003

D'Uva, G., Aharonov, A., Lauriola, M., Kain, D., Yahalom-Ronen, Y., Carvalho, S., et al. (2015). ERBB2 triggers mammalian heart regeneration by promoting cardiomyocyte dedifferentiation and proliferation. *Nat. Cell Biol.* 17, 627–638. doi: 10.1038/ncb3149

Erickson, J. R., Joiner, M. L., Guan, X., Kutschke, W., Yang, J., Oddis, C. V., et al. (2008). A dynamic pathway for calcium-independent activation of CaMKII by methionine oxidation. *Cell* 133, 462–474. doi: 10.1016/j.cell.2008.02.048

Eschenhagen, T., Force, T., Ewer, M. S., de Keulenaer, G. W., Suter, T. M., Anker, S. D., et al. (2011). Cardiovascular side effects of cancer therapies: a position statement from the heart failure association of the European Society of Cardiology. *Eur. J. Heart Fail.* 13, 1–10. doi: 10.1093/eurjhf/hfq213

Ewer, M. S., and Ewer, S. M. (2010). Troponin I provides insight into cardiotoxicity and the anthracycline-trastuzumab interaction. *J. Clin. Oncol.* 28, 3901–3904. doi: 10.1200/JCO.2010.30.6274

Fedele, C., Riccio, G., Coppola, C., Barbieri, A., Monti, M. G., Arra, C., et al. (2012). Comparison of preclinical cardiotoxic effects of different ErbB2 inhibitors. *Breast Cancer Res. Treat.* 133, 511–521. doi: 10.1007/s10549-011-1783-9

Ferroni, P., Della-Morte, D., Palmirotta, R., McClendon, M., Testa, G., Abete, P., et al. (2011). Platinum-based compounds and risk for cardiovascular toxicity in the elderly: role of the antioxidants in chemoprevention. *Rejuvenation Res.* 14, 293–308. doi: 10.1089/rej.2010.1141

Flenner, F., Friedrich, F. W., Ungeheuer, N., Christ, T., Geertz, B., Reischmann, S., et al. (2016). Ranolazine antagonizes catecholamine-induced dysfunction in isolated cardiomyocytes, but lacks long-term therapeutic effects in vivo in a mouse model of hypertrophic cardiomyopathy. *Cardiovasc Res.* 109, 90–102. doi: 10.1093/cvr/cvv247

Force, T., Krause, D. S., and Van Etten, R. A. (2007). Molecular mechanisms of cardiotoxicity of tyrosine kinase inhibition. *Nat. Rev. Cancer* 7, 332–344. doi: 10.1038/nrc2106

Gabrielson, K., Bedja, D., Pin, S., Tsao, A., Gama, L., Yuan, B., et al. (2007). Heat shock protein 90 and ErbB2 in the cardiac response to doxorubicin injury. *Cancer Res.* 67, 1436–1441. doi: 10.1158/0008-5472.CAN-06-3721

Ghigo, A., Li, M., and Hirsch, E. (2016). New signal transduction paradigms in anthracycline-induced cardiotoxicity. *Biochim. Biophys. Acta* 1863(7 Pt B), 1916–1925. doi: 10.1016/j.bbamcr.2016.01.021

Giordano, F. J. (2005). Oxygen, oxidative stress, hypoxia, and heart failure. *J. Clin. Invest.* 115, 500–508. doi: 10.1172/JCI200524408

Gordon, L. I., Burke, M. A., Singh, A. T., Prachand, S., Lieberman, E. D., Sun, L., et al. (2009). Blockade of the erbB2 receptor induces cardiomyocyte death through mitochondrial and reactive oxygen species-dependent pathways. *J. Biol. Chem.* 284, 2080–2087. doi: 10.1074/jbc.M804570200

Kandasamy, A. D., Chow, A. K., Ali, M. A., and Schulz, R. (2010). Matrix metalloproteinase-2 and myocardial oxidative stress injury: beyond the matrix. *Cardiovasc. Res.* 85, 413–423. doi: 10.1093/cvr/cvp268

Kohlhaas, M., Liu, T., Knopp, A., Zeller, T., Ong, M. F., Böhm, M., et al. (2010). Elevated cytosolic Na+ increases mitochondrial formation of reactive oxygen species in failing cardiac myocytes. *Circulation* 121, 1606–1613. doi: 10.1161/CIRCULATIONAHA.109.914911

Ky, B., Vejpongsa, P., Yeth, E. T., Force, T., and Moslehi, J. J. (2013). Emerging paradigms in cardiomyopathies associated with cancer therapies. Emerging paradigms in cardiomyopathies associated with cancer therapies. *Circ. Res.* 113, 754–764. doi: 10.1161/CIRCRESAHA.113.300218

Lim, S. L., Lam, C. S., Segers, V. F., Brutsaert, D. L., and De Keulenaer, G. W. (2015). Cardiac endothelium-myocyte interaction: clinical opportunities for new heart failure therapies regardless of ejection fraction. *Eur. Heart J.* 36, 2050–2060. doi: 10.1093/eurheartj/ehv132

Maack, C., Cortassa, S., Aon, M. A., Ganesan, A. N., Liu, T., and O'Rourke, B. (2006). Elevated cytosolic Na+ decreases mitochondrial Ca2+ uptake during excitation–contraction coupling and impairs energetic adaptation in cardiac myocytes. *Circ. Res.* 99, 172–182. doi: 10.1161/01.RES.0000232546.92777.05

Menna, P., Paz, O. G., Chello, M., Covino, E., Salvatorelli, E., and Minotti, G. (2012). Anthracycline cardiotoxicity. *Expert Opin. Drug Saf.* 11(Suppl. 1), S21–S36. doi: 10.1517/14740338.2011.589834

Mercurio, V., Pirozzi, F., Lazzarini, E., Marone, G., Rizzo, P., Agnetti, G., et al. (2016). Models of heart failure based on the cardiotoxicity of anticancer drugs. *J. Card. Fail.* 22, 449–458. doi: 10.1016/j.cardfail.2016.04.008

Minotti, G. (2013). Pharmacology at work for cardio-oncology: ranolazine to treat early cardiotoxicity induced by antitumor drugs. *J. Pharmacol. Exp. Ther.* 346, 343–349. doi: 10.1124/jpet.113.204057

Moslehi, J. J. (2016). Cardiovascular toxic effects of targeted cancer therapies. *N. Engl. J. Med.* 375, 1457–1467. doi: 10.1056/NEJMra1100265

Nediani, C., Raimondi, L., Borchi, E., and Cerbai, E. (2011). Nitric oxide/reactive oxygen species generation and nitroso/redox imbalance in heart failure: from molecular mechanisms to therapeutic implications. *Antioxid. Redox Signal.* 14, 289–331. doi: 10.1089/ars.2010.3198

Ozcelik, C., Erdmann, B., Pilz, B., Wettschureck, N., Britsch, S., Hüner, N., et al. (2002). Conditional mutation of the ErbB2 (HER2) receptor in cardiomyocytes leads to dilated cardiomyopathy. *Proc. Natl. Acad. Sci. U.S.A.* 99, 8880–8885. doi: 10.1073/pnas.122249299

Pieske, B., and Houser, S. R. (2003). [Na+]i handling in the failing human heart. *Cardiovasc. Res.* 57, 874–886. doi: 10.1016/S0008-6363(02)00841-6

Rastogi, S., Sharov, V. G., Mishra, S., Gupta, R. C., Blackburn, B., Belardinelli, L., et al. (2008). Ranolazine combined with enalapril or metoprolol prevents progressive LV dysfunction and remodeling in dogs with moderate heart failure. *Am. J. Physiol. Heart Circ. Physiol.* 295, H2149–H2155. doi: 10.1152/ajpheart.00728.2008

Reagan-Shaw, S., Nihal, M., and Ahmad, N. (2008). Dose translation from animal to human studies revisited. *FASEB J.* 22, 659–661. doi: 10.1096/fj.07-9574LSF

Riccio, G., Esposito, G., Leoncini, E., Contu, R., Condorelli, G., Chiariello, M., et al. (2009). Cardiotoxic effects, or lack thereof, of anti-ErbB2 immunoagents. *FASEB J.* 23, 3171–3178. doi: 10.1096/fj.09-131383

Sabbah, H. N., Chandler, M. P., Mishima, T., Suzuki, G., Chaudhry, P., Nass, O., et al. (2002). Ranolazine, a partial fatty acid oxidation (pFOX) inhibitor, improves left ventricular function in dogs with chronic heart failure. *J. Card. Fail.* 8, 416–422. doi: 10.1054/jcaf.2002.129232

Sawyer, D. B. (2013). Anthracyclines and heart failure. *N. Engl. J. Med.* 368, 1154–1115. doi: 10.1056/NEJMcibr1214975

Sawyer, D. B., Siwik, D. A., Xiao, L., Pimentel, D. R., Singh, K., and Colucci, W. S. (2002). Role of oxidative stress in myocardial hypertrophy and failure. *J. Mol. Cell. Cardiol.* 34, 379–388. doi: 10.1006/jmcc.2002.1526

Slamon, D. J., Clark, G. M., Wong, S. G., Levin, W. J., Ullrich, A., and McGuire, W. L. (1987). Human breast cancer: correlation of relapse and survival with amplification of the HER-2/neu oncogene. *Science* 235, 177–182. doi: 10.1126/science.3798106

Slamon, D. J., Leyland-Jones, B., Shak, S., Fuchs, H., Paton, V., Bajamonde, A., et al. (2001). Use of chemotherapy plus a monoclonal antibody against HER2 for metastatic breast cancer that overexpresses HER2. *N. Engl. J. Med.* 344, 783–792. doi: 10.1056/NEJM200103153441101

Song, Y., Shryock, J. C., Wagner, S., Maier, L. S., and Belardinelli, L. (2006). Blocking late sodium current reduces hydrogen peroxide-induced arrhythmogenic activity and contractile dysfunction. *J. Pharmacol. Exp. Ther.* 318, 214–222. doi: 10.1124/jpet.106.101832

Štěrba, M., Popelová, O., Vávrová, A., Jirkovský, E., Kovaríková, P., Geršl, V., et al. (2013). Oxidative stress, redox signaling, and metal chelation in anthracycline cardiotoxicity and pharmacological cardioprotection. *Antioxid. Redox Signal.* 18, 899–929. doi: 10.1089/ars.2012.4795

Suter, T. M., and Ewer, M. S. (2013). Cancer drugs and the heart: importance and management. *Eur. Heart J.* 34, 1102–1111. doi: 10.1093/eurheartj/ehs181

Suter, T. M., Procter, M., van Veldhuisen, D. J., Muscholl, M., Bergh, J., Carlomagno, C., et al. (2007). Trastuzumab-associated cardiac adverse effects in the herceptin adjuvant trial. *J. Clin. Oncol.* 25, 3859–3865. doi: 10.1200/JCO.2006.09.1611

Takimoto, E., and Kass, D. A. (2007). Role of oxidative stress in cardiac hypertrophy and remodeling. *Hypertension* 49, 241–248. doi: 10.1161/01.HYP.0000254415.31362.a7

Timolati, F., Ott, D., Pentassuglia, L., Giraud, M. N., Perriard, J. C., Suter, T. M., et al. (2006). Neuregulin-1 beta attenuates doxorubicin-induced alterations of excitation-contraction coupling and reduces oxidative stress in adult rat cardiomyocytes. *J. Mol. Cell. Cardiol.* 41, 845–854. doi: 10.1016/j.yjmcc.2006.08.002

Tocchetti, C. G., Caceres, V., Stanley, B. A., Xie, C., Shi, S., Watson, W. H., et al. (2012). GSH or palmitate preserves mitochondrial energetic/redox balance, preventing mechanical dysfunction in metabolically challenged myocytes/hearts from type 2 diabetic mice. *Diabetes* 61, 3094–3005. doi: 10.2337/db12-0072

Tocchetti, C. G., Cadeddu, C., Di Lisi, D., Femminò, S., Madonna, R., Mele, D., et al. (2017). From molecular mechanisms to clinical management of antineoplastic drug-induced cardiovascular toxicity: a translational overview. *Antioxid. Redox Signal.* doi: 10.1089/ars.2016.6930. [Epub ahead of print].

Tocchetti, C. G., Carpi, A., Coppola, C., Quintavalle, C., Rea, D., Campesan, M., et al. (2014). Ranolazine protects from doxorubicin-induced oxidative stress and cardiac dysfunction. *Eur. J. Heart Fail.* 16, 358–366. doi: 10.1002/ejhf.50

Wagner, S., Dybkova, N., Rasenack, E. C., Jacobshagen, C., Fabritz, L., Kirchhof, P., et al. (2006). Ca2+/calmodulindependent protein kinase II regulates cardiac Na+ channels. *J. Clin. Invest.* 116, 3127–3138. doi: 10.1172/JCI26620

Zamorano, J. L., Lancellotti, P., Rodriguez Muñoz, D., Aboyans, V., Asteggiano, R., Galderisi, M., et al. (2016). 2016 ESC Position Paper on cancer treatments and cardiovascular toxicity developed under the auspices of the ESC Committee for Practice Guidelines: the task force for cancer treatments and cardiovascular toxicity of the European Society of Cardiology (ESC). *Eur. Heart J.* 37, 2768–2801. doi: 10.1093/eurheartj/ehw211

Zeitz, O., Maass, A. E., VanNguyen, P., Hensmann, G., Kögler, H., Möller, K., et al. (2002). Hydroxyl radical-induced acute diastolic dysfunction is due to calcium overload via reverse-mode Na(+)–Ca(2+) exchange. *Circ. Res.* 90, 988–995. doi: 10.1161/01.RES.0000018625.25212.1E

Zhao, Y., McLaughlin, D., Robinson, E., Harvey, A. P., Hookham, M. B., Shah, A. M., et al. (2010). Nox2 NADPH oxidase promotes pathologic cardiac remodeling associated with Doxorubicin chemotherapy. *Cancer Res.* 70, 9287–9297. doi: 10.1158/0008-5472.CAN-10-2664

13

Sympathetic, Metabolic Adaptations and Oxidative Stress in Autism Spectrum Disorders: How Far From Physiology?

Antonietta Messina [1†], Vincenzo Monda [1†], Francesco Sessa [2], Anna Valenzano [2], Monica Salerno [2], Ilaria Bitetti [3], Francesco Precenzano [3], Rosa Marotta [4], Francesco Lavano [4], Serena M. Lavano [4], Margherita Salerno [5], Agata Maltese [5], Michele Roccella [5], Lucia Parisi [5], Roberta I. Ferrentino [3], Gabriele Tripi [6], Beatrice Gallai [7], Giuseppe Cibelli [2], Marcellino Monda [1], Giovanni Messina [2] and Marco Carotenuto [3]*

[1] Department of Experimental Medicine, Section of Human Physiology and Unit of Dietetics and Sports Medicine, Università degli Studi della Campania "Luigi Vanvitelli," Naples, Italy, [2] Department of Clinical and Experimental Medicine, University of Foggia, Foggia, Italy, [3] Clinic of Child and Adolescent Neuropsychiatry, Department of Mental Health, Physical and Preventive Medicine, Università degli Studi della Campania "Luigi Vanvitelli," Naples, Italy, [4] Department of Health Sciences, University "Magna Graecia," Catanzaro, Italy, [5] Child Neuropsychiatry, Department of Psychology and Pedagogical Sciences, University of Palermo, Palermo, Italy, [6] Childhood Psychiatric Service for Neurodevelopmentals Disorders, Chinon, France, [7] Department of Surgical and Biomedical Sciences, University of Perugia, Perugia, Italy

Edited by:
Mariarosaria Santillo,
University of Naples Federico II, Italy

Reviewed by:
Davide Viggiano,
University of Molise, Italy
Paolo Chieffi,
Università degli Studi della Campania "Luigi Vanvitelli" Caserta, Italy

***Correspondence:**
Giovanni Messina
giovanni.messina@unifig.it

†These authors have contributed equally to this work.

Autism spectrum disorders (ASD) is a complex and multifaceted neurobehavioral syndrome with no specific cause still identified, despite the worldwide increasing (prevalence for 1,000 children from 6.7 to 14.6, between 2000 and 2012). Many biological and instrumental markers have been suggested as potential predictive factors for the precocious diagnosis during infancy and/or pediatric age. Many studies reported structural and functional abnormalities in the autonomic system in subjects with ASD. Sleep problems in ASD are a prominent feature, having an impact on the social interaction of the patient. Considering the role of orexins (A and B) in wake-sleep circadian rhythm, we could speculate that ASD subjects may present a dysregulation in orexinergic neurotransmission. Conversely, oxidative stress is implicated in the pathophysiology of many neurological disorders. Nonetheless, little is known about the linkage between oxidative stress and the occurrence or the progress of autism and autonomic functioning; some markers, such as heart rate (HR), heart rate variability (HRV), body temperature, and galvanic skin response (GSR), may be altered in the patient with this so complex disorder. In the present paper, we analyzed an autism case report, focusing on the rule of the sympathetic activity with the aim to suggest that it may be considered an important tool in ASD evaluation. The results of this case confirm our hypothesis even if further studies needed.

Keywords: autism spectrum disorders (ASD), Orexin-A, oxidative stress, heart rate (HR), heart rate variability (HRV)

BACKGROUND

Autism spectrum disorders (ASD) is a complex and multifaceted neurobehavioral syndrome with no specific cause still identified, despite the worldwide increasing (prevalence for 1,000 children from 6.7 to 14.6, between 2000 and 2012). Many biological and instrumental markers have been suggested as potential predictive factors for the precocious diagnosis during infancy and/or pediatric age. Functional magnetic resonance imaging (fMRI) has shown the structural abnormalities in relevant brain structures such as the amygdala, cingulated anterior cortex, and cerebellum (Uddin and Menon, 2009). These alterations seem to be associated with neurotransmitters dysregulation with the imbalance between excitation and inhibition in neural circuits (Purcell et al., 2001a,b).

Many studies reported structural and functional abnormalities in the autonomic system in subjects with ASD (Neri et al., 2009a,b; Bujnakova et al., 2016; Bonaventure et al., 2017). As previously described, ASD patients show decreased levels of essential fatty acids. In this scenario, the assumption of polyunsaturated fatty acids (PUFA) can help the brain development and function (Brigandi et al., 2015).

On the other hand, ASD patients present sleep disorders, such as parasomnias, obstructive apnea sleep disorders syndrome (OSAS), disorders of initiating and maintaining of sleep, sleep-related movement disorders (Giallongo et al., 2011; Accetta et al., 2016; Precenzano et al., 2017). Considering the role of orexins (A and B) in wake-sleep circadian rhythm, we could speculate that ASD subjects may present a dysregulation in orexinergic neurotransmission also involved in various brain dysfunctions connected with numerous neuropsychiatric disorders including neurodevelopmental disorders. Sleep disturbance in ASD patients depending on the increased activity of the orexinergic system (probably due to amygdala dysfunction) associated with a reduction of 5-HT and melatonergic system activity (Kohyama, 2016; Mondola et al., 2016; Petito et al., 2016; Bertozzi et al., 2017). Orexin evaluation may be considered a new interesting biomarker in ASD pathogenesis, even if to date only associative studies were performed to demonstrate their relationship with health disturbances, such as obesity (Hao et al., 2017).

Conversely, oxidative stress is implicated in the pathophysiology of many neurological disorders (Essick and Sam, 2010). The diacron reactive oxygen metabolites (d-ROMs) test has been used in the clinics, to evaluate the oxidative stress. Particularly it could be considered an important atherosclerotic risk factor in type 2 diabetes mellitus (T2DM), in cardiac disease, neurological disorders, aging, and cancer (Kotani et al., 2013). Nonetheless, little is known about the linkage between oxidative stress and the occurrence or the progress of autism and autonomic functioning; some markers, such as heart rate (HR), heart rate variability (HRV), body temperature, and galvanic skin response (GSR), may be altered in patient with this so complex disorder (Bricout et al., 2017; Hufnagel et al., 2017; Kuiper et al., 2017; Oshodi et al., 2017).

HRV is considered, indeed, a standard noninvasive method for evaluating Autonomic Nervous System (ANS) function (Messina et al., 2012; Neri et al., 2013). It was frequently investigated in a large number of cardiology studies. Nowadays, recent scientific studies suggested the HRV as an important tool in the field of physiology, psychology, psychiatry, and occupational medicine. The HRV variations are linked with the sympathetic and parasympathetic activities directed to the sinus node characterized by each cardiac cycle. The high frequency (HF) component is associated solely with parasympathetic activity, while the low frequency (LF) component is associated with both sympathetic and parasympathetic activities, even if the sympathetic activity is the greater contributor.

In the present paper, we analyzed an autism case report, focusing on the rule of the sympathetic activity with the aim to suggest that it may be considered an important tool in ASD evaluation.

CASE PRESENTATION

We enrolled a male, a child 9 years old, height 1.33 m and weight 28 kg (normal BMI), in the Child Neuropsychiatry at the University of Palermo. The values of serum thyroid hormones levels, systolic and diastolic blood pressure have remained within the normal range.

Written informed consent was obtained from parents. At any time, they could choose to leave the study. All the investigation procedures were approved by the local Human Ethical Review Committee in accordance with the revised Declaration of Helsinki (2013).

The pregnancy was normally conducted and completed with a natural birth at 38 gestational weeks. The infant conditions were good. The development stages were achieved in time (walking at 11 months; first words at 12 months, two phrase sentences at 15 months). Between 15 and 18 months, there was no evolution of language. During this period, sleeping difficulties (rarely sleepwalking) and bizarre behaviors (hand flapping, turn on himself) were reported. At the age of about 3 years old, parents noticed the tendency to isolation, lack of expressive language, difficult eye contact, stereotyped movements of the body, hyperactivity.

At the age of 4 years the "Social Interaction Disorder" was diagnosed. The neuropsychomotor therapy (play-therapy) and speech therapy for 2 times per week were prescribed. These therapies helped the patient to improve his clinical situation.

At the age of 6 years, the complete diagnosis was done: "Cognitive disability in the subject with psychopathological aspects of autism spectrum and signs of immaturity." In this scenario, the FRAXA (Fragile X) test was performed, considering that it is a very important test for anyone with signs of autism or unexplained developmental delay. The genetic FRAXA test was negative.

Clinical evaluation, instrument examinations, plasma Orexin-A detection, and d-ROMs test were performed. All data were in accord with the diagnosis of autism in a subject with intellectual disability.

Clinical Evaluation

The patient had poor language skills: he communicated using one or two sentences of words even if he sang in full sentences (echolalics). The comprehension was good as he was able to hyperventilate for 3 min. Frequently, he related to others mostly by pointing. He showed self-stimulating behaviors in the form of rocking, manual rotation, and hand flapping. His motor skills were below normal. His sleep was good but he was defiant and unable to calm down at bedtime. He did not show any interest in other children and his eye contact is poor. He did not show aggressive behavior, but often he did afinalistic actions (turn around the room).

For the diagnosis, the ADOS-2 (Autism Diagnostic Observation Schedules, Second Edition) was performed. The total score of the "Module 1" was compatible with autistic spectrum, with a total score of 22 (cut-off for autistic spectrum = 8; cut-off for autism = 12). Comparison Scoring ADOS-2 also indicated that the children presented a high level of autism spectrum-related symptoms compared to children with ASDs of the same age and language level.

Furthermore, the semi-structured interview ADI-R was carried out. As summarized in **Table 1**, all results were compatible with ASD.

Finally, the (CarS-T) Infant Caring Assessment Scale was carried out: the patient had a total score of 45, that was indicative of a relation compromisation and it was compatible with "Severely Autistic."

LABORATORY INVESTIGATIONS AND DIAGNOSTIC TESTS

Electroencephalographic Evaluation (EEG)

The cerebral background rhythm during awake stage showed well-organized and well-developed average voltage 9–10 Hz alpha activity predominantly in the posterior regions. With eye-opening, it was bilaterally synchronous and symmetrical. No spike-and-wave discharges or any lateralizing abnormalities were observed. Photic stimulation did not produce any abnormalities. A brief drowsiness was seen in the later part of the recording. Hyperventilation was also performed for about 3 min; no abnormalities were seen during the procedure. In conclusion, the EEG test was normal and no epileptiform discharges or any other paroxysmal activities or focal abnormalities were observed.

Magnetic Resonance Imaging (MRI) of the Brain

The magnetic resonance imaging (MRIs) of the brain was performed: no any alteration of the brain was detected.

TABLE 1 | The results of semi-structured interview ADI-R.

	Patient score	Cut-off for autism
Qualitative abnormalities in mutual social interaction	15	10
Qualitative communication abnormalities	14	7
Constrained, repetitive and stereotyped behavior patterns	10	3

HR Measurement

The HR measurement was carried out with a chest strap wired to a digital R-R recorder (BTL08 SD ECG); the QRS-signal wave-form R-R signal was sampled at the resolution of 1 ms. The HR (beats min^{-1}) was calculated using the formula: HR = 60/R-R interval in seconds; the R-R interval was converted into seconds.

In the patient, the HR-value was higher (84 bpm) than the normal value of children (average normal value 70 bpm).

Power Spectral Analysis (PSA) of HRV

The Power spectral analysis (PSA) of HRV was evaluated by an electrocardiogram (ECG) for 5 min. The signals were acquired on a PC at 100 s/s by an electrocardiograph (delta-1 plus, Cardioline, Milan, Italy) connected to the serial port of a PC; a custom software made with LabView (National Instruments, Texas, USA) was used for data acquisition and analysis.

The R waves were automatically recognized, and the RR intervals were calculated and resampled to obtain a constant-time-based signal (100 ms). The Fourier transform was then applied to this signal and visualized in the form of power LF (0.04–0.15 Hz) and HF (0.15–0.40 Hz). The LF, HF, and the LF/HF ratio were used to estimate the sympathetic and parasympathetic activities. Although the time window for HRV recording is generally >5 min, the Task Force on HRV (1996) indicates that main spectral components are distinguished in a spectrum calculated from short-term recordings of 2–5 min.

In the patient, the LF (S^2/Hz) was higher (0.74 S^2/Hz) than the normal values (a.n.v. 0.44 S^2/Hz).

Galvanic Skin Response (GRS)

The GSR parameters were measured simultaneously using the SenseWear Pro Armband™ (version 3.0, BodyMedia, Inc. PA, USA), which was worn on the right arm over the triceps muscle at the midpoint between acromion and olecranon processes, as recommended by the manufacturer.

The GSR (μS) value in the patient was higher (1.79 μS) than the normal status (a.n.v. 1.11 μS).

Rectal Temperature

Rectal temperature was measured with electronic thermometer thermistor/thermocouple (Ellab A/S, Hilleroed, Denmark).

The body temperature changed in relationship with normal status. In the patient, the rectal temperature (°C) was higher (37.81°C) than the normal value (a.n.v. 37.01°C).

Plasma Orexin-A Detection

Blood sample was obtained at 8:00 a.m. after overnight fast into Vacutainer tubes (BD, Franklin Lakes, NJ) containing EDTA and 0.45 TIU/ml of aprotinin.

Each sample was mixed and then immediately centrifuged at 3,000 rpm for 12 min at 4°C.

Plasma was separated and stored at −80°C until analysis.

The plasma Orexin-A levels were measured with Hypocretin Orexin-A1 ELISA (Enzyme-Linked Immuno Assay) kit (Phoenix Pharmaceuticals). For this test, the minimal detectable concentration was 0.37 ng/ml, the intra-assay error <5% and the inter-assay error <14%.

Before ELISA test, the Orexin-A extraction was obtained with Sep-Pak C18 columns (Waters, Milford, MA) using the following protocol:

- 10 ml of methanol and 20 ml of H_2O were used to activate the columns;
- 1.5 ml of sample was added to the column and washing with 20 ml of water;
- the sample was eluted slowly with 80% acetonitrile and resulting volume was reduced to 400 μl under nitrogen flow;
- the aliquot obtained was led to exsiccation using Speedvac (Savant Instruments, Holbrook, NY).

To perform the ELISA test, the dry residue was dissolved in water.

There was no cross-reactivity of the antibody for hypocretin-1 (16–33), hypocretin-2, agouti-related protein (83–132)-amide.

The Orexin A-values (3,592 pg/mL) was higher in the patient than to the normal status (a.n.v. 2,100 pg/mL).

d-ROMs (Reactive Oxygen Metabolites) Test

The d-ROMs test is a simple assay marketed for analyzing the total amount of hydroperoxides in serum via the Fenton's reaction.

Hydroperoxides, consisting of lipids, carbonylated proteins, and oxidized nucleic acids, are one of the most important ROS involved in oxidative stress and their measurement is considered a reliable marker of oxidation in plasma.

The test was performed with the Free Radical Analytical System 4 (FRAS 4): this is a photometric analytical system developed for the assessment of oxidative stress that measures plasma hydroperoxides concentrations using the d-ROMs test with a single drop of peripheral (finger) blood.

The blood sample was collected by patient's finger (0.15 mL) in a heparinized microcuvette. Thanks to the centrifuge of the FRAS 4 Evolvo System, plasma was immediately isolated by centrifugation at 37°C for 60 s. The plasma was dissolved in an acidic buffer (pH 4.8) in which its hydroperoxides react with the transition metal ions liberated from the proteins in the acidic medium and was converted to alkoxy and peroxy radicals. Subsequently, a colorless chromogen was added (N,N-diethyl-para-phenylenediamine). These newly formed radicals oxidized this chromogen that changed into a radical cation producing a magenta colored derivative. This color is directly correlated with the concentration of hydroperoxides in the plasma sample that is proportional to the quantity of ROMs, according to the Lambert-Beer law. The photometer FRAS 4 Evolvo (absorption at 505 nm, Temperature 37°C) was used to measure the magenta color in order to measure the hydroperoxide concentration. The d-ROMs value was expressed in the arbitrary unit U. CARR (Units Carratelli), as established by the manufacturer (1 U. CARR corresponds to 0.08 mg of H_2O_2/dL). Normal values range between 250 and 300 U. CARR and values higher than 300 U. CARR suggest increased oxidative stress (Cornelli et al., 2001).

The results of the d-ROMs test showed different values: in the patient the value (532 U) was higher than to the normal status (a.n.v. 255 U); this finding suggests the increase of oxidative stress in ASD.

DISCUSSION

The present paper may suggest the need to broaden horizons and the study target on ASD, including oxidative stress, neurotransmitters evaluation, and sympathetic activity measurements. As summarized in **Table 2**, the parameters tested in the case study are adulterated observing the normal values.

The oxidative stress is implicated in the pathophysiology of many neurological disorders, such as anxiety, depression, schizophrenia, bipolar disorder (Salim, 2014).

Undoubtedly the ASD pathogenesis is complex and still not well-identified, hypothesizing that autism can be traced back to a single and univocal pathogenesis. On the other hand, there is increasing evidence that ASD patients show excessive ROS production as reported by many studies (Ghezzo et al., 2013; Bafunno et al., 2014; Anwar et al., 2016; El-Ansary et al., 2017; Howsmon et al., 2017; Khemakhem et al., 2017; Oshodi et al., 2017).

In this perspective, the PUFA administration may be justified in ASD children (Bramanti et al., 2016; Parletta et al., 2016; Sun et al., 2016; Weiser et al., 2016).

Moreover, also vitamin D and its metabolites have been recognized as lower in ASD children respect of typically developing children (Basheer et al., 2017; Berridge, 2017; Jia et al., 2018), pinpointing the role of neuroinflammation in ASD etiology (Mostafa and Al-Ayadhi, 2012; Macfabe, 2013; Salomone et al., 2014; Cianci et al., 2016).

Neuroinflammation may explain the dysregulation between GABA and Glutamate cortical neurocircuitry in ASD children, particularly in the frontostriatal system with functional network topology (Cerame et al., 2008; Jakab et al., 2013; Carvalho Pereira et al., 2017; Naaijen et al., 2017; Nardone et al., 2017).

TABLE 2 | Results of the parameters analyzed in the case study.

Parameters	Values
HR measurement	84 bpm (average normal value, a.v.n., 70 bpm)
Power spectral analysis (PSA) of HRV (LF)	0.74 S^2/Hz (a.n.v. 0.44 S^2/Hz)
Galvanic skin response (GRS)	1.79 μS (a.n.v. 1.11 μS)
Rectal temperature	37.81°C (a.n.v. 37.01°C)
Plasma Orexin-A detection	3,592 pg/mL (a.n.v. 2,100 pg/mL)
d-ROMs (reactive oxygen metabolites) test	532U (a.n.v. 255 U)

Conversely, these neurotransmitters alterations could explain also the sleep disorders such as nocturnal awakenings, insomnia, and parasomnias (Bramanti et al., 2012; Precenzano et al., 2017) and food selectivity in ASD children (Chistol et al., 2017; Li et al., 2017; Suarez, 2017). In this context may be explained the cerebral metabolism increasing (Mitelman et al., 2017) and the autonomic hyperfunctioning in ASD (Avola et al., 2004; Goodman, 2016; Parisi et al., 2017) sustained by high Orexin A levels (Messina et al., 2013, 2014, 2015; Kohyama, 2016; Messina A. et al., 2016; Messina G. et al., 2016).

Even if further studies needed, the findings of this study confirm the hypothesis that the markers of the sympathetic activity could become an important tool in ASD evaluation.

AUTHOR CONTRIBUTIONS

AnM, VM, IB, FP, MaS, AgM, MR, LP, and RF: substantial contributions to the conception or design of the work, or the acquisition, analysis, or interpretation of data for the work. AV, MoS, RM, FL, FS, and SL: drafting the work or revising it critically for important intellectual content. FS, GT, BG, GC, and MM: final approval of the version to be published. AgM, GM, and MC: agreement to be accountable for all aspects of the work in ensuring that questions related to the accuracy or integrity of any part of the work are appropriately investigated and resolved. All authors read and approved the final manuscript.

REFERENCES

Accetta, R., Damiano, S., Morano, A., Mondola, P., Paternò, R., Avvedimento, E. V., et al. (2016). Oxygen species derived from NOX3 and NOX5 drive differentiation of human oligodendrocytes. *Front. Cell. Neurosci.* 10:146. doi: 10.3389/fncel.2016.00146

Anwar, A., Marini, M., Abruzzo, P. M., Bolotta, A., Ghezzo, A., Visconti, P., et al. (2016). Quantitation of plasma thiamine, related metabolites and plasma protein oxidative damage markers in children with autism spectrum disorder and healthy controls. *Free Radic. Res.* 50, S85–S90. doi: 10.1080/10715762.2016.1239821

Avola, R., Di Tullio, M. A., Fisichella, A., Tayebati, S. K., and Tomassoni, D. (2004). Glial fibrillary acidic protein and vimentin expression is regulated by glucocorticoids and neurotrophic factors in primary rat astroglial cultures. *Clin. Exp. Hypertens* 26, 323–333. doi: 10.1081/CEH-120034137

Bafunno, V., Bury, L., Tiscia, G. L., Fierro, T., Favuzzi, G., Caliandro, R., et al. (2014). A novel congenital dysprothrombinemia leading to defective prothrombin maturation. *Thromb. Res.* 134, 1135–1141. doi: 10.1016/j.thromres.2014.08.028

Basheer, S., Natarajan, A., van Amelsvoort, T., Venkataswamy, M. M., Ravi, V., Srinath, S., et al. (2017). Vitamin D status of children with autism spectrum disorder: case-control study from India. *Asian J. Psychiatr.* 30, 200–201. doi: 10.1016/j.ajp.2017.10.031

Berridge, M. J. (2017). Vitamin D deficiency: infertility and neurodevelopmental diseases (attention deficit hyperactivity disorder, autism and schizophrenia). *Am. J. Physiol. Cell Physiol.* 314, C135–C151. doi: 10.1152/ajpcell.00188.2017

Bertozzi, G., Sessa, F., Albano, G. D., Sani, G., Maglietta, F., Roshan, M. H. K., et al. (2017). The role of anabolic androgenic steroids in disruption of the physiological function in discrete areas of the central nervous system. *Mol. Neurobiol.* 1–9. doi: 10.1007/s12035-017-0774-1. [Epub ahead of print].

Bonaventure, A., Harewood, R., Stiller, C. A., Gatta, G., Clavel, J., Stefan, D. C., et al. (2017). Worldwide comparison of survival from childhood leukaemia for 1995-2009, by subtype, age, and sex (CONCORD-2): a population-based study of individual data for 89 828 children from 198 registries in 53 countries. *Lancet Haematol.* 4, e202–e217. doi: 10.1016/S2352-3026(17)30052-2

Bramanti, V., Grasso, S., Tibullo, D., Giallongo, C., Pappa, R., Brundo, M. V., et al. (2016). Neuroactive molecules and growth factors modulate cytoskeletal protein expression during astroglial cell proliferation and differentiation in culture. *J. Neurosci. Res.* 94, 90–98. doi: 10.1002/jnr.23678

Bramanti, V., Tomassoni, D., Grasso, S., Bronzi, D., Napoli, M., Campisi, A., et al. (2012). Cholinergic precursors modulate the expression of heme oxigenase-1, p21 during astroglial cell proliferation and differentiation in culture. *Neurochem. Res.* 37, 2795–2804. doi: 10.1007/s11064-012-0873-3

Bricout, V.-A., Pace, M., Dumortier, L., Favre-Juvin, A., and Guinot, M. (2017). Autonomic responses to head-up tilt test in children with autism spectrum disorders. *J. Abnorm. Child Psychol.* doi: 10.1007/s10802-017-0339-9. [Epub ahead of print].

Brigandi, S. A., Shao, H., Qian, S. Y., Shen, Y., Wu, B.-L., and Kang, J. X. (2015). Autistic children exhibit decreased levels of essential fatty acids in red blood cells. *Int. J. Mol. Sci.* 16, 10061–10076. doi: 10.3390/ijms1605 10061

Bujnakova, I., Ondrejka, I., Mestanik, M., Visnovcova, Z., Mestanikova, A., Hrtanek, I., et al. (2016). Autism spectrum disorder is associated with autonomic underarousal. *Physiol. Res.* 65, S673–S682.

Carvalho Pereira, A., Violante, I. R., Mouga, S., Oliveira, G., and Castelo-Branco, M. (2017). Medial frontal lobe neurochemistry in autism spectrum disorder is marked by reduced N-acetylaspartate and unchanged gamma-aminobutyric acid and Glutamate + glutamine levels. *J. Autism Dev. Disord.* doi: 10.1007/s10803-017-3406-8. [Epub ahead of print].

Cerame, G., Meli, V., Vitale, F., Firenze, A., Viviano, E., Mazzucco, W., et al. (2008). A study to evaluate the lifestyle of medical students in Palermo (Italy) [Indagine sugli stili di vita degli studenti della Facoltà di Medicina di Palermo]. *Igiene Sanità Pubblica* 64, 469–484.

Chistol, L. T., Bandini, L. G., Must, A., Phillips, S., Cermak, S. A., and Curtin, C. (2017). Sensory sensitivity and food selectivity in children with autism spectrum disorder. *J. Autism Dev. Disord.* 48, 583–591. doi: 10.1007/s10803-017-3340-9

Cianci, P., Tartaglia, N., Altamura, A., Fersini, A., Vovola, F., Sanguedolce, F., et al. (2016). A recurrent epidermoid cyst of the spleen: report of a case and literature review. *World J. Surg. Oncol.* 14:98. doi: 10.1186/s12957-016-0857-x

Cornelli, U., Terranova, R., Luca, S., Cornelli, M., and Alberti, A. (2001). Bioavailability and antioxidant activity of some food supplements in men and women using the D-Roms test as a marker of oxidative stress. *J. Nutr.* 131, 3208–3211. doi: 10.1093/jn/131.12.3208

El-Ansary, A., Bjørklund, G., Chirumbolo, S., and Alnakhli, O. M. (2017). Predictive value of selected biomarkers related to metabolism and oxidative stress in children with autism spectrum disorder. *Metab. Brain Dis.* 32, 1209–1221. doi: 10.1007/s11011-017-0029-x

Essick, E. E., and Sam, F. (2010). Oxidative stress and autophagy in cardiac disease, neurological disorders, aging and cancer. *Oxid. Med. Cell. Longev.* 3, 168–177. doi: 10.4161/oxim.3.3.12106

Ghezzo, A., Visconti, P., Abruzzo, P. M., Bolotta, A., Ferreri, C., Gobbi, G., et al. (2013). Oxidative stress and erythrocyte membrane alterations in children with autism: correlation with clinical features. *PLoS ONE* 8:e66418. doi: 10.1371/journal.pone.0066418

Giallongo, C., Tibullo, D., La Cava, P., Branca, A., Parrinello, N., Spina, P., et al. (2011). BRIT1/MCPH1 expression in chronic myeloid leukemia and its regulation of the G2/M checkpoint. *Acta Haematol.* 126, 205–210. doi: 10.1159/000329911

Goodman, B. (2016). Autonomic dysfunction in Autism Spectrum Disorders (ASD) P5.117. *Neurology* 86(Suppl. 16).

Hao, Y., Yuan, H., Fang, P., Zhang, Y., Liao, Y. X., Shen, C., et al. (2017). Plasma orexin-A level associated with physical activity in obese people. *Eat. Weight Disord.* 22:69. doi: 10.1007/s40519-016-0271-y

Howsmon, D. P., Kruger, U., Melnyk, S., James, S. J., and Hahn, J. (2017). Classification and adaptive behavior prediction of children with autism spectrum disorder based upon multivariate data analysis of markers of oxidative stress and DNA methylation. *PLoS Comput. Biol.* 13:e1005385. doi: 10.1371/journal.pcbi.1005385

Hufnagel, C., Chambres, P., Bertrand, P. R., and Dutheil, F. (2017). The need for objective measures of stress in autism. *Front. Psychol.* 8:64. doi: 10.3389/fpsyg.2017.00064

Jakab, A., Beres, M., Berenyi, E., Emri, M., Spisak, T., Kis, S. A., et al. (2013). Autistic traits in neurotypical adults: correlates of graph theoretical functional network topology and white matter anisotropy patterns. *PLoS ONE* 8:e60982. doi: 10.1371/journal.pone.0060982

Jia, F., Shan, L., Wang, B., Li, H., Miao, C., Xu, Z., et al. (2018). Bench to bedside review: possible role of vitamin D in autism spectrum disorder. *Psychiatry Res.* 260, 360–365. doi: 10.1016/j.psychres.2017.12.005

Khemakhem, A. M., Frye, R. E., El-Ansary, A., Al-Ayadhi, L., and Bacha, A. B. (2017). Novel biomarkers of metabolic dysfunction is autism spectrum disorder: potential for biological diagnostic markers. *Metab. Brain Dis.* 32, 1983–1997. doi: 10.1007/s11011-017-0085-2

Kohyama, J. (2016). Possible neuronal mechanisms of sleep disturbances in patients with autism spectrum disorders and attention-deficit/hyperactivity disorder. *Med. Hypotheses* 97, 131–133. doi: 10.1016/j.mehy.2016.11.001

Kotani, K., Tsuzaki, K., Taniguchi, N., and Sakane, N. (2013). Correlation between reactive oxygen metabolites & atherosclerotic risk factors in patients with type 2 diabetes mellitus. *Indian J. Med. Res.* 137, 742–748.

Kuiper, M. W. M., Verhoeven, E. W. M., and Geurts, H. M. (2017). Heart rate variability predicts inhibitory control in adults with autism spectrum disorders. *Biol. Psychol.* 128, 141–152. doi: 10.1016/j.biopsycho.2017.07.006

Li, X. S., Pinto-Martin, J. A., Thompson, A., Chittams, J., and Kral, T. V. (2017). Weight status, diet quality, perceived stress, and functional health of caregivers of children with autism spectrum disorder. *J. Spec. Pediat. Nurs.* 23. doi: 10.1111/jspn.12205

Macfabe, D. (2013). Autism: metabolism, mitochondria, and the microbiome. *Glob. Adv. Health Med.* 2, 52–66. doi: 10.7453/gahmj.2013.089

Messina, A., De Fusco, C., Monda, V., Esposito, M., Moscatelli, F., Valenzano, A., et al. (2016). Role of the orexin system on the hypothalamus-pituitary-thyroid axis. *Front. Neural Circ.* 10:66. doi: 10.3389/fncir.2016.00066

Messina, G., De Luca, V., Viggiano, A., Ascione, A., Iannaccone, T., Chieffi, S., et al. (2013). Autonomic nervous system in the control of energy balance and body weight: personal contributions. *Neurol. Res. Int.* 2013:639280. doi: 10.1155/2013/639280

Messina, G., Dalia, C., Tafuri, D., Monda, V., Palmieri, F., Dato, A., et al. (2014). Orexin-A controls sympathetic activity and eating behavior. *Front. Psychol.* 5:997. doi: 10.3389/fpsyg.2014.00997

Messina, G., Di Bernardo, G., Viggiano, A., De Luca, V., Monda, V., Messina, A., et al. (2016). Exercise increases the level of plasma orexin A in humans. *J. Basic Clin. Physiol. Pharmacol.* 27, 611–616. doi: 10.1515/jbcpp-2015-0133

Messina, G., Monda, V., Moscatelli, F., Valenzano, A. A., Monda, G., Esposito, T., et al. (2015). Role of orexin system in obesity. *Biol. Med.* 7:248. doi: 10.4172/0974-8369.1000248

Messina, G., Vicidomini, C., Viggiano, A., Tafuri, D., Cozza, V., Cibelli, G., et al. (2012). Enhanced parasympathetic activity of sportive women is paradoxically associated to enhanced resting energy expenditure. *Auton. Neurosci. Basic Clin.* 169, 102–106. doi: 10.1016/j.autneu.2012.05.003

Mitelman, S. A., Buchsbaum, M. S., Young, D. S., Haznedar, M. M., Hollander, E., Shihabuddin, L., et al. (2017). Increased white matter metabolic rates in autism spectrum disorder and schizophrenia. *Brain Imaging Behav.* doi: 10.1007/s11682-017-9785-9. [Epub ahead of print].

Mondola, P., Damiano, S., Sasso, A., and Santillo, M. (2016). The Cu, Zn superoxide dismutase: not only a dismutase enzyme. *Front. Physiol.* 7:594. doi: 10.3389/fphys.2016.00594

Mostafa, G. A., and Al-Ayadhi, L. Y. (2012). Reduced serum concentrations of 25-hydroxy vitamin D in children with autism: relation to autoimmunity. *J. Neuroinflammation* 9:201. doi: 10.1186/1742-2094-9-201

Naaijen, J., Zwiers, M. P., Amiri, H., Williams, S. C. R., Durston, S., Oranje, B., et al. (2017). Fronto-striatal glutamate in autism spectrum disorder and obsessive compulsive disorder. *Neuropsychopharmacology* 42, 2456–2465. doi: 10.1038/npp.2016.260

Nardone, S., Sams, D. S., Zito, A., Reuveni, E., and Elliott, E. (2017). Dysregulation of cortical neuron DNA methylation profile in autism spectrum disorder. *Cereb. Cortex* 27, 5739–5754. doi: 10.1093/cercor/bhx250

Neri, V., Ambrosi, A., Fersini, A., Tartaglia, N., Lapolla, F., and Forlano, I. (2013). Severe acute pancreatitis: clinical forms of different gravity. *Ann. Ital. Chir.* 84, 47–53.

Neri, V., Fersini, A., Ambrosi, A., Tartaglia, N., and Valentino, T. P. (2009a). Diagnostic evaluation prior to chelecystectomy in mild-moderate acute biliary pancreatitis. *Ann. Ital. Chir.* 80, 363–367.

Neri, V., Fersini, A., Ambrosi, A., Tartaglia, N., and Valentino, T. P. (2009b). Mild-moderate acute biliary pancreatitis: role of magnetic resonance cholangiopancreatography in preparation of cholecystectomy. *Pancreas* 38:717. doi: 10.1097/MPA.0b013e3181a83087

Oshodi, Y., Ojewunmi, O., Oshodi, T. A., Ijarogbe, G. T., Ogun, O. C., Aina, O. F., et al. (2017). Oxidative stress markers and genetic polymorphisms of glutathione S-transferase T1, M1, and P1 in a subset of children with autism spectrum disorder in Lagos, Nigeria. *Niger. J. Clin. Pract.* 20, 1161–1167. doi: 10.4103/njcp.njcp_282_16

Parisi, L., Salerno, M., Maltese, A., Tripi, G., Romano, P., Folco, A. D., et al. (2017). Autonomic regulation in autism spectrum disorders. *Acta Med. Mediter.* 33, 491–494. doi: 10.19193/0393-6384_2017_3_073

Parletta, N., Niyonsenga, T., and Duff, J. (2016). Omega-3 and omega-6 polyunsaturated fatty acid levels and correlations with symptoms in children with attention deficit hyperactivity disorder, autistic spectrum disorder and typically developing controls. *PLoS ONE* 11:e0156432. doi: 10.1371/journal.pone.0156432

Petito, A., Altamura, M., Iuso, S., Padalino, F. A., Sessa, F., D'Andrea, G., et al. (2016). The relationship between personality traits, the 5HTT polymorphisms, and the occurrence of anxiety and depressive symptoms in elite athletes. *PLoS ONE* 11:e0156601. doi: 10.1371/journal.pone.0156601

Precenzano, F., Ruberto, M., Parisi, L., Salerno, M., Maltese, A., Verde, D., et al. (2017). Sleep habits in children affected by autism spectrum disorders: a preliminary case-control study. *Acta Med. Mediter.* 33, 405–409. doi: 10.19193/0393-6384_2017_3_059

Purcell, A. E., Jeon, O.-H., and Pevsner, J. (2001a). The abnormal regulation of gene expression in autistic brain tissue. *J. Autism Dev. Disord.* 31, 545–549. doi: 10.1023/A:1013290826504

Purcell, A. E., Jeon, O. H., Zimmerman, A. W., Blue, M. E., and Pevsner, J. (2001b). Postmortem brain abnormalities of the glutamate neurotransmitter system in autism. *Neurology* 57, 1618–1628. doi: 10.1212/WNL.57.9.1618

Salim, S. (2014). Oxidative stress and psychological disorders. *Curr. Neuropharmacol.* 12, 140–147. doi: 10.2174/1570159X11666131120230309

Salomone, F., Li Volti, G., Vitaglione, P., Morisco, F., Fogliano, V., Zappalà, A., et al. (2014). Coffee enhances the expression of chaperones and antioxidant proteins in rats with nonalcoholic fatty liver disease. *Transl. Res.* 163, 593–602. doi: 10.1016/j.trsl.2013.12.001

Suarez, M. A. (2017). Laboratory food acceptance in children with autism spectrum disorder compared with children with typical development. *Am. J. Occup. Ther.* 71. doi: 10.5014/ajot.2017.022152

Sun, G. Y., Simonyi, A., Fritsche, K. L., Chuang, D. Y., Hannink, M., Gu, Z., et al. (2016). Docosahexaenoic acid (DHA): an essential nutrient and a nutraceutical for brain health and diseases. *Prostaglandins Leukot. Essent. Fatty Acids.* doi: 10.1016/j.plefa.2017.03.006. [Epub ahead of print].

Uddin, L. Q., and Menon, V. (2009). The anterior insula in autism: under-connected and under-examined. *Neurosci. Biobehav. Rev.* 33, 1198–1203. doi: 10.1016/j.neubiorev.2009.06.002

Weiser, M. J., Mucha, B., Denheyer, H., Atkinson, D., Schanz, N., Vassiliou, E., et al. (2016). Dietary docosahexaenoic acid alleviates autistic-like behaviors resulting from maternal immune activation in mice. *Prostaglandins Leukot. Essent. Fatty Acids* 106, 27–37. doi: 10.1016/j.plefa.2015.10.005

14

Phosphodiesterase-5 Inhibition Alleviates Pulmonary Hypertension and Basal Lamina Thickening in Rats Challenged by Chronic Hypoxia

Coline Nydegger[1], *Carla Martinelli*[2], *Fabiano Di Marco*[2,3], *Gaetano Bulfamante*[2,3], *Ludwig von Segesser*[1], *Piergiorgio Tozzi*[1], *Michele Samaja*[2] *and Giuseppina Milano*[1*]

[1] *Laboratory of Cardiovascular Research, Department of Surgery and Anesthesiology, University Hospital of Lausanne, Lausanne, Switzerland,* [2] *Department of Health Science, University of Milan, Milan, Italy,* [3] *ASST Santi Paolo e Carlo, Milan, Italy*

Edited by:
Pasquale Pagliaro,
Università degli Studi di Torino, Italy

Reviewed by:
Valentina Mercurio,
University of Naples Federico II, Italy
Guido Iaccarino,
Università degli Studi di Salerno, Italy

***Correspondence:**
Giuseppina Milano
giuseppina.milano@chuv.ch

Background: Hypoxia represents both an outcome of cardiopulmonary diseases and a trigger for severe pulmonary complications as pulmonary hypertension. Because nitric oxide (NO) is a critical mediator in the development of pulmonary hypertension, the modulators of its downstream function may become target of pharmacological interventions aimed at alleviating the impact of this condition. Here, we investigate the effects of an early administration of phosphodiesterase-5 inhibitor in rats where pulmonary artery hypertension was induced by chronic exposure to hypoxia.

Methods: Rats were divided into three groups: normoxic control, hypoxic with no treatments (2 weeks breathing an atmosphere containing 10% oxygen), and hypoxic treated with sildenafil (1.4 mg/Kg per day in 0.3 mL i.p.). After sacrifice, hearts and lungs were removed and harvested for analyses.

Results: Sildenafil reduced hypoxia-induced right ventricle hypertrophy without effects in lung hypertrophy, and blunted the increase in right ventricle pressure without effects on left ventricle pressure. Furthermore, the NO-producing systems (i.e., the phosphorylation of the endothelial isoforms of NO synthase that was measured in both myocardial and lung tissues), and the blood NO stores (i.e., the plasma level of nitrates and nitrites) were up-regulated by sildenafil. We did not find significant effects of sildenafil on weight and hemoglobin concentration. Morphological analysis in lung biopsies revealed that 2-week hypoxia increased the frequency of small pulmonary vessels leaving large vessels unaffected. Finally, ultrastructural analysis showed that sildenafil down-regulated the hypoxia-induced increase in the thickness of the pulmonary basal lamina.

Conclusions: In this model of pulmonary hypertension, sildenafil contrasts the negative effects of hypoxia on pulmonary vascular and right ventricle remodeling. This action does not only encompass the canonical vasomodulatory effect, but involves several biochemical pathways. Although the human pathological model is certainly more complex than that described here (for example, the inflammatory issue), the potential role of phosphodiesterase-5 for long-term treatment, and perhaps prevention, of pulmonary hypertension is worthy of investigation.

Keywords: pulmonary hypertension, nitric oxide, phosphodiesterase 5, sildenafil, right heart failure, nitrites and nitrates, endothelial NO synthase, pulmonary vascular remodeling

INTRODUCTION

Pulmonary hypertension (PH), a devastating complication of several cardiopulmonary diseases such as chronic heart failure (CHF) and chronic obstructive pulmonary disease (COPD), arises from the progressive narrowing or destruction of the arteries that carry blood from the heart to the lungs. The raise in pulmonary arteries pressure strains the right ventricle (RV) causing hypertrophy and eventually leading to right heart failure. This pathobiology is complicated by hypoxia, which is at the same time an outcome of pulmonary diseases and an established trigger for PH as it was reported, for example, in rats breathing 10% O_2 for 2 weeks, which develop marked signs of RV hypertrophy (Milano et al., 2011). Impaired nitric oxide (NO) bioavailability is a key feature in most forms of clinical and experimental PH (Giaid and Saleh, 1995; Bueno et al., 2013). Classically, NO is believed to modulate the vascular function through stimulation of smooth muscle cell soluble guanylate cyclase that catalyzes the conversion of guanosine triphosphate into cyclic guanosine monophosphate (cGMP), which lowers cytoplasmic Ca^{2+} and mediates smooth muscle cell relaxation. Pharmacologically, this effect can be made more persistent and intense by selective inhibitors of phosphodiesterase type 5 (PDE5), an enzyme that degrades cGMP into inactive 5′GMP. The best known example of these inhibitors, sildenafil surged as a drug able to alleviate symptoms in several cardiopulmonary diseases including pulmonary arterial hypertension (PAH) (Guazzi and Samaja, 2007) and to correct hypoxia-induced RV hypertrophy (Milano et al., 2011). The underlying scenario reflects a situation where the sildenafil-induced increase in cGMP levels upregulates the phosphorylation of the endothelial isoform of NOS (eNOS), which increases the phosphorylation of Akt, thereby mitigating apoptosis in cardiomyocytes. Although we are far from definite data due to the controversy of available results, in some cases the administration of sildenafil revealed to be useful for the treatment of cardiac heart failure devoid of remarkable adverse effects (Guazzi et al., 2007). The same NO/cGMP pathway is used by the drug riociguat that stimulates the activity of soluble guanylate cyclase independently of NO and acts in synergy with NO to produce anti-proliferative and vasodilatory effects (Lang et al., 2012). However, sildenafil may also have effects not mediated by modulation of vasoconstriction, and in lungs it has been shown to improve pulmonary hemodynamic by modulating the recruitment of bone marrow-derived c-kit+ cells (Favre et al., 2017).

The basal lamina, a layer of extracellular matrix secreted by epithelial cells, acts both as an attachment point for cells and as a permeability barrier. Degenerative pathologies like diabetes mellitus, but also primary respiratory diseases such as asthma and COPD, are known to induce a thickening of the pulmonary basal lamina (Weynand et al., 1999; Liesker et al., 2009), whose thickness represents a compromise between two opposite needs, providing mechanical resistance against excessive pressure buildup, and facilitating the diffusion of gasses across the alveolar-capillary barrier (West and Mathieu-Costello, 1999). This compromise may be overruled in several instances, and hypoxia-induced pulmonary edema has been attributed to stress failure of pulmonary capillaries, which may be due by un-matching the delicate balance between basal lamina strengthening and increased pulmonary hypertension (West et al., 1995). However, direct measurement of the basal lamina thickness as a function of hypoxia is still lacking, consequently it may become difficult to assess whether acute alterations of the thickness and strength of the basal lamina may make part of hypoxia adaptation and pulmonary hypertension development. Aim of this study was to test the impact of sildenafil, a PDE5 inhibitor, on right heart and pulmonary vessels in an experimental model of hypoxia-induced PH.

METHODS

Animal Experiments

We used 42 male 8-week old Sprague-Dawley rats (200–250 g initial nominal weight). Rats were randomly divided into three groups: control, exposed to hypoxia (10% O_2) for 2 weeks, and exposed to hypoxia and treated with sildenafil (1.4 mg/Kg per day in 0.3 mL i.p.). Each group was composed of two subgroups of 6 rats/each. Rats from the first and second subgroup were used for morphometry/hemodynamics, and biochemical measurements, respectively. Hypoxia was administered in specially designed chambers that enable all treatments, including drug administration and animals handling, avoiding any exposure of animals to atmospheric air (Milano et al., 2002, 2004). Sacrifice was performed 24 h after the last administration. Rats were anesthetized (80 mg/kg xylazine, 100 mg/kg ketasol and 1,500 IU heparin i.p.) in the compensation chamber kept at 10% O_2. This study was carried out in accordance with the recommendations of the National Institutes

Abbreviations: PD, chronic obstructive pulmonary disease. eNOS, endothelial isoform of NO synthase. LV, left ventricle. LVSP, LV systolic pressure. NO, nitric oxide, NOx, nitrates and nitrites. PAH, pulmonary arterial hypertension. PDE-5, phosphodiesterase-5. p-eNOS, phosphorylated isoform of eNOS. PH, pulmonary hypertension. RV, right ventricle. RVSP, RV systolic pressure. TEM, transmission electron microscope. VEGF, vascular endothelial factor. VEGFR1, receptor of VEGF.

of Health (NIH Publication No. 85–23, Revised 1996). The protocol was approved y the Government Veterinary Office (Lausanne, Switzerland; authorization Nr VD2467.1).

Hemodynamic Monitoring

At the end of study, the left ventricle (LV) and right ventricle (RV) systolic pressures (RVSP and LVSP, respectively) were measured by placing a Millar Mikro-Tip conductance catheter (SPR-838, 2F catheter, Millar Instruments Inc., Oxford, UK, coupled to a MPVS Ultra system Millar Instruments, Oxford, UK) as described (Favre et al., 2017). Briefly, anesthetized rats were placed on a heating pad at 37°C and ventilated at 50 cycles·min^{-1} with a tidal volume of 2.5 ml (Harvard Apparatus model 683, Holliston, MA, USA) with either room air or hypoxic atmosphere for normoxic and hypoxic groups, respectively. To evaluate the LVPS, the Millar catheter was introduced into the LV via right carotid artery. To evaluate the RVSP, the chest cavity was opened and the Millar catheter was introduced in the RV cavity using a 24-gauge needle.

Blood Measurements

A blood sample was taken into heparinized tubes after euthanasia from the descending abdominal aorta for measurement of blood hemoglobin (Servomex Oxygen Analyzer 570 A, Zurich, Switzerland) and plasma nitrates and nitrites (colorimetric Griess reaction).

Animal Sacrifice and Pulmonary and Cardiac Hypertrophy

After the hemodynamic measurements, lungs and hearts were perfused en-block with PBS via the RV with efflux through a small opening in the left atrium as reported (Favre et al., 2017). Then, lungs and hearts were placed in PBS solution and kept on ice. After removing the atria from the ventricles, the RV was separated from the LV and the septum (S), blotted dry and weighed to obtain the ratio of RV/(LV+S).

Pulmonary Vascular Remodeling

The degree of muscularization of pulmonary arterioles was assessed from immunohistochemical staining of the small pulmonary artery, as previously described (Favre et al., 2017). Briefly, paraffin-embedded lungs were serially sectioned at 8 μm thickness. Following citrate-based antigen retrieval, the sections were blocked with 5% (v/v) goat serum for 1 h. Then, sections were incubated with an antibody against smooth muscle α-actin (α-SMA 1:250, clone 1A4, Sigma-Aldrich) overnight at 4°C, followed by a goat anti-mouse IgG secondary antibody (1/500, DAKO). Pulmonary arterioles were divided by outer vessel diameter in four categories: small (0–50 μm), medium (50–100 μm), large (100–200 μm) and very large (>200 μm) diameters. Pulmonary vascular remodeling was assessed by the percent medial wall thickness. Ten vessels were analyzed for each rat, in seven rats per group per time-point, except for very large (>200 μm) vessels, where the number of analyzed vessels was 2–3. Morphological analyses were conducted in a double-blind method.

Protein Extraction and Western Blot Analysis

In a subset of experiment animals, standard Western blotting analysis was performed using lung and cardiac lysates, as described previously (Favre et al., 2017). The membranes were incubated overnight at 4°C with antibodies against p-eNOS (Ser^{1177}, 1:1,000, Cell Signaling Technology) and e-NOS (1:1,000, Santa Cruz Biotechnology, Santa Cruz). Secondary HRP-conjugated antibodies were applied for 1 h at room temperature (1:4,000). Signals were detected by using the enhanced chemiluminescence system (Amersham, Arlington Heights, IL, USA) of a commercial ECL kit. Quantification of the band intensities was performed using NIH ImageJ.

ELISA

VEGF and VEGF-R1 protein levels were quantified in lung lysates by ELISA (ELISA kit, Assay Designs, Inc., MI). All assays were made in duplicate and performed according to the manufacturer's instruction.

RT-PCR

Total RNA of lung tissues was extracted using the TRIzol method as described (Favre et al., 2017). The relative amount of mRNA expression for vascular endothelial growth factor (VEGF) was represented using the 2-ΔΔCt value. The primer pairs for VEGF (109 bp) were designed (sense: 5′ -AGTACCTGTTCTGGCTAA TGG-3′; anti-sense: 5′-TCACTTTCGTGCGCTCGTAG-3′) and

TABLE 1 | Whole animal data expressed as mean ± SEM.

	Normoxia	Hypoxia	Hypoxia + sildenafil	1-way ANOVA
Body weight initial, g	248.1 ± 3.0	246.5 ± 8.5	254.5 ± 9.1	NS
Body weight final, g	340.3 ± 7.9	252.2 ± 10.4§	271.8 ± 5.1§	<0.0001
Heart weight, g	1.303 ± 0.047	1.383 ± 0.058	1.161 ± 0.054	0.0484
Lungs weight, g	1.545 ± 0.071	1.990 ± 0.058§	1.957 ± 0.063§	<0.0001
Hematocrit, %	50.7 ± 1.5	66.0 ± 2.4§	64.7 ± 1.3§	<0.0001
Hemoglobin, g/L	158.18 ± 3.58	200.25 ± 7.25§	201.53 ± 5.15§	<0.0001
RBC/fl	8.65 ± 0.36	10.45 ± 0.43§	10.05 ± 0.29§	<0.0001

§*P* < 0.05 vs. normoxia (Tukey's multiple comparison test). No significant differences have been observed between hypoxia and hypoxia + sildenafil.

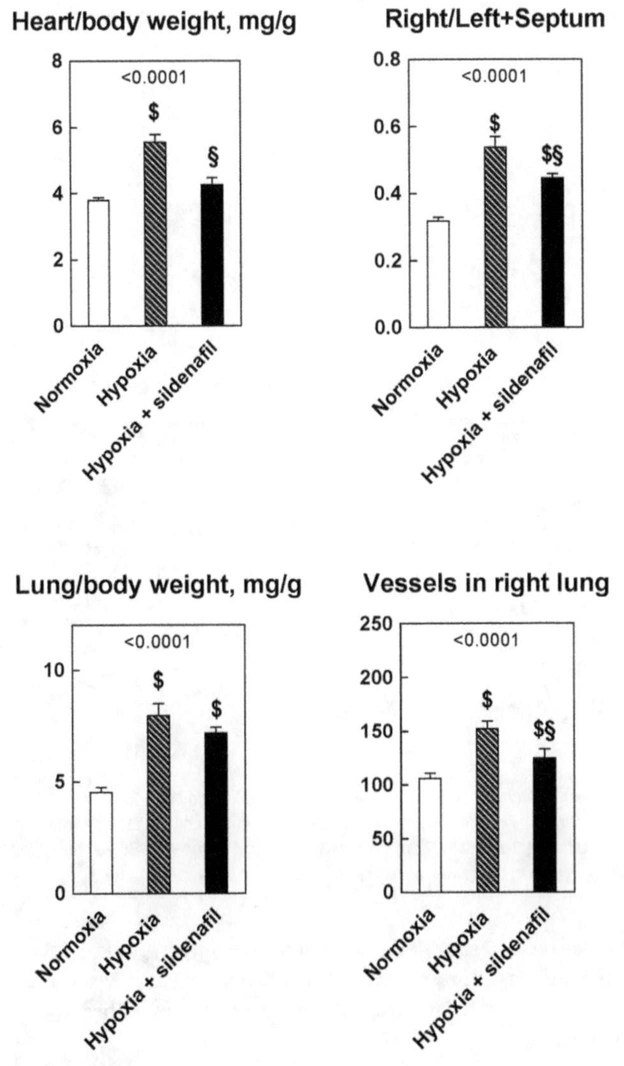

FIGURE 1 | Effects of 2-week hypoxia (10% O_2) and hypoxia + sildenafil on the heart/body weight ratio, right ventricle hypertrophy, lung/body weight ratio, and number of vessels in the right lung. Data are expressed as mean ± SEM. The 1-way ANOVA value is reported for each variable. $^{\$}P < 0.05$ vs. normoxia, $^{\S}P < 0.05$ between hypoxia and hypoxia + sildenafil (Tukey's multiple comparison test).

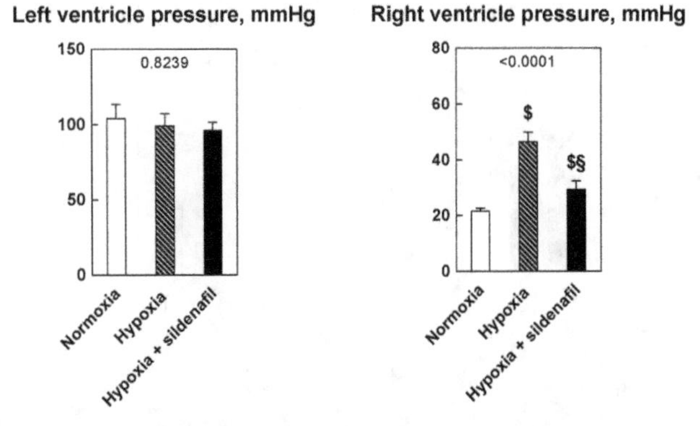

FIGURE 2 | Effects of 2-week hypoxia (10% O_2) and hypoxia + sildenafil on the pressures developed by the left and right ventricles. Data are expressed as mean ± SEM. The 1-way ANOVA value is reported for each variable. $^{\$}P < 0.05$ vs. normoxia, $^{\S}P < 0.05$ between hypoxia and hypoxia + sildenafil (Tukey's multiple comparison test).

for the housekeeping gene GAPDH (359 bp) were (forward) 5′-TGAAGGTCGGTGTGAACGGATTTG-3′ and (reverse) 5′-GGCGGAGATGATGACCCTTTTG-3′, respectively.

Transmission Electron Microscopy (TEM)

Lung biopsies were fixed in 2.5% (v/v) glutaraldehyde dissolved in 0.13 M phosphate buffer (pH 7.2–7.4). Five specimens for each biopsy were post-fixed in 1% OsO_4, dehydrated in ethanol plus propylene oxide and embedded in epoxy resin. Ultrathin 50–60 nm sections were routinely counterstained with uranyl acetate (10 min, Merck, Darmstadt, Germany) and lead citrate (5 min, Merck, Darmstadt, Germany), and examined with a JEM 1010 (Jeol, Tokyo, Japan) electron microscope. To determine the median basal lamina thickness, the Marquez simplified method was applied in printed 18 × 24 cm micrographs taken at 24,000 × magnification using 10 areas at a fixed 4 mm distance from one to another. The average thickness measured in the 10 areas was considered as the final value. To determine the mitochondrial size, the areas of 30 randomly selected mitochondria for each condition was calculated.

Statistics

Data are expressed as mean ± SEM. To measure the effects of hypoxia and sildenafil, we performed one-way analysis of variance followed by the Tukey's multiple comparison test if significant. The significance level was set at $P = 0.05$.

RESULTS

Whole Animal Data

All animals survived the experimental protocol without signs of discomfort. Whole animal data are reported in **Table 1**. Exposure to hypoxia for 2 weeks decreased body weight. Likewise, hypoxia increased blood hemoglobin, hematocrit and red cell count. No changes were observed in heart weight, but hypoxia increased the wet weight in both lungs. None of these variables was affected by sildenafil.

Sildenafil Reduced Hypoxia-Induced Right Ventricle Hypertrophy Without Effects in Lung Morphology

Although the heart weight was apparently unaffected by neither hypoxia, nor sildenafil, the simultaneous decrease in body weight led to varied heart/body weight ratios, which is an index of myocardial hypertrophy (**Figure 1**). This ratio increased markedly in untreated rats upon hypoxia, but the administration of sildenafil markedly blunted this effect. The RV/(LV+S) ratio is a reliable index of RV hypertrophy. This ratio increased markedly after 2-week hypoxia, but the increase was less in sildenafil-treated rats. The lung/body wet weight was also markedly increased by hypoxia, and sildenafil was unable to alleviate

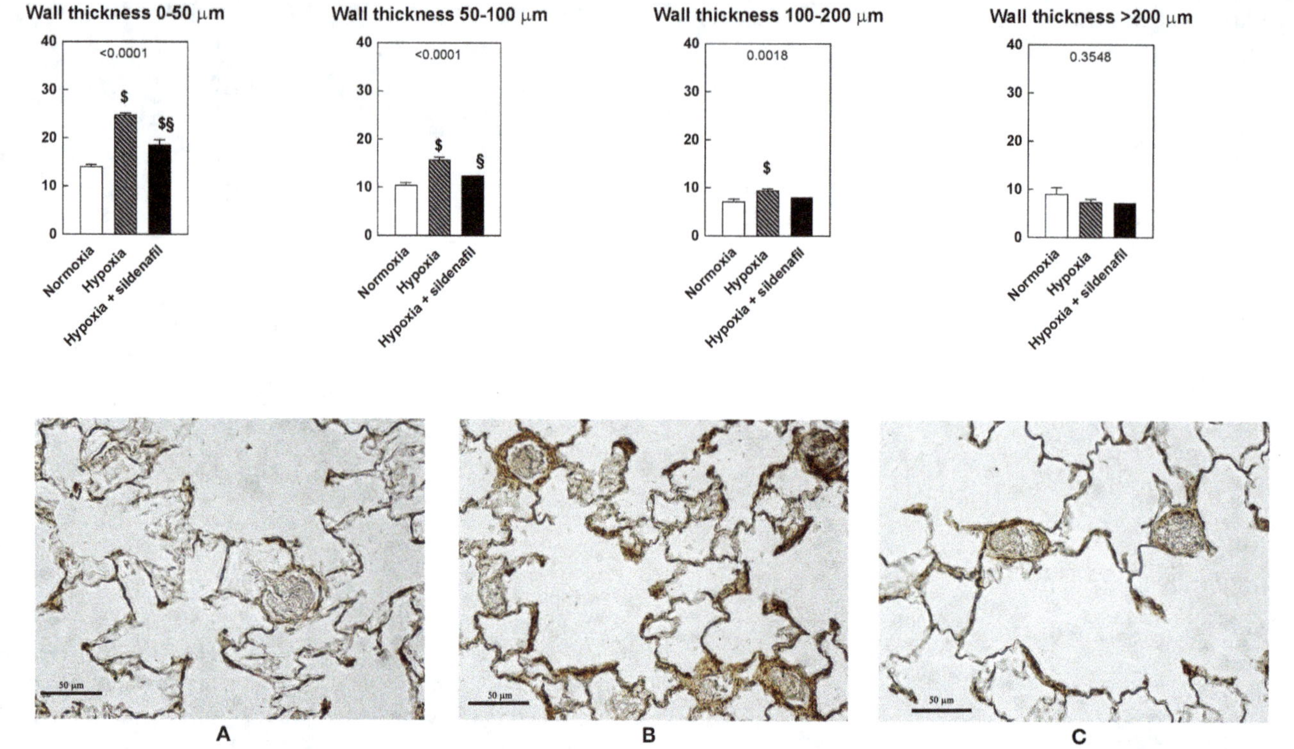

FIGURE 3 | Effects of 2-week hypoxia (10% O_2) and hypoxia + sildenafil on the wall thickness of small (0–50 μm), medium (50–100 μm), large (100–200 μm), and very large (>200 μm) pulmonary vessels determined as explained in the Materials and Methods section. The lower row shows representative images taken from each group. Notations **(A-C)** refer to normoxia, hypoxia, and hypoxia + sildenafil, respectively. The bar represents 100 μm. Data are expressed as mean ± SEM. The 1-way ANOVA value is reported for each variable. $^{\$}P < 0.05$ vs. normoxia, $^{\S}P < 0.05$ between hypoxia and hypoxia + sildenafil (Tukey's multiple comparison test).

this increase. Likewise, the number of vessels in the right lung increased during hypoxia and sildenafil corrected this increase.

Sildenafil Blunted the Increase in Right Ventricle Pressure Without Effects on Left Ventricle Pressure

Figure 2 shows the left and right ventricle pressure as measured as explained in the Materials and Methods section. The pressure developed by the left ventricle was not affected by neither hypoxia nor sildenafil. By contrast, the pressure developed by the right ventricle was increased by hypoxia, indicative of PAH development. This increase was markedly blunted in sildenafil-treated rats.

Two-Week Hypoxia Increases the Frequency of Small Pulmonary Vessels Leaving Large Vessels Unaffected

As shown in **Figure 1**, hypoxia increased the number of pulmonary vessels. To ascertain whether this increase was shared to both newly formed and mature vessels, we measured the frequency of vessels in four categories of wall thickness, arbitrarily divided into small (0–50 μm), medium (50–100 μm), large (100–200 μm), and very large (>200 μm) diameters (**Figure 3**). It appears that the effect of hypoxia was more pronounced for small vessels and progressively diminished with the vessels diameter. As a result, the anti-hypoxic effect of sildenafil was more marked in small than in large vessels. The frequency of very large vessels was unaffected by either hypoxia or sildenafil.

NO-producing Systems Are Up-Regulated by Sildenafil

The p-eNOS/eNOS ratio highlights the activation of NO-producing enzymes. In both heart and lung biopsies, hypoxia decreased this ratio, while sildenafil promoted eNOS phosphorylation (**Figure 4**). The plasma level of nitrates and nitrites (NOx) marks the NO stores level. While hypoxia produced an increase in plasma NO stores, sildenafil was able to further increases it. However, neither hypoxia nor sildenafil were able to affect none of the factors linked to the vascular endothelial growth factor (VEGF). Indeed, the protein expression of VEGF and VEGF-R, as well as VEGF mRNA remained constant in the three groups.

Sildenafil Efficiently Down-Regulates the Hypoxia-Induced Increase in the Thickness of the Pulmonary Basal Lamina

Figure 5 shows some representative electron microscope images highlighting the effects of 2-week hypoxia (10% O_2) and sildenafil on mitochondrial size and the thickness of the basal lamina.

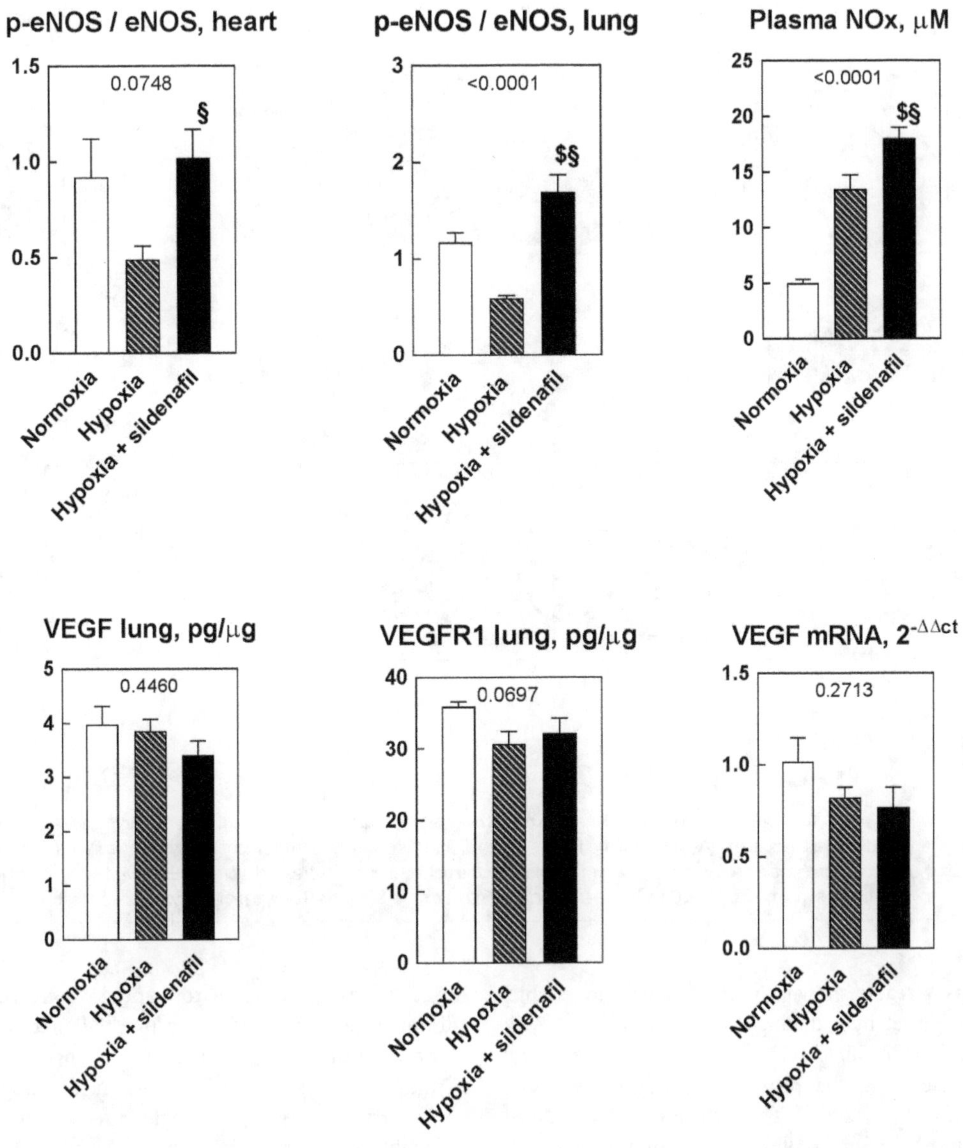

FIGURE 4 | Effects of 2-week hypoxia (10% O_2) and hypoxia + sildenafil on the phosphorylation and activation of NO-generating enzymes as well as on the level of nitrites and nitrates in plasma **(Upper row)**, and VEGF-related parameters **(Lower row)**. Data are expressed as mean ± SEM. The 1-way ANOVA value is reported for each variable. $^{\$}P < 0.05$ vs. normoxia, $^{§}P < 0.05$ between hypoxia and hypoxia + sildenafil (Tukey's multiple comparison test).

Averaged data obtained in all available samples are shown on the right panel. As expected, hypoxia increased the mitochondrial size, and sildenafil contrasted this effect. Likewise, while hypoxia increased the thickness of the basal lamina, sildenafil down-regulated this increase.

DISCUSSION

In this study, we report some cardiopulmonary responses to 2-week chronic hypoxia. The severity of the hypoxia challenge, 10% O_2, is known to induce molecular and cellular alterations without becoming lethal even after 4 weeks in mice (Terraneo et al., 2017). In the rat, breathing 10% O_2 for 2 weeks impairs the myocardial tolerance to ischemia/reperfusion (Milano et al., 2002), induces RV hypertrophy (Corno et al., 2004), impairs K^{+}_{ATP} channels opening (Milano et al., 2004), activates hypoxic signaling and apoptosis (Bianciardi et al., 2006), modulates differentially the expression of mitogen-activated protein kinases (Caretti et al., 2007) and increases the immunoreactivity against the 70 kDa heat shock proteins (Tarricone et al., 2008). Furthermore, 2-week hypoxia also reduces the myocardial p-eNOS/eNOS ratio while increasing plasma NOx in a mechanism resembling that underlying intermittent hypoxia (Milano et al., 2010, 2011). Here, we show that most of the hypoxia-induced changes that regard NO handling in the lungs may be strongly modulated by sildenafil.

Despite its short plasma half-life of sildenafil of 4–6 h (Boolell et al., 1996), the selected dose and timing for sildenafil

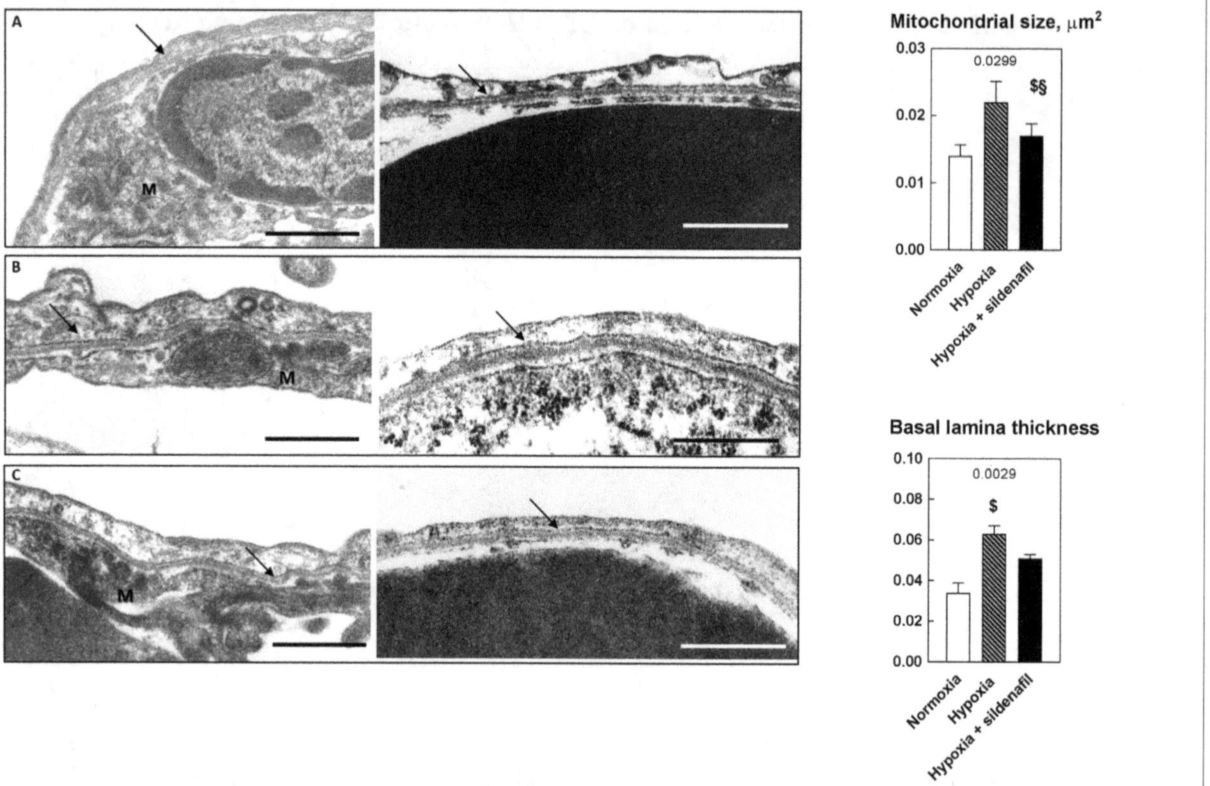

FIGURE 5 | Effects of 2-week hypoxia (10% O_2) and hypoxia + sildenafil on mitochondrial size and the thickness of the pulmonary basal lamina. Two representative micrographs for each group are displayed. Notations **(A-C)** refer to normoxia, hypoxia, and hypoxia + sildenafil, respectively. Arrows indicate the basal lamina, while the notation M indicates the mitochondria (scale bars = 0.5 μm). Averaged data on the right panel are expressed as mean ± SEM. The 1-way ANOVA value is reported for each variable. $^{\$}P < 0.05$ vs. normoxia, $^{\S}P < 0.05$ between hypoxia and hypoxia + sildenafil (Tukey's multiple comparison test).

administration was already shown to be sufficient to enable sildenafil to hit its target by inducing a x4 increase in cGMP in heart tissue (Milano et al., 2011). Sildenafil was shown to protect tissue by elevating the protein level of both iNOS and eNOS (Salloum et al., 2003). The activation of the NO-producing system by eNOS Ser^{1177} phosphorylation was reported to be a key step through which sildenafil exerts cardioprotective effects in chronically hypoxic hearts (Baker et al., 2001) by reducing apoptosis, enhancing protein kinase B activation (Milano et al., 2011), down-regulating intracellular calcium by mitochondrial K^{+}ATP channels opening (Fitzpatrick et al., 2005), and attenuating the recruitment of bone-marrow-derived c-kit(+) cells (Favre et al., 2017). Remarkably, we were unable to document a similar effect on VEGF and VEGF-R1 expression that were reviewed to be upregulated by sildenafil in an attempt to improve angiogenesis to restore the hypoxia-challenged viability (Liu and Simon, 2004). However, the situation in lungs that are exposed directly to atmospheric air may be quite different from that in other internal organs where angiogenesis is the key way to transfer the oxygen brought by capillary blood. Because sildenafil did not affect the blood hemoglobin concentration, the increased activation of eNOS reflects into higher plasma NO stores or NOx.

The total number of vessels in both lungs appear to follow the same pattern described for eNOS phosphorylation and NO stores: whereas exposure to hypoxia increases the value, the administration of sildenafil can markedly reduce, and sometimes blunt, such increase. However, the changes in size distribution of pulmonary vessels is dependent on the vessel diameter. Small pulmonary vessels are strongly affected by hypoxia and by sildenafil. By contrast, larger pulmonary vessels are less affected by hypoxia and sildenafil. If the size of the pulmonary vessels is associated with their degree of maturation, then this may be attributed to the vessel maturation process. The thickness of the basal lamina may be another key to understand the effects of PDE-5 inhibition in lungs. As mentioned above, the pulmonary blood-gas barrier represents a compromise between two opposite needs: a reduced thickness favors oxygen diffusion, while its increase contributes to strengthen the barrier. If hypoxia involves high RVSP, and sildenafil reduces it, this translates into less demand to improve pulmonary resistance against circulatory stress by tightening the basal lamina, thus favoring oxygen diffusion. As such, sildenafil may be considered an "anti-hypoxic" drug.

PH is an important complication in the natural history of cardiopulmonary diseases, such as COPD. Its presence is associated with reduced survival and greater use of healthcare resources. In COPD, pulmonary vascular remodeling, due to inflammation and/or hypoxia, affects small and precapillary arteries, and has been identified at different degrees of disease severity. Patients with end-stage COPD and PH show deposition of longitudinal muscle, fibrosis and elastosis that enlarge the intima in pulmonary muscular arteries (Barberà and Blanco, 2009). Impairment of endothelial function may be associated with or result from changes in the expression or balanced release of vasoactive mediators with vasodilator properties, such as NO or prostacyclin, and mediators with vasoconstrictive properties, such as endothelin-1 or angiotensin. Indeed, eNOS expression in pulmonary arteries, which is diminished in patients with idiopathic PAH (Giaid and Saleh, 1995) is also reduced in COPD patients (Yang et al., 2012) and in smokers without airflow obstruction (Barberà et al., 2001). In COPD, pulmonary vasodilation can lead to deterioration of gas exchange due to the high ventilation/perfusion ratio mismatch areas. Inhaled prostanoids may acutely reduce pulmonary arterial pressure while largely maintaining gas exchange; however, long-term clinical trials have not been reported. Robust data for the clinical beneficial effect of endothelin receptor antagonists (ERAs) on pulmonary hemodynamics and exercise tolerance in COPD with pulmonary hypertension are lacking. Finally, there is definitely a lack of evidence of a long-term clinical beneficial effect of PDE5 inhibitors in COPD patients (Seeger et al., 2013), even if a recently published study demonstrated that treatment with sildenafil is able to reduce pulmonary vascular resistance and improve the BODE index (a multidimensional grading system that predict mortality in COPD) and quality of life, without a significant effect on gas exchange, in a cohort of patients with severe pulmonary hypertension and COPD (Vitulo et al., 2017). In this context, the result of the present study, which demonstrates that sildenafil affects the negative effects of hypoxia on right ventricle through its impact on NO-pathway, may be of interest because one can speculate a protective effect of sildenafil, or other drugs active on the NO-pathway such as riociguat, on vessels remodeling leading and pulmonary hypertension and right ventricle hypertrophy.

CONCLUSIONS

In the described model of pulmonary hypertension induced by chronic exposure to hypoxia, PDE-5 inhibition by sildenafil contrasts the negative effects of hypoxia on pulmonary and right ventricle remodeling. This action does not only encompass the canonical vasomodulatory effect, but involves several cell pathways. Although the human pathological model is certainly more complex than that described here (for example, by including marked pro-inflammatory issues), PDE-5 inhibition may become an appreciable target for long-term treatment of pulmonary hypertension, and perhaps also for the prevention of this debilitating disease.

ETHICS STATEMENT

Experimental protocols conformed to Swiss law. The local ethical committee for animal research (Service de la Consommation et des Affaire Vétérinaires, SCAV) approved the protocol (authorization VD2467.1).

AUTHOR CONTRIBUTIONS

CN performed the experiments and the statistical analysis. CM performed the TEM analyses and participated to the discussion of the results of this manuscript. FD contributed for the clinical impact of the described data and participated to the discussion of the results of this manuscript. GB contributed for the TEM analyses. LvS and PT participated to the discussion of the results of this manuscript. MS performed the statistical analyses, participated to the discussion of the results of this manuscript and wrote the manuscript. GM supervised all the phases of this study.

ACKNOWLEDGMENTS

This work was supported in part by the Swiss Heart Foundation and the Department of Health Science, University of Milan, Italy.

REFERENCES

Baker, J., Contney, S., Singh, R., Kalyanaraman, B., Gross, G., and Bosnjak, Z. (2001). Nitric oxide activates the sarcolemmal KATP channel in normoxic and chronically hypoxic hearts by a cyclic GMP-dependent mechanism. *J. Mol. Cell Cardiol.* 33, 331–341. doi: 10.1006/jmcc.2000.1305

Barberà, J. A., and Blanco, I. (2009). Pulmonary hypertension in patients with chronic obstructive pulmonary disease: advances in pathophysiology and management. *Drugs* 69, 1153–1171. doi: 10.2165/00003495-200969090-00002

Barberà, J. A., Peinado, V. I., Santos, S., Ramirez, J., Roca, J., and Rodriguez-Roisin, R. (2001). Reduced expression of endothelial nitric oxide synthase in pulmonary arteries of smokers. *Am. J. Respir. Crit. Care Med.* 164, 709–713. doi: 10.1164/ajrccm.164.4.2101023

Bianciardi, P., Fantacci, M., Caretti, A., Ronchi, R., Milano, G., Morel, S., et al. (2006). Chronic *in vivo* hypoxia in various organs: hypoxia-inducible factor-1alpha and apoptosis. *Biochem. Biophys. Res. Commun.* 342, 875–880. doi: 10.1016/j.bbrc.2006.02.042

Boolell, M., Allen, M. J., Ballard, S. A., Gepi-Attee, S., Muirhead, G. J., Naylor, A. M., et al. (1996). Sildenafil: an orally active type 5 cyclic GMP-specific phosphodiesterase inhibitor for the treatment of penile erectile dysfunction. *Int. J. Impot. Res.* 8, 47–52.

Bueno, M., Wang, J., Mora, A. L., and Gladwin, M. T. (2013). Nitrite signaling in pulmonary hypertension: mechanisms of bioactivation, signaling, and therapeutics. *Antioxid. Redox Signal.* 18, 1797–1809. doi: 10.1089/ars.2012.4833

Caretti, A., Morel, S., Milano, G., Fantacci, M., Bianciardi, P., Ronchi, R., et al. (2007). Heart HIF-1α and MAP kinases during hypoxia: are they associated *in vivo*? *Exp. Biol. Med.* 232, 887–894.

Corno, A. F., Milano, G., Morel, S., Tozzi, P., Genton, C. Y., Samaja, M., et al. (2004). Hypoxia: unique myocardial morphology? *J. Thorac. Cardiovasc. Surg.* 127, 1301–1308. doi: 10.1016/j.jtcvs.2003.06.012

Favre, S., Gambini, E., Nigro, P., Scopece, A., Bianciardi, P., Caretti, A., et al. (2017). Sildenafil attenuates hypoxic pulmonary remodelling by inhibiting bone marrow progenitor cells. *J. Cell. Mol. Med.* 21, 871–880. doi: 10.1111/jcmm.13026

Fitzpatrick, C. M., Shi, Y., Hutchins, W. C., Su, J., Gross, G. J., Ostadal, B., et al. (2005). Cardioprotection in chronically hypoxic rabbits persists on exposure to normoxia: role of NOS and KATP channels. *Am. J. Physiol. Heart Circ. Physiol.* 288, H62–H68. doi: 10.1152/ajpheart.00701.2004

Giaid, A., and Saleh, D. (1995). Reduced expression of endothelial nitric oxide synthase in the lungs of patients with pulmonary hypertension. *N. Engl. J. Med.* 333, 214–221. doi: 10.1056/NEJM199507273330403

Guazzi, M., and Samaja, M. (2007). The role of PDE5-inhibitors in cardiopulmonary disorders: from basic evidence to clinical development. *Curr. Med. Chem.* 14, 1893–1910. doi: 10.2174/092986707781389619

Guazzi, M., Samaja, M., Arena, R., Vicenzi, M., and Guazzi, M. D. (2007). Long-term use of sildenafil in the therapeutic management of heart failure. *J. Am. Coll. Cardiol.* 50, 2136–2144. doi: 10.1016/j.jacc.2007.07.078

Lang, M., Kojonazarov, B., Tian, X., Kalymbetov, A., Weissmann, N., Grimminger, F., et al. (2012). The soluble guanylate cyclase stimulator riociguat ameliorates pulmonary hypertension induced by hypoxia and SU5416 in rats. *PLoS ONE* 7:e43433. doi: 10.1371/journal.pone.0043433

Liesker, J. J., Ten Hacken, N. H., Zeinstra-Smith, M., Rutgers, S. R., Postma, D. S., and Timens, W. (2009). Reticular basement membrane in asthma and COPD: similar thickness, yet different composition. *Int. J. Chron. Obstruct. Pulmon. Dis.* 4, 127–135. doi: 10.2147/COPD.S4639

Liu, L., and Simon, M. C. (2004). Regulation of transcription and translation by hypoxia. *Cancer Biol. Ther.* 3, 492–497. doi: 10.4161/cbt.3.6.1010

Milano, G., Bianciardi, P., Corno, A. F., Raddatz, E., Morel, S., von Segesser, L. K., et al. (2004). Myocardial impairment in chronic hypoxia is abolished by short aeration episodes: involvement of K+ATP channels. *Exp. Biol. Med.* 229, 1196–1205. doi: 10.1177/153537020422901115

Milano, G., Bianciardi, P., Rochemont, V., Vassalli, G., Segesser, L. K., Corno, A. F., et al. (2011). Phosphodiesterase-5 inhibition mimics intermittent reoxygenation and improves cardioprotection in the hypoxic myocardium. *PLoS ONE* 6:e27910. doi: 10.1371/journal.pone.0027910

Milano, G., Corno, A. F., Lippa, S., Von Segesser, L. K., and Samaja, M. (2002). Chronic and intermittent hypoxia induce different degrees of myocardial tolerance to hypoxia-induced dysfunction. *Exp. Biol. Med.* 227, 389–397. doi: 10.1177/153537020222700604

Milano, G., Corno, A. F., Samaja, M., Morel, S., Vassalli, G., and von Segesser, L. K. (2010). Daily reoxygenation decreases myocardial injury and improves post-ischaemic recovery after chronic hypoxia. *Eur. J. Cardiothorac. Surg.* 37, 942–949. doi: 10.1016/j.ejcts.2009.10.030

Salloum, F., Yin, C., Xi, L., and Kukreja, R. C. (2003). Sildenafil induces delayed preconditioning through inducible nitric oxide synthase-dependent pathway in mouse heart. *Circ. Res.* 92, 595–597. doi: 10.1161/01.RES.0000066853.09821.98

Seeger, W., Adir, Y., Barbera, J. A., Champion, H., Coghlan, J. G., Cottin, V., et al. (2013). Pulmonary hypertension in chronic lung diseases. *J. Am. Coll. Cardiol.* 62(25 Suppl), D109–D116. doi: 10.1016/j.jacc.2013.10.036

Tarricone, E., Scapin, C., Vitadello, M., Esposito, F., Margonato, V., Milano, G., et al. (2008). Cellular distribution of Hsp70 expression in rat skeletal muscles. Effects of moderate exercise training and chronic hypoxia. *Cell Stress Chaperones* 13, 483–495. doi: 10.1007/s12192-008-0048-y

Terraneo, L., Paroni, R., Bianciardi, P., Giallongo, T., Carelli, S., Gorio, A., et al. (2017). Brain adaptation to hypoxia and hyperoxia in mice. *Redox Biol.* 11, 12–20. doi: 10.1016/j.redox.2016.10.018

Vitulo, P., Stanziola, A., Confalonieri, M., Libertucci, D., Oggionni, T., Rottoli, P., et al. (2017). Sildenafil in severe pulmonary hypertension associated with chronic obstructive pulmonary disease: a randomized controlled multicenter clinical trial. *J. Heart Lung Transplant.* 36, 166–174. doi: 10.1016/j.healun.2016.04.010

West, J. B., and Mathieu-Costello, O. (1999). Structure, strength, failure, and remodeling of the pulmonary blood-gas barrier. *Annu. Rev. Physiol.* 61, 543–572. doi: 10.1146/annurev.physiol.61.1.543

West, J. B., Colice, G. L., Lee, Y. J., Namba, Y., Kurdak, S. S., Fu, Z., et al. (1995). Pathogenesis of high-altitude pulmonary oedema: direct evidence of stress failure of pulmonary capillaries. *Eur Respir. J.* 8, 523–529.

Weynand, B., Jonckheere, A., Frans, A., and Rahier, J. (1999). Diabetes mellitus induces a thickening of the pulmonary basal lamina. *Respiration* 66, 14–19. doi: 10.1159/000029331

Yang, Q., Shigemura, N., Underwood, M. J., Hsin, M., Xue, H. M., Huang, Y., et al. (2012). NO and EDHF pathways in pulmonary arteries and veins are impaired in COPD patients. *Vasc. Pharmacol.* 57, 113–118. doi: 10.1016/j.vph.2012.05.004

15

The Antioxidant Therapy: New Insights in the Treatment of Hypertension

Daniela Sorriento [1], Nicola De Luca [1], Bruno Trimarco [1] and Guido Iaccarino [2*]

[1] Dipartimento di Scienze Biomediche Avanzate, Università Federico II, Napoli, Italy, [2] Dipartimento di Medicina, Chirurgia e Odontoiatria, Università degli Studi di Salerno, Baronissi, Italy

Edited by:
Pasquale Pagliaro,
Università degli Studi di Torino, Italy

Reviewed by:
Ioanna Andreadou,
National and Kapodistrian University of Athens, Greece
Claudio Molinari,
Università degli Studi del Piemonte Orientale, Italy

***Correspondence:**
Guido Iaccarino
giaccarino@unisa.it

Reactive oxygen species (ROS) and reactive nitrogen species (RNS) play a key role in the regulation of the physiological and pathological signaling within the vasculature. In physiological conditions, a delicate balance between oxidants and antioxidants protects cells from the detrimental effects of ROS/RNS. Indeed, the imbalance between ROS/RNS production and antioxidant defense mechanisms leads to oxidative and nitrosative stress within the cell. These processes promote the vascular damage observed in chronic conditions, such as hypertension. The strong implication of ROS/RNS in the etiology of hypertension suggest that antioxidants could be effective in the treatment of this pathology. Indeed, in animal models of hypertension, the overexpression of antioxidants and the genetic modulation of oxidant systems have provided an encouraging proof of concept. Nevertheless, the translation of these strategies to human disease did not reach the expected success. This could be due to the complexity of this condition, whose etiology depends on multiple factors (smoking, diet, life styles, genetics, family history, comorbidities). Indeed, 95% of reported high blood pressure cases are deemed “essential hypertension,” and at the molecular level, oxidative stress seems to be a common feature of hypertensive states. In this scenario, new therapies are emerging that could be useful to reduce oxidative stress in hypertension. It is now ascertained the role of Vitamin D deficiency in the development of essential hypertension and it has been shown that an appropriate high dose of Vitamin D significantly reduces blood pressure in hypertensive cohorts with vitamin D deficiency. Moreover, new drugs are emerging which have both antihypertensive action and antioxidant properties, such as celiprolol, carvedilol, nebivolol. Indeed, besides adrenergic desensitization, these kind of drugs are able to interfere with ROS/RNS generation and/or signaling, and are therefore considered promising therapeutics in the management of hypertension. In the present review we have dealt with the effectiveness of the antioxidant therapy in the management of hypertension. In particular, we discuss about Vitamin D and anti-hypertensive drugs with antioxidant properties.

Keywords: hypertension, oxidative stress, nitrosative stress, antioxidants, ROS

OXIDATIVE AND NITROSATIVE STRESS: PHYSIO-PATHOLOGICAL IMPLICATIONS

Reactive oxygen species (ROS) are produced in several cellular systems within the cell: plasma membrane, cytosol, peroxisomes, mitochondria, lysosomes and endoplasmic reticulum (Di Meo et al., 2016). The enzymes involved in ROS generation are: nitric oxide synthase, peroxidases, NADPH oxidase, NADPH oxidase isoforms (NOX), xanthine oxidase (XO), lipoxygenases (LOXs), glucose oxidase, cyclooxygenases (COXs), and myeloperoxidase (MPO) (Bhattacharyya et al., 2014). Moreover, exogenous sources of ROS also exists that include air pollution, smoking, ionizing radiations, foods and drugs, chemical agents, heavy metals, organic solvents, pesticides (Bhattacharyya et al., 2014). ROS derive from oxygen reduction which produces, through several steps, important intermediate products: superoxide anion, hydrogen peroxide, and hydroxyl radical. Superoxide anion ($O_2^{\bullet -}$) is the most common ROS, which is generated in mitochondria by the electron transport chain (ETC) through the partial reduction of oxygen (Bolisetty and Jaimes, 2013). Superoxide dismutase (SOD) is responsible of H_2O_2 production from superoxide anion by means of amino acid and xanthine oxidase or a dismutation reaction. In the presence of metal ions and superoxide anion, H_2O_2 can produce the hydroxyl radical (·OH), that is the most reactive and dangerous one (Quinlan et al., 2013; Ogun, 2015).

RNS derives from nitric oxide (NO) that is generated during the breakdown of arginine to citrulline by the NADPH-dependent enzyme nitric oxide synthase (Drew and Leeuwenburgh, 2002). NO is a neurotransmitter and a blood pressure regulator; it is a free radical but is not a very reactive one. NO is able to form other nitrogen reactive intermediates (nitrate, peroxynitrite, and 3-nitrotyrosine), which affect cell function (Ramchandra et al., 2005; Ogun, 2015). NO competes with O2 for the binding at the binuclear center of cytochrome *c* oxidoreductase, leading to the inhibition of cytochrome c oxidase activity (Cleeter et al., 1994). In mitochondria it increases the production of ROS and RNS which affect several processes such as mitochondrial biogenesis, respiration, and oxidative stress (Bolisetty and Jaimes, 2013; Ogun, 2015). NO reacts with O_2^-, which derives from mitochondrial respiratory chain, to give peroxynitrite ($OONO^-$), which spontaneously decompose to $NO_2^{\cdot}$ and hydroxyl radical (.OH). Peroxynitrite is cytotoxic, oxidizes low-density lipoprotein and inhibits mitochondrial function (Radi et al., 2002; Halliwell, 2007). Nitrogen dioxide (NO_2) derives from the reaction of peroxyl radical and NO, triggers lipid peroxidation and oxidizes ascorbic acid (Patel et al., 1999).

ROS and RNS play a key role in both health and disease acting as signaling molecules (Di Meo et al., 2016). Indeed, they are involved in several physiologic processes (proliferation, growth, differentiation, apoptosis, migration, contraction, and cytoskeletal regulation,) but, when in excess, they also trigger the development of pathologic conditions (chronic inflammation and autoimmune diseases, sensory impairment, cardiovascular diseases, cancer, fibrotic disease, obesity, insulin resistance, neurological disorders, and infectious diseases; Mittler et al., 2011; Sena and Chandel, 2012; Brown and Griendling, 2015). In physiological conditions, a delicate balance between oxidants and antioxidants exists that allow cells to conduct their physiological functions and to improve the systemic defense mechanisms (**Figure 1**; Ristow and Schmeisser, 2014; Ogun, 2015). However, when this balance is impaired leading to an excessive production of ROS/RNS, oxidative and nitrosative stress occurs and causes extensive cellular damage. This dual effect of ROS has been named mitohormesis, indicating a non-linear dose-response relationship between ROS levels and mortality (Ristow and Schmeisser, 2014).

THE INVOLVEMENT OF ROS/RNS IN THE ETIOLOGY OF HYPERTENSION

Hypertension is a complex condition whose etiology depends on several factors (smoking, diet, genetics, family history, pre-existing pathologies) and, in most cases, it is difficult to determine the main cause ("essential hypertension"). Besides the complex etiology of this disease, oxidative and nitrosative stress appear to be a common feature within hypertensive disorders (Harrison et al., 2007; Harrison and Gongora, 2009; Baradaran et al., 2014). Even if it is still debated whether excessive ROS/RNS production is the cause or the consequence of hypertension, several *in vitro* and *in vivo* evidence suggest that ROS/RNS trigger the activation of specific molecular mechanisms which in turn increase blood pressure levels (Ward and Croft, 2006).

In Vitro Evidence in Cultured Vascular Cells

Vascular cell types (endothelialcells, smooth muscle cells, adventitial fibroblasts, and perivascular adipocytes) are able to produce ROS through the activity of many enzymes (Touyz and Briones, 2011; Kim and Byzova, 2014). Among these latter, mitochondrial enzymes and nicotinamide adenine dinucleotide phosphate (NADPH) oxidase (Nox) are the major sources of ROS in the vascular wall that trigger mitochondrial dysfunction and consequently oxidative stress. Angiotensin II has been shown to induce mitochondrial ROS production through the activation of NADPH oxidase (Doughan et al., 2008; **Figure 2**). The vascular production of ROS/RNS causes a significant reduction of NO production and eNOS activity (Rodrigo et al., 2011). Indeed, when the levels of superoxide anion increase, nitric oxide is rapidly degraded causing endothelial dysfunction (McIntyre et al., 1999; Touyz and Schiffrin, 2004). The peroxynitrite oxidizes BH4, an important NO synthase cofactor, and inducing an increase of superoxide production leading to the development of oxidative stress (Laursen et al., 2001). Through lipid peroxidation, ROS can also cause the generation of secondary products (lipid-derived aldehydes) that contributes to endothelial dysfunction and hypertension (Cracowski et al., 2002).

In hypertension, ROS affected several processes which in turn trigger endothelial dysfunction (apoptosis, angiogenesis, inflammation). Indeed, in endothelial cells, the increase of ROS production in response to pro-inflammatory and pro-atherosclerotic factors (Ang II, oxLDL, TNFalpha), activates apoptotic events which are prevented by the treatment with

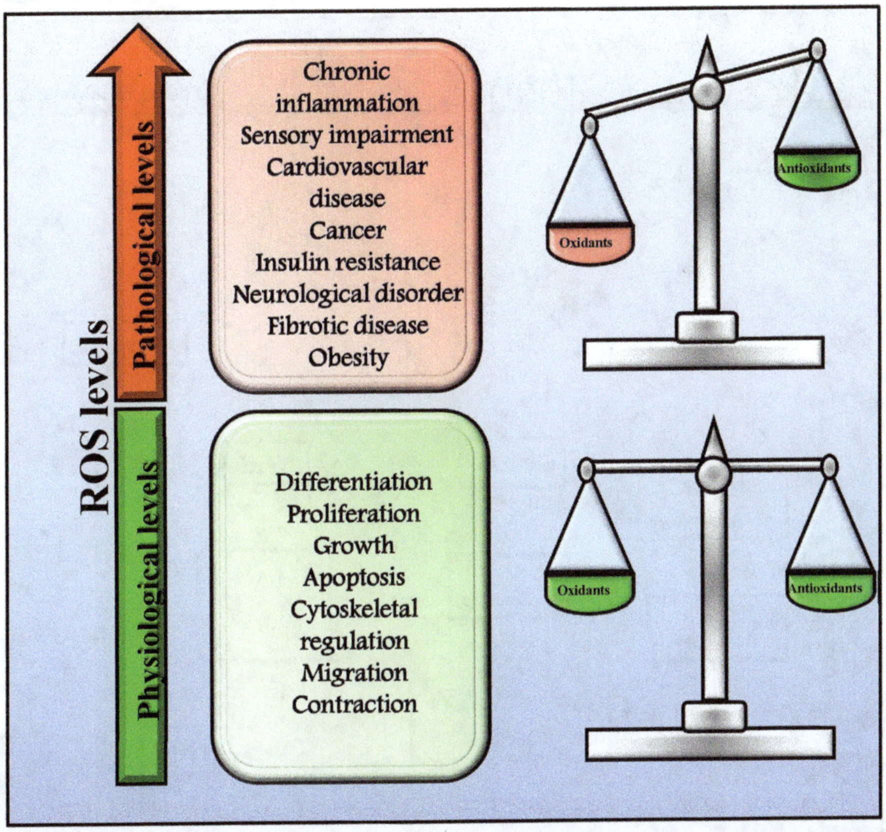

FIGURE 1 | Physiological and pathological ROS levels. In physiological conditions, there is a delicate balance between oxidants and antioxidants that allow cells to conduct their physiological functions and to improve systemic defense mechanisms by inducing an adaptive response. In this conditions ROS production is physiologic and not dangerous. However, when the balance between oxidants and antioxidants is impaired and ROS production increase over the physiological threshold, excessive ROS levels trigger the development of pathologic conditions.

antioxidants (Dimmeler and Zeiher, 2000). The pro-apoptotic effects of ROS in endothelial cells derives from the impairment of mitochondrial membrane permeability followed by cytochrome c release and caspase activation (Breitschopf et al., 2000; Lee et al., 2009).

In the endothelium, the expression of some adhesion molecules (vascular cell adhesion molecule-1 and intracellular adhesion molecule-1) is ROS-dependent, suggesting that ROS promote adhesion of inflammatory cells (Marui et al., 1993; Khan et al., 1996).

It has been demonstrated that ROS-dependent angiogenesis is associated with VEGF expression (Kim and Byzova, 2014). Indeed, hydrogen peroxide increases VEGF expression both in vascular smooth muscle cells and in endothelial cells, thus promoting angiogenic responses (Ruef et al., 1997; Chua et al., 1998). ROS also affect the dimerization and autophosphorylation of VEGFR2 in response to VEGF, and subsequent angiogenesis induced by VEGFR2 activation (Colavitti et al., 2002; Ushio-Fukai et al., 2002; Kim and Byzova, 2014). Recent studies also identified novel mechanisms of ROS-dependent angiogenesis which are VEGF-independent (Kim et al., 2013; Kim and Byzova, 2014). Indeed, ROS are involved in the generation of new lipid oxidation products with proangiogenic activities through TLR-2 dependent NFkappaB activation. Also, ROS-dependent NFkappaB activation induces the expression of pro-inflammatory genes (Malinin et al., 2011; Kim et al., 2013; Kim and Byzova, 2014).

In Vivo Evidence in Animal Models of Hypertension

The involvement of ROS in the etiology of hypertension has been demonstrated in several animal models of hypertension: spontaneously hypertensive rat (Kerr et al., 1999), the angiotensin II-infused rat (Haugen et al., 2000), renovascular hypertension (Lerman et al., 2001), the deoxycorticosterone acetate-salt model (Wu et al., 2001), and obesity-related hypertension (Dobrian et al., 2001). These studies associate oxidative stress with the mechanisms of hypertension, including vascular and organ damage. A further confirmation of ROS involvement in hypertension derives from the finding that in animal models of hypertension the increased ROS production causes endothelial dysfunction that is reversed by SOD (Laursen et al., 1997; Bauersachs et al., 1999; Somers et al., 2000).

In Vivo Evidence in Humans

In smooth muscle cells from arteries of hypertensive patients the treatment with Angiotensin II induces ROS production, as demonstrated by the increase of several parameters that

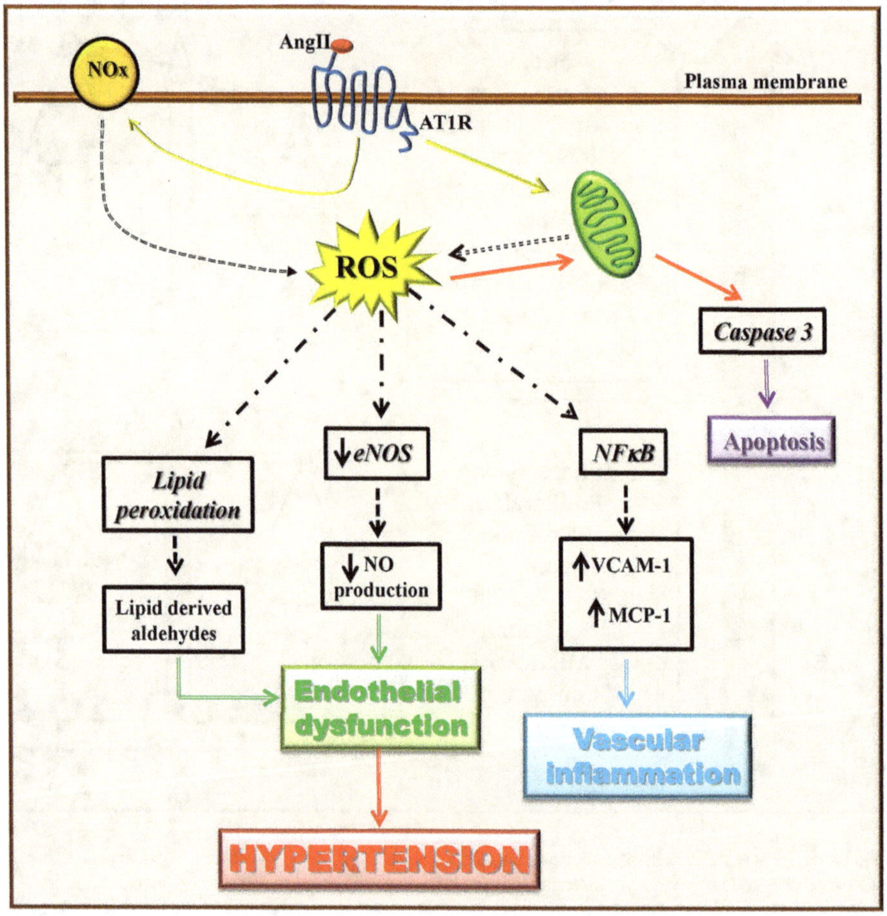

FIGURE 2 | Angiotensin II-dependent ROS production induces hypertension. Angiotensin II induces ROS production through the activation of mitochondrial enzymes and nicotinamide adenine dinucleotide phosphate (NADPH) oxidase (Nox). Angiotensin II-dependent ROS production causes in turn a significant reduction of eNOS activity and NO production, lipid peroxidation, induction of apoptotic signaling, and NFκB activation. These all lead to endothelial dysfunction and vascular inflammation that trigger the development of the hypertensive state.

are related to ROS (Touyz and Schiffrin, 2001; Ahmad et al., 2017). Furthermore, in hypertensive patients a strong association exists between blood pressure and the elevated oxidative stress biomarkers such as malondialdehyde, F2-isoprostanes, GSSG, and the DNA oxidation marker 8-oxo-7,8-dihydro-2′-deoxyguanosine (8-oxo-dG) (Rodrigo et al., 2007; Ahmad et al., 2017).

THE ANTIOXIDANT THERAPY IN HYPERTENSION

Given the above discussed involvement of oxidative and nitrosative stress in the etiology of hypertension, the antioxidant therapy seems to be a useful strategy to restore the impaired balance between oxidants and antioxidants in hypertensive conditions. Indeed, the treatment with antioxidants has been successfully used in animal models of hypertension. The oral treatment with Lazaroid, a ROS scavenger, in spontaneously hypertensive rats (SHR) improved NO viability and reduced blood pressure (Vaziri et al., 2000). Similarly, treatment with the antioxidant N-acetylcysteine (NAC) inhibited ROS production and improved NOS activity and accordingly reduced blood pressure (Ahmad et al., 2017). The same results were found also in SHR treated with the xanthine oxidase inhibitor, allopurinol (Mazzali et al., 2001). Moreover, successful results were also obtained by targeting antioxidant peptides to the vasculature to increase the antioxidant effect, reduce vascular resistances and lower BP. For instance, the antioxidant peptide gp91ds affects the assembly of NAD(P)H oxidase and consequently reduces superoxide production (Greig et al., 2010). This peptide was engineered to target vasculature and chronically administered to a preclinical model of endothelial dysfunction and more severe hypertension, the stroke-prone SHR. The treatment significantly improved nitric oxide bioavailability and attenuated the time-dependent and progressive increase in systolic blood pressure (Greig et al., 2010).

Opposite to preclinical models, however, antioxidant strategies for the treatment of hypertension in clinic did not reach the expected success. Indeed, literature is quite discordant on the effect of antioxidant therapy in hypertension as demonstrated by data from clinical trials (Kizhakekuttu and Widlansky, 2010). This could be due to the complexity of this condition. Indeed, while we call hypertensives all patients with blood pressure values above a given threshold (Mancia et al., 2013; Whelton et al., 2017) indeed within this generic definition a much diversified range of phenotypes are included, ranging from the young lean to the obese, to the postmenopausal women or the elderly hypertensives. For each of this phenotype, indeed, it is expected to recognize different etiology, depending on several risk factors (genetics, family history), lifestyles (smoking, diet, sedentary lifestyle), concomitant conditions (chronic kidney disease, diabetes). In each of these phenotypes, the role of oxidants might be different, and therefore diluted within clinical trials that do not select the appropriate patient. Moreover, it is to be considered that the effectiveness of antioxidants can be lowered by the cross-talk with other substances. For instance, it has been shown that Vitamin C alone reduced both systolic and diastolic blood pressure (BP) vs. placebo (Ward et al., 2005) through the down-regulation of NADPH oxidase and up-regulation of eNOS (Briones and Touyz, 2010; Juraschek et al., 2012). However, the same vitamin, in combination with Polyphenols, increases BP, while in combination with other antioxidants (Vitamin E, beta-carotene, and zinc) modestly reduces systolic BP and does not modify diastolic BP (Ardalan and Rafieian-Kopaei, 2014). Furthermore, ineffective dosing regimens and inadequate selection of subjects recruited in the studies could also have affected the effectiveness of the treatment. **Table 1** summarize the main common natural antioxidants (e.g., vitamins and mitochondrial related antioxidants), other potential antioxidants (e.g., vitamin D), and anti-hypertensive drugs that also exert antioxidant effects.

Among natural antioxidants, here we focused on Vitamin D, whose levels has been recently associated with hypertension, since it has great potentiality to be used for therapeutic treatments. Among the other antioxidants listed in **Table 1**, we discuss the ability of some anti-hypertensive drugs to reduce oxidative stress. This latter property of anti-hypertensive drugs enforces the proof of concept about the key role of oxidative stress in the development and progression of hypertensive states and the benefit of antioxidants as therapeutic strategy.

Vitamin D

Among antioxidants, Vitamin D is recently emerging as anti-hypertensive effector through the activation of antioxidant mechanisms. In human, most vitamin D (~80%) is naturally synthesized in the skin from 7-dehydrocholesterol in response to ultraviolet (UV) B radiation but it can also derive from dietary sources. Vitamin D is metabolized in the liver to 25-hydroxyvitamin D (25(OH)D) that is converted by 1α-hydroxylase into 1,25-dihydroxyvitamin D3, the biologically active agonist for the Vitamin D receptor (VDR) (**Figure 3**; Chen et al., 2015). Serum levels of Vitamin D are regulated by calcium homeostasis and parathyroid hormone (PTH) level since low calcium and high PTH levels induce Vitamin D synthesis by increasing 1α-hydroxylase activity (Chen et al., 2015).

A large part of western population is thought to have a Vitamin D deficiency/insufficiency, which has been associated with an increased risk for cardiovascular diseases (McGreevy and Williams, 2011; Tamez et al., 2013). The reason for this deficiency can be probably due to a decreased exposure to sun as a prevention for melanoma (Holick, 2007), although nutritional aspects are also being considered and posed a the base of replacement therapy strategies.

Recently, an association between low Vitamin D serum levels and hypertension have been suggested (Ullah et al., 2010; Kota et al., 2011). Indeed, 1-alpha-hydroxylase deficient mice, which cannot synthesize Vitamin D3, develop high blood pressure and left ventricular hypertrophy (Zhou et al., 2008). Vitamin D can affect blood pressure through several mechanisms. Indeed, in both animals and humans it has been shown that vitamin D decreases renin-angiotensin-aldosterone system (RAAS) activity (Li et al., 2002; Tomaschitz et al., 2010), modulates endothelial function (Wong et al., 2010; Pittarella et al., 2015; Molinari et al., 2018) and regulates vascular oxidative stress (Argacha et al., 2011).

Clinical studies demonstrated an inverse, dose-response relationship between plasma Vitamin D3 concentration and blood pressure or renin activity in both normotensive and hypertensive patients (Nigwekar and Thadhani, 2013; Grubler et al., 2017). High levels of Vitamin D in humans, for instance, are associated with lower blood pressure (Vimaleswaran et al., 2014). All these reports suggest that Vitamin D levels are associated with BP also in humans. Based on such findings, it is likely to believe that Vitamin D supplementation could be an effective therapy for hypertension. This hypothesis was confirmed in animal models of hypertension. Indeed, Vitamin

TABLE 1 | Known and potential antioxidants.

Antioxidant vitamins	Mitochondrial related antioxidants	Enzymatic antioxidants	Other potential antioxidants	Anti-hypertensive drugs
Vitamin A	Coenzyme Q10	Glutathione peroxidase	Vitamin D	Propanolol
Vitamin C	Acetyl-L-Carnitine	Catalase	Glutamate	Nebivilol
Vitamin E	α-Lipoic Acid	Superoxide dismutase	N-acetylcysteine	Carvedilol
L-Arginin			Sour milk	Celiprolol
Flavonoids			Garlic	Amlodipine
				Enalapril

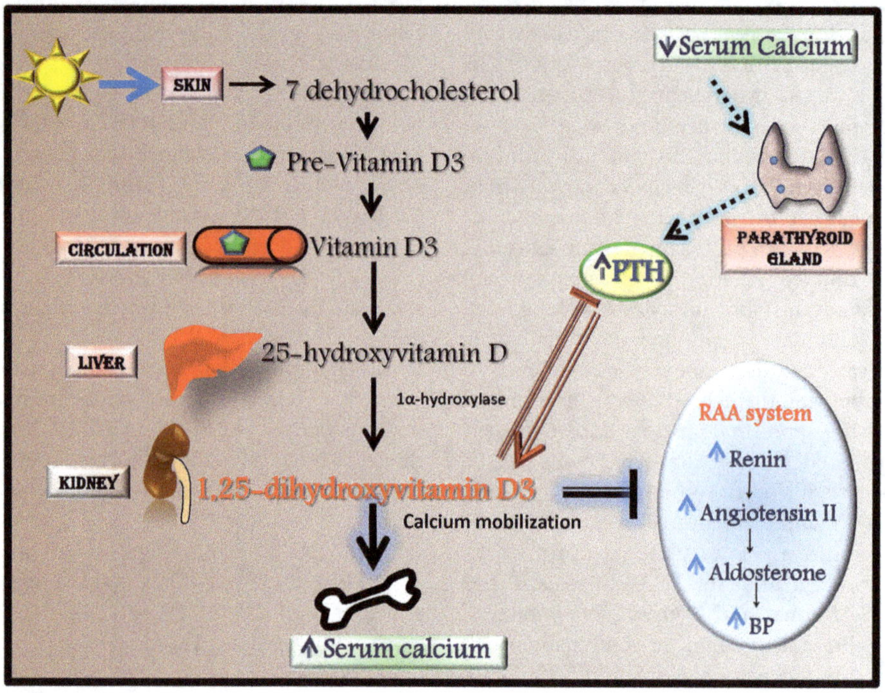

FIGURE 3 | Vitamin D synthesis and effects. Most vitamin D is naturally synthesized in the skin from 7-dehydrocholesterol in response to ultraviolet radiation. 7-dehydrocholesterol is converted to Pre-Vitamin D3 that through the circulation reach the liver where it is metabolized to 25-hydroxyvitamin D (25(OH)D). This latter is then converted in the kidney by 1α-hydroxylase into 1,25-dihydroxyvitamin D3, the biologically active agonist for the Vitamin D receptor. The synthesis of 1,25-dihydroxyvitamin D3 is mainly regulated by PTH and serum calcium levels. 1,25-dihydroxyvitamin D3 has a several effects since it increases serum calcium levels by inducing calcium mobilization from bone, decreases renin-angiotensin-aldosterone system (RAAS) activity and inhibits PTH production.

D supplementation ameliorates pathological right ventricular hypertrophy in rats with pulmonary hypertension (Tanaka et al., 2017) and reduces blood pressure levels in SHR rats (Wong et al., 2010). Accordingly, several clinical trials show the effectiveness of natural vitamin D, Vitamin D3 or its analog supplementation on BP levels in those patients with essential hypertension that is dependent on Vitamin D-deficiency (Kimura et al., 1999; Pfeifer et al., 2001; Judd et al., 2010; Goel and Lal, 2011; Bernini et al., 2013; Forman et al., 2013; Carrara et al., 2014; Mozaffari-Khosravi et al., 2015). Vitamin D supplementation therapy also in pregnancy is able to reduce the incidence of gestational hypertension/preeclampsia (Behjat Sasan et al., 2017). Moreover, Vitamin D have beneficial effects on BP also in patients affected by other pathologies, such as type 2 diabetes (de Paula et al., 2017).

However, other randomized controlled trials show that Vitamin D supplementation results ineffective as anti-hypertensive agent (Li et al., 2004; Michos and Melamed, 2008; Beveridge et al., 2015; Grubler et al., 2017; Wu and Sun, 2017). Thus, literature seems to be quite discordant on the effectiveness of Vitamin D supplementation in the treatment of the hypertensive condition. However, this discrepancy could be dependent on several variables in study population (Vitamin D-deficiency levels, gender, ethnicity, BP levels, age, parathormone levels). Indeed, a recent study show that the relationship between serum levels of Vitamin D and BP differs according to ethnicity and gender with a significant inverse association among non-hispanic whites (NHW) and females, NHW females and non-hispanic black females (Vishnu and Ahuja, 2017). Data from this study suggest a non-linear relationship between Vitamin D and hypertension with significant decline in hypertension only up to a physiological level of Vitamin D that is different depending on race/ethnicity and gender (Vishnu and Ahuja, 2017). Among the putative mechanisms involved in the association between Vitamin D deficiency and increased blood pressure levels, anti-oxidant effects of Vitamin D have been implicated. Nevertheless, it has also to consider that Vitamin D is inversely correlated with the calcium modulator paratohormone (PTH). The vascular effects of such hormone, as well as the mechanisms associated with the reduced kidney function are both possible mechanisms of increased vascular resistance and blood volume, two determinants of hypertension. Indeed, increased PTH has been demonstrated to correlates better than Vitamin D deficiency with blood pressure and cardiovascular risk, including hypertension, in a large population in Southern Italy (Pascale et al., 2018) suggesting that also PTH levels could be a discriminating parameter in the selection of patients that could be sensitive to Vitamin D supplementation. Thus, future researches on this issue should take into account these parameters and, accordingly, identify an ideal population which result more sensitive to this kind of treatment.

Anti-hypertensive Drugs With Antioxidant Properties

To date, several molecules have been discovered that are effective anti-hypertensive drugs with antioxidant properties. Indeed, some beta-blockers, apart from their ability to inhibit adrenaline/noradrenaline dependent activation of beta adrenergic receptors (Iaccarino et al., 2006; Sorriento et al., 2011; Galasso et al., 2013), are also able to reduce oxidative stress. Among them, Propanolol, Nebivilol, Carvedilol, and Celiprolol are the most studied (Yao et al., 2008). Propranolol inhibits oxidative stress and reduces tissue lipid peroxidation (Mak and Weglicki, 1988; Yao et al., 2008). Carvedilol reduces lipid peroxidation in patients with heart failure by acting as a free radical scavenger (Kukin et al., 1999; Yao et al., 2008). Celiprolol reduces superoxide anions generation in patients with essential hypertension and improves endothelial function (Mehta et al., 1994; Kobayashi et al., 2001; Yao et al., 2008). However, this antioxidant effects are not a common feature of all beta-blockers since it has been shown that Atenolol has no effect on ROS production in endothelial cells (Fratta Pasini et al., 2005).

At the molecular level, the beta-blocking effect is itself important to reduce ROS production by blocking catecholamines that are known to induce oxidative stress in the myocardium. Furthermore, some beta-blockers have also direct antioxidant effects which are different depending on the modulation of specific intracellular signaling.

Indeed, Nebivolol exerts its effects by increasing NO levels, NOS activity, and expression of eNOS, as well as by reducing ROS production and Nox expression (Wang et al., 2017). Carvedilol inhibits 4-hydroxy-2-nonenal (HNE)-induced intracellular Ca^{2+}overload (Nakamura et al., 2011). Celiprolol significantly suppresses BP levels and ameliorates hypoxia-induced LV remodeling in mice, by restoring eNOS expression via stimulation of PI3K-AKT signaling pathway (Kobayashi et al., 2003; Nishioka et al., 2013).

Besides these beta-blockers, also Amlodipine, a calcium channel blocker, shares the same anti-hypertensive and antioxidant properties. Indeed, Amlodipine is able to decrease blood pressure as well as oxidative stress as shown by a decrease of malondialdehyde and an increase of Na^+ K^+ ATPase and SOD levels in essential hypertensive patients (Mahajan et al., 2007). This effect is further increased by Vitamin C supplementation (Mahajan et al., 2007).

Furthermore, Enalapril, an ACE-inhibitor, reduces the expression of oxidant stress markers and antioxidant enzymes in the heart and kidney of SHR rats (Chandran et al., 2014; Yusoff et al., 2017) and of diabetic rats (de Cavanagh et al., 2001). Also in hypertensive patients, 3 months of Enalapril therapy are beneficial to prevent oxidative stress compared with Atenolol treated patients (Deoghare and Kantharia, 2013). Similarly, the antioxidant beneficial effects on vascular biology, including nitrix oxide availability, has been demonstrated for SH- containing ACE inhibitors (Captopril, Lisinopril, zofenopril) due to the free radical scavenging properties of the tiol residues contained in the drug sequence (Chopra et al., 1990; Buikema et al., 2000; Donnarumma et al., 2016).

CONCLUSIONS AND FUTURE DIRECTIONS

Several diseases have been associated with oxidative stress suggesting that this latter could be a trigger for diseases and that antioxidant therapy could be an effective therapeutic treatment. However, while basic research and pre-clinical studies support this point of view, clinical studies still produce controversial results. This could probably be dependent on the pathophysiological complexity of ROS/RNS signaling in humans with comorbidities (Pagliaro and Penna, 2015, 2017; Egea et al., 2017). Here, in particular, we have discussed about the role of oxidative stress in the development and progression of hypertensive states even if the idea that antioxidant therapy is effective against this disease by inhibiting or destroying free radicals is not accepted yet. Indeed, the promising results in pre-clinical model of hypertension are not always support by data from patients. A great discrepancy exists among results from different clinical trials. Actually, limitations to the effectiveness of antioxidant therapy in the management of hypertension could be due to numerous variables. First of all, the half-life of the particular antioxidant administered affects its effectiveness in long-term treatments. Moreover, the cross-talks with other substances in some cases reduce the anti-hypertensive effects. Finally, the inadequate homogeneity of patients characteristics in study population is probably the most important limitation of clinical trials. To date, the use of anti-hypertensive drugs with antioxidants properties seems to be the most effective treatment in the management of hypertension since they are able to reduce blood pressure by affecting molecular mechanisms which are involved in the regulation of both vascular function and oxidative state. Despite the discordant results of clinical trials, Vitamin D supplementation could also be a promising therapeutic treatment for hypertension that is worthwhile to further investigate considering not only the rate of Vitamin D deficiency, but also PTH levels, as discriminating factors in the selection of patients. For the future improvement of antioxidant therapy the above proposed potential limitations should be taken into account. Moreover, further studies are needed to better clarify the sources and targets of ROS/RNS and their harmful or beneficial roles, the specific molecular mechanisms and their cross-talks, and to identify the ideal patient which could be sensitive to specific antioxidant therapies.

AUTHOR CONTRIBUTIONS

DS, ND, BT, and GI conceived and designed the work, drafted the work and revisited it critically.

REFERENCES

Ahmad, K. A., Yuan Yuan, D., Nawaz, W., Ze, H., Zhuo, C. X., Talal, B., et al. (2017). Antioxidant therapy for management of oxidative stress induced hypertension. *Free Radic. Res.* 51, 428–438. doi: 10.1080/10715762.2017.1322205

Ardalan, M. R., and Rafieian-Kopaei, M. (2014). Antioxidant supplementation in hypertension. *J. Renal Inj. Prev.* 3, 39–40. doi: 10.12861/jrip.2014.13

Argacha, J. F., Egrise, D., Pochet, S., Fontaine, D., Lefort, A., Libert, F., et al. (2011). Vitamin D deficiency-induced hypertension is associated with vascular oxidative stress and altered heart gene expression. *J. Cardiovasc. Pharmacol.* 58, 65–71. doi: 10.1097/FJC.0b013e31821c832f

Baradaran, A., Nasri, H., and Rafieian-Kopaei, M. (2014). Oxidative stress and hypertension: possibility of hypertension therapy with antioxidants. *J. Res. Med. Sci.* 19, 358–367.

Bauersachs, J., Bouloumié, A., Fraccarollo, D., Hu, K., Busse, R., and Ertl, G. (1999). Endothelial dysfunction in chronic myocardial infarction despite increased vascular endothelial nitric oxide synthase and soluble guanylate cyclase expression: role of enhanced vascular superoxide production. *Circulation* 100, 292–298. doi: 10.1161/01.CIR.100.3.292

Behjat Sasan, S., Zandvakili, F., Soufizadeh, N., and Baybordi, E. (2017). The effects of Vitamin D supplement on prevention of recurrence of preeclampsia in pregnant women with a history of preeclampsia. *Obstet. Gynecol. Int.* 2017:8249264. doi: 10.1155/2017/8249264

Bernini, G., Carrara, D., Bacca, A., Carli, V., Virdis, A., Rugani, I., et al. (2013). Effect of acute and chronic Vitamin D administration on systemic renin angiotensin system in essential hypertensives and controls. *J. Endocrinol. Invest.* 36, 216–220. doi: 10.1007/BF03347275

Beveridge, L. A., Struthers, A. D., Khan, F., Jorde, R., Scragg, R., Macdonald, H. M., et al. (2015). Effect of Vitamin D supplementation on blood pressure: a systematic review and meta-analysis incorporating individual patient data. *JAMA Intern. Med.* 175, 745–754. doi: 10.1001/jamainternmed.2015.0237

Bhattacharyya, A., Chattopadhyay, R., Mitra, S., and Crowe, S. E. (2014). Oxidative stress: an essential factor in the pathogenesis of gastrointestinal mucosal diseases. *Physiol. Rev.* 94, 329–354. doi: 10.1152/physrev.00040.2012

Bolisetty, S., and Jaimes, E. A. (2013). Mitochondria and reactive oxygen species: physiology and pathophysiology. *Int. J. Mol. Sci.* 14, 6306–6344. doi: 10.3390/ijms14036306

Breitschopf, K., Haendeler, J., Malchow, P., Zeiher, A. M., and Dimmeler, S. (2000). Posttranslational modification of Bcl-2 facilitates its proteasome-dependent degradation: molecular characterization of the involved signaling pathway. *Mol. Cell. Biol.* 20, 1886–1896. doi: 10.1128/MCB.20.5.1886-1896.2000

Briones, A. M., and Touyz, R. M. (2010). Oxidative stress and hypertension: current concepts. *Curr. Hypertens. Rep.* 12, 135–142. doi: 10.1007/s11906-010-0100-z

Brown, D. I., and Griendling, K. K. (2015). Regulation of signal transduction by reactive oxygen species in the cardiovascular system. *Circ. Res.* 116, 531–549. doi: 10.1161/CIRCRESAHA.116.303584

Buikema, H., Monnink, S. H., Tio, R. A., Crijns, H. J., de Zeeuw, D., and van Gilst, W. H. (2000). Comparison of zofenopril and lisinopril to study the role of the sulfhydryl-group in improvement of endothelial dysfunction with ACE-inhibitors in experimental heart failure. *Br. J. Pharmacol.* 130, 1999–2007. doi: 10.1038/sj.bjp.0703498

Carrara, D., Bernini, M., Bacca, A., Rugani, I., Duranti, E., Virdis, A., et al. (2014). Cholecalciferol administration blunts the systemic renin-angiotensin system in essential hypertensives with hypovitaminosis D. *J. Renin Angiotensin Aldosterone Syst.* 15, 82–87. doi: 10.1177/1470320312471149

Chandran, G., Sirajudeen, K. N., Yusoff, N. S., Swamy, M., and Samarendra, M. S. (2014). Effect of the antihypertensive drug enalapril on oxidative stress markers and antioxidant enzymes in kidney of spontaneously hypertensive rat. *Oxid. Med. Cell. Longev.* 2014:608512. doi: 10.1155/2014/608512

Chen, S., Sun, Y., and Agrawal, D. K. (2015). Vitamin D deficiency and essential hypertension. *J. Am. Soc. Hypertens.* 9, 885–901. doi: 10.1016/j.jash.2015.08.009

Chopra, M., McMurray, J., Stewart, J., Dargie, H. J., and Smith, W. E. (1990). Free radical scavenging: a potentially beneficial action of thiol-containing angiotensin converting enzyme inhibitors. *Biochem. Soc. Trans.* 18, 1184–1185. doi: 10.1042/bst0181184

Chua, C. C., Hamdy, R. C., and Chua, B. H. (1998). Upregulation of vascular endothelial growth factor by H_2O_2 in rat heart endothelial cells. *Free Radic. Biol. Med.* 25, 891–897. doi: 10.1016/S0891-5849(98)00115-4

Cleeter, M. W., Cooper, J. M., Darley-Usmar, V. M., Moncada, S., and Schapira, A. H. (1994). Reversible inhibition of cytochrome c oxidase, the terminal enzyme of the mitochondrial respiratory chain, by nitric oxide. Implcations for neurodegenerative diseases. *FEBS Lett.* 345, 50–54. doi: 10.1016/0014-5793(94)00424-2

Colavitti, R., Pani, G., Bedogni, B., Anzevino, R., Borrello, S., Waltenberger, J., et al. (2002). Reactive oxygen species as downstream mediators of angiogenic signaling by vascular endothelial growth factor receptor-2/KDR. *J. Biol. Chem.* 277, 3101–3108. doi: 10.1074/jbc.M107711200

Cracowski, J. L., Durand, T., and Bessard, G. (2002). Isoprostanes as a biomarker of lipid peroxidation in humans: physiology, pharmacology and clinical implications. *Trends Pharmacol. Sci.* 23, 360–366. doi: 10.1016/S0165-6147(02)02053-9

de Cavanagh, E. M., Inserra, F., Toblli, J., Stella, I., Fraga, C. G., and Ferder, L. (2001). Enalapril attenuates oxidative stress in diabetic rats. *Hypertension* 38, 1130–1136. doi: 10.1161/hy1101.092845

de Paula, T. P., Kramer, C. K., Viana, L. V., and Azevedo, M. J. (2017). Effects of individual micronutrients on blood pressure in patients with type 2 diabetes: a systematic review and meta-analysis of randomized clinical trials. *Sci. Rep.* 7:40751. doi: 10.1038/srep40751

Deoghare, S., and Kantharia. N. D. (2013). Effect of atenolol and enalapril treatment on oxidative stress parameters in patients with essential hypertension. *Int. J. Basic Clin. Pharmacol.* 2, 252–256. doi: 10.5455/2319-2003.ijbcp20130604

Di Meo, S., Reed, T. T., Venditti, P., and Victor, V. M. (2016). Role of ROS and RNS sources in physiological and pathological conditions. *Oxid. Med. Cell. Longev.* 2016:1245049. doi: 10.1155/2016/1245049

Dimmeler, S., and Zeiher, A. M. (2000). Reactive oxygen species and vascular cell apoptosis in response to angiotensin II and pro-atherosclerotic factors. *Regul. Pept.* 90, 19–25. doi: 10.1016/S0167-0115(00)00105-1

Dobrian, A. D., Davies, M. J., Schriver, S. D., Lauterio, T. J., and Prewitt, R. L. (2001). Oxidative stress in a rat model of obesity-induced hypertension. *Hypertension* 37(2 Pt 2), 554–560. doi: 10.1161/01.HYP.37.2.554

Donnarumma, E., Ali, M. J., Rushing, A. M., Scarborough, A. L., Bradley, J. M., Organ, C. L., et al. (2016). Zofenopril protects against myocardial ischemia-reperfusion injury by increasing nitric oxide and hydrogen sulfide bioavailability. *J. Am. Heart Assoc.* 5:e003531. doi: 10.1161/JAHA.116.003531

Doughan, A. K., Harrison, D. G., and Dikalov, S. I. (2008). Molecular mechanisms of angiotensin II-mediated mitochondrial dysfunction: linking mitochondrial oxidative damage and vascular endothelial dysfunction. *Circ. Res.* 102, 488–496. doi: 10.1161/CIRCRESAHA.107.162800

Drew, B., and Leeuwenburgh, C. (2002). Aging and the role of reactive nitrogen species. *Ann. N.Y. Acad. Sci.* 959, 66–81. doi: 10.1111/j.1749-6632.2002.tb02084.x

Egea, J., Fabregat, I., Frapart, Y. M., Ghezzi, P., Görlach, A., Kietzmann, T., et al. (2017). European contribution to the study of ROS: a summary of the findings and prospects for the future from the COST action BM1203 (EU-ROS). *Redox Biol.* 13, 94–162. doi: 10.1016/j.redox.2017.05.007

Forman, J. P., Scott, J. B., Ng, K., Drake, B. F., Suarez, E. G., Hayden, D. L., et al. (2013). Effect of vitamin D supplementation on blood pressure in blacks. *Hypertension* 61, 779–785. doi: 10.1161/HYPERTENSIONAHA.111.00659

Fratta Pasini, A., Garbin, U., Nava, M. C., Stranieri, C., Davoli, A., Sawamura, T., et al. (2005). Nebivolol decreases oxidative stress in essential hypertensive patients and increases nitric oxide by reducing its oxidative inactivation. *J. Hypertens.* 23, 589–596. doi: 10.1097/01.hjh.0000160216.86597.ff

Galasso, G., De Rosa, R., Ciccarelli, M., Sorriento, D., Del Giudice, C., Strisciuglio, T., et al. (2013). β2-adrenergic receptor stimulation improves endothelial progenitor cell-mediated ischemic neoangiogenesis. *Circ. Res.* 112, 1026–1034. doi: 10.1161/CIRCRESAHA.111.300152

Goel, R. K., and Lal, H. (2011). Role of Vitamin D supplementation in hypertension. *Indian J. Clin. Biochem.* 26, 88–90. doi: 10.1007/s12291-010-0092-0

Greig, J. A., Shirley, R., Graham, D., Denby, L., Dominiczak, A. F., Work, L. M., et al. (2010). Vascular-targeting antioxidant therapy in a model of hypertension and stroke. *J. Cardiovasc. Pharmacol.* 56, 642–650. doi: 10.1097/FJC.0b013e3181f8f19f

Grübler, M. R., März, W., Pilz, S., Grammer, T. B., Trummer, C., Müllner, C., et al. (2017). Vitamin-D concentrations, cardiovascular risk and events - a review of epidemiological evidence. *Rev. Endocr. Metab. Disord.* 18, 259–272. doi: 10.1007/s11154-017-9417-0

Halliwell, B. (2007). Biochemistry of oxidative stress. *Biochem. Soc. Trans.* 35(Pt 5), 1147–1150. doi: 10.1042/BST0351147

Harrison, D. G., and Gongora, M. C. (2009). Oxidative stress and hypertension. *Med. Clin. North Am.* 93, 621–635. doi: 10.1016/j.mcna.2009.02.015

Harrison, D. G., Gongora, M. C., Guzik, T. J., and Widder, J. (2007). Oxidative stress and hypertension. *J. Am. Soc. Hypertens.* 1, 30–44. doi: 10.1016/j.jash.2006.11.006

Haugen, E. N., Croatt, A. J., and Nath, K. A. (2000). Angiotensin II induces renal oxidant stress *in vivo* and heme oxygenase-1 *in vivo* and *in vitro*. *Kidney Int.* 58, 144–152. doi: 10.1046/j.1523-1755.2000.00150.x

Holick, M. F. (2007). Vitamin D deficiency. *N. Engl. J. Med.* 357, 266–281. doi: 10.1056/NEJMra070553

Iaccarino, G., Izzo, R., Trimarco, V., Cipolletta, E., Lanni, F., Sorriento, D., et al. (2006). β_2-adrenergic receptor polymorphisms and treatment-induced regression of left ventricular hypertrophy in hypertension. *Clin. Pharmacol. Ther.* 80, 633–645. doi: 10.1016/j.clpt.2006.09.006

Judd, S. E., Raiser, S. N., Kumari, M., and Tangpricha, V. (2010). 1,25-dihydroxyvitamin D3 reduces systolic blood pressure in hypertensive adults: a pilot feasibility study. *J. Steroid Biochem. Mol. Biol.* 121, 445–447. doi: 10.1016/j.jsbmb.2010.04.013

Juraschek, S. P., Guallar, E., Appel, L. J., and Miller, E. R. III. (2012). Effects of vitamin C supplementation on blood pressure: a meta-analysis of randomized controlled trials. *Am. J. Clin. Nutr.* 95, 1079–1088. doi: 10.3945/ajcn.111.027995

Kerr, S., Brosnan, M. J., McIntyre, M., Reid, J. L., Dominiczak, A. F., and Hamilton, C. A. (1999). Superoxide anion production is increased in a model of genetic hypertension: role of the endothelium. *Hypertension* 33, 1353–1358. doi: 10.1161/01.HYP.33.6.1353

Khan, B. V., Harrison, D. G., Olbrych, M. T., Alexander, R. W., and Medford, R. M. (1996). Nitric oxide regulates vascular cell adhesion molecule 1 gene expression and redox-sensitive transcriptional events in human vascular endothelial cells. *Proc. Natl. Acad. Sci. U.S.A.* 93, 9114–9119. doi: 10.1073/pnas.93.17.9114

Kim, Y. W., and Byzova, T. V. (2014). Oxidative stress in angiogenesis and vascular disease. *Blood* 123, 625–631. doi: 10.1182/blood-2013-09-512749

Kim, Y. W., West, X. Z., and Byzova, T. V. (2013). Inflammation and oxidative stress in angiogenesis and vascular disease. *J. Mol. Med.* 91, 323–328. doi: 10.1007/s00109-013-1007-3

Kimura, Y., Kawamura, M., Owada, M., Oshima, T., Murooka, M., Fujiwara, T., et al. (1999). Effectiveness of 1,25-dihydroxyvitamin D supplementation on blood pressure reduction in a pseudohypoparathyroidism patient with high renin activity. *Intern. Med.* 38, 31–35. doi: 10.2169/internalmedicine.38.31

Kizhakekuttu, T. J., and Widlansky, M. E. (2010). Natural antioxidants and hypertension: promise and challenges. *Cardiovasc. Ther.* 28, e20–e32. doi: 10.1111/j.1755-5922.2010.00137.x

Kobayashi, N., Mita, S., Yoshida, K., Honda, T., Kobayashi, T., Hara, K., et al. (2003). Celiprolol activates eNOS through the PI3K-Akt pathway and inhibits VCAM-1 Via NF-κB induced by oxidative stress. *Hypertension* 42, 1004–1013. doi: 10.1161/01.HYP.0000097547.35570.70

Kobayashi, N., Mori, Y., Nakano, S., Tsubokou, Y., Shirataki, H., and Matsuoka, H. (2001). Celiprolol stimulates endothelial nitric oxide synthase expression and improves myocardial remodeling in deoxycorticosterone acetate-salt hypertensive rats. *J. Hypertens.* 19, 795–801. doi: 10.1097/00004872-200104000-00017

Kota, S. K., Kota, S. K., Jammula, S., Meher, L. K., Panda, S., Tripathy, P. R., et al. (2011). Renin-angiotensin system activity in vitamin D deficient, obese individuals with hypertension: an urban Indian study. *Indian J. Endocrinol. Metab.* 15(Suppl. 4), S395–S401. doi: 10.4103/2230-8210.86985

Kukin, M. L., Kalman, J., Charney, R. H., Levy, D. K., Buchholz-Varley, C., Ocampo, O. N., et al. (1999). Prospective, randomized comparison of effect of long-term treatment with metoprolol or carvedilol on symptoms, exercise, ejection fraction, and oxidative stress in heart failure. *Circulation* 99, 2645–2651. doi: 10.1161/01.CIR.99.20.2645

Laursen, J. B., Rajagopalan, S., Galis, Z., Tarpey, M., Freeman, B. A., and Harrison, D. G. (1997). Role of superoxide in angiotensin II-induced but not catecholamine-induced hypertension. *Circulation* 95, 588–593. doi: 10.1161/01.CIR.95.3.588

Laursen, J. B., Somers, M., Kurz, S., McCann, L., Warnholtz, A., Freeman, B. A., et al. (2001). Endothelial regulation of vasomotion in apoE-deficient mice: implications for interactions between peroxynitrite and tetrahydrobiopterin. *Circulation* 103, 1282–1288. doi: 10.1161/01.CIR.103.9.1282

Lee, W. J., Ou, H. C., Wu, C. M., Lee, I. T., Lin, S. Y., Lin, L. Y., et al. (2009). Sesamin mitigates inflammation and oxidative stress in endothelial cells exposed to oxidized low-density lipoprotein. *J. Agric. Food Chem.* 57, 11406–11417. doi: 10.1021/jf902876p

Lerman, L. O., Nath, K. A., Rodriguez-Porcel, M., Krier, J. D., Schwartz, R. S., Napoli, C., et al. (2001). Increased oxidative stress in experimental renovascular hypertension. *Hypertension* 37(2 Pt 2), 541–546. doi: 10.1161/01.HYP.37.2.541

Li, Y. C., Kong, J., Wei, M., Chen, Z. F., Liu, S. Q., and Cao, L. P. (2002). 1,25-Dihydroxyvitamin D(3) is a negative endocrine regulator of the renin-angiotensin system. *J. Clin. Invest.* 110, 229–238. doi: 10.1172/JCI0215219

Li, Y. C., Qiao, G., Uskokovic, M., Xiang, W., Zheng, W., and Kong, J. (2004). Vitamin D: a negative endocrine regulator of the renin-angiotensin system and blood pressure. *J. Steroid Biochem. Mol. Biol.* 89–90, 387–392. doi: 10.1016/j.jsbmb.2004.03.004

Mahajan, A. S., Babbar, R., Kansal, N., Agarwal, S. K., and Ray, P. C. (2007). Antihypertensive and antioxidant action of amlodipine and vitamin C in patients of essential hypertension. *J. Clin. Biochem. Nutr.* 40, 141–147. doi: 10.3164/jcbn.40.141

Mak, I. T., and Weglicki, W. B. (1988). Protection by beta-blocking agents against free radical-mediated sarcolemmal lipid peroxidation. *Circ. Res.* 63, 262–266. doi: 10.1161/01.RES.63.1.262

Malinin, N. L., West, X. Z., and Byzova, T. V. (2011). Oxidation as "the stress of life" *Aging* 3, 906–910. doi: 10.18632/aging.100385

Mancia, G., Fagard, R., Narkiewicz, K., Redon, J., Zanchetti, A., Böhm, M., et al. (2013). 2013 ESH/ESC guidelines for the management of arterial hypertension: the Task Force for the Management of Arterial Hypertension of the European Society of Hypertension (ESH) and of the European Society of Cardiology (ESC). *Eur. Heart J.* 34, 2159–2219. doi: 10.1093/eurheartj/eht151

Marui, N., Offermann, M. K., Swerlick, R., Kunsch, C., Rosen, C. A., Ahmad, M., et al. (1993). Vascular cell adhesion molecule-1 (VCAM-1) gene transcription and expression are regulated through an antioxidant-sensitive mechanism in human vascular endothelial cells. *J. Clin. Invest.* 92, 1866–1874. doi: 10.1172/JCI116778

Mazzali, M., Hughes, J., Kim, Y. G., Jefferson, J. A., Kang, D. H., Gordon, K. L., et al. (2001). Elevated uric acid increases blood pressure in the rat by a novel crystal-independent mechanism. *Hypertension* 38, 1101–1106. doi: 10.1161/hy1101.092839

McGreevy, C., and Williams, D. (2011). New insights about vitamin D and cardiovascular disease: a narrative review. *Ann. Intern. Med.* 155, 820–826. doi: 10.7326/0003-4819-155-12-201112200-00004

McIntyre, M., Bohr, D. F., and Dominiczak, A. F. (1999). Endothelial function in hypertension: the role of superoxide anion. *Hypertension* 34(4 Pt 1), 539–545. doi: 10.1161/01.HYP.34.4.539

Mehta, J. L., Lopez, L. M., Chen, L., and Cox, O. E. (1994). Alterations in nitric oxide synthase activity, superoxide anion generation, and platelet aggregation in systemic hypertension, and effects of celiprolol. *Am. J. Cardiol.* 74, 901–905. doi: 10.1016/0002-9149(94)90583-5

Michos, E. D., and Melamed, M. L. (2008). Vitamin D and cardiovascular disease risk. *Curr. Opin. Clin. Nutr. Metab. Care* 11, 7–12. doi: 10.1097/MCO.0b013e3282f2f4dd

Mittler, R., Vanderauwera, S., Suzuki, N., Miller, G., Tognetti, V. B., Vandepoele, K., et al. (2011). ROS signaling: the new wave? *Trends Plant Sci.* 16, 300–309. doi: 10.1016/j.tplants.2011.03.007

Molinari, C., Morsanuto, V., Polli, S., and Uberti, F. (2018). Cooperative effects of Q10, Vitamin D3, and L-arginine on cardiac and endothelial cells. *J. Vasc. Res.* 55, 47–60. doi: 10.1159/000484928

Mozaffari-Khosravi, H., Loloei, S., Mirjalili, M. R., and Barzegar, K. (2015). The effect of vitamin D supplementation on blood pressure in patients with elevated blood pressure and vitamin D deficiency: a randomized, double-blind, placebo-controlled trial. *Blood Press Monit.* 20, 83–91. doi: 10.1097/MBP.0000000000000091

Nakamura, K., Murakami, M., Miura, D., Yunoki, K., Enko, K., Tanaka, M., et al. (2011). β-blockers and oxidative stress in patients with heart failure. *Pharmaceuticals* 4, 1088–1100. doi: 10.3390/ph4081088

Nigwekar, S. U., and Thadhani, R. (2013). Vitamin D receptor activation: cardiovascular and renal implications. *Kidney Int. Suppl.* 3, 427–430. doi: 10.1038/kisup.2013.89

Nishioka, S., Yoshioka, T., Nomura, A., Kato, R., Miyamura, M., Okada, Y., et al. (2013). Celiprolol reduces oxidative stress and attenuates left ventricular remodeling induced by hypoxic stress in mice. *Hypertens. Res.* 36, 934–939. doi: 10.1038/hr.2013.60

Ogun, A. O. (2015). *Biochemistry of Reactive Oxygen and Nitrogen Species, Basic Principles and Clinical Significance of Oxidative Stress.* Available online at: https://www.intechopen.com/books/basic-principles-and-clinical-significance-of-oxidative-stress/biochemistry-of-reactive-oxygen-and-nitrogen-species

Pagliaro, P., and Penna, C. (2015). Redox signalling and cardioprotection: translatability and mechanism. *Br. J. Pharmacol.* 172, 1974–1995. doi: 10.1111/bph.12975

Pagliaro, P., and Penna, C. (2017). Hypertension, hypertrophy, and reperfusion injury. *J. Cardiovasc. Med.* 18, 131–135. doi: 10.2459/JCM.0000000000000435

Pascale, A. V., Finelli, R., Giannotti, R., Visco, V., Fabbricatore, D., Matula, I., et al. (2018). Vitamin D, parathyroid hormone and cardiovascular risk: the good, the bad and the ugly. *J. Cardiovasc. Med.* 19, 62–66. doi: 10.2459/JCM.0000000000000614

Patel, R. P., McAndrew, J., Sellak, H., White, C. R., Jo, H., Freeman, B. A., et al. (1999). Biological aspects of reactive nitrogen species. *Biochim. Biophys. Acta* 1411, 385–400. doi: 10.1016/S0005-2728(99)00028-6

Pfeifer, M., Begerow, B., Minne, H. W., Nachtigall, D., and Hansen, C. (2001). Effects of a short-term vitamin D(3) and calcium supplementation on blood pressure and parathyroid hormone levels in elderly women. *J. Clin. Endocrinol. Metab.* 86, 1633–1637. doi: 10.1210/jcem.86.4.7393

Pittarella, P., Squarzanti, D. F., Molinari, C., Invernizzi, M., Uberti, F., and Renò, F. (2015). NO-dependent proliferation and migration induced by Vitamin D in HUVEC. *J. Steroid Biochem. Mol. Biol.* 149, 35–42. doi: 10.1016/j.jsbmb.2014.12.012

Quinlan, C. L., Perevoshchikova, I. V., Hey-Mogensen, M., Orr, A. L., and Brand, M. D. (2013). Sites of reactive oxygen species generation by mitochondria oxidizing different substrates. *Redox Biol.* 1, 304–312. doi: 10.1016/j.redox.2013.04.005

Radi, R., Cassina, A., Hodara, R., Quijano, C., and Castro, L. (2002). Peroxynitrite reactions and formation in mitochondria. *Free Radic Biol. Med.* 33, 1451–1464. doi: 10.1016/S0891-5849(02)01111-5

Ramchandra, R., Barrett, C. J., and Malpas, S. C. (2005). Nitric oxide and sympathetic nerve activity in the control of blood pressure. *Clin. Exp. Pharmacol. Physiol.* 32, 440–446. doi: 10.1111/j.1440-1681.2005.04208.x

Ristow, M., and Schmeisser, K. (2014). Mitohormesis: promoting health and lifespan by increased levels of Reactive Oxygen Species (ROS). *Dose Response* 12, 288–341. doi: 10.2203/dose-response.13-035.Ristow

Rodrigo, R., González, J., and Paoletto, F. (2011). The role of oxidative stress in the pathophysiology of hypertension. *Hypertens. Res.* 34, 431–440. doi: 10.1038/hr.2010.264

Rodrigo, R., Prat, H., Passalacqua, W., Araya, J., Guichard, C., and Bächler, J. P. (2007). Relationship between oxidative stress and essential hypertension. *Hypertens. Res.* 30, 1159–1167. doi: 10.1291/hypres.30.1159

Ruef, J., Hu, Z. Y., Yin, L. Y., Wu, Y., Hanson, S. R., Kelly, A. B., et al. (1997). Induction of vascular endothelial growth factor in balloon-injured baboon arteries. A novel role for reactive oxygen species in atherosclerosis. *Circ. Res.* 81, 24–33. doi: 10.1161/01.RES.81.1.24

Sena, L. A., and Chandel, N. S. (2012). Physiological roles of mitochondrial reactive oxygen species. *Mol. Cell* 48, 158–167. doi: 10.1016/j.molcel.2012.09.025

Somers, M. J., Mavromatis, K., Galis, Z. S., and Harrison, D. G. (2000). Vascular superoxide production and vasomotor function in hypertension induced by deoxycorticosterone acetate-salt. *Circulation* 101, 1722–1728. doi: 10.1161/01.CIR.101.14.1722

Sorriento, D., Trimarco, B., and Iaccarino, G. (2011). Adrenergic mechanism in the control of endothelial function. *Transl. Med. UniSa.* 1, 213–228.

Tamez, H., Kalim, S., and Thadhani, R. I. (2013). Does vitamin D modulate blood pressure? *Curr. Opin. Nephrol. Hypertens.* 22, 204–209. doi: 10.1097/MNH.0b013e32835d919b

Tanaka, H., Kataoka, M., Isobe, S., Yamamoto, T., Shirakawa, K., Endo, J., et al. (2017). Therapeutic impact of dietary vitamin D supplementation for preventing right ventricular remodeling and improving survival in pulmonary hypertension. *PLoS ONE* 12:e0180615. doi: 10.1371/journal.pone.0180615

Tomaschitz, A., Pilz, S., Ritz, E., Grammer, T., Drechsler, C., Boehm, B. O., et al. (2010). Independent association between 1,25-dihydroxyvitamin D, 25-hydroxyvitamin D and the renin-angiotensin system: the Ludwigshafen Risk and Cardiovascular Health (LURIC) study. *Clin. Chim. Acta* 411, 1354–1360. doi: 10.1016/j.cca.2010.05.037

Touyz, R. M., and Briones, A. M. (2011). Reactive oxygen species and vascular biology: implications in human hypertension. *Hypertens. Res.* 34, 5–14. doi: 10.1038/hr.2010.201

Touyz, R. M., and Schiffrin, E. L. (2001). Increased generation of superoxide by angiotensin II in smooth muscle cells from resistance arteries of hypertensive patients: role of phospholipase D-dependent NAD(P)H oxidase-sensitive pathways. *J. Hypertens.* 19, 1245–1254. doi: 10.1097/00004872-200107000-00009

Touyz, R. M., and Schiffrin, E. L. (2004). Reactive oxygen species in vascular biology: implications in hypertension. *Histochem. Cell Biol.* 122, 339–352. doi: 10.1007/s00418-004-0696-7

Ullah, M. I., Uwaifo, G. I., Nicholas, W. C., and Koch, C. A. (2010). Does vitamin d deficiency cause hypertension? Current evidence from clinical studies and potential mechanisms. *Int. J. Endocrinol.* 2010:579640. doi: 10.1155/2010/579640

Ushio-Fukai, M., Tang, Y., Fukai, T., Dikalov, S. I., Ma, Y., Fujimoto, M., et al. (2002). Novel role of gp91(phox)-containing NAD(P)H oxidase in vascular endothelial growth factor-induced signaling and angiogenesis. *Circ. Res.* 91, 1160–1167. doi: 10.1161/01.RES.0000046227.65158.F8

Vaziri, N. D., Ni, Z., Oveisi, F., and Trnavsky-Hobbs, D. L. (2000). Effect of antioxidant therapy on blood pressure and NO synthase expression in hypertensive rats. *Hypertension* 36, 957–964. doi: 10.1161/01.HYP.36.6.957

Vimaleswaran, K. S., Cavadino, A., Berry, D. J., LifeLines Cohort, Study, i, Jorde, R., Dieffenbach, A. K., et al. (2014). Association of vitamin D status with arterial blood pressure and hypertension risk: a mendelian randomisation study. *Lancet Diabetes Endocrinol.* 2, 719–729. doi: 10.1016/S2213-8587(14)70113-5

Vishnu, A., and Ahuja, V. (2017). Vitamin D and blood pressure among U.S. adults: a cross-sectional examination by race/ethnicity and gender. *Am. J. Prev. Med.* 53, 670–679 doi: 10.1016/j.amepre.2017.07.006

Wang, Y., Zhang, F., Liu, Y., Yin, S., Pang, X., Li, Z., et al. (2017). Nebivolol alleviates aortic remodeling through eNOS upregulation and inhibition of oxidative stress in l-NAME-induced hypertensive rats. *Clin. Exp. Hypertens.* 39, 628–639. doi: 10.1080/10641963.2017.1306539

Ward, N. C., and Croft, K. D. (2006). Hypertension and oxidative stress. *Clin. Exp. Pharmacol. Physiol.* 33, 872–876. doi: 10.1111/j.1440-1681.2006.04457.x

Ward, N. C., Hodgson, J. M., Croft, K. D., Burke, V., Beilin, L. J., and Puddey, I. B. (2005). The combination of vitamin C and grape-seed polyphenols increases blood pressure: a randomized, double-blind, placebo-controlled trial. *J. Hypertens.* 23, 427–434. doi: 10.1097/00004872-200502000-00026

Whelton, P. K., Carey, R. M., Aronow, W. S., Casey, D. E. Jr., Collins, K. J., Dennison Himmelfarb, C., et al. (2017). 2017 ACC/AHA/AAPA/ABC/ACPM/AGS/APhA/ASH/ASPC/NMA/PCNA guideline for the prevention, detection, evaluation, and management of high blood pressure in adults: a report of the American College of Cardiology/American Heart Association Task Force on clinical practice guidelines. *Hypertension.* 12, 238. doi: 10.1016/j.jacc.2017.11.006

Wong, M. S., Delansorne, R., Man, R. Y., Svenningsen, P., and Vanhoutte, P. M. (2010). Chronic treatment with vitamin D lowers arterial blood pressure and reduces endothelium-dependent contractions in the aorta of the spontaneously hypertensive rat. *Am. J. Physiol. Heart. Circ. Physiol.* 299, H1226–H1234. doi: 10.1152/ajpheart.00288.2010

Wu, L., and Sun, D. (2017). Effects of calcium plus vitamin D supplementation on blood pressure: a systematic review and meta-analysis of randomized controlled trials. *J. Hum. Hypertens.* 31, 547–554. doi: 10.1038/jhh.2017.12

Wu, R., Millette, E., Wu, L., and de Champlain, J. (2001). Enhanced superoxide anion formation in vascular tissues from spontaneously hypertensive and desoxycorticosterone acetate-salt hypertensive rats. *J. Hypertens.* 19, 741–748. doi: 10.1097/00004872-200104000-00011

Yao, E. H., Fukuda, N., Matsumoto, T., Katakawa, M., Yamamoto, C., Han, Y., et al. (2008). Effects of the antioxidative beta-blocker celiprolol on endothelial progenitor cells in hypertensive rats. *Am. J. Hypertens.* 21, 1062–1068. doi: 10.1038/ajh.2008.233

Yusoff, N. S. N., Mustapha, Z., Sharif, S. E. T., Govindasamy, C., and Sirajudeen, K. N. S. (2017). Effect of antihypertensive drug treatment on oxidative stress markers in heart of spontaneously hypertensive rat models. *J. Environ. Pathol. Toxicol. Oncol.* 36, 43–53. doi: 10.1615/JEnvironPatholToxicolOncol.2017014521

Zhou, C., Lu, F., Cao, K., Xu, D., Goltzman, D., and Miao, D. (2008). Calcium-independent and $1{,}25(OH)_2D_3$-dependent regulation of the renin-angiotensin system in 1α-hydroxylase knockout mice. *Kidney Int.* 74, 170–179. doi: 10.1038/ki.2008.101

16

Rat Pial Microvascular Changes During Cerebral Blood Flow Decrease and Recovery: Effects of Cyanidin Administration

Teresa Mastantuono [1], Martina Di Maro [1], Martina Chiurazzi [1], Laura Battiloro [1], Espedita Muscariello [1], Gilda Nasti [1], Noemy Starita [2], Antonio Colantuoni [1] and Dominga Lapi [1]*

[1] Department of Clinical Medicine and Surgery, "Federico II" University Medical School, Naples, Italy, [2] Molecular Biology and Viral Oncology Unit, Istituto Nazionale Tumori IRCCS - "Fond. G. Pascale", Naples, Italy

Edited by:
Pasquale Pagliaro,
Università degli Studi di Torino, Italy

Reviewed by:
Francesco Moccia,
University of Pavia, Italy
Maria Carmela Cerra,
University of Calabria, Italy

***Correspondence:**
Teresa Mastantuono
teresa.mastantuono@libero.it

The reactive oxygen species (ROS) are known to play a major role in many pathophysiological conditions, such as ischemia and reperfusion injury. The present study was aimed to evaluate the *in vivo* cyanidin (anthocyanin) effects on damages induced by rat pial microvascular hypoperfusion-reperfusion injury by cerebral blood flow decrease (CBFD) and subsequent cerebral blood flow recovery (CBFR). In particular, the main purpose was to detect changes in ROS production after cyanidin administration. Rat pial microvasculature was investigated using fluorescence microscopy through a cranial window (closed); Strahler's method was utilized to define the geometric features of pial vessels. ROS production was investigated *in vivo* by 2′-7′-dichlorofluorescein-diacetate assay and neuronal damage was measured on isolated brain sections by 2,3,5-triphenyltetrazolium chloride staining. After 30 min of CBFD, induced by bilateral common carotid artery occlusion, and 60 min of CBFR, rats showed decrease of arteriolar diameter and capillary perfusion; furthermore, increase in microvascular leakage and leukocyte adhesion was observed. Conversely, cyanidin administration induced dose-related arteriolar dilation, reduction in microvascular permeability as well as leukocyte adhesion when compared to animals subjected to restriction of cerebral blood flow; moreover, capillary perfusion was protected. ROS generation increase and marked neuronal damage were detected in animals subjected to CBFD and CBFR. On the other hand, cyanidin was able to reduce ROS generation and neuronal damage. In conclusion, cyanidin treatment showed dose-related protective effects on rat pial microcirculation during CBFD and subsequent CBFR, inducing arteriolar dilation by nitric oxide release and inhibiting ROS formation, consequently preserving the blood brain barrier integrity.

Keywords: cyanidin, cerebral blood flow reduction, reperfusion, pial microcirculation, reactive oxygen species, neuronal damage

INTRODUCTION

Many evidences indicate that a diet rich in antioxidants is associate to a decreased incidence of cardiovascular diseases, such as stroke, acute myocardial disease or cancer (Galvano et al., 2004; Lapi et al., 2016). Anthocyanins, belonging to polyphenol family, are one of the natural antioxidants responsible of fruit and flower colors (red, orange and blue) and play an important role in counteracting the oxidative stress induced by reactive oxygen species (ROS). These radicals have been related to different pathophysiological conditions (Serraino et al., 2003; Accetta et al., 2016; Mondola et al., 2016). Higher ROS production, indeed, appears to be associated to the pathogenesis of ischemia/reperfusion injury (Tsuda et al., 1999). On the other hand, the protective role of natural anthocyanins has been demonstrated to be effective against ischemia/reperfusion injury in different organs, such as kidney, heart and intestine (Jakesevic et al., 2013; Quintieri et al., 2013; Isaak et al., 2017). Moreover, we previously demonstrated the protective effects of Vaccinium myrtillus extract supplementation to the diet (containing 34.7% of anthocyanins) on hamster pial microcirculation during brain hypoperfusion-reperfusion. In particular, after 2, 4, and 6 months of oral supplementation, anthocyanins were able to counteract microvascular changes such as arteriolar vasoconstriction, increase of microvascular permeability and leukocyte adhesion (Mastantuono et al., 2016).

Cyanidin, belonging to the anthocyanin family, has been widely studied in *in vivo* and *in vitro* models (Galvano et al., 2004). In particular, Aguirre et al. and Fratantonio et al. observed that Cyanidin-3-O-glucoside presents many properties, such as anti-inflammatory and anti-tumor effects (Fratantonio et al., 2016; Olivas-Aguirre et al., 2016). Furthermore, this substance appears to enhance the release of nitric oxide (NO) and other vasodilating factors, thereby improving endothelial-dependent vasodilation (Sivasinprasasn et al., 2016). It is worth noting that ORAC (oxygen radical absorbance capacity) activity is highest for cyanidin compared to other anthocyanins (Zheng and Wang, 2003). Tsuda et al. have demonstrated that rats, treated with an orally administered Cyanidin-3-O-glucoside for 14 days, were preserved from hepatic I/R damage (Tsuda et al., 1999).

The aim of this study was to investigate the *in vivo* effects of cyanidin on oxidative stress and changes in rat pial microvasculature determined by 30 min of cerebral blood flow decrease (CBFD) and 60 min of cerebral blood flow recovery (CBFR). To do this, we evaluated ROS production during CBFD and CBFR, respectively, and assessed the antioxidant properties of cyanidin using 2′-7′-dichlorofluorescein-diacetate (DCFH-DA) assay. Finally, the neuronal damage was quantified by 2,3,5-triphenyltetrazolium chloride (TTC) staining.

MATERIALS AND METHODS

Experimental Groups

Experiments were carried out utilizing male Wistar rats, 250–300g (Harlan, Italy), randomly assigned to three groups, as reported in **Table 1**: (1) sham group (SO group), subjected to the same surgical procedure of the other experimental groups without changes in cerebral blood flow; (2) reduced blood flow group (RF group) and (3) cyanidin-treated group (Cy group) underwent 30 min CBFD plus 60 min CBFR.

SO animals were divided in subgroups: (a) SO-Na subgroup ($n = 14$) was injected with intravenous (i.v.) saline solution (0.9% NaCl); (b) SO-Cy subgroup ($n = 10$), successively divided in SO-Cy_1 ($n = 5$) and SO-Cy_2 ($n = 5$) subgroups, received i.v. cyanidin, 10 mg/kg body weight (b.w.) or 20 mg/kg b.w., respectively; (c) SO-L subgroup ($n = 5$) was infused with i.v. N5-(1-iminoethyl)-L-ornithine (L-NIO), 10 mg/kg b.w. The animals of each subgroup received the substances twice within 40 min interval.

RF group ($n = 14$) was injected with i.v. saline solution (0.9% NaCl), 10 min before the CBFD and at the beginning of CBFR.

Cy group was differentiated in the following subgroups: (a) Cy_1 ($n = 14$) and Cy_2 ($n = 14$), administered with i.v. cyanidin, 10 mg/kg b.w. or 20 mg/kg b.w., respectively, 10 min before the CBFD and at the beginning of CBFR; (b) L/Cy_2 subgroup ($n = 14$) was administered with i.v. L-NIO, 10 mg/kg b.w., prior to i.v. higher dosage cyanidin (20 mg/kg b.w.).

Five animals for SO-Na subgroup, RF and Cy groups were investigated by *in vivo* fluorescence microscopy, to detect microcirculation damage; six rats were utilized to assess oxidative stress by DCFH-DA assay after CBFD ($n = 3$) and after CBFR ($n = 3$); in three animals tissue damage was evaluated by TTC staining. The rats belonging to the SO-Cy_2 and SO-L subgroups were utilized only for microcirculation investigations.

Drug Administration

Each utilized drug (cyanidin or L-NIO) was dissolved in 0.5 mL saline solution and, successively, i.v. injected to rats within 3 min, 10 min before CBFD and at the beginning of CBFR.

We tested the effects of two cyanidin doses: 10 or 20 mg/kg b.w. Pilot experiments indicated that cyanidin dosages below 10 mg/kg b.w. were ineffective on the pial microvasculature; on the other hand, dosages higher than 20 mg/kg b.w. did not improve microvascular protection detected in the animals administered with 20 mg/kg b.w cyanidin before and after CBFD. In **Table 2** we reported the data about animals treated with cyanidin at a dosage of 5 mg/kg or 30 mg/kg b.w (chosen as reference values) administered 10 min before CBFD and at the beginning of CBFR.

Moreover, L-NIO, known to inhibit the NO release (Moreau et al., 1995; Lapi et al., 2012), was administered at the dosage of 10 mg/kg b.w., 10 min before i.v. infusion of higher dosage cyanidin (20 mg/kg b.w.). In pilot experiments L-NIO, 10 mg/kg b.w., was effective in blunting arteriolar dilation determined by i.v. injection of 10 mg/4 min L-arginine (diameter increase by 22.8 $\pm$ 2.0%, compared to basal values) or in abolishing vasodilation due to topical administration of 100 μM acetylcholine (diameter increase by 5.0 $\pm$ 1.5%, compared to basal values).

The protocol of drug administration was previously described (Lapi et al., 2016). Appropriately mixing 2′-7′-dichlorofluorescein-diacetate (DCFH-DA) and artificial cerebrospinal fluid (aCSF) allowed us to superfuse the pial layer with 250 mM DCFH-DA solution (Watanabe, 1998) for 30 min after CBFD. Sigma Chemical, St. Louis, MO, USA supplied all drugs.

TABLE 1 | Number of animals (N), experimental protocol and treatment of each group.

Group	Subgroup	N	Experimental protocol	Treatment
SO	SO-Na	14	Same surgical procedure as in the other experimental groups without changes in cerebral blood flow	saline solution, twice within 40 min interval
	SO-Cy_1	5	Same surgical procedure as in the other experimental groups without changes in cerebral blood flow	10 mg/kg b.w. cyanidin, twice within 40 min interval
	SO-Cy_2	5	Same surgical procedure as in the other experimental groups without changes in cerebral blood flow	20 mg/kg b.w. cyanidin, twice within 40 min interval
	SO-L	5	Same surgical procedure as in the other experimental groups without changes in cerebral blood flow	10 mg/kg b.w. L-NIO, twice within 40 min interval
RF		14	30 min CBFD plus 60 min CBFR	saline solution,10 min before CBFD and CBFR
Cy	Cy_1	14	30 min CBFD plus 60 min CBFR	10 mg/kg b.w. cyanidin,10 min before CBFD and CBFR
	Cy_2	14	30 min CBFD plus 60 min CBFR	20 mg/kg b.w. cyanidin,10 min before CBFD and CBFR
	L/Cy_2	14	30 min CBFD plus 60 min CBFR	10 mg/kg b.w. L-NIO, prior to higher dosage cyanidin

TABLE 2 | Variations of the main parameters in the two pilot groups: Cy_A and Cy_B subgroup (rats treated with cyanidin at the doses of 5 mg/kg b.w. or 30 mg/kg b.w) and subjected to 30 min CBFR and 60 min CBFR, compared with RF group and Cy_2 subgroup.

Groups	Number of animals/ arterioles (n)	Percent diameter changes (%)		Microvascular leakage (NGL)	Leukocyte adhesion (number of leukocyte/100 μm of venular length/30s)	Capillary perfusion (BFCL) (% reduction compared to baseline)
		After 30 min CBFD	After 60 min CBFR	After 60 min CBFR		
RF group	5/25	$85.0 \pm 2.5^{\#}$	$75 \pm 3^{\#}$	$0.48 \pm 0.03^{\#}$	$10 \pm 2^{\#}$	$48 \pm 4^{\#}$
Cy_A subgroup	5/25	$90.5 \pm 3.0^{\#}$	$80.0 \pm 2.5^{\#}$	$0.40 \pm 0.02^{\#}$	$8 \pm 2^{\#}$	$40 \pm 5^{\#}$
Cy_B subgroup	5/25	$134 \pm 3.5^{\wedge}$	$140 \pm 4^{\wedge}$	$0.24 \pm 0.02^{\wedge}$	$4 \pm 1^{\wedge}$	$12 \pm 2^{\wedge}$
Cy_2 subgroup	5/25	$130 \pm 3^{\wedge}$	$138.0 \pm 3.5^{\wedge}$	$0.25 \pm 0.03^{\wedge}$	$5 \pm 2^{\wedge}$	$14 \pm 3^{\wedge}$

Data are reported as Mean ± SEM; $^{\#}p < 0.01$ vs. Cy_A and Cy_2 subgroup, $^{\wedge}p < 0.01$ vs. RF group and Cy_B subgroup.

Rat Preparation

All experiments conform to the Guide for the Care and Use of Laboratory Animals published by the US National Institutes of Health (NIH Publication No. 85-23, revised 1996) and to institutional rules for the care and handling of experimental animals, as previously reported (Lapi et al., 2012). The protocol was approved by the "Federico II" University Medical School of Naples, Ethical Committee (n° 2011/0059997, 24/05/2011).

Rats were anesthetized with intra peritoneal (i.p.) injection of α-chloralose, (60 mg/kg b.w. for induction; afterward 30 mg/kg b.w.) and mechanically ventilated after tracheotomy, according to the protocol previously reported (Lapi et al., 2012). Briefly, two catheters were placed, one in the right femoral artery and the other in the left femoral vein, respectively, for the measurement of arterial blood pressure and to inject the fluorescent tracers [fluorescein isothiocyanate bound to dextran, molecular weight 70 kDa (FD 70), 50 mg/100 g b.w., as 5% wt/vol solution in 3 min just once at the start of experiment after 30 min of the preparation stabilization; rhodamine 6G, 1 mg/100 g b.w. in 0.3 mL, as a bolus with supplemental injection throughout CBFD and CBFR (final volume 0.3 mL·100 g−1·h−1) to label leukocytes for adhesion evaluation]. Both carotid arteries were prepared for clamping.

Blood gases were measured on arterial blood samples at 30 min intervals (ABL5; Radiometer, Copenhagen, Denmark). The parameters monitored in all animals were: heart rate, mean arterial blood pressure, respiratory CO_2 and blood gases values. They were stable within physiological ranges. Rectal temperature was recorded and maintained at 37.0 ± 0.5°C, as previously reported (Lapi et al., 2016).

The visualization of pial microvasculature was carried out as previously reported (Morii et al., 1986; Ngai et al., 1988; Lapi et al., 2012). Briefly, a closed cranial window was positioned at the level of the left frontoparietal cortex through an incision in the skin to operate a craniotomy. Cerebral cortex was preserved by overheating caused by drilling with saline solution superfusion of the skull. The dura mater was gently cut and displayed on the corner; a quarz microscope coverglass was bound to the skull bone. Artificial cerebrospinal fluid was superfused the cerebral surface with a rate of 0.5 mL/min. The composition of the aCSF was 119.0 mM NaCl, 2.5 mM KCl, 1.3 mM MgSO4•7H2O, 1.0 mM NaH2PO4, 26.2 mM NaHCO3, 2.5 mM CaCl2 and 11.0 mM glucose (equilibrated with 10.0% O2, 6.0% CO2 and 84.0% N2; pH 7.38 ± 0.02).

The decrease in cerebral blood flow (CBFD) was produced by clamping both common carotid arteries, previously prepared. The clamping was removed after 30 min; thereafter the pial microvasculature was investigated during the recovery of cerebral blood flow (CBFR), lasting 60 min (Hudetz et al., 1985).

Fluorescence Microscopy

A fluorescence microscope was utilized to study pial microvascular networks as previously described

(Lapi et al., 2012). In brief, the microscope (Leitz Orthoplan, Wetzlar, Germany) was equipped with long-distance objectives (2.5 x, numerical aperture (NA) 0.08; 10 x, NA 0.20; 20 x, NA 0.25; 32 x, NA 0.40) a 10x eyepiece. Moreover, a x10 eyepiece and a filter block (Ploemopak, Leitz) were used. A 100-Watt mercury lamp was used for epiillumination with the corresponding filters for FITC and rhodamine 6G. A heat filter prevented overheating of the preparations (Leitz KG1). Pial microvascular networks were televised with a DAGE MTI 300 low-light level camera and stored through a computer-based frame grabber (Pinnacle DC 10 plus, Avid Technology, Burlington, MA, USA).

Geometric Detection of Microvascular Network

In each animal, first we characterized the arteriolar network by stop-frame images and pial arterioles were assigned order according to Strahler's method, starting from capillaries to the largest arterioles (centripetal method), as previously reported (Kassab et al., 1993; Lapi et al., 2008). In each experiment we studied one order 4 arteriole, two order 3 and two order 2 arterioles. Furthermore, we assessed the functional changes of each arteriolar order under the experimental conditions. We report, however, the results detected in order 2 arterioles.

Microvascular Parameter Assessment

Microvascular parameters were measured off-line utilizing a computerized imaging technique, previously described in details by Lapi et al. (2012) and Lapi et al. (2016). Concisely, arteriolar diameters were measured with a computerized method, Microvascular Imaging Program (MIP), frame by frame. The increase in permeability was measured by evaluating fluorescent dextran extravasation from venules and expressed as normalized gray levels (NGL): NGL = (I − Ir)/Ir, where Ir is the baseline gray level at the microvasculature filling with fluorescence, and I is the value at the end of CBFD or CBFR. Gray levels were obtained using the MIP image program by average of 5 windows, measuring 50 × 50 mM (10x objective) and located outside the venules. During recordings the same regions of interest were localized by a computer-assisted device for XY movement of the microscope table.

Leukocytes sticking to the vessel walls (45 venules for every group) over a 30-s time-period were reported as number of adherent cells/100 μm of venular length (v.l.)/30 s, utilizing appropriate magnification (20 x and 32 x, objectives) (Lapi et al., 2012). Perfused capillaries were evaluated as the length of the capillaries showing blood flow (BFCL), assessed by MIP image in an area of 150 × 150 μm (Lapi et al., 2016).

A Gould Windograf recorder (model 13-6615-10S, Gould, OH, USA) was utilized to record arterial blood pressure (mean), by Viggo-Spectramed P10E2 transducer; Oxnard, CA, USA, linked to catheterized femoral artery, and heart rate, as previously reported (Lapi et al., 2012). We measured the arterial blood gases (ABL5; Radiometer, Copenhagen, Denmark) at 30 min intervals, as previously reported (Lapi et al., 2012), as well as the hematocrit in basal conditions, at the end of CBFD and CBFR.

ROS Production Evaluation

Superfusion of the pial layer with artificial cerebrospinal fluid, containing 250 mM 2′-7′-dichlorofluorescein-diacetate (DCFH-DA) at 37.0 ± 0.5°, was carried out after 30 min CBFD ($n = 3$) or 60 min CBFR ($n = 3$), as previously reported (Lapi et al., 2013). DCFH-DA is widely used as a marker for oxidative stress of the cells and tissues (Wang and Joseph, 1999). DCF fluorescence intensity, related to the intracellular ROS level, was assessed using an appropriate filter (522 nm) and measured by NGL (Watanabe, 1998).

Tissue Damage Estimation

At the end of CBFR, rats were sacrificed to evaluate tissue damage. The brains were isolated and rostro-caudally cut into coronal sections (1 mm) with a vibratome (Campden Instrument, 752 M; Lafayette, IN, USA). Slices were incubated in 2% 2,3,5-triphenyltetrazolium chloride (TTC) (20 min) at 37°C and in 10% formalin overnight, as previously reported (Lapi et al., 2013). TTC, a white salt, is reduced to red 1,3,5-triphenylformazan by dehydrogenases in living cells. The location and extent of necrotic areas were assessed by computerized image analysis (Image-Pro Plus; Rockville, MD, USA). Moreover, the infarct size was quantified by manual measurements, according to the following formula: [(area of nonhypoperfused, or area not subjected to cerebral blood flow decrease, cortex or striatum − area of remaining hypoperfused, or area subjected to cerebral blood flow decrease, cortex or striatum)/area of nonhypoprfused cortex or striatum] × 100 (Bederson et al., 1986).

Statistical Analysis

All data were reported as mean ± SEM. Normal distribution of data was assessed with the Kolmogorov-Smirnov test. Parametric (Student's t-tests, ANOVA and Bonferroni post hoc test) or nonparametric tests (Wilcoxon, Mann-Whitney and Kruskal-Wallis tests) were utilized, according to data distribution; diameter and length data among experimental groups were compared with nonparametric tests, as previously reported (Lapi et al., 2016). Data derived from DCFH-DA treated rats were analyzed with non-parametric tests. SPSS 14.0 statistical package (IBM Italia, Segrate, MI, Italy) was used. Statistical significance was set at $p < 0.05$.

RESULTS

Under baseline conditions, Sthraler's method was used to differentiate arterioles in pial microvascular networks of all animals according to a centripetal scheme (Lapi et al., 2008). In particular, five orders of arterioles were observed, assigning order 5 to the largest vessels (mean diameter 62.6 ± 4.5 μm) up to the smallest ones, identified as order 1 (mean diameter: 15.8 ± 2.0 μm). Order 0 was assigned to the capillaries, sprouting from order 1 arterioles.

SO Group

After the investigation period, no differences in microvascular parameters were detected in SO-Na subgroup, as reported in **Table 3** and **Figure 1**. Furthermore, DCF fluorescence intensity

TABLE 3 | Variations of the main parameters at the end of reperfusion in SO-Na subgroup (SO-Na), reduced blood flow group (RF), lower dosage cyanidin-treated subgroup (Cy_1), higher dosage cyanidin-treated subgroup (Cy_2) and higher dosage cyanidin plus L-NIO-treated subgroup (L/Cy_2).

Groups	Number of animals/arterioles (n)	Microvascular leakage (NGL)	Leukocyte adhesion (number of leukocyte/100 μm of venular length/30 s)	Capillary perfusion (BFCL) (% reduction compared to baseline)
SO-Na subgroup	5/25	0.02 ± 0.01	2 ± 1	0 ± 5
RF group	5/25	$0.48 \pm 0.03^{\S\circ}$	$10 \pm 2^{\S\circ}$	$48 \pm 4^{\S\circ}$
Cy_1 subgroup	5/25	$0.36 \pm 0.02^{\S\circ *}$	$7 \pm 1^{\S\circ *}$	$22 \pm 6^{\S\circ *}$
Cy_2 subgroup	5/25	$0.25 \pm 0.03^{\S\circ *}$	$5 \pm 2^{*}$	$14 \pm 3^{\S\circ *}$
L/Cy_2 subgroup	5/25	$0.27 \pm 0.02^{\S\circ *}$	$6 \pm 1^{*}$	$17 \pm 5^{\S\circ *}$

Leukocyte adhesion: n = 45 venules for each entry. Data are reported as Mean ± SEM; $^{\S}p < 0.01$ vs. baseline; $^{\circ}p < 0.01$ vs. SO-Na subgroup; $^{*}p < 0.01$ vs. RF group.

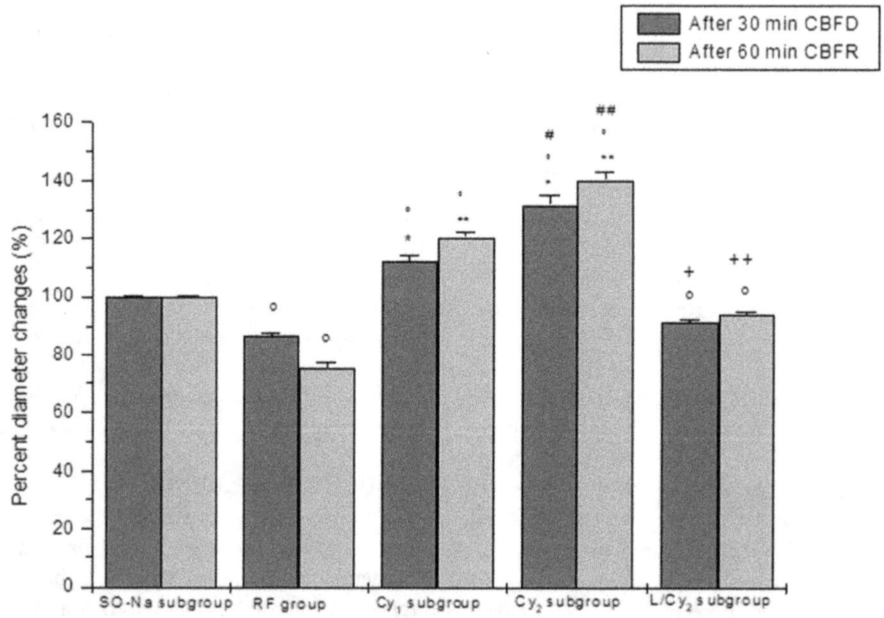

FIGURE 1 | Diameter changes of order 2 arterioles, expressed in percent of baseline after 30 min cerebral blood flow reduction (CBFD) and after 60 min cerebral blood flow recovery (CBFR), in SO-Na subgroup (SO-Na), reduced blood flow group (RF), lower dosage cyanidin-treated subgroup (Cy_1), higher dosage cyanidin-treated subgroup (Cy_2) and higher dosage cyanidin plus L-NIO-treated subgroup (L/Cy_2). Data are reported as Mean ± SEM. $^{\circ}p < 0.01$ vs. SO-Na subgroup; $^{*}p < 0.01$ vs. RF group after 30 min CBFD; $^{**}p < 0.01$ vs. RF group after 60 min CBFR; $^{+}p < 0.01$ vs. Cy_2 subgroup after 30 min CBFD; $^{++}p < 0.01$ vs. Cy_2 subgroup after 60 min CBFR; $^{\#}p < 0.01$ vs. Cy_1 subgroup after 30 min CBFD; $^{\#\#}p < 0.01$ vs. Cy_1 subgroup after 60 min CBFR.

did not change (0.04 ± 0.02 NGL) in the animals belonging to the SO-Na subgroup, superfused with DCFH-DA (**Figure 3A**).

Cyanidin injection caused arteriolar dilation in dose-related manner: order 2 arteriole diameter increased by 15.1 ± 1.8 and 34.6 ± 2.4% of baseline ($p < 0.01$ vs. baseline) in the rats of SO-Cy_1 and SO-Cy_2 subgroups, respectively. However, no significant changes in the other microvascular parameters and DCF fluorescence intensity were observed. Furthermore, after L-NIO injection, no significant variations of all parameters were detected in the animals of the SO-L subgroup.

RF Group

The decrease in cerebral blood flow for 30 min was accompanied by a reduction in diameter of all arteriolar orders with a decrease by 13.8 ± 1.5% of baseline in order 2 arterioles ($p < 0.01$ vs. baseline: mean diameter 25.6 ± 2.2 μm, and SO-Na subgroup; **Figure 1**). Leakage of fluorescent dextran was detected along the venules, indicating increased microvascular permeability (0.27 ± 0.02 NGL; $p < 0.01$ vs. baseline and SO-Na subgroup). Furthermore, fluorescence intensity increase was observed in animals subjected to DCFH-DA superfusion, demonstrating an increased ROS generation (**Figure 3A**).

At the end of CBFR, all arteriolar orders presented a decrease in diameter when compared to baseline. Order 2 arteriole diameter diminished by 24.5 ± 2.0% of baseline ($p < 0.01$ vs. baseline and SO-Na subgroup; **Figure 1**). Moreover, dextran leakage significantly increased indicating marked microvascular permeability (0.48 ± 0.03 NGL; $p < 0.01$ vs. baseline and SO-Na subgroup); there was also increase in leukocytes adhesion (10 ± 2/100 μm v.l./30 s; $p < 0.01$ vs. baseline and SO-Na subgroup; **Figures 2A,B**). BFCL was reduced by 48.0 ± 4.0% of baseline

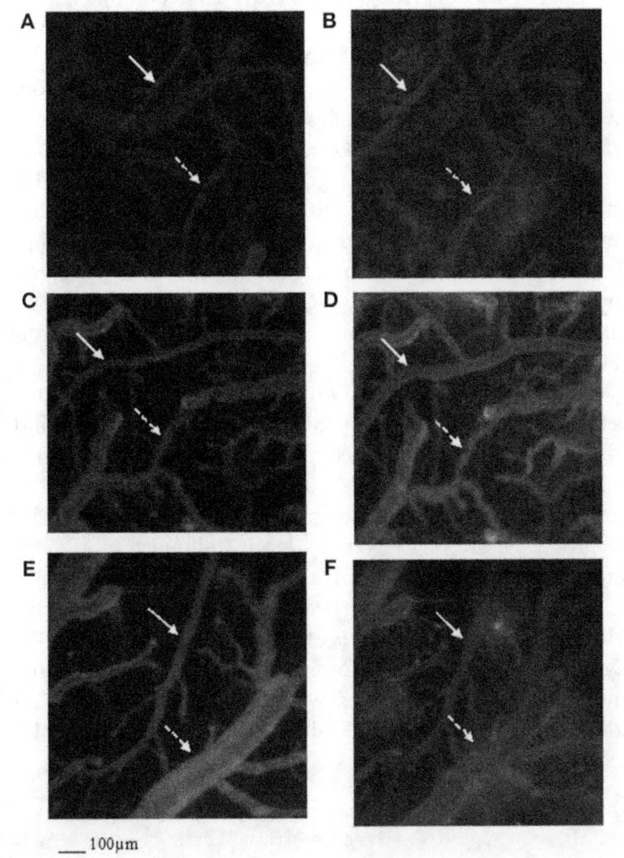

FIGURE 2 | Computer-assisted images of the pial microvascular network under baseline conditions **(A)** and after cerebral blood flow decrease and recovery **(B)** in a rat of RF group: the increase in microvascular leakage is outlined by the marked change in the color of interstitium (from black to white). Computer-assisted images of the pial microvascular network under baseline conditions **(C)** and after cerebral blood flow decrease and recovery **(D)** in a higher dosage cyanidin-treated animal: no leakage of fluorescent-dextran was detected. Computer-assisted images of the pial microvascular network under baseline conditions **(E)** and after cerebral blood flow decrease and recovery **(F)** in a higher dosage cyanidin-treated plus L-NIO-treated rat. The arterioles are indicated by the white arrows, while the venules are outlined by dashed white arrows.

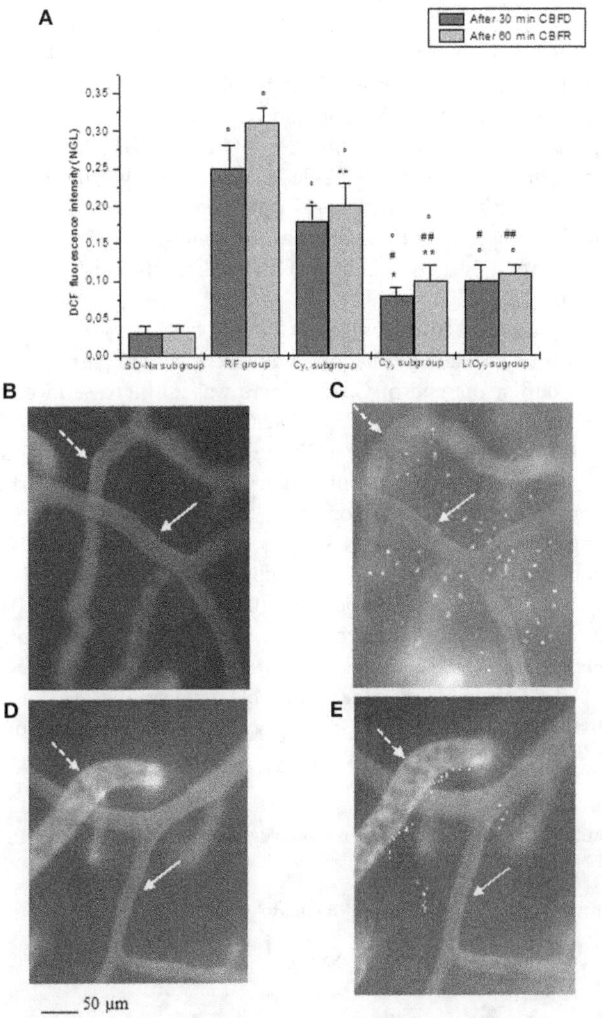

FIGURE 3 | DCF fluorescence intensity after 30 min cerebral blood flow reduction (CBFD) and after 60 min cerebral blood flow recovery (CBFR) in the experimental groups **(A)**: SO-Na subgroup (SO-Na), reduced blood flow group (RF), lower dosage cyanidin-treated subgroup (Cy_1), higher dosage cyanidin-treated subgroup (Cy_2) and higher dosage cyanidin plus L-NIO-treated subgroup (L/Cy_2). Data are reported as Mean ± SEM. $^{\circ}p < 0.01$ vs. SO-Na subgroup; $^{*}p < 0.01$ vs. RF group after 30 min CBFD; $^{**}p < 0.01$ vs. RF group after 60 min CBFR; $^{+}p < 0.01$ vs. Cy_2 subgroup after 30 min CBFD; $^{++}p < 0.01$ vs. Cy_2 subgroup after 60 min CBFR; $^{\#}p < 0.01$ vs. Cy_1 subgroup after 30 min CBFD; $^{\#\#}p < 0.01$ vs. Cy_1 subgroup after 60 min CBFR. Computer-assisted images of the pial microvascular network under baseline conditions **(B)** and after cerebral blood flow decrease and recovery **(C)** in a rat of RF group: several fluorescent spots are outlined by the marked change in the color of interstitium (from black to white). Computer-assisted images of the pial microvascular network under baseline conditions **(D)** and after cerebral blood flow decrease and recovery **(E)** in a higher dosage cyanidin-treated animal: decreased number of fluorescent spots are detected. The arterioles are indicated by the white arrows, while the venules are outlined by dashed white arrows.

($p < 0.01$ vs. baseline and SO-Na subgroup) (**Table 3**). Finally, DCF fluorescence intensity was marked in the rats subjected to DCFH-DA perfusion, indicating a further increase in ROS formation: NGL were 0.31 ± 0.02 ($p < 0.01$ vs. SO-Na subgroup; **Figures 3A–C**).

Cy Group

Cyanidin, at 10 mg/kg b.w. dosage (Cy_1 subgroup), prevented damage of the microvascular networks, inducing an increase in arteriolar diameter at the end of CBFD. In particular, order 2 arterioles dilated by $12.5 \pm 1.8\%$ of baseline ($p < 0.01$ vs. baseline: mean diameter $25.2 \pm 2.3\,\mu m$, SO-Na subgroup and RF group; **Figure 1**). Microvascular permeability significantly decreased compared to RF group (0.22 ± 0.03 NGL; $p < 0.01$ vs. baseline, SO-Na subgroup and RF group) as well as DCF fluorescence intensity (0.18 ± 0.02 NGL; **Figure 3A**) ($p < 0.01$ vs. baseline, SO-Na subgroup and RF group).

After 60 min CBFR, all pial arterioles dilated: order 2 arteriole diameter increased by $20.5 \pm 1.5\%$ of baseline ($p < 0.01$ vs. baseline, SO-Na subgroup and RF group; **Figure 1**).

Furthermore, fluorescent dextran leakage was significantly reduced compared to RF group (0.36 ± 0.02 NGL; $p < 0.01$ vs. baseline, SO-Na subgroup and RF group) as well as leukocytes adhering to venular walls (7 ± 1/100 μm v.l./30 s; $p < 0.01$ vs. baseline, SO-Na subgroup and RF group). BFCL decreased by 22.0 ± 2.2% of baseline ($p < 0.01$ vs. baseline, SO-Na subgroup and RF group) (**Table 3**). Finally, a slight increase in DCF fluorescence intensity was observed in rats belonging to the Cy_1 subgroup, after DCFH-DA superfusion: NGL were 0.20 ± 0.03 ($p < 0.01$ vs. baseline, SO-Na subgroup and RF group) (**Figure 3A**).

Cyanidin, at the dosage 20 mg/kg b.w. (Cy_2 subgroup), determined a marked dilation in all arterioles compared to Cy_1 subgroup at the end of CBFD. There was an increase in order 2 arteriole diameter by 31.7 ± 3.0% of baseline ($p < 0.01$ vs. baseline: mean diameter 27.0 ±1.5 μm, SO-Na subgroup, RF group and Cy_1 subgroup; **Figure 1**). Microvascular leakage appeared to be blunted compared to animals of RF and Cy_1 subgroup (0.16 ± 0.02 NGL; $p < 0.01$ vs. baseline, SO-Na subgroup, RF group and Cy_1 subgroup). Intensity in DCF fluorescence appeared to be slight (0.08 ± 0.01 NGL; $p < 0.01$ vs. baseline, SO-Na subgroup, RF group and Cy_1 subgroup) (**Figure 3A**).

After 60 min CBFR, order 2 arteriole diameter increased up to 40.5 ± 2.8% of baseline ($p < 0.01$ vs. baseline, SO-Na subgroup, RF group and Cy_1 subgroup; **Figure 1**). Additionally, there was a significant decrease in fluorescent dextran leakage when compared to RF and Cy_1 subgroup (0.25 ± 0.03 NGL; $p < 0.01$ vs. baseline, SO-Na subgroup, RF group and Cy_1 subgroup). Leukocyte adherent to venules were 5 ± 2/100 μm v.l./30 s, while BFCL decreased by 14.0 ± 2.0% of baseline ($p < 0.01$ vs. baseline, SO-Na subgroup, RF group and Cy_1 subgroup) (**Table 3** and **Figures 2C,D**). Finally, ROS production was completely counteracted by higher dosage cyanidin administration, as detected by reduction in fluorescence intensity in Cy_2 subgroup, superfused with DCFH-DA: NGL were 0.10 ± 0.02 ($p < 0.01$ vs. baseline, SO-Na subgroup, RF group and Cy_1 subgroup) (**Figures 3A,D,E**).

In L/Cy_2 subgroup, L-NIO injection (10 mg/kg b.w.) 10 min before cyanidin treatment at the higher dose, blunted cyanidin effects on arteriolar diameter within 30 min of CBFD. In particular, diameter of order 2 arterioles was reduced by 8.7 ± 1.2% of baseline (mean diameter: 24.3 ± 1.7 μm; $p < 0.01$ vs. Cy_2 subgroup; **Figure 1**). Conversely, L-NIO administration did not alter cyanidin effects on microvascular permeability (**Table 3**).

At the end of CBFR, all order 2 pial arterioles constricted with a decrease by 6.2 ± 1.0% of baseline diameter ($p < 0.01$ vs. Cy_2 subgroup; **Figure 1**). However, microvascular permeability and adhesion of leukocytes were not influenced by L-NIO administration (**Figures 2E,F**). BFCL decreased by 17.0 ± 1.5%

TABLE 4 | (A) Mean arterial blood pressure (MABP), heart rate, respiratory CO_2 and (B) blood gases (pCO_2 and pO_2) under baseline conditions, at the end of CBFD and CBFR in all subgroups.

Groups	MAPB (mmHg)			Heart rate (bpm)			Respiratory CO_2 (mmHg)		
	Baseline	CBFD	CBFR	Baseline	CBFD	CBFR	Baseline	CBFD	CBFR
A									
SO-Na	100.0 ± 1.5	–	–	328.5 ± 1.8	–	–	30.5 ± 1.5	–	–
SO-Cy_1	101.0 ± 1.6	–	–	330.0 ± 1.5	–	–	30.8 ± 1.6	–	–
SO-Cy_2	101.0 ± 1.4	–	–	325.0 ± 1.3	–	–	30.6 ± 1.8	–	–
SO-L	102.0 ± 1.5	–	–	327.0 ± 1.9	–	–	29.8 ± 2.0	–	–
RF	101.0 ± 1.7	92.5 ± 1.6*	97.5 ± 1.8	320.0 ± 1.5	315.5 ± 1.7	324.0 ± 2.0	30.2 ± 1.8	29.3± 1.5	30.8 ± 1.4
Cy_1	102.0 ± 1.8	93.7 ± 1.5*	99.7 ± 1.6	321.5 ± 1.7	318.0 ± 1.5	325.0 ± 2.0	30.5 ± 1.5	30.5 ± 1.4	31.0 ± 1.6
Cy_2	104.0 ± 2.8	95.8 ± 1.4*	100.0 ± 2.5	328.0 ± 1.6	320.5 ± 1.8	330.0 ± 1.5	30.6 ± 1.8	30.5 ± 1.7	30.9 ± 1.5
L/Cy_2	106.0 ± 2.5	97.5 ± 1.6*	101.5 ± 2.0	320.8 ± 1.8	318.0 ± 1.4	320 ± 2.5	30.8 ± 2.0	31.0 ± 1.7	30.8 ± 1.8

Groups	pCO_2 (mmHg)			pO_2 (mmHg)		
	Baseline	CBFD	CBFR	Baseline	CBFD	CBFR
B						
SO-Na	41.5 ± 2.0	–	–	96.5 ± 2.0	–	–
SO-Cy_1	41.8 ± 1.8	–	–	97.0 ± 1.8	–	–
SO-Cy_2	41.0 ± 1.5	–	–	97.2 ± 1.7	–	–
SO-L	42.0 ± 1.6	–	–	96.0 ± 2.2	–	–
RF	40.2 ± 2.1	40.1 ± 1.8	40.1 ± 2.1	96.8 ± 2.0	96.1 ± 1.8	96.0 ± 1.8
Cy_1	40.8 ± 1.7	40.8 ± 1.6	40.5 ± 1.5	97.1 ± 1.7	98.0 ± 1.8	98.0 ± 1.5
Cy_2	40.6 ± 2.0	41.0 ± 1.9	40.9 ± 1.7	97.0 ± 1.8	97.5 ± 1.7	97.0 ± 2.0
L/Cy_2	40.8 ± 2.2	40.5 ± 2.0	40.4 ± 1.9	96.4 ± 2.1	96.0 ± 1.9	96.0 ± 1.7

*Data are reported as Mean ± SEM; *$p < 0.01$ vs. baseline.*

of baseline ($p < 0.01$ vs. baseline, SO-Na and RF groups; **Table 3**). No differences in DCF fluorescence were observed in L/Cy_2 subgroup when compared to Cy_2 subgroup animals: NGL were 0.10 ± 0.02 and 0.11 ± 0.01 at 30 min CBFD and 60 min CBFR, respectively ($p < 0.01$ vs. Rf group; **Figure 3A**).

No significant changes in MABP, heart rate, respiratory CO_2 and blood gases were detected among the different subgroups under baseline conditions, at the end of CBFD and CBFR (as reported in **Table 4**).

2,3,5-triphenyltetrazolium Chloride (TTC) staining

CBFD and CBFR caused damage in cortex and striatum cerebral tissue of both hemispheres in RF animals, compared to SO-Na subgroup (**Figure 4A**). Cortex infarct size was $8.6 \pm 2.0\%$ ($p < 0.01$ vs. nonhypoperfused cortex), while in the striatum the damage was more marked (striatum infarct size $30.5 \pm 3.2\%$, $p < 0.01$ vs. nonhypoperfused cortex).

Conversely, neuronal damage drastically diminished in rats undergoing CBFD and CBFR treated with cyanidin (Cy_1 and Cy_2 subgroups), when compared to the previous subgroups (**Figure 4B**); in particular, the injury was limited to the striatum (infarct sizes were $25 \pm 2\%$ and $16.3 \pm 1.8\%$ in rats treated with low or high cyanidin dosage, respectively, $p < 0.01$ vs. hypoperfused striatum).

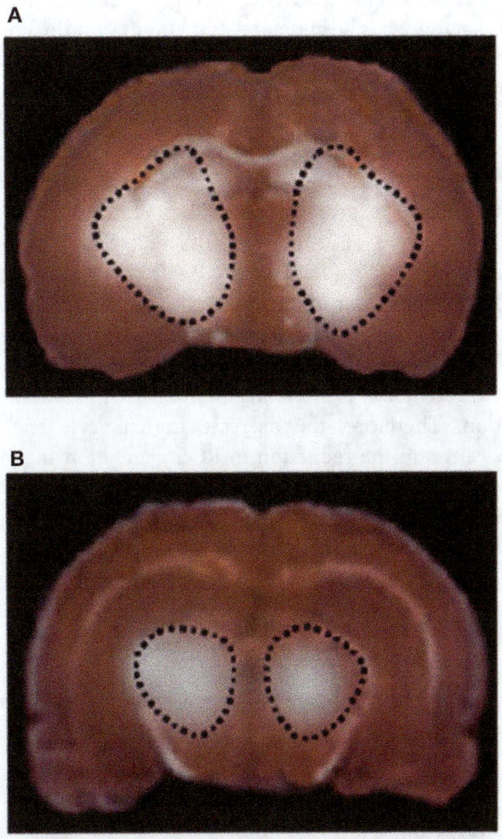

FIGURE 4 | TTC staining of coronal brain slices from a rat of RF group **(A)** and higher dosage cyanidin-treated subgroup **(B)** after 30 min CBFD and 60 min CBFR. The lesion in the striatum is outlined by the dashed black line.

DISCUSSION

The present data indicate that cyanidin, a polyphenol widely diffused in nature, was able to counteract oxidative stress and microvascular changes induced by 30 min of cerebral blood flow decrease, caused by bilateral occlusion of common carotid arteries, and 60 min of cerebral blood flow recovery. These data are the first evidence of ROS reduction in rat pial networks during cyanidin administration under conditions of reduced blood flow and reperfusion. We characterized the pial microcirculation by fluorescence microscopy to study microvascular responses after acute injury. The alterations caused by the reduction in cerebral blood flow and subsequent reperfusion were characterized by arteriolar constriction, venular permeability increase, leukocyte adhesion to venular walls and capillary rarefaction, as previously reported (Lapi et al., 2016; Mastantuono et al., 2016). Moreover, we observed a dramatic increase in ROS production, as detected by DCFH-DA assay.

Interestingly, cyanidin protected rat pial microcirculation during the decrease in cerebral blood flow and consequent reperfusion in a dose-related manner. We chose to analyze cyanidin effects on arteriolar responses, because these vessels were mainly involved in the regulation of tissue perfusion (Martinez-Lemus, 2012). At the end of the restriction in blood flow, cyanidin prevented the decrease in diameter of order 2 arterioles, compared with RF group. Moreover, at the end of the time-period of blood flow recovery, higher dosage cyanidin induced a vasodilation by 40.5% of baseline in order 2 arterioles. These vasodilatory effects were accompanied by preservation of capillary perfusion, significant decrease in venular leakage as well as in leukocyte adhesion to venular walls. The latter effects may be related to the reduction in ROS formation induced by cyanidin, because ROS have been shown to play a crucial role in the regulation of vessel wall permeability and adhesion of leukocyte to venular walls (Accetta et al., 2016; Mondola et al., 2016). It is worth noting, indeed, that ROS formation was marked in RF group, but resulted lower in cyanidin-treated animals.

Arteriolar vasodilation was counteracted by L-NIO, an inhibitor of the endothelial isoform of nitric oxide synthase (NOS), injected 10 min before cyanidin; therefore, it is possible to hypothesize that cyanidin vasodilatory properties may be due to NO release from vascular endothelial cells. These data are in agreement with previous studies indicating that this polyphenol was able to enhance the release of NO and other vasodilating factors, improving the endothelial-dependent vasodilation (Sivasinprasasn et al., 2016). Interestingly, cyanidin protective effects on leakage were not abolished by L-NIO infusion, suggesting that this polyphenol is able to protect the blood brain barrier integrity mainly through its scavenger activity rather than through its vasodilatory properties.

The biochemical properties of cyanidin have been widely studied; this molecule showed several antioxidant and anti-inflammatory activities (Olivas-Aguirre et al., 2016). In particular, the highest ORAC (oxygen radical absorbance capacity) activity has been demonstrated for cyanidin, compared to other anthocyanins (Zheng and Wang, 2003). Moreover, this polyphenol down-regulates plasminogen activator inhibitor-1 and pro-inflammatory cytokine IL-6, ameliorating human adipocytokine profile (Tsuda et al., 2006). It is interesting to note that isolated rat hearts are protected by oxidative stress, increased in several cardiovascular diseases, after treatment with cyanidin (Ziberna et al., 2012) as well as rat hepatic I/R damage is decreased by cyanidin (Tsuda et al., 1999). In the present study, cyanidin showed a strong antioxidant activity reducing ROS production, but at the same time was able to decrease adhesion of leukocytes to vessel walls blunting the damage induced by leukocyte activation, a mechanism effective in promoting ROS generation. Therefore, the decrease in leukocyte sticking to vessels walls and the reduction in ROS generation merged and reduced the effects of ROS on vessel wall leakage. These effects were effective in preventing marked microvascular damage, avoiding the disruption of blood-brain barrier and tissue edema. All together these vasodilatory and antioxidant properties preserved cerebral perfusion and prevented neuronal loss at the end of blood flow recovery in cyanidin-treated animals. Consequently, there was a reduction of the infarct size in cortical and striatal zones, compared to the rats subjected to decrease in cerebral blood flow and subsequent recovery.

Our data are in agreement with previous observations by Di Giacomo et al. who have observed the effects of Cyanidin-3-O-glucoside injection before the bilateral common carotid artery occlusion and during reperfusion. Their data indicate that cyanidin is able to reduce the lipid hydroperoxides and the expression of neuronal and inducible NOS and to increase the expression in endothelial nitric oxide synthase (eNOS) (Di Giacomo et al., 2012).

In conclusion, our data are the first evidence in an *in vivo* study that rat pial microcirculation was protected against different mechanisms of damage: cyanidin was able to induce arteriolar dilation, to reduce oxidative stress and prevent neuronal loss. All these activities resulted in the protection of cerebral perfusion, blood brain barrier integrity and brain function. Therefore, cyanidin appears to be useful in counteracting ROS generation in brain circulation and to protect cerebral tissues.

AUTHOR CONTRIBUTIONS

Conceived and designed the experiments: TM, AC, and DL. Performed the experiments and the animal treatments: TM, MD, MC, LB, NS, AC, and DL. Analyzed the data: TM, MD, MC, LB, EM, GN, AC, and DL. Wrote the paper: TM, MD, MC, AC, and DL.

REFERENCES

Accetta, R., Damiano, S., Morano, A., Mondola, P., Paternò, R., Avvedimento, E. V., et al. (2016). Reactive oxygen species derived from NOX3 and NOX5 drive differentiation of human oligodendrocytes. *Front. Cell Neurosci.* 10:146. doi: 10.3389/fncel.2016.00146

Bederson, J. B., Pitts, L. H., Germano, S. M., Nishimura, M. C., Davis, R. L., and Bartkowski, H. M. (1986). Evaluation of 2,3,5-triphenyltetrazolium chloride as a stain for detection and quantification of experimental cerebral infarction in rats. *Stroke* 17, 1304–1308.

Di Giacomo, C., Acquaviva, R., Santangelo, R., Sorrenti, V., Vanella, L., Li Volti, G., et al. (2012). Effect of treatment with cyanidin-3-O-β-D-glucoside on rat ischemic/reperfusion brain damage. *Evid. Based Comp. Alternat. Med.* 2012:285750. doi: 10.1155/2012/285750

Fratantonio, D., Cimino, F., Molonia, M. S., Ferrari, D., Saija, A., Virgili, F., et al. (2016). Cyanidin-3-O-glucoside ameliorates palmitate-induced insulin resistance by modulating IRS-1 phosphorylation and release of endothelial derived vasoactive factors. *Biochim. Biophys. Acta* 1862, 351–357. doi: 10.1016/j.bbalip.2016.12.008

Galvano, F., La Fauci, L., Lazzarino, G., Fogliano, V., Ritieni, A., Ciappellano, S., et al. (2004). Cyanidins: metabolism and biological properties. *J. Nutr. Biochem.* 15, 2–11. doi: 10.1016/j.jnutbio.2003.07.004

Hudetz, A. G., Fehér, G., Weigle, C. G., Knuese, D. E., and Kampine, J. P. (1985). Video microscopy of cerebrocortical capillary flow: response to hypotension and intracranial hypertension. *Am. J. Physiol.* 268, H2202–H2210.

Isaak, C. K., Wang, P., Prashar, S., O, K., Brown, D. C., Debnath, S. C., et al. (2017). Supplementing diet with Manitoba lingonberry juice reduces kidney ischemia-reperfusion injury. *J. Sci. Food Agric.* 97, 3065–3076. doi: 10.1002/jsfa.8200

Jakesevic, M., Xu, J., Aaby, K., Jeppsson, B., Ahrn,é, S., and Molin, G. (2013). Effects of bilberry (*Vaccinium myrtillus*) in combination with lactic acid bacteria on intestinal oxidative stress induced by ischemia-reperfusion in mouse. *J. Agric. Food Chem.* 61, 3468–3478. doi: 10.1021/jf400203h

Kassab, G. S., Rider, C. A., Tang, N. J., and Fung, Y. C. (1993). Morphometry of pig coronary arterial trees. *Am. J. Physiol.* 265, H350–H365.

Lapi, D., Chiurazzi, M., Di Maro, M., Mastantuono, T., Battiloro, L., Sabatino, L., et al. (2016). Malvidin's effects on rat pial microvascular permeability changes due to hypoperfusion and reperfusion injury. *Front. Cell Neurosci.* 10:153. doi: 10.3389/fncel.2016.00153

Lapi, D., Marchiafava, P. L., and Colantuoni, A. (2008). Geometric Characteristics of arterial network of rat pial microcirculation. *J. Vasc. Res.* 45, 69–77. doi: 10.1159/000109078

Lapi, D., Mastantuono, T., Sapio, D., Paterni, M., and Colantuoni, A. (2013). Pial Microvascular responses induced by transient bilateral common carotid artery occlusion in Zucker rats. *Clin. Hemorheol. Microcirc.* 54, 415–429. doi: 10.3233/CH-131763

Lapi, D., Vagnani, S., Pignataro, G., Esposito, E., Paterni, M., and Colantuoni, A. (2012). Protective effects of quercetin on rat pial microvascular changes during transient bilateral common carotid artery oclusion and reperfusion. *Front. Physiol.* 32, 1–12. doi: 10.3389/phys.2012.00032

Martinez-Lemus, L. A. (2012). The dynamic structure of arterioles. *Basic Clin. Pharmacol. Toxicol.* 110, 5–11. doi: 10.1111/j.1742-7843.2011.00813.x

Mastantuono, T., Starita, N., Sapio, D., D'Avanzo, S. A., Di Maro, M., Muscariello, E., et al. (2016). The effects of *Vaccinium myrtillus* extract on hamster pial microcirculation during hypoperfusion-reperfusion injury. *PLoS ONE* 11:e0150659. doi: 10.1371/journal.pone.0150659

Mondola, P., Damiano, S., Sasso, A., and Santillo, M. (2016). The Cu, Zn superoxide dismutase: not only a dismutase enzyme. *Front. Physiol.* 7:594. doi: 10.3389/fphys.2016.00594

Moreau, P., Takasa, H., Küng, C. F., van Rooijen, M. M., Schaffner, T., and Lüscher, T. F. (1995). Structure and function of the rat asilar artery during chronic nitric oxide synthase inhibition. *Stroke* 26, 1922–1928.

Morii, S., Ngai, A. C., and Winn, H. R. (1986). Reactivity of rat pial arterioles and venules to adenosine and carbon dioxine: with detailed description of the closed cranial window technique in rats. *J. Cereb. Blood Flow Metab.* 6, 34–41. doi: 10.1038/jcbfm.1986.5

Ngai, A. C., Ko, K. R., Morii, S., and Winn, H. R. (1988). Effect of sciatic nerve stimulation on pial arterioles in rats. *Am. J. Physiol.* 254, H133–H139.

Olivas-Aguirre, F. J., Rodrigo-García, J., Martínez-Ruiz, N. D., Cárdenas-Robles, A. I., Mendoza-Díaz, S. O., Álvarez-Parrilla, E., et al. (2016). Cyanidin-3-O-glucoside: physical-chemistry, foodomics and health effects. *Molecules* 21:E1264. doi: 10.3390/molecules21091264

Quintieri, A. M., Baldino, N., Filice, E., Seta, L., Vitetti, A., Tota, B., et al. (2013). Malvidin, a red wine polyphenol, modulates mammalian myocardial and coronary performance and protects the heart against ischemia/reperfusion injury. *J. Nutr. Biochem.* 24, 1221–1231. doi: 10.1016/j.jnutbio.2012.09.006

Serraino, I., Dugo, L., Dugo, P., Mondello, L., Mazzon, E., Dugo, G., et al. (2003). Protective effects of cyanidin-3-O-glucoside from blackberry extract against peroxynitrite-induced endothelial dysfunction and vascular failure. *Life Sci.* 73, 1097–1114. doi: 10.1016/S0024-3205(03)00356-4

Sivasinprasasn, S., Pantan, R., Thummayot, S., Tocharus, J., Suksamrarn, A., and Tocharus, C. (2016). Cyanidin-3-glucoside attenuates angiotensin II-induced oxidative stress and inflammation in vascular endothelial cells. *Chem Biol Interact.* 260, 67–74. doi: 10.1016/j.cbi.2016.10.022

Tsuda, T., Horio, F., Kitoh, J., and Osawa, T. (1999). Protective Effects of Dietary Cyanidin 3-O-β-d-Glucoside on Liver Ischemia–Reperfusion Injury in Rats. *Arch. Biochem. Biophys.* 368, 361–366.

Tsuda, T., Ueno, Y., Yoshikawa, T., Kojo, H., and Osawa, T. (2006). Microarray profiling of gene expression in human adipocytes in response to anthocyanins. *Biochem. Pharmacol.* 71, 1184–1197. doi: 10.1016/j.bcp.2005.12.042

Wang, H., and Joseph, J. A. (1999). Quantifying cellular oxidative stress by dichlorofluorescein assay using microplate reader. *Free Radic Biol Med.* 27, 612–616.

Watanabe, S. (1998). *In vivo* fluorometric measurement of cerebral oxidative stress using 2'-7'- dichlorofluorescein (DCF). *Keio J Med.* 47, 92–98.

Zheng, W., and Wang, S.Y. (2003). Oxygen radical absorbing capacity of phenolics in blueberries, cranberries, chokeberries, and lingonberries. *J. Agric. Food Chem.* 51, 502–509. doi: 10.1021/jf020728u

Ziberna, L., Tramer, F., Moze, S., Vrhovsek, U., Mattivi, F., and Passamonti, S. (2012). Transport and bioactivity of cyaniding 3-glucoside into the vascular endothelium. *Free Radic. Biol. Med.* 52, 1750–1759. doi: 10.1016/j.freeradbiomed.2012.02.027

17

Impact of Nitric Oxide Bioavailability on the Progressive Cerebral and Peripheral Circulatory Impairments During Aging and Alzheimer's Disease

Massimo Venturelli[1], Anna Pedrinolla[2], Ilaria Boscolo Galazzo[3], Cristina Fonte[1,4], Nicola Smania[1,4], Stefano Tamburin[1], Ettore Muti[5], Lucia Crispoltoni[6], Annamaria Stabile[6], Alessandra Pistilli[6], Mario Rende[6], Francesca B. Pizzini[7] and Federico Schena[1]*

[1] Department of Neurosciences, Biomedicine and Movement Sciences, University of Verona, Verona, Italy, [2] Department of Medicine, University of Verona, Verona, Italy, [3] Department of Computer Science, University of Verona, Verona, Italy, [4] Neuromotor and Cognitive Rehabilitation Research Centre, University of Verona, Verona, Italy, [5] Mons. Mazzali Foundation, Mantua, Italy, [6] Department of Surgical and Biomedical Sciences, Section of Human Anatomy, School of Medicine, University of Perugia, Perugia, Italy, [7] Neuroradiology, Department of Diagnostics and Pathology, Verona University Hospital, Verona, Italy

Edited by:
Pasquale Pagliaro,
Università degli Studi di Torino, Italy

Reviewed by:
Tommaso Angelone,
University of Calabria, Italy
Antonio Crisafulli,
Università degli studi di Cagliari, Italy

***Correspondence:**
Massimo Venturelli
massimo.venturelli@univr.it

Advanced aging, vascular dysfunction, and nitric oxide (NO) bioavailability are recognized risk factors for Alzheimer's disease (AD). However, the contribution of AD, *per se*, to this putative pathophysiological mechanism is still unclear. To better answer this point, we quantified cortical perfusion with arterial spin labeling (PVC-CBF), measured ultrasound internal carotid (ICA), and femoral (FA) artery blood flow in a group of patients with similar age (~78 years) but different cognitive impairment (i.e., mild cognitive impairment MCI, mild AD-AD1, moderate AD-AD2, and severe AD-AD3) and compared them to young and healthy old (aged-matched) controls. NO-metabolites and passive leg-movement (PLM) induced hyperemia were used to assess systemic vascular function. Ninety-eight individuals were recruited for this study. PVC-CBF, ICA, and FA blood flow were markedly (range of 9–17%) and significantly (all $p < 0.05$) reduced across the spectrum from YG to OLD, MCI, AD1, AD2, AD3 subjects. Similarly, plasma level of nitrates and the values of PLM were significantly reduced (range of 8–26%; $p < 0.05$) among the six groups. Significant correlations were retrieved between plasma nitrates, PLM and PVC-CBF, CA, and FA blood flow. This integrative and comprehensive approach to vascular changes in aging and AD showed progressive changes in NO bioavailability and cortical, extracranial, and peripheral circulation in patients with AD and suggested that they are directly associated with AD and not to aging. Moreover, these results suggest that AD-related impairments of circulation are progressive and not confined to the brain. The link between cardiovascular and the central nervous systems degenerative processes in patients at different severity of AD is likely related to the depletion of NO.

Keywords: circulation, aging, Alzheimer's disease, nitric oxide, vascular dysfunction

INTRODUCTION

Alzheimer's disease (AD) is the most common form of dementia, with an attested prevalence of ~24 million which is predicted to quadruplicate by 2050 (Reitz et al., 2011). Pathophysiological mechanisms of AD are well-defined, including diffuse neuritic extracellular amyloid (Aβ) plaques and intracellular neurofibrillary tangles coupled with reactive microgliosis, loss of neurons and synapses in the cortex (Reitz and Mayeux, 2014). From the vascular point of view, Aβ peptide accumulation in the tunica media and adventitia of cerebral blood vessels, a condition termed cerebral amyloid angiopathy (CAA), is associated with vessel smooth muscle cell degeneration, resulting in impaired cerebral circulation (Maier et al., 2014).

Apart from this direct effect of Aβ accumulation in the cortical neurons and vessels, there is increasing evidence that AD is associated with several dysregulated processes, which affect brain and systemic circulation, suggesting that vascular dysfunction may play a role in the pathogenesis of AD (Iturria-Medina et al., 2016). These pieces of evidence pose the question whether AD is an age-related neurodegenerative disorder with vascular consequences, or a vascular disorder with neurodegenerative sequels (De La Torre, 2010). Indeed, both aging and AD appear to be involved in the decline of the systemic and cerebral vascular function (De La Torre, 2009). However, the contribution of AD, *per se*, to vascular changes is still unclear. Additionally, the cardiovascular and the central nervous system (CNS) changes have been postulated to occur in parallel during the progression of AD (Picano et al., 2014).

In the brain of patients with AD, diffuse cortical changes have been demonstrated (Dallaire-Theroux et al., 2017), coupled with a reduced perfusion of the temporo-parietal association cortices, mesial temporal structures and the frontal association cortex (Herholz, 2011). However, potential reduction of blood flow availability inward from extracranial conduit arteries (i.e., internal carotid artery (ICA), vertebral artery) may also contribute to the onset of AD (Liu et al., 2014; Clark et al., 2017). In this scenario, nitric oxide (NO) is considered the most important vasodilator factor responsible for the preservation of vasomotor function (Katusic and Austin, 2014). Indeed, reduced availability of NO in both cerebral and peripheral vessels results in major detrimental alterations of vascular function (Katusic and Austin, 2014). However, the role of NO bioavailability in the control of extracranial blood flow, cerebral, and systemic circulation in patients with different AD severity have not been so far fully elucidated.

Therefore, the aims of the present study were two-fold. The first was to evaluate if the NO bioavailability, cerebral perfusion, extracranial, peripheral blood flow and systemic vascular function are reduced in AD in comparison to healthy young and old individuals. The second was to compare these measures in patients with different AD severity. Specifically, we have assessed cortical perfusion with arterial spin labeling (ASL) Magnetic Resonance Imaging (MRI), and measured ICA and femoral (FA) artery blood flow in young (YG) and old (OLD) healthy controls, patients with mild cognitive impairment (MCI) and AD of different severity: mild AD (AD1), moderate AD (AD2), and severe AD (AD3). NO bioavailability was determined in the six groups via plasma NO metabolites (nitrite and nitrate). Passive leg-movement (PLM) induced hyperemia was used to assess both endothelial NO availability and systemic vascular function. We hypothesized that (a) the severity of AD would impact on cortical perfusion, as well as ICA and FA blood flow, and (b) brain and systemic impairment of circulation would be associated with a depletion of NO bioavailability.

METHODS

Participants

Patients with MCI and AD were recruited from the Neuromotor and Cognitive Rehabilitation Research Center Azienda Ospedaliera Universitaria Integrata of Verona, and the Geriatric Institute Mons. Arrigo Mazzali Foundation (Mantua, Italy). Clinical diagnosis of MCI and probable AD was established according to the National Institute on Aging-Alzheimer's Association diagnostic guideline for MCI due to AD and AD (Albert et al., 2011; Mckhann et al., 2011). All patients had a previous neuroimaging study (MRI or CT) to support the diagnosis of MCI and/or probable AD.

Dementia severity was assessed by means of the Mini Mental State Examination (MMSE) (Folstein et al., 1975) and the Clinical Dementia Rating scale (CDR) (Morris, 1993). According to the severity of dementia, patients with AD were divided in three groups: AD1 with MMSE scores between 20 and 24 and CDR 1, AD2 with MMSE scores between 10 and 19 and CDR 2, and AD3 with MMSE scores lower than 10 and CDR 3. Two additional healthy control groups (i.e., YG and OLD) were recruited from the same geographical area, after a physician's assessment of negligible cardiovascular and musculoskeletal diseases. This screening included health history, physical examination, blood pressure assessment, blood sample, and familiarization with the study procedures. OLD had to have a MMSE $\geq$ 24. As reported in the AD diagnostic guidelines (Mckhann et al., 2011), individuals with a diagnosis of vascular dementia (VaD) were not included in the study. Other exclusion criteria were: history of depression or psychosis, alcohol or drug abuse, other neurological (e.g., Parkinson's disease, traumatic brain injury, stroke, multiple sclerosis), cardiac, orthopedic (e.g., osteoarthrosis) or respiratory conditions (e.g., chronic obstructive pulmonary disease). All experiments were conducted after informed and written consent was obtained from the patients and their relatives and healthy individuals in accordance with the Declaration of Helsinki, as part of a protocol approved by the Institutional Review Board of the Azienda Ospedaliera Universitaria Integrata (Approval #2389).

Assessment Procedure

Neurologists and clinical neuropsychologists with a specific expertise in dementia investigated the cognitive profile of the patients with a full neuropsychological profile and the following tests were performed. The MMSE (Folstein et al., 1975) was used to assess the global cognitive status. The CDR (Morris, 1993) scale was administered to quantify the severity of dementia.

The Italian version of the Frontal Assessment Battery (FAB) (Appollonio et al., 2005) was used to assess executive functions.

Level of Physical Activity

The International Physical Activity Questionnaire (IPAQ) (Booth, 2000) was used to estimate the level of physical activity of the participants. Each question was administered to the healthy volunteers and to the patient's caregivers.

Volume Anthropometry Assessment

Thigh and lower leg volume were calculated based on leg circumferences (three sites: distal, middle, and proximal), thigh and lower leg length, and skinfold measurements using the following formula:

$$V = \frac{L}{12\pi} \cdot \left(C1^2 + C2^2 + C3^2\right) - \frac{S - 0.4}{2} \cdot L \cdot \frac{C1 + C2 + C3}{3}$$

where L refers to the length; C1, C2, and C3 refer to the proximal, middle, and distal circumferences, respectively; and S is skinfold thickness of either the thigh or the lower leg. The length of the leg was measured from the greater trochanter to the lateral femoral epicondyle (thigh) and from the head of the fibula to the lateral malleolus (lower leg). The length and circumference were measured to the nearest 1 mm using a flexible standard measuring tape. Skinfold thickness was measured using skinfold calipers (Beta Technology Incorporated, Cambridge, MD) at three sites at the midpoint of each limb segment (Layec et al., 2014).

Resting Oxygen Uptake Assessment

Briefly, oxygen uptake was recorded with the subjects supine and at rest for 20 min. Expired gases were analyzed on a breath-by-breath basis by a metabolimeter (K4 b^2, Cosmed, Rome, Italy).

Cortical Perfusion Assessment

A subgroup of the total population underwent MRI to assess non-invasively cerebral blood flow (CBF) with ASL (Detre et al., 1992). In details, forty-three subjects (YG: 10, OLD: 7, MCI: 6, AD1: 5, AD2: 9, AD3: 6) were scanned on a 3T Philips Achieva system equipped with an 8-channel head coil. They were instructed to lie as still as possible in the scanner, to keep their eyes closed but not to fall asleep while images were collected. For ASL data, pseudo-continuous (pCASL) labeling was acquired using the following parameters: TR/TE = 4,400/11 ms; label duration/post-label delay = 1,650/1,800 ms; 45 Control/Label volumes; 26 slices, $3 \times 3 \times 3$ mm^3, slice gap = 1 mm; two background suppression pulses at 1,700 and 2,926 ms from the start of the scan. A calibration scan with the same parameters as the ASL sequence but longer TR (10 s) and no background suppression was also acquired to estimate the equilibrium magnetization. Finally, a 3D T1-weighted turbo field echo anatomical scan was also acquired for each subject (TR/TE = 8.16/3.73 ms; 180 slices, $1 \times 1 \times 1$ mm^3).

ASL data were preprocessed and analyzed using FSL 5.0.9 (FMRIB, Oxford, UK) and Matlab 7.14 (MathWorks, Natick, MA). ASL data were first corrected for nuisance effects (head motion profiles, cerebrospinal fluid (CSF) and white matter (WM) signals) by using linear regression that minimizes the sum of squares of the residuals. The ASL calibration scan was used for estimating the coregistration parameters from ASL to the individual T1-weighted image by applying a 3D rigid-body registration with a normalized mutual-information cost function and 7 degrees of freedom.

Pre-processed Control and Label volumes were then surround subtracted and averaged to obtain perfusion-weighted images. These perfusion-weighted maps were quantified into CBF [ml/100 g/min] applying the general kinetic model (Buxton et al., 1998) as follows:

$$CBF = \frac{6000 \cdot \lambda \cdot \Delta M \cdot e^{\frac{PLD}{T_{1b}}}}{2 \cdot \alpha \cdot \alpha_{inv} \cdot T_{1b} \cdot M_{0t} \cdot \left(1 - e^{-\frac{\tau}{T_{1b}}}\right)}$$

where λ is the brain-blood partition coefficient (0.9 mL/g), ΔM represents the difference images (perfusion-weighted maps), PLD is the post-labeling delay, T_{1b} is the longitudinal relaxation time of arterial blood (1,650 ms), α is the labeling efficiency (0.85 for pCASL), where α_{inv} corrects for the decrease in labeling efficiency due to two background suppression pulses (0.83). M_{0t} is the tissue equilibrium magnetization, voxel-wise estimated from the calibration scan, and τ represents the labeling duration (Alsop et al., 2015). The increase in label decay in the ascending slices acquired with 2D readout was accounted for.

In order to perform partial volume effects-correction (PVC) mainly related to the low ASL spatial resolution and brain atrophy, partial volume-corrected cortical and WM flow maps were created for each subject. In details, high resolution gray matter (GM) and WM probability maps from the segmentation of the 3D T1-weighted image were first smoothed with a $3 \times 3 \times 3$ mm^3 kernel to mimic the ASL resolution. These smoothed maps were then down sampled to the ASL space using the inverse of the previously estimated transformation matrix and finally applied to the CBF maps for PVC following the equation $I_{corr} = I_{uncorr}/(P_{gm} + 0.4 \cdot P_{wm})$ (Du et al., 2006). For each subject, the mean corrected CBF value within the GM mask was calculated and used as individual representative measure of the whole cortical perfusion.

To provide group CBF maps, individual T1-weighted images were registered to the Montreal Neurological Institute (MNI) space with $1 \times 1 \times 1$ mm^3 resolution using a non-linear method (FNIRT tool in FSL) and the joint ASL/T1-weighted and T1-weighted/MNI space transformation parameters were used to spatially normalize the subject specific CBF maps in this common space. Representative mean uncorrected (whole brain) and PVC cortical (GM only) CBF maps in MNI space were finally derived for each of the six groups.

ICA and FA Blood Flow Assessment With Doppler Ultrasound Imaging

ICA, and FA artery diameters and blood velocities were recorded with the subjects supine and at rest for 20 min. When the blood flow was stable, 1-min video of the above-mentioned arteries was recorded on the ultrasound system. Specifically, the Doppler probe was positioned at the level of ICA ~1 cm above the common carotid bifurcation, and at the level of the common FA, distal to the inguinal ligament and proximal to the deep and superficial femoral bifurcation. Triplex Doppler clips were recorded with a Logiq-7 ultrasound Doppler system (General Electric Medical Systems, Milwaukee, WI, USA). The ultrasound Doppler system was equipped with a 12-14 MHz linear array transducer. Artery diameter was determined at a 90° angle along the central axis of the scanned area. Blood velocity (V_{mean}) was measured using the same probe utilizing a frequency of 5 MHz. Measurements of V_{mean} were obtained with the probe positioned to maintain an insonation angle of 60° or less and the sample volume was centered and maximized according to vessel size. Utilizing arterial diameter and V_{mean}, blood flow was calculated as:

$$\text{Blood flow} = V_{mean} \cdot \pi \cdot (\text{vessel diameter}/2)^2 \cdot 60$$

where blood flow is in milliliters per minute. To perform muscle and brain volume effect-corrections, mostly related to the lower limb muscle and brain atrophy, FA and ICA blood flow were normalized to leg muscle volume (thigh + lower leg volume) and total brain tissue volume (cortical, subcortical GM and WM volumes, including the brainstem and cerebellum), respectively (Liu et al., 2014; Venturelli et al., 2014). All scanning and blinded analyses were performed by experienced and skilled sonographers.

NO Bioavailability via Plasma Nitrates Assessments

It is important to note, that all the participants were asked to refrain from oral intake of supplements or nutrients with elevated levels of nitrates. Specifically, on the 3 days before the assessments strawberries, lettuce, beets, and carrots were not included in the participants diet. Venous peripheral blood (25 mL) was collected between 9:00 and 10:00 am from patients and healthy controls in a fasted state and processed within 2 h to obtain measurements of blood glucose, number of red blood cells (RBC), hemoglobin (Hb), high- and low-density lipoprotein (HDL, LDL). From a different vacutainer, plasma was separated from peripheral blood by centrifugation (1,200 rpm for 20 min at 4°C) and kept at −80°C until analysis. Plasma samples were ultrafiltrated through a 30 kDa molecular weight cut-off filter (cat. No UFC503096) (Millipore, Molseheim, France) to reduce background absorbance. Nitrate concentration was detected by nitrate/nitrite colorimetric assay kit (cat. No 780001) (Cayman Chemical Co, Ann Arbor, MI, USA) according to the manufacturer's protocol. The detection limit of nitrate was 2.5 μM. The nitrate concentration was analyzed in duplicate and read against the manufacturer standard curve.

Endothelial NO Bioavailability and Systemic Vascular Function via PLM

Recent investigations have revealed that PLM-induced hyperemia is predominantly a consequence of NO mediated vasodilation (Trinity et al., 2012). Therefore, we have adopted this noninvasive and reliable method to determine endothelial NO bioavailability. Moreover, the PLM protocol has been successfully adopted to determine systemic vascular function in healthy young (Mcdaniel et al., 2010a), elderly (Mcdaniel et al., 2010b), patients with spinal cord injury (Venturelli et al., 2014), and heart failure (Ives et al., 2016). During this evaluation, the subjects rested in the upright-seated position for 20 min before the start of data collection and remained in this position throughout this part of the study. The PLM protocol consisted of 60 s of resting baseline femoral blood flow data collection, followed by 60 s of passive knee extension and flexion with the same measure. PLM was performed by a member of the research team, who moved the subject's lower leg through a 90° range of motion (180-90° knee joint angle) at 1 Hz. Blood V_{mean} was analyzed with 1 Hz resolution on the Doppler ultrasound system (GE Logiq-7) for 60 s at rest and second by second for the first 60 s following the initiation of PLM. Relative changes (Δpeak) from rest of femoral blood flow was determined for each subject. To perform muscle volume effect-correction related to the skeletal muscle atrophy, Δpeak blood flow was normalized by thigh muscle volume (Venturelli et al., 2014).

Data Analysis and Interpretation

The representative outcomes from each assessment were analyzed using a statistical software package (StatPlus:mac, AnalystSoft Inc.,-statistical analysis program for Mac OS®. Version v6.). The normal distribution of the sampling was checked by the Shapiro-Wilk test. A one-way analysis of variance (ANOVA), and, where indicated, a Tukey *post hoc* test, were used to determine the group differences. A chi-square (χ^2) analysis was used to establish differences between categorical variables. Pearson correlation test was used to examine the correlation between variables. Significance was set at an α level of 0.05 (two-tailed), and the results are presented as mean ± SE.

RESULTS

Characteristics of the Participants

Demographic and clinical characteristics of the study participants are displayed in **Table 1**. Ninety-eight individuals (YG:10, OLD:14, MCI:19, AD:55) were recruited for this study. Except for the YG, all groups were matched for age, sex, body mass, thigh muscle volume, lower leg muscle volume, coexisting chronic conditions. Drugs for AD and other medications taken by the four groups of MCI/AD patients and the two groups of healthy individuals are displayed in **Table 1**.

Resting Metabolism, and Level of Physical Activity

Resting oxygen uptake, expired carbon dioxide ($ExpCO_2$) and the values of IPAQ, taken as marker of basal metabolism and level of physical activity, respectively, are illustrated in **Table 1**. Interestingly, any statistical difference was retrieved among the six groups in terms of basal metabolism (all $p > 0.2$). In comparison to the YG, the level of physical activity was significantly reduced in OLD ($p < 0.01$), MCI ($p < 0.01$), AD1 ($p < 0.01$), AD2 ($p < 0.01$), and AD3 ($p < 0.01$). However, the

TABLE 1 | Demographic and clinical characteristics of the study participants.

	YG ($N = 10$)	OLD ($N = 14$)	MCI ($N = 19$)	AD1 ($N = 24$)	AD2 ($N = 20$)	AD3 ($N = 11$)
Sex	4♂-6♀	6♂-6♀	9♂-10♀	9♂-15♀	6♂-14♀	2♂-9♀
Age (years)	28 ± 2	76 ± 6*	77 ± 4*	78 ± 7*	80 ± 8*	80 ± 7*
Weight (kg)	68 ± 20	73 ± 12	75 ± 19	63 ± 12	73 ± 13	62 ± 4§
Height (m)	1.69 ± 0.3	1.67 ± 0.1	1.65 ± 0.1	1.58 ± 0.1	1.62 ± 0.1	1.62 ± 0.2
Lower limb volume (l)	8.3 ± 1.7	8.3 ± 1.5	7.8 ± 1.6	7.4 ± 1.4	7.4 ± 1.1	7.3 ± 1.3
Thigh volume (l)	5.9 ± 1.5	6.2 ± 1.3	5.7 ± 1.4	5.4 ± 0.9	5.1 ± 2.0	5.3 ± 1.3
Leg volume (l)	2.4 ± 0.7	2.1 ± 0.6	2.1 ± 0.9	2.0 ± 0.5	2.3 ± 1.1	2.0 ± 0.7
SBP (mm Hg)	118 ± 20	129 ± 33	136 ± 37	132 ± 12*	130 ± 9*	125 ± 9*
DBP (mm Hg)	85 ± 10	90 ± 24	92 ± 12	86 ± 10	90 ± 5	82± 10
Glucose ($mg{\cdot}dl^{-1}$)	88 ± 12	95 ± 32	107 ± 21*	91 ± 8§	95 ± 47§	89 ± 15§
RBC ($10^6{\cdot}\mu l^{-1}$)	5.2 ± 0.9	5.0 ± 0.6	4.8 ± 0.4	4.8 ± 0.6	4.5 ± 0.5*†§	4.3 ± 0.3*†§
Hb ($g{\cdot}dl^{-1}$)	15 ± 2	15 ± 3	13 ± 1*†	13 ± 2*†	13 ± 2*†	12 ± 0.6*†
HDL ($mg{\cdot}dl^{-1}$)	49 ± 24	50 ± 17	58 ± 19	57 ± 21	57 ± 11	64± 17*†‡¶
LDL ($mg{\cdot}dl^{-1}$)	99 ± 30	100 ± 23	102 ± 15*	122 ± 32*§	110 ± 12*‡	136 ± 18*§
Education (years)	19 ± 2	10 ± 6*	10 ± 4*	9 ± 5*	7 ± 4*	7 ± 4*
IPAQ ($METs{\cdot}min{\cdot}week^{-1}$)	12,340 ± 832	4,043 ± 548*	3,874 ± 655*	4,129 ± 438*	3,784 ± 732*	3,833 ± 543*
Resting oxygen uptake ($ml{\cdot}m^{-1}{\cdot}kg^{-1}$)	4.4 ± 1.8	3.9 ± 1.8	3.6 ± 1.1	4.5 ± 1.2	3.5 ± 1.8	3.7 ± 1.5
$ExpCO_2$ (ml)	27.5 ± 7.8	23.2 ± 9.2	17.8 ± 9.8	21.9 ± 14.3	15.0 ± 5.5	19.5 ± 7.8
CLINICAL CHARACTERISTICS						
Time since diagnose of MCI or AD (years)	–	–	2 ± 1	6 ± 2 §	8 ± 3§‡	8 ± 2§‡
MMSE (0-30)	–	28 ± 1	27 ± 2†	22 ± 3†§	16 ± 3†§‡	11 ± 4*†§‡¶
CDR (0-3)	–	–	0.5	1§	2§‡	3§‡¶
FAB (0-18)	–	–	12 ± 2	9 ± 3§	8 ± 3§	4 ± 4§‡¶
PHARMACOLOGICAL TREATMENT n. (%)						
Cholinesterase Inhibitors	0	0	2 (10)	10 (42)*†	5 (25)*†	3 (27)*†
Antipsychotics	0	0	0	1 (4)	1 (5)	1 (9)
Antidepressants	0	0	0	2 (8)	4 (20)*†	2 (18)*†
Benzodiazepines	0	0	0	0	1 (5)	1 (5)
COMORBIDITY n. (%)						
Cardiovascular diseases	0	0	1 (5)	4 (16)*†	2 (10)*†	3 (27)*†
Diabetes	0	0	1 (5)	0	1 (5)	1 (9)
Arthrosis	0	0	1 (5)	2 (8)	1 (5)	1 (9)

*♂, male; ♀, female; MCI, Mild Cognitive Impairment; AD, Alzheimer's Disease; SBP, systolic blood pressure; DBP, diastolic blood pressure; RBC, red blood cells; Hb, hemoglobin; HDL, high-density lipoprotein; LDL low-density lipoprotein; IPAQ, international physical activity questionnaire; $ExpCO_2$, expired carbon dioxide; MET, metabolic equivalent; MMSE, Mini Mental State Examination; CDR, Clinical Dementia Rating Scale; FAB, Frontal Assessment Battery. Values are expressed as mean ±standard deviation (or percentage in brackets). *$p < 0.05$ vs. YG; †$p < 0.05$ vs. OLD; §$p < 0.05$ vs. MCI; ‡$p < 0.05$ vs. AD1; ¶$p < 0.05$ vs. AD2.*

differences in IPAQ values among OLD, MCI, AD1, AD2, and AD3 were not significant and negligible.

Cortical Perfusion

Representative mean CBF images for the six groups are shown in **Figure 1**, reporting both whole brain uncorrected (**Figure 1A**) and PVC cortical (**Figure 1B**) CBF maps at the same anatomical level. As clearly visible, there was a marked and progressive reduction in the CBF parameter, confirmed after PVC, across the spectrum from YG to OLD, MCI, AD1, AD2, and AD3 subjects. Quantitative analysis supported these visual impressions ($p < 0.05$ among the six groups) with average PVC-CBF levels of 57.7 ± 1.7 $ml{\cdot}100\ g^{-1}{\cdot}min^{-1}$ in YG, 48.6 ± 1.0 $ml{\cdot}100\ g^{-1}{\cdot}min^{-1}$ in OLD, 44.7 ± 1.0 $ml{\cdot}100\ g^{-1}{\cdot}min^{-1}$ in MCI, 40.8 ± 2.0 $ml{\cdot}100\ g^{-1}{\cdot}min^{-1}$ in AD1, 34.5 ± 1.5 $ml{\cdot}100\ g^{-1}{\cdot}min^{-1}$ in AD2, and 30.1 ± 2.5 $ml{\cdot}100\ g^{-1}{\cdot}min^{-1}$ in AD3 and significant post-hoc comparisons across MCI and different AD stages (**Figure 1C**).

ICA Blood Flow

Resting blood flow in the ICA normalized to total brain tissue volume, taken as marker of extracranial blood flow, is illustrated in **Figure 2**. Among the six groups there was a progressive significant reduction in ICA blood flow ($p < 0.05$). Specifically, blood flow in the ICA was 0.34 ± 0.02 $ml{\cdot}min^{-1}{\cdot}100\ ml^{-1}$ in YG, 0.30 ± 0.03 $ml{\cdot}min^{-1}{\cdot}100\ ml^{-1}$ in OLD, 0.24 ± 0.01 $ml{\cdot}min^{-1}{\cdot}100\ ml^{-1}$ in MCI, 0.22 ± 0.01 $ml{\cdot}min^{-1}{\cdot}100\ ml^{-1}$ in AD1, 0.20 ± 0.01 $ml{\cdot}min^{-1}{\cdot}100\ ml^{-1}$ in AD2, and 0.17 ± 0.01 $ml{\cdot}min^{-1}{\cdot}100\ ml^{-1}$ in AD3 subjects (**Figure 2**). Post-hoc

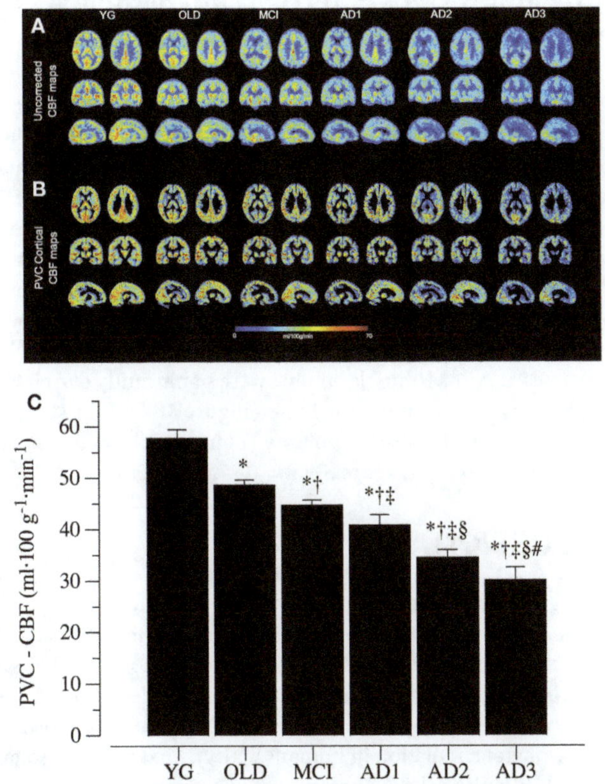

FIGURE 1 | Cortical perfusion data. **(A)** Group whole brain uncorrected cerebral blood flow (CBF) maps, calculated as average across the individual subjects belonging to healthy young (YG) and healthy old (OLD) controls, patients with mild cognitive impairment (MCI) and with different severity of AD, namely mild AD (AD1), moderate AD (AD2), and severe AD (AD3). Two representative sections are reported for each of the three views (axial, coronal, and sagittal). **(B)** Group mean cortical CBF maps after partial volume correction (PVC cortical), reported for the same anatomical levels as before. **(C)** reports group mean PVC cortical CBF levels (mean ± S.E). *Significantly different vs. YG group; †Significantly different vs. OLD group. ‡Significantly different vs. MCI group. §Significantly different vs. AD1 group. #Significantly different vs. AD2 group.

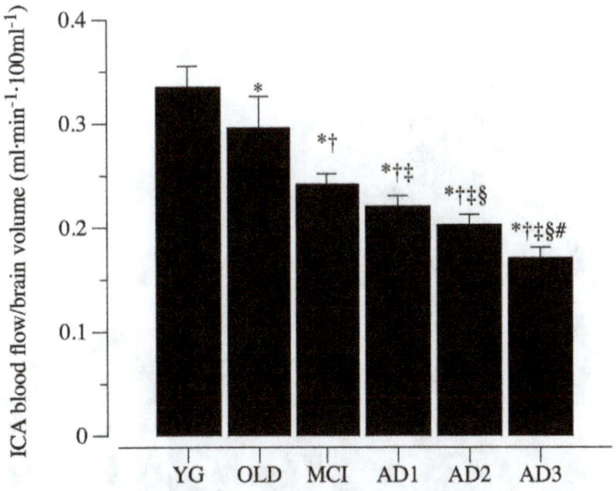

FIGURE 2 | Internal carotid artery blood flow normalized to brain volume. Internal carotid artery (ICA) blood flow normalized to brain volume in healthy young (YG) and healthy old (OLD) controls, patients with mild cognitive impairment (MCI), and with different severity of AD, namely mild AD (AD1), moderate AD (AD2), and severe AD (AD3). Data are presented as mean ±S.E.; *significantly different vs. YG group. †Significantly different vs. OLD group. ‡Significantly different vs. MCI group. §Significantly different vs. AD1 group. #Significantly different vs. AD2 group.

comparisons were significant across MCI and different AD stages.

FA Blood Flow

Resting blood flow in the FA normalized to the lower limb muscle volume, is illustrated in **Figure 3**. With a similar trend of the ICA blood flow, the FA hemodynamic was significantly attenuated ($p < 0.05$) compared to the YG (45 ± 2 ml·min^{-1}·l^{-1}) in the OLD (39 ± 3 ml·min^{-1}·l^{-1}) and even more so in the MCI, AD1, AD2 and AD3 (35 ± 2 ml·min^{-1}·l^{-1}, 31 ± 3 ml·min^{-1}·l^{-1}, 27 ± 3 ml·min^{-1}·l^{-1}, and 23 ± 2 ml·min^{-1}·l^{-1}) respectively (**Figure 3**). Post-hoc comparisons were significant across MCI and different AD stages.

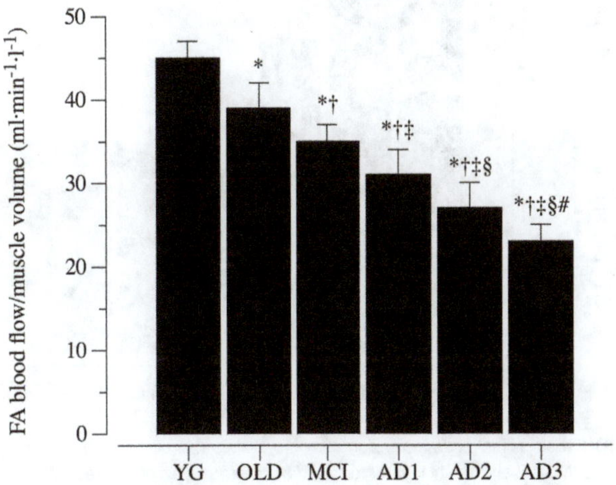

FIGURE 3 | Femoral artery blood flow normalized to muscle limb volume. Femoral artery (FA) blood flow normalized for lower limb muscle volume in healthy young (YG) and healthy old (OLD) controls, patients with mild cognitive impairment (MCI), and with different severity of AD, namely mild AD (AD1), moderate AD (AD2), and severe AD (AD3). Data are presented as mean ±S.E.; *Significantly different vs. YG group. †Significantly different vs. OLD group. ‡Significantly different vs. MCI group. §Significantly different vs. AD1 group. #Significantly different vs. AD2 group.

NO Bioavailability and Systemic Vascular Function

Plasma levels of nitrates and PLM induced hyperemia, which were used as markers of NO bioavailability and systemic vascular function, are illustrated in **Figure 4**. Both these markers of NO bioavailability showed a clear and progressive reduction across the groups. Specifically, plasma level of nitrates was significantly reduced ($p < 0.05$) from YG to OLD, MCI and through AD stages, with values of $67.8 \pm 4.2\,\mu$M in the YG, $58.1 \pm 5.1\,\mu$M in OLD, $51.1 \pm 3.0\,\mu$M in MCI, $45.1 \pm 3.7\,\mu$M in AD1, $39.2 \pm 3.7\,\mu$M in AD2, and $36.1 \pm 23.3\,\mu$M in AD3

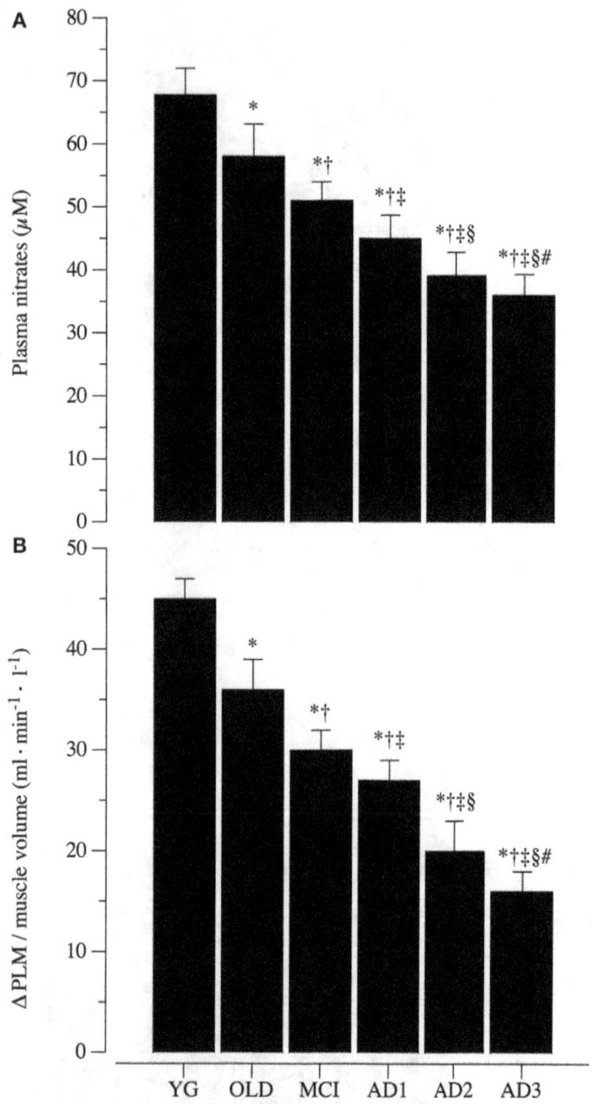

FIGURE 4 | Nitric oxide bioavailability and systemic vascular function. Nitric oxide (NO) bioavailability was determined by plasma levels of nitrates **(A)** and passive limb movement induced hyperemia normalized for muscle volume (ΔPLM; **B**). Systemic vascular function determined via ΔPLM/muscle volume is represented in **(B)** in healthy young (YG) and healthy old (OLD) controls, patients with mild cognitive impairment (MCI), and with different severity of AD, namely mild AD (AD1), moderate AD (AD2), and severe AD (AD3). Data are presented as mean ±S.E.; *Significantly different vs. YG group. †Significantly different vs. OLD group. ‡Significantly different vs. MCI group. §Significantly different vs. AD1 group. #Significantly different vs. AD2 group.

(**Figure 4A**). Similarly, ΔPLM hyperemia normalized for the muscle volume was significantly reduced ($p < 0.05$) among the 6 groups, with values of 45 ± 2 ml·min^{-1}·l^{-1} in YG, 36 ± 3 ml·min^{-1}·l^{-1} in OLD, 30 ± 2 ml·min^{-1}·l^{-1} in MCI, 27 ± 2 ml·min^{-1}·l^{-1} in AD1, 20 ± 3 ml·min^{-1}·l^{-1} in AD2, and 16 ± 2 ml·min^{-1}·l^{-1} in AD3 (**Figure 4B**). Post-hoc comparisons were significant across MCI and different AD stages for both measures.

Correlation Between NO Bioavailability, Systemic Vascular Function and Cortical, Extracranial, and Peripheral Blood Flow

Correlations between plasma levels of nitrates, PLM-induced hyperemia, which were used as markers of NO bioavailability and systemic vascular function, cortical perfusion, extracranial blood flow, and peripheral circulation are illustrated in **Figure 5**. Specifically, significant correlations were found between plasma levels of nitrates and FA blood flow normalized to the limb muscle volume (**Figure 5A**; $r = 0.48$, $p < 0.05$), ICA blood flow normalized for brain volume (**Figure 5C**; $r = 0.61$, $p < 0.05$), and PVC–CBF (**Figure 5E**; $r = 0.45$, $p < 0.05$). Interestingly, also values of ΔPLM/muscle volume were significantly correlated with FA blood flow/muscle volume (**Figure 5B**; $r = 0.71$, $p < 0.05$), ICA blood flow/brain volume (**Figure 5D**; $r = 0.82$, $p < 0.05$), and PVC–CBF (**Figure 5F**; $r = 0.77$, $p < 0.05$).

DISCUSSION

Although the association between reduction of NO bioavailability, cortical hypoperfusion and systemic vascular dysfunction has been already investigated in relation to AD onset in murine models, the mechanistic role of NO depletion in the reduction of extracranial blood flow and impairment of cortical and peripheral circulation in humans with AD has received so far only little attention. In the present study, we assessed ICA blood flow, cortical perfusion, and peripheral circulation in patients with MCI and different stages of AD and compared them to young and old healthy controls. Additionally, NO bioavailability was determined in the six groups of participants via plasma NO metabolites. A further indicator of endothelial NO bioavailability and systemic vascular function was estimated with PLM induced hyperemia. The main finding of this study was that ICA blood flow, cortical perfusion, peripheral circulation, and systemic vascular function were reduced in OLD vs. YG controls, and progressively further decreased in parallel to MCI and AD severity. These data suggest a pivotal role of AD, *per se,* to these vascular abnormalities. Though the causative relationship between NO bioavailability, central and peripheral circulation is still matter of debate, according to our hypothesis, circulation impairment was associated with NO depletion (**Figures 5, 6**).

Evidence That AD, *per se*, Affects NO Bioavailability and Blood Flow

Indeed, the first risk factor for AD is advanced age (Reitz et al., 2011; Reitz and Mayeux, 2014). It should also be noted that, independent of AD, reduced availability of NO, which is dramatically decreased in the aged population, results in major detrimental alterations of vascular function, including vasoconstriction and hypertension, leading to atherosclerosis. On the other hand, recent literature highlighted that AD is highly correlated to systemic vascular dysfunction (Iturria-Medina et al., 2016). Interestingly, current literature suggests the key role of NO depletion in the pathogenesis of neurodegenerative disease (Katusic and Austin, 2014). Therefore, we may speculate that both age and AD appear to be involved in the decline

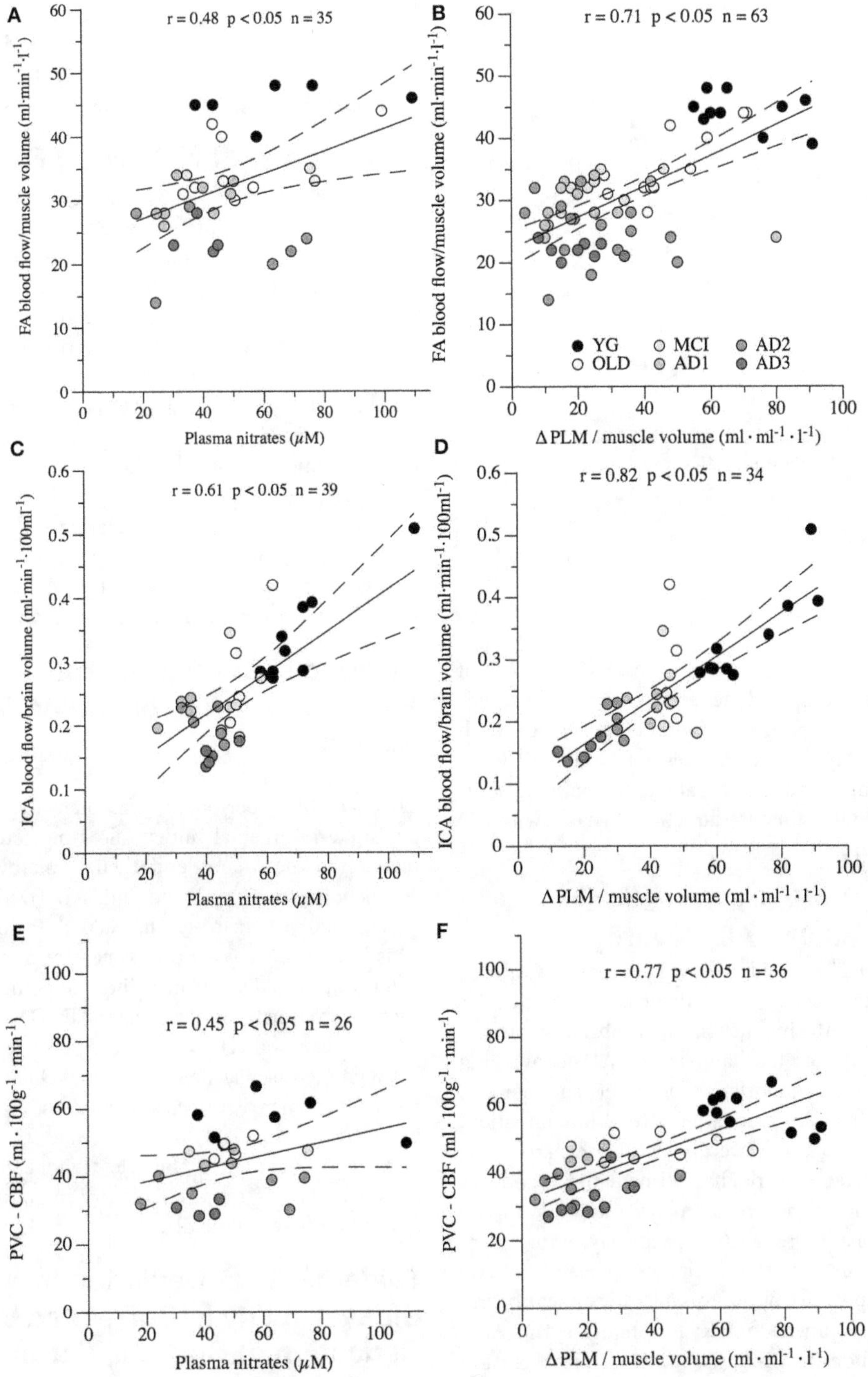

FIGURE 5 | Correlations between nitric oxide bioavailability, systemic vascular function and cortical (PVC–CBF), internal carotid artery (ICA) and femoral artery (FA) blood flow normalized for brain and muscle volume, respectively. Nitric oxide (NO) bioavailability was determined by plasma levels of nitrates **(A,C,E)** and passive limb movement induced hyperemia normalized to muscle volume (ΔPLM; **B,D,F**). Systemic vascular function determined via ΔPLM/muscle volume is represented in **B,D,F** in healthy young (YG) and healthy old (OLD) controls, and patients with mild cognitive impairment (MCI), and with different severity of AD, namely mild AD (AD1), moderate AD (AD2), and severe AD (AD3). Each point represents a single subject, dashed lines represents interval of confidence.

of the systemic and cerebral vascular function likely because of endogenous NO reduced bioavailability. However, the contribution of AD, *per se*, to this putative pathophysiological mechanism is still unclear. To better answer this point, we explored NO bioavailability, and cortical, ICA and peripheral blood flow in a group of patients with similar age (~78

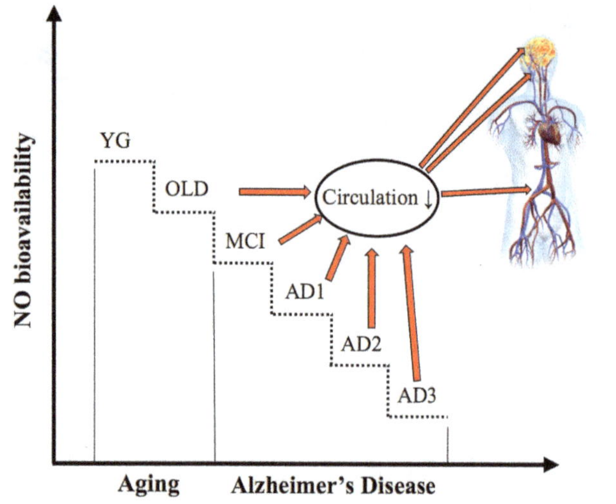

FIGURE 6 | schematic illustration: Impact of nitric oxide bioavailability on the progressive cerebral and peripheral circulatory impairments during aging and Alzheimer's disease.

years) but different cognitive impairment (i.e., MCI and AD of increasing severity) and compared them to young and old (aged-matched) controls. This integrative and comprehensive approach to vascular changes in AD showed changes in NO bioavailability and cortical, extracranial, and peripheral circulation in patients with AD and suggested that they are directly associated with AD and not to aging (**Figure 6**).

Evidence That Cortical Circulation Is Impaired in Parallel to AD Severity

Although the traditional "amyloid cascade hypothesis" proposed by Hardy and Higgins (Hardy and Higgins, 1992) indicates cortical deposition of Aβ fragments, neurofibrillary tangles and reactive microgliosis as the hallmark of AD, converging evidence underscores the importance of other pathogenetic mechanisms in AD, including oxidative stress, inflammation, and mitochondrial dysfunction (Swerdlow, 2011; Zenaro et al., 2016). In this multifaceted scenario, has germane the hypothesis that vascular dysfunction in the cortex plays a key role in AD pathophysiology (De La Torre, 2010). Specifically, impairment of cortical perfusion appears to be highly correlated to AD onset, implicating a pivotal role of vascular dysfunction and CAA. The recent development in MRI techniques led to ASL, a new advanced and non-invasive approach to brain perfusion measurement, coupled with more precise post-processing analysis. Our data are in agreement with and extend previous knowledge in this field (Detre et al., 1992), indicating that cortical hypoperfusion is not only associated with the presence of AD, but most important, is well correlated with the severity of dementia, NO bioavailability, and systemic vascular dysfunction (**Figures 1, 5**). The relevance of this result is particularly important because current biomarkers of AD, such as cerebrospinal fluid tau/Aβ fragments and positron emission tomography amyloid imaging, are known to change non-linearly throughout the progression of AD (Jack et al., 2013). We may speculate that cognitive impairment might be more related to cortical perfusion, while Aβ deposition takes place in the early/preclinical phases of AD. If confirmed in longitudinal studies, this hypothesis might indicate new therapeutic strategies for AD.

Evidence That ICA Blood Flow Is Impaired in Parallel to AD Severity

Indeed, most of the literature related to circulatory dysfunction associated with AD was focused on the cortical areas, which are primarily affected in AD (Du et al., 2006). Our data (**Figures 2, 3**) are in agreement with recent reports of a coupling between cortical hypoperfusion and a reduction of blood flow from ICA (Maalikjy Akkawi et al., 2003; Liu et al., 2014; Clark et al., 2017), and highlight that AD-related circulation impairment is not confined to the cortex, but is more likely the effect of a systemic vascular dysfunction (De La Torre, 2009, 2010). Moreover, the recognition of ICA blood flow reduction in parallel to AD severity implies an exacerbated cortical hypo perfusion in this population. These findings suggest that cortical perfusion changes measured via ASL are strongly dependent on abnormal inflow from extracranial arteries (Clark et al., 2017).

Evidence That Peripheral Vascular Function Is Impaired in Parallel to AD Severity

Along with cortical alteration of blood flow, few studies reported evidence that peripheral vascular dysfunction determined by ankle-to-brachial index, flow-mediated dilation, intima-media thickness, and endothelial microvascular response to acetylcholine are associated with AD (Dede et al., 2007; Khalil et al., 2007; Laurin et al., 2007; Tachibana et al., 2016). This literature suggests that systemic vascular impairments are determined by AD, or from a different point of view, that systemic vascular dysfunctions may trigger AD (De La Torre, 2004). In this complex cause-effect scenario, the peripheral vascular difference between the vascular dementia and AD has been accounted, and AD appears, *per se*, to be associated with a significant reduction of systemic vascular function. Data from the current study (**Figures 3–5**) confirm this view and extend the relationship between AD onset and circulatory impairment up to the more advanced phases of the disease.

Evidence That Depletion in NO Bioavailability Is Correlated With Reduction of Cortical, Extracranial, and Peripheral Blood Flow

Nitric oxide, an unstable free radical endogenously synthesized by several cell-types, exerts various biological regulatory functions at peripheral level in the nervous and cardiovascular systems (Loscalzo and Welch, 1995; Calabrese et al., 2007). Indeed, depletion of NO and endothelial nitric oxide synthase enzymatic activity, as a major endogenous source of NO, are one of the mechanisms in the pathogenesis of endothelial dysfunction in both cerebral and peripheral blood vessels (Katusic and Austin, 2014). Interestingly, recent literature has underlined the key role of NO depletion in the early stage of neurodegenerative disorders, as well as in their progression (Katusic and Austin, 2014). In a recent murine study, Merlini and coauthors (Merlini et al., 2017) revealed that reduced NO bioavailability mediates cerebro-arterial and peripheral dysfunction independently from CAA. Interestingly, and similarly to the data retrieved in our human model, endothelium-dependent vasorelaxation was significantly impaired in both basilar and femoral arteries of 15-month-old Swedish arctic (SweArc) transgenic AD mice compared with that of age-matched wild-type and 6-month-old SweArc. This vascular impairment was accompanied by significantly reduced levels of cyclic GMP, demonstrating the central role of NO bioavailability in the pathogenesis and development of AD. Due to the transitory and unstable nature of this free radical, several studies have determined the bioavailability of NO via plasma levels of nitrite and nitrate (Casey et al., 2007, 2010). Interestingly, this literature indicates a strong positive relationship between plasma level of nitrite and nitrate and systemic vascular function (Casey et al., 2007, 2010). The present data are in agreement with the above-mentioned animal and human studies, and support the hypothesis that, in humans, the depletion in NO bioavailability is correlated with reduction of cortical, extracranial, and peripheral blood flow during aging and in parallel to AD severity (**Figures 4–6**).

Other Physiological Considerations

The recent literature underlined that augmenting physical activity and fitness can protect NO bioavailability, attenuating the deleterious effects of advancing age on vascular function (Groot et al., 2016). Therefore, particular attention on the determination of the physical activity level is needed in order to better describe the net effect of aging and AD to the systemic vascular function. As expected, our results indicate that in comparison to the YG, healthy elderly and patients with AD, were more sedentary (**Table 1**). These data suggest that the reduction of systemic vascular function and NO bioavailability of these groups are likely affected by their low-level of physical activity. However, it is important to note that the IPAQ values among OLD, MCI, AD1, AD2, and AD3 were similar, implicating that in these age-matched groups, aging and level of physical activity are not responsible of the progressive reduction of NO bioavailability and vascular dysfunction. Another physiological factor important to mention in relation to the cerebral blood flow assessment is the level of CO_2. In fact, due to its vasodilatory effect on the conduit intra- and extracranial arteries, hypercapnia is routinely utilized for the evaluation of maximal cerebral perfusion. Therefore, the determination of $ExpCO_2$ is required in order to normalize the cerebral blood flow. The data of resting $ExpCO_2$ (**Table 1**) were similar in the 6 groups, implicating that $ExpCO_2$ did not play a role in the changes of cerebral blood flow in our subjects. Indeed, resting blood flow to a specific organ is affected by its volume of metabolically active tissue. As previously described in the text, partial volume-corrected cortical and WM flow maps were created for each subject, and FA and ICA blood flow were normalized to leg muscle volume (thigh + lower leg volume) and total brain tissue volume (cortical, subcortical gray matter and white matter volumes including the brainstem and cerebellum), respectively (Liu et al., 2014; Venturelli et al., 2014). Indeed, basal metabolism is another important physiological factor affected by aging (Venturelli et al., 2013) and AD (Venturelli et al., 2016), that may contribute to the resting blood flow changes during aging and AD. Interestingly, our data of resting oxygen uptake (**Table 1**) indicate similar basal metabolism in the six groups of subjects, suggesting that this physiological factor is not playing a direct role in the progressive changes of brain and skeletal muscle blood flow. It is important to mention that NO is a free radical playing several positive regulatory functions at cellular and systemic level. However, it is well established that elevated levels of free radicals have a plethora of deleterious effects on the vascular and nervous system during aging and AD, primarily associated with mitochondrial dysfunction. Indeed, Sewrdlow and Khan (Swerdlow, 2011) hypothesized the "*mitochondrial cascade hypothesis*" in AD, whereby mitochondrial dysfunction accumulates over the disease course, resulting in both symptoms and neuropathological aspects of AD (Swerdlow et al., 2010). It is believed that mitochondrial dysfunction precedes Aβ formation, increasing reactive oxygen species (ROS) and oxidative stress, which, in turn, may facilitate overproduction of Aβ (Morris et al., 2014). In AD, mitochondrial damage is characterized by decreased respiratory chain complexes activities, where complexes III and IV are typically involved, causing ROS overproduction and reduced ATP synthesis (Marques-Aleixo et al., 2012; Cadonic et al., 2016; Pedrinolla et al., 2017). In this regard, brain tissues are metabolically very active and are particularly susceptible to the damaging effects by ROS. In case of AD, ROS have been reported within those brain regions, such as the cerebral cortex and hippocampus, which undergo selective neurodegeneration (Bhat et al., 2015). Interestingly, a large body of evidence shows that AD patients have oxidative metabolism dysfunction in both the central nervous system (CNS) and peripheral tissues (i.e., vascular endothelial cells, platelets) suggesting that pathological changes co-exist in brain and non-neural tissues (Morris et al., 2014; Cadonic et al., 2016). Moreover, recent studies suggest that mitochondria ROS overproduction contribute to accelerate the development of the senescent phenotype in endothelial cells, impairing regenerative and angiogenic capacity of the endothelium, promoting atherosclerosis by altering the secretion of cytokines, growth factors, and protease in the vascular wall (Dai et al., 2012; El Assar et al., 2013).

Other potential confounding factors that may have influenced, at least in part, our findings include the deconditioning due to AD, the age-related aortic stiffness and progressive impairment in diastolic heart functions (Pase et al., 2016).

AUTHOR CONTRIBUTIONS

MV performed the experiments, analyzed the data, prepared the figures, and drafted the manuscript. APe performed the experiments, analyzed the data, and drafted the manuscript. IB performed the experiments, analyzed the data, and drafted the manuscript. CF performed the experiments, analyzed the data, and drafted the manuscript. NS interpreted the results of experiments, and drafted the manuscript. ST performed the experiments, interpreted the results of experiments, and drafted the manuscript. EM performed the experiments, interpreted the results of experiments, and drafted the manuscript. LC performed the experiments, interpreted the results of experiments, and drafted the manuscript. AS performed the experiments, interpreted the results of experiments, and drafted the manuscript. APi performed the experiments, interpreted the results of experiments, and drafted the manuscript. MR interpreted the results of experiments, and drafted the manuscript. FP interpreted the results of experiments, and drafted the manuscript. FS edited, revised, and approved the final version of manuscript.

FUNDING

The study was supported by the grant 2010KL2Y73_004 awarded to FS from the Italian Ministry for Research (PRIN 2010).

ACKNOWLEDGMENTS

We thank all the study participants and Dr. Scarsini R. for their support and dedication to the research project.

REFERENCES

Albert, M. S., Dekosky, S. T., Dickson, D., Dubois, B., Feldman, H. H., Fox, N. C., et al. (2011). The diagnosis of mild cognitive impairment due to Alzheimer's disease: recommendations from the National Institute on Aging-Alzheimer's Association workgroups on diagnostic guidelines for Alzheimer's disease. *Alzheimers Dement.* 7, 270–279. doi: 10.1016/j.jalz.2011.03.008

Alsop, D. C., Detre, J. A., Golay, X., Gunther, M., Hendrikse, J., Hernandez-Garcia, L., et al. (2015). Recommended implementation of arterial spin-labeled perfusion MRI for clinical applications: a consensus of the ISMRM perfusion study group and the European consortium for ASL in dementia. *Magn. Reson. Med.* 73, 102–116. doi: 10.1002/mrm.25197

Appollonio, I., Leone, M., Isella, V., Piamarta, F., Consoli, T., Villa, M. L., et al. (2005). The Frontal Assessment Battery (FAB): normative values in an Italian population sample. *Neurol. Sci.* 26, 108–116. doi: 10.1007/s10072-005-0443-4

Bhat, A. H., Dar, K. B., Anees, S., Zargar, M. A., Masood, A., Sofi, M. A., et al. (2015). Oxidative stress, mitochondrial dysfunction and neurodegenerative diseases; a mechanistic insight. *Biomed. Pharmacother.* 74, 101–110. doi: 10.1016/j.biopha.2015.07.025

Booth, M. (2000). Assessment of physical activity: an international perspective. *Res. Q. Exerc. Sport* 71(Suppl. 2), 114–120. doi: 10.1080/02701367.2000.11082794

Buxton, R. B., Frank, L. R., Wong, E. C., Siewert, B., Warach, S., and Edelman, R. R. (1998). A general kinetic model for quantitative perfusion imaging with arterial spin labeling. *Magn. Reson. Med.* 40, 383–396. doi: 10.1002/mrm.1910400308

Cadonic, C., Sabbir, M. G., and Albensi, B. C. (2016). Mechanisms of mitochondrial dysfunction in Alzheimer's disease. *Mol. Neurobiol.* 53, 6078–6090. doi: 10.1007/s12035-015-9515-5

Calabrese, V., Mancuso, C., Calvani, M., Rizzarelli, E., Butterfield, D. A., and Stella, A. M. (2007). Nitric oxide in the central nervous system: neuroprotection versus neurotoxicity. *Nat. Rev. Neurosci.* 8, 766–775. doi: 10.1038/nrn2214

Casey, D. P., Beck, D. T., and Braith, R. W. (2007). Systemic plasma levels of nitrite/nitrate (NOx) reflect brachial flow-mediated dilation responses in young men and women. *Clin. Exp. Pharmacol. Physiol.* 34, 1291–1293. doi: 10.1111/j.1440-1681.2007.04715.x

Casey, D. P., Nichols, W. W., Conti, C. R., and Braith, R. W. (2010). Relationship between endogenous concentrations of vasoactive substances and measures of peripheral vasodilator function in patients with coronary artery disease. *Clin. Exp. Pharmacol. Physiol.* 37, 24–28. doi: 10.1111/j.1440-1681.2009.05225.x

Clark, L. R., Berman, S. E., Rivera-Rivera, L. A., Hoscheidt, S. M., Darst, B. F., Engelman, C. D., et al. (2017). Macrovascular and microvascular cerebral blood flow in adults at risk for Alzheimer's disease. *Alzheimers Dement.* 7, 48–55. doi: 10.1016/j.dadm.2017.01.002

Dai, D. F., Rabinovitch, P. S., and Ungvari, Z. (2012). Mitochondria and cardiovascular aging. *Circ. Res.* 110, 1109–1124. doi: 10.1161/CIRCRESAHA.111.246140

Dallaire-Theroux, C., Callahan, B. L., Potvin, O., Saikali, S., and Duchesne, S. (2017). Radiological-pathological correlation in Alzheimer's Disease: systematic review of antemortem magnetic resonance imaging findings. *J. Alzheimers Dis.* 57, 575–601. doi: 10.3233/JAD-161028

Dede, D. S., Yavuz, B., Yavuz, B. B., Cankurtaran, M., Halil, M., Ulger, Z., et al. (2007). Assessment of endothelial function in Alzheimer's disease: is Alzheimer's disease a vascular disease? *J. Am. Geriatr. Soc.* 55, 1613–1617. doi: 10.1111/j.1532-5415.2007.01378.x

De La Torre, J. C. (2004). Alzheimer's disease is a vasocognopathy: a new term to describe its nature. *Neurol. Res.* 26, 517–524. doi: 10.1179/016164104225016254

De La Torre, J. C. (2009). Cerebrovascular and cardiovascular pathology in Alzheimer's disease. *Int. Rev. Neurobiol.* 84, 35–48. doi: 10.1016/S0074-7742(09)00403-6

De La Torre, J. C. (2010). The vascular hypothesis of Alzheimer's disease: bench to bedside and beyond. *Neurodegener. Dis.* 7, 116–121. doi: 10.1159/000285520

Detre, J. A., Leigh, J. S., Williams, D. S., and Koretsky, A. P. (1992). Perfusion imaging. *Magn. Reson. Med.* 23, 37–45. doi: 10.1002/mrm.19102 30106

Du, A. T., Jahng, G. H., Hayasaka, S., Kramer, J. H., Rosen, H. J., Gorno-Tempini, M. L., et al. (2006). Hypoperfusion in frontotemporal dementia and Alzheimer disease by arterial spin labeling MRI. *Neurology* 67, 1215–1220. doi: 10.1212/01.wnl.0000238163.71349.78

El Assar, M., Angulo, J., and Rodriguez-Manas, L. (2013). Oxidative stress and vascular inflammation in aging. *Free Radic. Biol. Med.* 65, 380–401. doi: 10.1016/j.freeradbiomed.2013.07.003

Folstein, M. F., Folstein, S. E., and Mchugh, P. R. (1975). "Mini-mental state". A practical method for grading the cognitive state of patients for the clinician. *J. Psychiatr. Res.* 12, 189–198. doi: 10.1016/0022-3956(75)90026-6

Groot, H. J., Rossman, M. J., Garten, R. S., Wang, E., Hoff, J., Helgerud, J., et al. (2016). The effect of physical activity on passive leg movement-induced vasodilation with age. *Med. Sci. Sports Exerc.* 48, 1548–1557. doi: 10.1249/MSS.0000000000000936

Hardy, J. A., and Higgins, G. A. (1992). Alzheimer's disease: the amyloid cascade hypothesis. *Science* 256, 184–185. doi: 10.1126/science.1566067

Herholz, K. (2011). Perfusion SPECT and FDG-PET. *Int. Psychogeriatr.* 23 (Suppl. 2), S25–S31. doi: 10.1017/S1041610211000937

Iturria-Medina, Y., Sotero, R. C., Toussaint, P. J., Mateos-Perez, J. M., Evans, A. C., and Alzheimer's Disease Neuroimaging, I. (2016). Early role of vascular dysregulation on late-onset Alzheimer's disease based on multifactorial data-driven analysis. *Nat. Commun.* 7:11934. doi: 10.1038/ncomms11934

Ives, S. J., Amann, M., Venturelli, M., Witman, M. A., Groot, H. J., Wray, D. W., et al. (2016). The mechanoreflex and hemodynamic response to passive leg movement in heart failure. *Med. Sci. Sports Exerc.* 48, 368–376. doi: 10.1249/MSS.0000000000000782

Jack, C. R. Jr., Knopman, D. S., Jagust, W. J., Petersen, R. C., Weiner, M. W., Aisen, P. S., et al. (2013). Tracking pathophysiological processes in Alzheimer's disease: an updated hypothetical model of dynamic biomarkers. *Lancet Neurol.* 12, 207–216. doi: 10.1016/S1474-4422(12)70291-0

Katusic, Z. S., and Austin, S. A. (2014). Endothelial nitric oxide: protector of a healthy mind. *Eur. Heart J.* 35, 888–894. doi: 10.1093/eurheartj/eht544

Khalil, Z., Logiudice, D., Khodr, B., Maruff, P., and Masters, C. (2007). Impaired peripheral endothelial microvascular responsiveness in Alzheimer's disease. *J. Alzheimers Dis.* 11, 25–32. doi: 10.3233/JAD-2007-11106

Laurin, D., Masaki, K. H., White, L. R., and Launer, L. J. (2007). Ankle-to-brachial index and dementia: the Honolulu-Asia aging study. *Circulation* 116, 2269–2274. doi: 10.1161/CIRCULATIONAHA.106.686477

Layec, G., Venturelli, M., Jeong, E. K., and Richardson, R. S. (2014). The validity of anthropometric leg muscle volume estimation across a wide spectrum: from able-bodied adults to individuals with a spinal cord injury. *J. Appl. Physiol. (1985)* 116, 1142–1147. doi: 10.1152/japplphysiol.01120.2013

Liu, J., Zhu, Y. S., Khan, M. A., Brunk, E., Martin-Cook, K., Weiner, M. F., et al. (2014). Global brain hypoperfusion and oxygenation in amnestic mild cognitive impairment. *Alzheimers Dement.* 10, 162–170. doi: 10.1016/j.jalz.2013.04.507

Loscalzo, J., and Welch, G. (1995). Nitric oxide and its role in the cardiovascular system. *Prog. Cardiovasc. Dis.* 38, 87–104. doi: 10.1016/S0033-0620(05)80001-5

Maalikjy Akkawi, N., Borroni, B., Agosti, C., Pezzini, A., Magoni, M., Rozzini, L., et al. (2003). Volume reduction in cerebral blood flow in patients with Alzheimer's disease: a sonographic study. *Dement. Geriatr. Cogn. Disord.* 16, 163–169. doi: 10.1159/000071005

Maier, F. C., Wehrl, H. F., Schmid, A. M., Mannheim, J. G., Wiehr, S., Lerdkrai, C., et al. (2014). Longitudinal PET-MRI reveals beta-amyloid deposition and rCBF dynamics and connects vascular amyloidosis to quantitative loss of perfusion. *Nat. Med.* 20, 1485–1492. doi: 10.1038/nm.3734

Marques-Aleixo, I., Oliveira, P. J., Moreira, P. I., Magalhaes, J., and Ascensao, A. (2012). Physical exercise as a possible strategy for brain protection: evidence from mitochondrial-mediated mechanisms. *Prog. Neurobiol.* 99, 149–162. doi: 10.1016/j.pneurobio.2012.08.002

Mcdaniel, J., Fjeldstad, A. S., Ives, S., Hayman, M., Kithas, P., and Richardson, R. S. (2010a). Central and peripheral contributors to skeletal muscle hyperemia: response to passive limb movement. *J. Appl. Physiol. (1985)* 108, 76–84. doi: 10.1152/japplphysiol.00895.2009

Mcdaniel, J., Hayman, M. A., Ives, S., Fjeldstad, A. S., Trinity, J. D., Wray, D. W., et al. (2010b). Attenuated exercise induced hyperaemia with age: mechanistic insight from passive limb movement. *J. Physiol. (Lond).* 588, 4507–4517. doi: 10.1113/jphysiol.2010.198770.

Mckhann, G. M., Knopman, D. S., Chertkow, H., Hyman, B. T., Jack, C. R. Jr., Kawas, C. H., et al. (2011). The diagnosis of dementia due to Alzheimer's disease: recommendations from the National Institute on Aging-Alzheimer's Association workgroups on diagnostic guidelines for Alzheimer's disease. *Alzheimers. Dement.* 7, 263–269. doi: 10.1016/j.jalz.2011.03.005

Merlini, M., Shi, Y., Keller, S., Savarese, G., Akhmedov, A., Derungs, R., et al. (2017). Reduced nitric oxide bioavailability mediates cerebroarterial dysfunction independent of cerebral amyloid angiopathy in a mouse model of Alzheimer's disease. *Am. J. Physiol. Heart Circ. Physiol.* 312, H232–H238. doi: 10.1152/ajpheart.00607.2016

Morris, J. C. (1993). The Clinical Dementia Rating (CDR): current version and scoring rules. *Neurology* 43, 2412–2414. doi: 10.1212/WNL.43.11.2412-a

Morris, J. K., Honea, R. A., Vidoni, E. D., Swerdlow, R. H., and Burns, J. M. (2014). Is Alzheimer's disease a systemic disease? *Biochim. Biophys. Acta* 1842, 1340–1349. doi: 10.1016/j.bbadis.2014.04.012

Pase, M. P., Beiser, A., Himali, J. J., Tsao, C., Satizabal, C. L., Vasan, R. S., et al. (2016). Aortic Stiffness and the Risk of Incident Mild Cognitive Impairment and Dementia. *Stroke* 47, 2256–2261. doi: 10.1161/STROKEAHA.116.013508

Pedrinolla, A., Schena, F., and Venturelli, M. (2017). Resilience to Alzheimer's disease: the role of physical activity. *Curr. Alzheimer Res.* 14, 546–553. doi: 10.2174/1567205014666170111145817

Picano, E., Bruno, R. M., Ferrari, G. F., and Bonuccelli, U. (2014). Cognitive impairment and cardiovascular disease: so near, so far. *Int. J. Cardiol.* 175, 21–29. doi: 10.1016/j.ijcard.2014.05.004

Reitz, C., Brayne, C., and Mayeux, R. (2011). Epidemiology of Alzheimer disease. *Nat. Rev. Neurol.* 7, 137–152. doi: 10.1038/nrneurol.2011.2

Reitz, C., and Mayeux, R. (2014). Alzheimer disease: epidemiology, diagnostic criteria, risk factors and biomarkers. *Biochem. Pharmacol.* 88, 640–651. doi: 10.1016/j.bcp.2013.12.024

Swerdlow, R. H. (2011). Brain aging, Alzheimer's disease, and mitochondria. *Biochim. Biophys. Acta* 1812, 1630–1639. doi: 10.1016/j.bbadis.2011.08.012

Swerdlow, R. H., Burns, J. M., and Khan, S. M. (2010). The Alzheimer's disease mitochondrial cascade hypothesis. *J Alzheimers Dis* 20(Suppl. 2), S265–279. doi: 10.3233/JAD-2010-100339

Tachibana, H., Washida, K., Kowa, H., Kanda, F., and Toda, T. (2016). Vascular function in Alzheimer's disease and vascular dementia. *Am. J. Alzheimers Dis. Other Demen.* 31, 437–442. doi: 10.1177/1533317516653820

Trinity, J. D., Groot, H. J., Layec, G., Rossman, M. J., Ives, S. J., Runnels, S., et al. (2012). Nitric oxide and passive limb movement: a new approach to assess vascular function. *J. Physiol.* 590, 1413–1425. doi: 10.1113/jphysiol.2011.224741

Venturelli, M., Amann, M., Layec, G., Mcdaniel, J., Trinity, J. D., Fjeldstad, A. S., et al. (2014). Passive leg movement-induced hyperaemia with a spinal cord lesion: evidence of preserved vascular function. *Acta Physiol. (Oxf).* 210, 429–439. doi: 10.1111/apha.12173

Venturelli, M., Ce, E., Limonta, E., Muti, E., Scarsini, R., Brasioli, A., et al. (2016). Possible predictors of involuntary weight loss in patients with Alzheimer's disease. *PLoS ONE* 11:e0157384. doi: 10.1371/journal.pone.0157384

Venturelli, M., Schena, F., Scarsini, R., Muti, E., and Richardson, R. S. (2013). Limitations to exercise in female centenarians: evidence that muscular efficiency tempers the impact of failing lungs. *Age (Dordr).* 35, 861–870. doi: 10.1007/s11357-011-9379-1

Zenaro, E., Piacentino, G., and Constantin, G. (2016). The blood-brain barrier in Alzheimer's disease. *Neurobiol. Dis.* 107, 41–56. doi: 10.1016/j.nbd.2016.07.007

18

Notch1 Mediates Preconditioning Protection Induced by GPER in Normotensive and Hypertensive Female Rat Hearts

Carmine Rocca[1†], Saveria Femminò[2†], Giorgio Aquila[3†], Maria C. Granieri[1], Ernestina M. De Francesco[4], Teresa Pasqua[1], Damiano C. Rigiracciolo[4], Francesca Fortini[3,5], Maria C. Cerra[1,6], Marcello Maggiolini[4], Pasquale Pagliaro[2,6], Paola Rizzo[5,7,8], Tommaso Angelone[1,6†] and Claudia Penna[2,6*†]*

[1] Laboratory of Molecular and Cellular Cardiac Physiology, Department of Biology, Ecology and E.S., University of Calabria, Rende, Italy, [2] Department of Biological and Clinical Sciences, University of Turin, Turin, Italy, [3] Department of Medical Sciences, University of Ferrara, Ferrara, Italy, [4] Department of Pharmacy, Health and Nutritional Sciences, University of Calabria, Rende, Italy, [5] Maria Cecilia Hospital, GVM Care & Research, E.S. Health Science Foundation, Cotignola, Italy, [6] National Institute for Cardiovascular Research, Bologna, Italy, [7] Department of Morphology, Surgery and Experimental Medicine, University of Ferrara, Ferrara, Italy, [8] Laboratory for Technologies of Advanced Therapies, University of Ferrara, Ferrara, Italy

Edited by:
Antonio Colantuoni,
University of Naples Federico II, Italy

Reviewed by:
Claudio Molinari,
Università degli Studi del Piemonte Orientale, Italy
Ioanna Andreadou,
National and Kapodistrian University of Athens, Greece

***Correspondence:**
Tommaso Angelone
tommaso.angelone@unical.it
Claudia Penna
claudia.penna@unito.it

† These authors have contributed equally to this work.

G protein-coupled estrogen receptor (GPER) is an estrogen receptor expressed in the cardiovascular system. G1, a selective GPER ligand, exerts cardiovascular effects through activation of the PI3K-Akt pathway and Notch signaling in normotensive animals. Here, we investigated whether the G1/GPER interaction is involved in the limitation of infarct size, and improvement of post-ischemic contractile function in female spontaneous hypertensive rat (SHR) hearts. In this model, we also studied Notch signaling and key components of survival pathway, namely PI3K-Akt, nitric oxide synthase (NOS) and mitochondrial K^+-ATP (MitoKATP) channels. Rat hearts isolated from female SHR underwent 30 min of global, normothermic ischemia and 120 min of reperfusion. G1 (10 nM) alone or specific inhibitors of GPER, PI3K/NOS and MitoKATP channels co-infused with G1, just before I/R, were studied. The involvement of Notch1 was studied by Western blotting. Infarct size and left ventricular pressure were measured. To confirm endothelial-independent G1-induced protection by Notch signaling, H9c2 cells were studied with specific inhibitor, *N*-[*N*-(3,5 difluorophenacetyl)-L-alanyl]-*S*-phenylglycine *t*-butyl ester (DAPT, 5 μM), of this signaling. Using DAPT, we confirmed the involvement of G1/Notch signaling in limiting infarct size in heart of normotensive animals. In the hypertensive model, G1-induced reduction in infarct size and improvement of cardiac function were prevented by the inhibition of GPER, PI3K/NOS, and MitoKATP channels. The involvement of Notch was confirmed by western blot in the hypertensive model and by the specific inhibitor in the normotensive model and cardiac cell line. Our results suggest that GPERs play a pivotal role in mediating preconditioning cardioprotection in normotensive and hypertensive conditions. The G1-induced protection involves Notch1 and is able to activate the survival pathway in the presence of comorbidity. Several pathological conditions, including hypertension, reduce the efficacy of ischemic conditioning strategies. However, G1-induced protection can result in significant reduction of I/R injury also female in hypertensive animals. Further studies may ascertain the clinical translation of the present results.

Keywords: cardioprotection, preconditioning, H9c2, isolated rat hearts, reperfusion injury salvage kinases, PI3K/Akt, NOS

INTRODUCTION

The G protein-coupled estrogen receptor (GPR30/GPER) is expressed in the heart and it mediates non-genomic effects of estrogen. It has been suggested that GPER activation mediates beneficial effects in the cardiovascular system, as demonstrated using pharmacological agonists/antagonists of GPER (Dennis et al., 2009). In this regard, the synthetic and selective GPER agonist, G1 (Bologa et al., 2006), has been shown to activate signaling pathways involved in cardiomyocytes survival, thus improving cardiovascular function both in normal and stressful conditions. Yet, the synthetic and selective GPER antagonist, G15 (Dennis et al., 2009), prevented these beneficial effects (De Francesco et al., 2013, 2017). To obtain its effect, GPER cross-reacts with a number of cell signaling systems, including the epidermal growth factor receptor, the mitogen-activated protein kinases and the Notch signaling pathway (Pupo et al., 2016).

In the normotensive rat, GPER activation improves contractile recovery and limits infarct size in isolated rat hearts following ischemia/reperfusion (I/R) through a gender-independent and PI3K-dependent mechanism (Deschamps and Murphy, 2009).

The potential of ischemic preconditioning to reduce I/R injury has been recognized more than 30 years ago (Hausenloy et al., 2016). Preconditioning limits I/R injury *via* multiple pathways. However, the effectiveness of this cardioprotective intervention is noticeably reduced in pathological animal models, such as hypertensive animals (Ferdinandy et al., 2007).

Several data demonstrated that in both normotensive male and female rodent models, the GPER activation plays a role as pre- and post-conditioning cardioprotective agent *in vitro* and *ex vivo* (Deschamps and Murphy, 2009; Bopassa et al., 2010; Deschamps et al., 2010; Li et al., 2015; Feng et al., 2017; Menazza et al., 2017). These GPER-dependent cardioprotective effects are displayed by its ability to improve the functional recovery, to preserve the mitochondrial structural integrity and function and to reduce mitophagy.

However, the potential of GPER to mediate beneficial effects in hypertensive conditions has not yet been fully investigated.

In male spontaneously hypertensive rats (SHRs) hearts, we have reported that the activation of GPER reduced the expression of apoptotic and fibrotic factors and induced negative inotropic and lusitropic effects (De Francesco et al., 2013). In these hearts, GPER induced activation Akt/PKB, ERK1/2, GSK-3β, c-Jun and endothelial nitric oxide (NO) synthase (eNOS) signaling. Also, GPER prevents the detrimental cardiac effects of certain anti-cancer agents like Doxorubicin (De Francesco et al., 2017). Hence, GPER may represent a novel pharmacological target in the treatment of some cardiovascular pathologies associated with stressful conditions, such as hypertension (De Francesco et al., 2013).

Besides cross-talking with GPER in breast cancer cell lines (Pupo et al., 2014), Notch signaling pathway plays an important role in regulating cell death, differentiation, and angiogenesis (Lubecka et al., 2016). Moreover, it is associated with cardioprotection. Indeed, Notch signaling pathway activation reduces I/R injury and modulates cardiac repair after myocardial infarction (Li et al., 2010). Importantly, Notch drives cell survival signaling contributing to cardioprotection by ischemic conditioning protocols in healthy animals (Zhou et al., 2013). Therefore, we hypothesized that GPER/Notch pathway may be involved in the cardioprotection mediated by GPER-agonist in hypertensive female models. To ascertain this hypothesis, we studied GPER/Notch pathway in the heart of hypertensive model, firstly using the two synthetic molecules G1 and G15, which act as selective and potent agonist and antagonist of GPER, respectively. These allowed to discriminate the selective GPER activation from the estrogen effects mediated by the classical intracellular estrogen receptors (ER α/β). In addition, in order to further explore the mechanism of action GPER-dependent, specific inhibitors of PI3K/NOS pathway and mitoKATP channels were used. The Notch involvement was studied by Western blot analysis. For comparative purpose, we confirmed the role of GPER/Notch pathway in hearts of normotensive animals using specif inhibitors of GPER and Notch pathway. To further analyze a direct cardioprotective effect of GPER agonist, we studied its effect in an *in vitro* model of injury: we subjected rat embryonic-heart derived cardiomyoblasts (H9c2) to hypoxia/reoxygenation with and without inhibitors of PI3K/NOS pathway and MitoKATP channels.

MATERIALS AND METHODS

Animals

Female normotensive Wistar rats (n = 25; body weight: 250–300 g; Harlan Laboratories, Udine, Italy) and Female SHRs (n = 28; body weight: 250–300; Harlan Laboratories, Udine, Italy) received humane care in compliance with the Guide for the Care and Use of Laboratory Animals published by the United States National Institutes of Health (NIH Publication No. 85-23, revised 1996). Two normotensive Wistar rat hearts and one SHR heart were discarded due to their very low left ventricular developed pressure or other technical issues after connection to the perfusion line. In accordance with the Italian law in force (DL n. 116, January 27, 1992), regarding animal protection, the scientific project has been approved by the Italian Ministry of Health (Rome, Italy). All animals were identically housed under controlled light and temperature conditions with access to food and water *ad libitum*. SHR female rats, used in this paper for hemodynamic studies, are part of a set of hypertensive animals whose male counterpart was employed in previous works (De Francesco et al., 2013; Pasqua et al., 2015). The basal blood pressure of female animals (recorded before experiments by the tail-cuff method) displayed the same trend of male rats (data not shown).

Experimental Models

Isolated Perfused Heart

The methods were similar to those previously described (Penna et al., 2009, 2011; Pasqua et al., 2015). Briefly, each animal was heparinized (800 U/100 g b.w., i.m.) and after 10 min rats were anesthetized with i.p. injection of ethyl carbamate (2 g/kg rat), then hearts were rapidly excised and immediately arrested in ice-cold buffered Krebs–Henseleit solution (KHS) for subsequent aorta cannulation. Hearts were then perfused at constant retrograde flow (12 ml/min) and constant temperature of 37°C. Perfusion medium was a modified Krebs–Henseleit Solution (KHS; pH 7.4) gassed with 95% O_2 and 5% CO_2 containing (in mM): 113.0 NaCl; 4.7 KCl; 1.2 $MgSO_4$; 25.0 $NaHCO_3$; 1.2 KH_2PO_4; 1.8 $CaCl_2$; 11.0 glucose; 1.1 mannitol; 5.0 Na-pyruvate (Pasqua et al., 2015). A water-filled latex balloon was connected to a pressure transducer (BLPR, WRI, Inc., Saratota, FL, United States) and pushed into the left ventricle (LV) through the mitral valve. Another pressure transducer connected with perfusion cannula was used to measure coronary pressure (CP). The developed left ventricular pressure (dLVP; mmHg, index of contractile activity) and the left ventricular end diastolic pressure (LVEDP; mmHg, index of contracture) were measured to evaluate cardiac function. The LVEDP was set to obtain a 5–8 mmHg pressure. Cardiac performance was recorded by using the PowerLab data acquisition system. Parameters were quantified by using Chart Software (ADInstruments, Oxford, United Kingdom) (Pasqua et al., 2015).

After stabilization, reference parameters were recorded and each heart was assigned in random order to one of the following experimental groups described below (**Figure 1A**).

Normotensive Heart Model

Four groups of hearts isolated from normotensive animals were subjected to the following protocols:

(1) Sham group (n = 3): hearts were stabilized for 30 min and then subjected to 150 min of perfusion only.
(2) I/R group (n = 8): after a 30 min stabilization period, the perfusion was completely stopped (global no-flow ischemia) for a duration of 30 min. Thereafter, hearts were reperfused for 120 min.
(3) GPER agonist G1 (G1) group (n = 7): hearts were pre-treated with G1 (10 nM), a GPER selective agonist for 20 min. Thereafter the hearts were subjected to I/R protocol, as above (De Francesco et al., 2013).
(4) G1+Notch inhibitor group (n = 5): hearts were pre-treated with a co-infusion of G1 and a selective inhibitor of Notch pathway, namely *N*-[*N*-(3,5 difluorophenacetyl)-L-alanyl]-*S*-phenylglycine *t*-butyl ester (DAPT, 5 μM) (Boccalini et al., 2015), and then four hearts were subjected to I/R.

Hypertensive Heart Model

In the following groups: Sham (n = 3), I/R (n = 3), G1 (n = 5), hearts isolated from female SHR were subjected to the protocols described above for normotensive animals.

Moreover, to deepen the signaling pathway involved in protection, the following groups were studied in the hypertensive model:

(8) G1+G15 group (n = 4): hearts were pre-treated with a co-infusion of the selective GPER agonist, G1 (10 nM), and the selective GPER antagonist G15 (100 nM) (De Francesco et al., 2013) and then subjected to I/R.
(9) G1+ WT group (n = 4): after stabilization, hearts were pretreated with a co-infusion of G1 (10 nM) and WT (100 nM) (Deschamps and Murphy, 2009; Penna et al., 2017).
(10) G1+L-NIO group (n = 4): after stabilization, hearts were pretreated with a co-infusion of G1 (10 nM) and L-NIO (10 μM) (El-Mas et al., 2009; De Francesco et al., 2013).
(11) G1+5HD group (n = 4): after stabilization, hearts were pretreated with a co-infusion of G1 (10 nM) and 5HD (100 μM) (Ajmani et al., 2011; Perrelli et al., 2013).

G1 concentration was selected on the basis of previous experiments (De Francesco et al., 2013).

The concentration for each pharmacological inhibitor was selected on the basis of preliminary dose–response curves, and according to the literature, as the first dose that did not significantly affect cardiac performance (De Francesco et al., 2013; Perrelli et al., 2013; Boccalini et al., 2015; Penna et al., 2017). The stability of the preparations was previously assessed by measuring each variable considered every 10 min. The stability of the preparation was on average 180 min.

In line with 3R principle for more ethical use of animals, we used less than four animals in those groups in which we have previous evidence of similar results (Penna et al., 2009, 2010, 2012; Rocca et al., 2018).

Cell Culture

The cardiac myoblast H9c2 cell line (ATCC, CRL-1446) was maintained in DMEM supplemented with 10% heat-inactivated fetal bovine serum (FBS) and 1% (v/v) streptomycin/penicillin in a humidified incubator at 37°C under 5% CO_2 air prior to use (Hescheler et al., 1991).

In all sets of experiments, 80% confluent flasks were detached, counted in the Burker chamber and plated in 96 wells plate at a density of 5000 cells/well. Cells were then left for 24-h in standard culture conditions before applying the hypoxia/reoxygenation (H/R) protocols.

Hypoxia/Reoxygenation (H/R) Protocol

In this set of experiments, performed for comparative purposes, cells were cultured in normoxic conditions (21% O_2 and 5% CO_2)

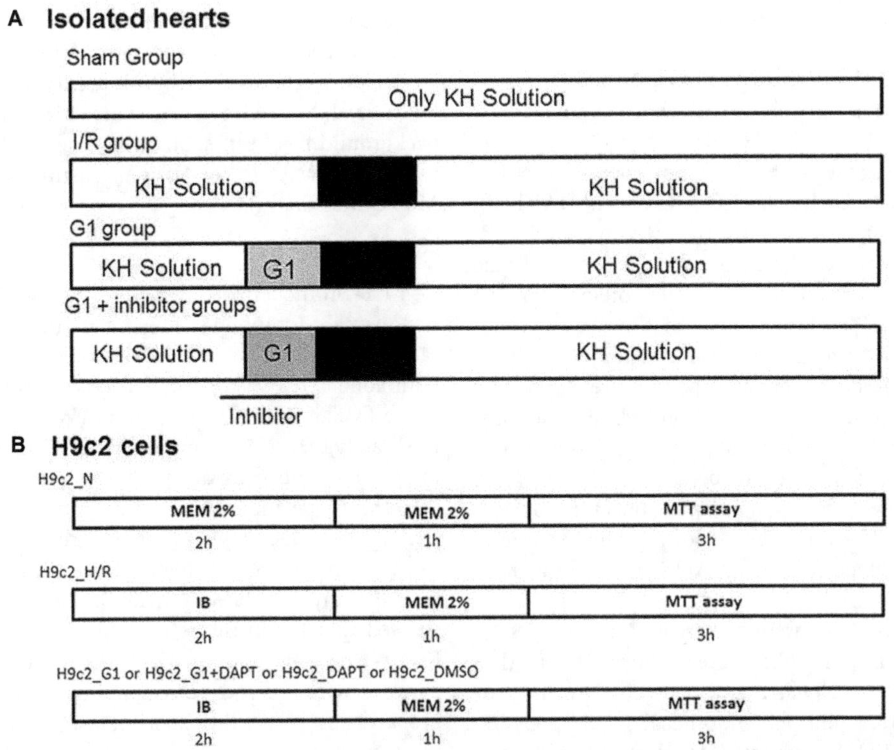

FIGURE 1 | Timeline of experimental protocols. **(A)** Protocols of ischemia/reperfusion (I/R) in isolated rat hearts and Sham group. G1 was given for 20 min before ischemia and inhibitors (DAPT, inhibitor of Notch or G15, selective GPER antagonist or Wortmannin, a specific inhibitor of PI3K activity or L-N5-(1-iminoethyl)ornithine (L-NIO), a specific inhibitor of nitric oxide synthase (NOS), or 5-hydroxydecanoate (5HD), a specific inhibitor of mitochondrial ATP-sensitive potassium [MitoK(ATP)]) were given 5 min before G1 and was stopped at the end of the 20 min of infusion of G1. **(B)** Protocols of normoxia and hypoxia/reoxygenation (H/R) in H9c2 cells. G1 or G1+DAPT or DMSO were given before hypoxia/reoxygenation protocol. MTT: 3-(4,5-dimethylthiazol-2-yl)-2,5-diphenyltetrazolium bromide dye is used as colorimetric assay for assessing cell metabolic activity, reflecting the number of viable cells present. IB, ischemic buffer.

or in conditions of Hypoxia/Reoxygenation (1% O_2 and 5% CO_2 for 2 h, and subsequently 21% O_2 and 5% CO_2 for 1 h).

As Normoxia (N) we considered cell survival studied during standard H9c2 culture conditions.

As Hypoxia/Reoxygenation (H/R) we considered cell survival studied with for 2-h and a subsequent reoxygenation for 1-h. H/R protocol was obtained in a hypoxic chamber (INVIVO2 200, Belsar, Varese, Italy) and with an "Ischemic Buffer" (IB) containing (in mM): 137 NaCl; 12 KCl; 0.49 $MgCl_2$; 0.9 $CaCl_2$; 4 HEPES; 20 sodium lactate (pH 6.2) (Yin et al., 2013).

Before hypoxia, cells were pre-treated with G1 (10 nM) (De Francesco et al., 2013), or G1+ DAPT, (5 μM); (Boccalini et al., 2015) dissolved in DMEM-2% FBS in normoxic conditions and in IB in hypoxic conditions. Experimental groups, recapitulated in **Figure 1B**, are as follows:

(a) Control Groups, untreated cells cultured in normoxic conditions (H9c2-N); untreated cells subjected to H/R (H9c2-H/R).
(b) G1 Group, cells pre-treated with G1 (10 nM) and then subject to H/R protocol (H9c2_G1_H/R).
(c) G1+DAPT Group, cells pre-treated with G1 + DAPT (5 μM) and then subject to H/R protocol (H9c2_G1+DAPT_H/R).
(d) DAPT Group, cells pre-treated with DAPT and then subject to H/R protocol (H9c2_DAPT_H/R).
(e) DMSO Group, cells pre-treated with DMSO (0.1%) and then subject to H/R protocol (H9c2_DMSO_H/R).

Assessment of Myocardial Injury

Infarct mass was measured as usual in our laboratories (Penna et al., 2014; Pasqua et al., 2015). In short, the hearts were detached from the perfusion system at the end of the reperfusion and the left ventricles cut into circumferential sections about 2 mm thick. The heart slices were incubated for 20 min at 37°C in a 0.1% nitro-blue tetrazolium solution with phosphate buffer. The non-colored necrotic tissue was carefully separated from the vital tissue colored by an observer who was unaware of the studied protocol. The necrotic mass was gravimetrically weighed and expressed as a percentage of total left ventricular mass that was considered to be a risk area for global ischemia (Penna et al., 2014).

MTT Assay

At the end of all experiments, cell viability was assessed using the 3-(4,5-Dimethylthiazol-2-yl)-2,5-diphenyltetrazolium bromide (MTT) kit (Pasqua et al., 2015). The absorbance was measured at 570 nm using a microplate reader and the results were expressed as a percentage of control.

Western Blotting and Densitometric Analysis

Immunoblot procedures and analyses were conducted as previously described (Rocca et al., 2018). Immediately after the hearts had undergone the specific protocols described above (Sham, I/R, I/R+DAPT, I/R+G1, I/R+G1+DAPT for normotensive group and Sham, I/R, G1, and G1+G15 for hypertensive group), the cardiac apices were frozen in liquid nitrogen before being stored at −80°C until protein extraction (Penna et al., 2014). Myocardial tissues of the above groups were homogenized in a frozen RIPA lysis buffer (Sigma-Aldrich, St. Louis, MO, United States) containing a mixture of protease inhibitors (1 mM of aprotinin, 20 mM of phenylmethylsulfonyl fluoride, and 200 mM of sodium orthovanadate). Subsequently, myocardial homogenates were centrifuged at 15,000 × *g* for 25 min at 4°C for debris removal. Protein concentration was assessed using a Bradford reagent following the procedure described by the manufacturer (Sigma-Aldrich, St. Louis, MO, United States).

30 μg of total protein were separated on 10% SDS-PAGE gel [for β-actin, phospho-protein kinase B (p-Akt), total Akt (t-Akt), total Notch1, and cleaved Notch1)] or 8% Gel SDS-PAGE [for phospho-endothelial NOS (p-eNOS) and total eNOS (t-eNOS)], subjected to electrophoresis and transferred to polyvinyl-fluoride membranes (PVDFs). The non-specific binding was blocked by incubating the membranes with a buffered saline solution (TBS)/Tween 0.1%, pH 7.6 (TBST), containing 5% of fat-free dried milk and 0.5% BSA, for 1 h at room temperature. The PVDF membranes were incubated overnight at 4°C with a goat polyclonal antibody for Notch1 (C-20; Santa Cruz, CA, United States), which recognizes the carboxy-terminal of the Notch1 receptor, to detect the precursor of Notch1 (Notch1-PR, 250 kDa) (Caliceti et al., 2013; Fortini et al., 2017) or rabbit monoclonal antibody against cleaved Notch (Cell Signaling Technology, Inc., Danvers, MA, United States), which detects endogenous levels of intracellular Notch1 domain (NICD) when released from the cleavage between Gly1753 and Val1754. Samples were also incubated with rabbit polyclonal antibody against p-Akt, Akt, or eNOS (Santa Cruz Biotechnology, Inc., Dallas, TX, United States), with monoclonal goat antibody against p-eNOS (Santa Cruz Biotechnology, Inc., Dallas, TX, United States), with mouse monoclonal antibody against β-actin (Santa Cruz Biotechnology, Inc., Dallas, TX, United States), or with mouse monoclonal antibodies to GAPDH (Cell Signaling Technology, Inc., Danvers, TX, United States). The antibodies were diluted 1:1000 in TBST containing 5% BSA (TBSTM). Antibodies against Akt, eNOS, GAPDH, and β-actin were used as loading controls. After washing them with TBST three times, the membranes were incubated for about 1 h at room temperature with antibodies conjugated with secondary peroxidase (1:1000) in TBSTM. Immunodetection was done using the enhanced chemiluminescence kit ECL PLUS (GE Healthcare, Amersham, United Kingdom). Autoradiographs were obtained by exposing the membrane films to X-ray (Hyperfilm ECL, Amersham, United Kingdom). We then proceeded to digitize the immunoblots that were subjected to densitometric analysis of the bands. The analysis was performed by evaluating the areas and the intensity of the pixels represented by 256 values of Gray (0 = white; 256 = black). As usual, the background has been subtracted. The analyses were performed using NIH IMAGE 1.6 (National Institutes of Health, Bethesda, MD, United States).

Chemicals

1-[4-(-6-Bromobenzol[1,3]diodo-5-yl)-3a,4,5,9-btetrahydro-3H-cyclopenta[c-]quinolin8yl]ethanone (G-1) and (3aS,4R,9bR) -4-(6-bromo-1,3-benzodioxol-5-yl)-3a,4,5,9b-3H-cyclopenta[c] quinolone (G15) were from Tocris Bioscience, distributed by Space (Milan, Italy). Wortmannin (WT), a specific inhibitor of PI3K activity, L-N5-(1-iminoethyl)ornithine (L-NIO), a specific inhibitor of nitric oxide synthase (NOS), 5-hydroxydecanoate (5HD), a specific inhibitor of MitoK(ATP) channels, and DAPT, a γ-secretase complex inhibitor, were purchased from Sigma-Aldrich (Milan, Italy). Reagents were dissolved in dimethylsulfoxide (DMSO). Preliminary experiments showed that the presence of equivalent amounts of DMSO in Krebs–Henseleit solution (KHs) did not modify basal cardiac performance. All drug-containing solutions were freshly prepared just before the experiments.

Statistical Analysis

All data were reported as mean ± SEM and analyzed by one-way analysis of variance (ANOVA). Non-parametric Newman–Keuls multiple comparison test (for post-ANOVA comparisons) was used for western blot and hemodynamic analyses. Differences at $^{*}p = < 0.05$, $^{**}p = < 0.01$, $^{***}p = < 0.001$, $^{****}p = < 0.0001$ were considered statistically significant. The statistical analyses were carried out using GraphPad Prism5.

RESULTS

The cardioprotective effects of G1 in isolated heart models were studied by comparing the effects elicited by I/R protocols with those induced by the GPER-agonist, G1, used as a pre-conditioning factor (PreC).

Normotensive Rat Model

Cardioprotective Effect of GPER

Infarct size reduction by G1 preconditioning

Here we confirmed the cardioprotective effect of GPER estrogen agonist, G1 (Bopassa et al., 2010; Li et al., 2015; Menazza et al., 2017). In particular, using an isolated rat heart model, infarct size was reduced from 63 ± 4% of risk area in I/R group to 48 ± 2% of risk area in G1 pretreated hearts ($p < 0.01$) (**Figure 2A**).

Involvement of Notch pathway in cardioprotective effect of GPER

The G1 cardioprotective effect was nullified by treatment with DAPT, an inhibitor of the γ-secretase, the enzyme required for the Notch1 cleavage and activation, co-infused with G1 (infarct

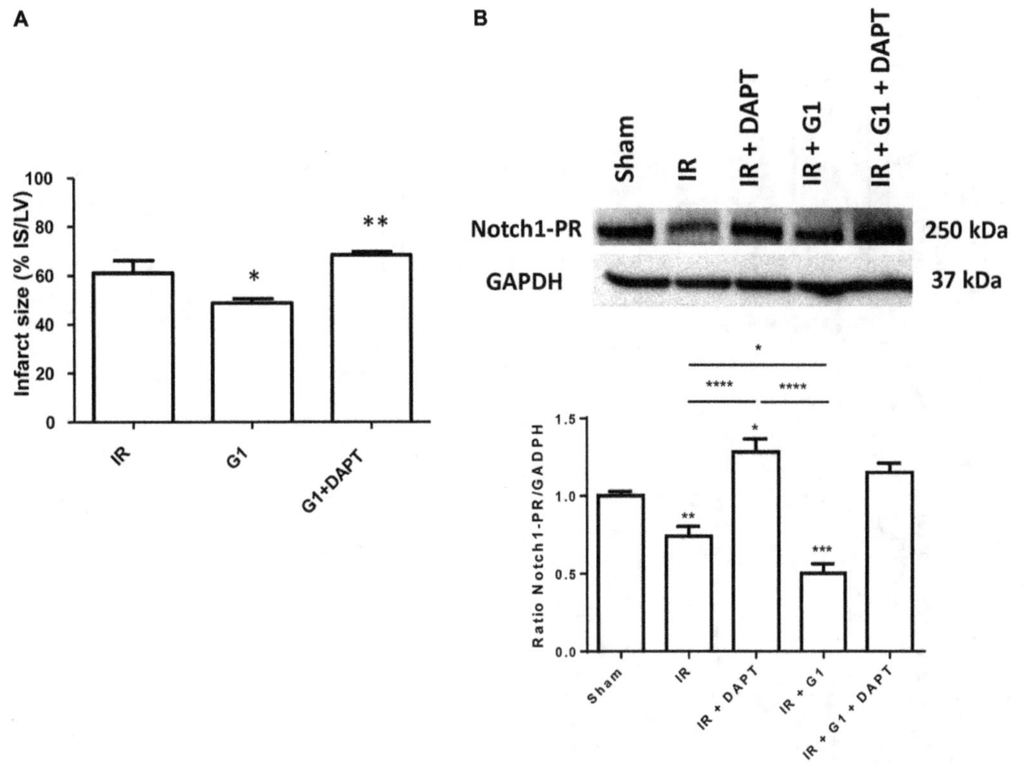

FIGURE 2 | Cardioprotective effects of G1 in normotensive female rats were abolished by Notch1 inhibitor. **(A)** Infarct size. The amount of necrotic tissue measured after I/R protocols (30-min global ischemia and 120-min reperfusion) is reported as percent of the left ventricle mass (LV; % IS/LV) for I/R (n = 8), G1 (n = 7), and G1+DAPT groups (n = 4). **(B)** Western blotting (upper panel) of rat heart homogenates electrophoresed and immunoblotted with Notch1 C-20 antibody. GAPDH was used as loading control. Histograms (bottom panel) represent the ratio of densitometric analysis of protein/loading control normalized to Sham. The level of Notch1-PR was reduced in heart after I/R injury, compared to Sham group, indicating activation of Notch1, activation further increased by G1 treatment. DAPT treatment increased Notch1-PR protein level in heart subjected to I/R injury, both in the presence and absence of G1, suggestive of an inhibition of Notch1 activation. ****$p < 0.0001$ IR vs. IR+DAPT and IR+G1 vs. IR+DAPT; ***$p < 0.001$ IR+G1 vs. SHAM; **$p < 0.01$ IR vs. SHAM; *$p < 0.05$ IR+DAPT vs. SHAM and IR vs. IR+G1.

size 68 ± 1%; $p < 0.05$ spect to G1 group; p = NS respect to I/R group) (**Figure 2A**). To confirm the involvement of Notch downstream of GPER during I/R, we performed Western blot analyses on heart homogenates from different treatment groups and showed that I/R induces the activation of Notch1, as indicated by the reduction of the precursor form (PR) of the receptor (**Figure 2B**). G1 treatment further induced Notch1 processing and this effect was blocked by DAPT (**Figure 2B**). The full unedited gel is showed in the Supplementary Figure 1.

Hypertensive Rat Model

After we demonstrated the involvement of the GPER/Notch pathway in normotensive hearts, we focused on studying the G1 cardioprotective pathway in the hypertensive model in the detail.

Cardioprotective Effect of GPER

Infarct size is reduced by G1 preconditioning

Infarct size was reduced from 80 ± 9.6% of risk area in I/R group to 42 ± 2.5% of risk area in G1 pretreated hearts ($p < 0.01$) (**Figure 3A**). Moreover, when G1 was co-infused with the direct inhibitor of GPER, G15, hearts showed an infarct size similar to that found for I/R group (**Figure 3A**).

Post-ischemic diastolic and systolic functions are improved by G1 preconditioning

The effects mediated by G1 on diastolic and systolic functions were analyzed as previously described (De Francesco et al., 2013).

It is known that an increase in post-ischemic left ventricular end-diastolic pressure (LVEDP) of 4 mmHg or more above the pre-ischemic level indicates an important index of cardiac contracture. The 30 min ischemia and the subsequent reperfusion caused a sustained increase in LVEDP in I/R group (**Figure 3B**) (Pagliaro et al., 2003; Pasqua et al., 2015). Conversely, the preconditioning with G1 was able to abolish the contracture (**Figure 3B**), indicating that G1 significantly reduces the heart damage after I/R. Similar to the reduction in infarct size, the limitation of contracture was suppressed when G1 was co-infused with the direct inhibitor of GPER, G15.

Systolic function was evaluated by the level of dLVP recovery during reperfusion (i.e., inotropic index). SHR hearts from I/R group showed a limited dLVP recovery, while G1, administered before ischemia induction, significantly improved this function (**Figure 3C**). The co-infusion with the GPER-antagonist, G15, abolished the post-systolic recovery, indicating that G1 exerts a selective action on its receptor.

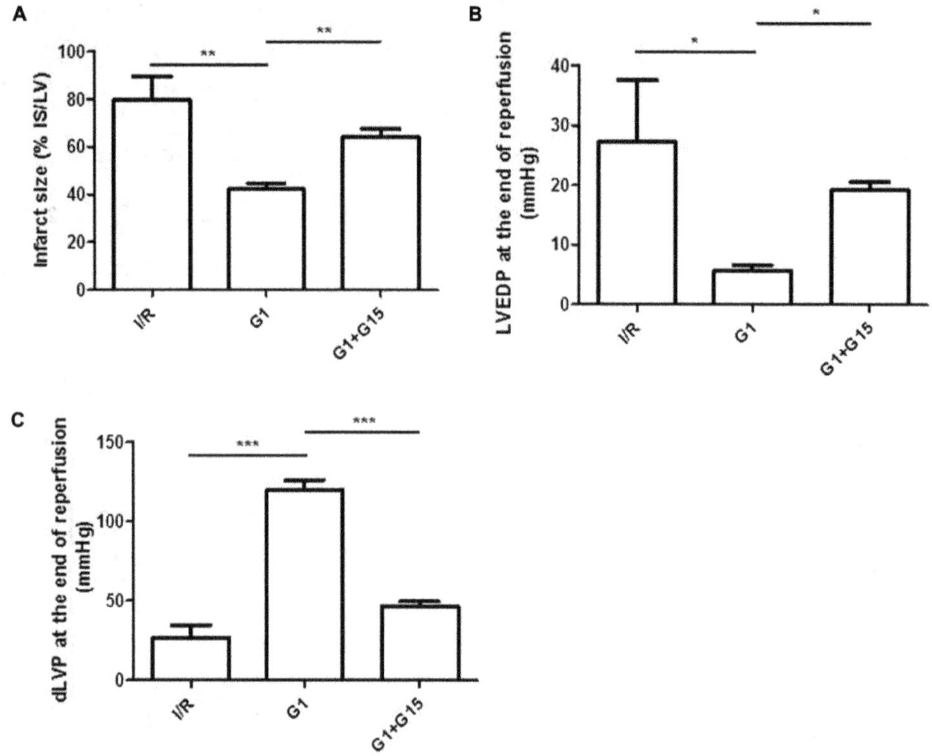

FIGURE 3 | Cardioprotective effects of G1 in Hypertensive Female Rats (SHR) were abolished by GPER antagonistic specific inhibitor. **(A)** Infarct size. The amount of necrotic tissue measured after I/R protocols (30-min global ischemia and 120-min reperfusion) is reported as percentage of the left ventricle mass (LV; % IS/LV) for I/R (n = 3), G1 (n = 5), and G1+G15 groups (n = 4). **(B,C)** LVEDP and dLVP variations at the end of reperfusion. Data are expressed as changes of dLVP and LVEDP values (mmHg) at the end of the 120-min of reperfusion for I/R (n = 3), G1 (n = 5), and G1+G15 groups (n = 4). Changes were evaluated as mean ± SEM. Significant difference (one-way ANOVA, Newman–Keuls test): $^*p < 0.05$, $^{**}p < 0.01$, $^{***}p < 0.001$.

G1-induced infarct size limitation and improvement of post-ischemic contractile recovery is mediated by PI3K/NO/mKATP channels

In order to estimate the mechanism of action by which G1 exerted the cardioprotective effects in SHR hearts, the isolated and perfused hearts were co-treated with G1 plus specific inhibitors of survival signaling pathways involved in cardioprotection (i.e., WT to block PI3K, L-NIO to inhibit NOS, and 5HD to antagonize MitoKATP channels). **Figure 4** shows that all inhibitors abrogate the beneficial effects of G1 on all analyzed parameters. Indeed, G1-dependent reduction of infarct size was abolished in hearts co-treated with all the cardioprotective signaling antagonists (**Figure 4A**). Moreover, these inhibitors limited the post-ischemic systolic recovery elicited by G1, as demonstrated by the low values of dLVP reached at the end of reperfusion (**Figure 4B**). Similarly, the contracture limitation induced by G1 was suppressed in the presence of the above blockers (data not shown).

Effects of G1 as preconditioning agent on Notch and PI3K/Akt/NOS pathways

The involvement of the kinase Akt, the endothelial form of NOS (eNOS) and cleaved Notch1 in the G1-induced cardioprotection was evaluated by Western blot analysis. Representative bands and densitometric analyses for these markers are shown in **Figure 5**. In post-ischemic SHR hearts preconditioned with G1, the levels of phosphorylated Akt (**Figure 5A**) and eNOS (**Figure 5B**), and the levels of cleaved Notch1 (**Figure 5C**) were significantly higher, compared to the control counterparts I/R. On the contrary, p-Akt, p-eNOS, and cleaved Notch1 expression levels were significantly reduced by G15 co-treatment (**Figure 5**). The full unedited gels are showed in the Supplementary Figures 2–4, respectively.

H9c2 Hypoxia/Reoxygenation (H/R) Protocol

G1 induces cardiac cell protection via Notch signaling pathway

In **Figure 6** the effects of H/R in G1 treated cells and after G1 + DAPT pre-treatment compared to normoxic and hypoxic controls (H9c2_N and H9c2_H/R) are reported. DAPT abolished the protective effect induced by G1 pre-treatment against cell death induced by H/R protocol ($p < 0.001$ vs. H9c2_H/R). These results suggest that G1 is an important protective factor during hypoxia able to trigger the Notch1 signaling in cardiac cells.

DISCUSSION

In this study, we confirm that the cardioprotective role of GPER is Notch1 dependent in normotensive female rats. Importantly,

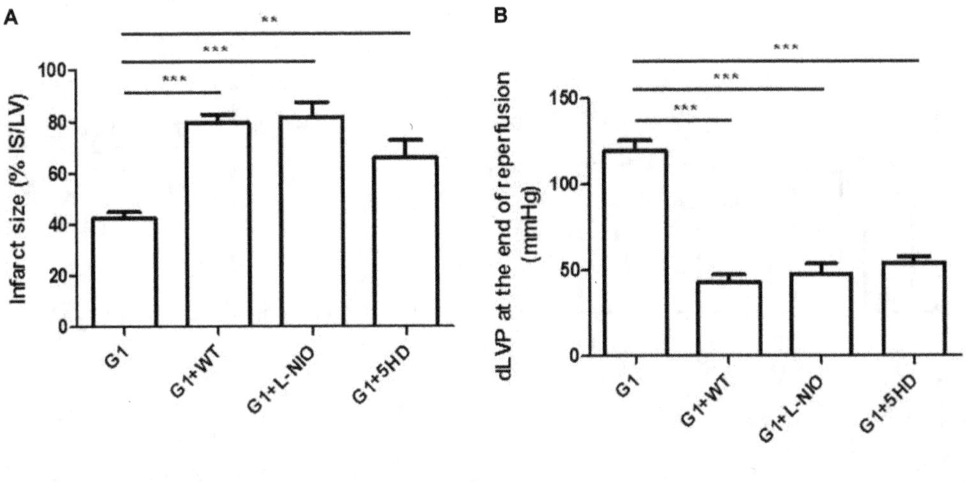

FIGURE 4 | Cardioprotective effects of G1 in Hypertensive Female Rats (SHR) were abolished by specific inhibitors of PI3K/Akt-eNOS-MitoKATP channels. **(A)** Infarct size. The amount of necrotic tissue measured after I/R protocols (30-min global ischemia and 120-min reperfusion) is reported as percentage of the left ventricle mass (LV; % IS/LV) for G1 ($n = 5$) and G1+inhibitors (WT, L-NIO, and 5HD) groups ($n = 4$). **(B)** dLVP variations. Data are expressed as changes of dLVP values (mmHg) at the end of the 120-min of reperfusion for G1 ($n = 5$) and G1+inhibitors (WT, L-NIO, and 5HD) groups ($n = 4$). Changes were evaluated as mean ± SEM. Significant difference (one-way ANOVA, Newman–Keuls test): $^{**}p < 0.01$, $^{***}p < 0.001$.

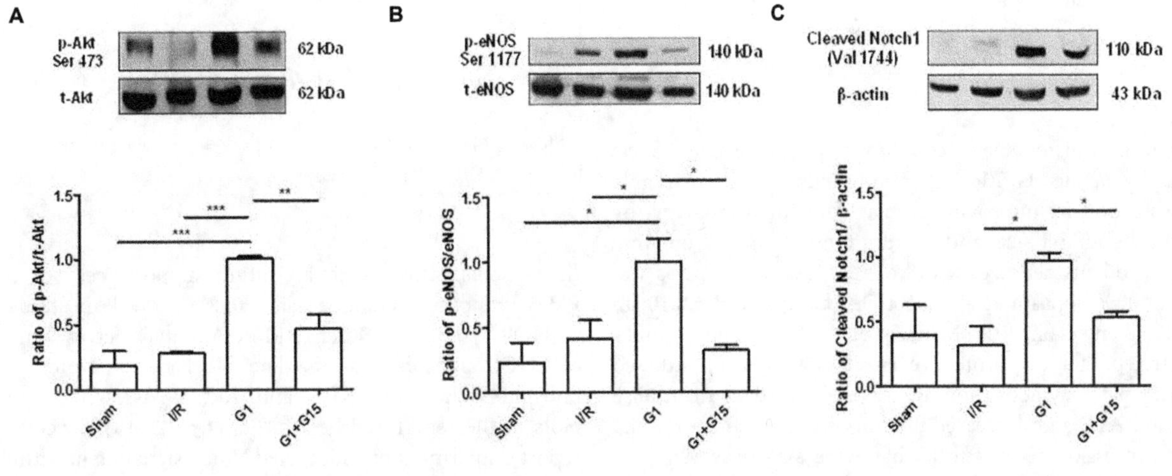

FIGURE 5 | Effects of G1 given as preconditioning agent on Notch, PI3K/Akt/NOS Pathway Western Blot analysis of **(A)** p-Akt, **(B)** p-eNOS, and **(C)** cleaved Notch1 expression in cardiac extracts of Sham, I/R, G1, and G1+G15 groups ($n = 3$ hearts/group). Histograms represent the ratio of densitometric analysis of protein/loading control. Significant difference (one-way ANOVA, Newman–Keuls test): $^{*}p < 0.05$, $^{**}p < 0.01$, $^{***}p < 0.001$.

the preconditioning activation of GPER with the selective agonist, G1, significantly reduces I/R injury in the hypertensive female rat heart model. Moreover, in this model G1 is able to activate PI3K/Akt/NOS/MitoKATP channel and Notch1 pathways. The protective effect induced by GPER activation is mediated by Notch1, as also suggested by reduction of cell mortality in the H9c2 model. These results obtained in cardiac cells suggest that the G1 protective effects do not require an endothelial mediation.

The main novel finding of the present study is that the activation of GPER by its selective ligand, G1, protects the heart against I/R injury not only in a normotensive model but also in a model of comorbidity, namely female SHR. In these hypertensive female rats, Notch1 signaling and PI3K/NOS/MitoKATP channel pathways are activated by preconditioning treatment with the GPER agonist G1.

It is well-known that estrogens act through two nuclear receptors: estrogen receptor-alpha (ER-α) or estrogen receptor-beta (ER-β); yet, a third, membrane-bound receptor G protein-coupled estrogen receptor (GPER), has been discovered. GPER has been shown to bind estrogen with high affinity (Zimmerman et al., 2016) and to be localized in the different internal and external cellular localization (Bopassa et al., 2010).

G1 demonstrated high specificity to GPER with little to no binding to other estrogen receptors, either ER-β or ER-α.

Treating acutely animals or perfusing the hearts with 17 beta-estradiol (E2), it has been demonstrated that E2/GPER interaction reduces I/R injury (Deschamps and Murphy, 2009).

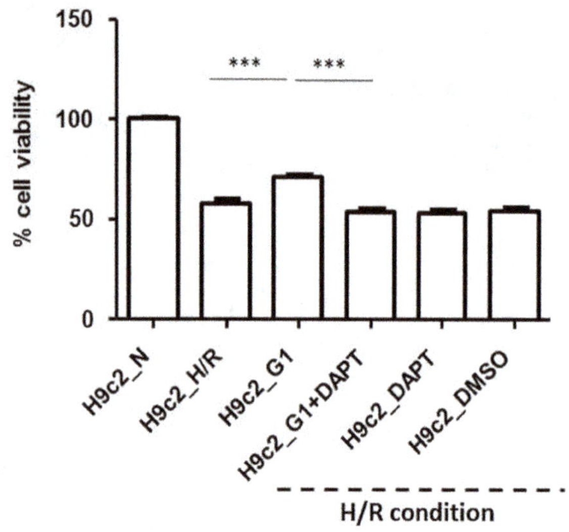

FIGURE 6 | Cell vitality in Normoxia (N) and Hypoxia/Reoxygenation (H/R) conditions. Data are presented as percentage variation with respect to mean value of cell count in normoxia, in control group. Treatment with G1 or G1 in the presence of Notch inhibitor (DAPT) in H/R conditions. Data of control I/R groups with DAPT and DMS are also reported. For acronyms see the text. ***$p < 0.001$ vs. H9c2_N; ***$p < 0.001$ H9c2_G1 vs. all other H/R conditions.

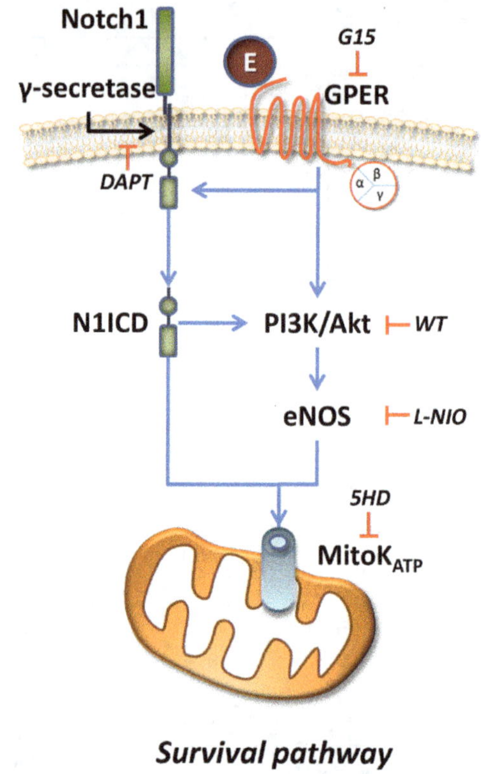

FIGURE 7 | Representative scheme of intracellular pathway involved in the GPER/Notch1 cardioprotection.

Moreover, in normotensive condition, the protective effects induced by acute GPER activation induce a remarkable cardioprotection by improving cardiac functional recovery, by reduction the infarct size, and by inhibiting the mPTP opening in isolated rodents hearts exposed to I/R stress (Deschamps and Murphy, 2009; Bopassa et al., 2010; Deschamps et al., 2010; Li et al., 2015; Feng et al., 2017; Menazza et al., 2017). These studies demonstrated that the protective effect of GPER is mediated by the Erk pathway activation, increased superoxide dismutase (SOD), and ATP and decreased the tumor necrosis factor alpha (TNFα) expression level, effects that were also observed in a cardiac cell model subjected to simulated I/R protocols (Li et al., 2015). These results are in agreement with the findings of our study.

As post-conditioning agent, Feng et al. (2017) reported that the cardioprotection of GPER displays via the protection of the mitochondrial structural integrity; moreover, the activation of MEK/Erk signaling leads to the reduction of mitochondrial protein ubiquitination and protection of mitochondrial membrane potential dissipation; these alterations are normally responsible of mitophagy, ROS generation and apoptosis typically of I/R damage (Feng et al., 2017).

Notch signaling pathway seems indispensable for functional activities controlling tissue formation in cardiogenesis (Kratsios et al., 2010). Moreover, it is an important cell–cell communication system and its activation after the damage has been demonstrated in several tissues (Kratsios et al., 2010; Rizzo et al., 2017). It has been reported that Notch signaling plays a regulatory role in adult cardiac damage and in the cardioprotection preserving cardiac function after ischemia. In particular, this Notch activation supports cell survival *via* PI3K induction (Gude et al., 2008). Indeed, in the control of NOS system by Notch1, PI3K/Akt may act as a mediator of eNOS phosphorylation. The blockade of Notch reduced phosphorylation of eNOS and Akt as assessed by western blots in the reperfused hearts (Pei et al., 2013). Several studies report impairment of endothelial Notch signaling in pathological conditions, e.g., heart failure (Pannella et al., 2016), inflammation (Fortini et al., 2017), and dyslipidemia (Briot et al., 2015). Notch signaling can be also impaired by anti-cancer drugs and this may represent an unwanted side effect (Rizzo et al., 2015). The relation of GPER/Notch is demonstrated in other cellular models (Pupo et al., 2016). In particular, we have recently observed that certain non-genomic estrogenic signals are mediated by a functional crosstalk between the Notch signaling pathway and GPER (Pupo et al., 2016). Moreover, we reported that this Notch/GPER crosstalk is involved in proliferative and migratory effects by estrogen, in breast cancer cells and cancer-associated fibroblasts (Pupo et al., 2014).

Here, for the first time, Notch signaling, nitric oxide, and cell survival pathway are linked to preconditioning protection by GPER activation (**Figure 7**).

Estrogens are hormones regulating physiological and pathological processes in both women and men. Endogenous estrogens affect importantly cardiovascular homeostasis in pre-menopausal women and interfere with the development of hypertension and coronary artery disease. Indeed, the gender differences in cardiovascular risk are surely correlated to hormonal specificity. The estrogens cardioprotective effects are widely reported in several animal and human studies; they are mostly mediated through ERα and/or ERβ, both expressed in the heart and involved in regulating cardioprotection, both in genomic and non-genomic mechanisms (Mendelsohn and Karas, 2005; Wang et al., 2006, 2009; Deschamps et al., 2010).

In addition to the classic ERs, the role exerted by GPER in acute cardioprotection and in the modulation of cardiovascular function is increasingly consolidating (Deschamps et al., 2010).

Our results support the possibility that acute pre-ischemic activation of GPER might protect female hypertensive animals against I/R injury. These results may pave the way for protective approaches in models with risk factors and comorbidities, which are much needed to translate successful animal experiments on cardioprotection beyond that by reperfusion to clinical practice.

CONCLUSION

Here, we have shown that GPER plays a pivotal role in mediating preconditioning cardioprotection in both normotensive and hypertensive conditions. This protection requires the involvement of Notch-1 in cardiac cells and is mediated by PI3K/NOS/MitoKATP channels.

CLINICAL PERSPECTIVES

The pathways here studied may represent novel targets and are particularly intriguing for the advancement in the field of cardioprotection, considering the paucity of studies in female hearts. These results may contribute to better understand the preconditioning GPER protection following ischemia/reperfusion stress in the normotensive and hypertensive heart, an important target tissue for estrogen-mediated signaling. Additionally, the present study may provide more insights for the potential development of a therapy application based on a selective transmembrane estrogen receptor modulator able to induces cardioprotection, without affecting the cancer risk.

AUTHOR CONTRIBUTIONS

CP, PR, and TA have devised and coordinated the experiments. CR, SF, GA, MG, EDF, TP, DR, and FF have performed the experiments and analyzed the results. CP and TA have written the first draft. PR and PP revised critically the manuscript. SF, CR, GA, and MG made the figures. CP, PP, PR, MC, MM, and TA finalized the manuscript. All authors approved the final version of the manuscript.

FUNDING

This research was supported by "Dottorato di Ricerca in Scienze della Vita" and University of Calabria (MIUR ex 60%), by the University of Turin, Ricerca Locale Ex-60% (Grant No. PAGP_RILO_16_01), by University of Ferrara [Fondo per l'Incentivazione alla Ricerca (FIR) - 2016] and by Associazione Italiana per la Ricerca sul Cancro (IG 16719/2015).

REFERENCES

Ajmani, P., Yadav, H. N., Singh, M., and Sharma, P. L. (2011). Possible involvement of caveolin in attenuation of cardioprotective effect of ischemic preconditioning in diabetic rat heart. *BMC Cardiovasc. Disord.* 12:43. doi: 10.1186/1471-2261-11-43

Boccalini, G., Sassoli, C., Formigli, L., Bani, D., and Nistri, S. (2015). Relaxin protects cardiac muscle cells from hypoxia/reoxygenation injury: involvement of the Notch-1 pathway. *FASEB J.* 29, 239–249. doi: 10.1096/fj.14-254854

Bologa, C. G., Revankar, C. M., Young, S. M., Edwards, B. S., Arterburn, J. B., Kiselyov, A. S., et al. (2006). Virtual and biomolecular screening converge on a selective agonist for GPR30. *Nat. Chem. Biol.* 2, 207–212. doi: 10.1038/nchembio775

Bopassa, J. C., Eghbali, M., Toro, L., and Stefani, E. (2010). A novel estrogen receptor GPER inhibits mitochondria permeability transition pore opening and protects the heart against ischemia-reperfusion injury. *Am. J. Physiol. Heart Circ. Physiol.* 298, H16–H23. doi: 10.1152/ajpheart.00588.2009

Briot, A., Civelek, M., Seki, A., Hoi, K., Mack, J. J., Lee, S. D., et al. (2015). Endothelial NOTCH1 is suppressed by circulating lipids and antagonizes inflammation during atherosclerosis. *J. Exp. Med.* 212, 2147–2163. doi: 10.1084/jem.20150603

Caliceti, C., Aquila, G., Pannella, M., Morelli, M. B., Fortini, C., Pinton, P., et al. (2013). 17β-estradiol enhances signalling mediated by VEGF-A-delta-like ligand 4-notch1 axis in human endothelial cells. *PLoS One* 8:e71440. doi: 10.1371/journal.pone.0071440

De Francesco, E. M., Angelone, T., Pasqua, T., Pupo, M., Cerra, M. C., and Maggiolini, M. (2013). GPER mediates cardiotropic effects in spontaneously hypertensive rat hearts. *PLoS One* 8:e69322. doi: 10.1371/journal.pone.0069322

De Francesco, E. M., Rocca, C., Scavello, F., Amelio, D., Pasqua, T., Rigiracciolo, D. C., et al. (2017). Protective role of GPER agonist G-1 on cardiotoxicity induced by doxorubicin. *J. Cell. Physiol.* 232, 1640–1649. doi: 10.1002/jcp.25585

Dennis, M. K., Burai, R., Ramesh, C., Petrie, W. K., Alcon, S. N., Nayak, T. K., et al. (2009). In vivo effects of a GPR30 antagonist. *Nat. Chem. Biol.* 5, 421–427. doi: 10.1038/nchembio.168

Deschamps, A. M., and Murphy, E. (2009). Activation of a novel estrogen receptor, GPER, is cardioprotective in male and female rats. *Am. J. Physiol. Heart Circ. Physiol.* 297, H1806–H1813. doi: 10.1152/ajpheart.00283.2009

Deschamps, A. M., Murphy, E., and Sun, J. (2010). Estrogen receptor activation and cardioprotection in ischemia reperfusion injury. *Trends Cardiovasc. Med.* 20, 73–78. doi: 10.1016/j.tcm.2010.05.001

El-Mas, M. M., Fan, M., and Abdel-Rahman, A. A. (2009). Facilitation of myocardial PI3K/Akt/nNOS signaling contributes to ethanol-evoked hypotension in female rats. *Alcohol. Clin. Exp. Res.* 33, 1158–1168. doi: 10.1111/j.1530-0277.2009.00939.x

Feng, Y., Madungwe, N. B., da Cruz Junho, C. V., and Bopassa, J. C. (2017). Activation of G protein-coupled oestrogen receptor 1 at the onset of reperfusion protects the myocardium against ischemia/reperfusion injury by reducing mitochondrial dysfunction and mitophagy. *Br. J. Pharmacol.* 174, 4329–4344. doi: 10.1111/bph.14033

Ferdinandy, P., Schulz, R., and Baxter, G. F. (2007). Interaction of cardiovascular risk factors with myocardial ischemia/reperfusion injury, preconditioning, and postconditioning. *Pharmacol. Rev.* 59, 418–458. doi: 10.1124/pr.107.06002

Fortini, F., Vieceli Dalla Sega, F., Caliceti, C., Aquila, G., Pannella, M., Pannuti, A., et al. (2017). Estrogen receptor β-dependent Notch1 activation protects vascular endothelium against tumor necrosis factor α (TNFα)-induced apoptosis. *J. Biol. Chem.* 292, 18178–18191. doi: 10.1074/jbc.M117.790121

Gude, N. A., Emmanuel, G., Wu, W., Cottage, C. T., Fischer, K., Quijada, P., et al. (2008). Activation of Notch-mediated protective signaling in the myocardium. *Circ. Res.* 102, 1025–1035. doi: 10.1161/CIRCRESAHA.107.164749

Hausenloy, D. J., Barrabes, J. A., Botker, H. E., Davidson, S. M., Di Lisa, F., Downey, J., et al. (2016). Ischaemic conditioning and targeting reperfusion injury: a 30 year voyage of discovery. *Basic Res. Cardiol.* 111:70. doi: 10.1007/s00395-016-0588-8

Hescheler, J., Meyer, R., Plant, S., Krautwurst, D., Rosenthal, W., and Schultz, G. (1991). Morphological, biochemical, and electrophysiological characterization of a clonal cell (H9c2) line from rat heart. *Circ. Res.* 69, 1476–1486.doi: 10.1161/01.RES.69.6.1476

Kratsios, P., Catela, C., Salimova, E., Huth, M., Berno, V., Rosenthal, N., et al. (2010). Distinct roles for cell-autonomous Notch signaling in cardiomyocytes of the embryonic and adult heart. *Circ. Res.* 106, 559–572. doi: 10.1161/CIRCRESAHA.109.203034

Li, W. L., Xiang, W., and Ping, Y. (2015). Activation of novel estrogen receptor GPER results in inhibition of cardiocyte apoptosis and cardioprotection. *Mol. Med. Rep.* 12, 2425–2430. doi: 10.3892/mmr.2015.3674

Li, Y., Hiroi, Y., and Liao, J. K. (2010). Notch signaling as an important mediator of cardiac repair and regeneration after myocardial infarction. *Trends Cardiovasc. Med.* 20, 228–231. doi: 10.1016/j.tcm.2011.11.006

Lubecka, K., Kurzava, L., Flower, K., Buvala, H., Zhang, H., Teegarden, D., et al. (2016). Stilbenoids remodel the DNA methylation patterns in breast cancer cells and inhibit oncogenic NOTCH signaling through epigenetic regulation of MAML2 transcriptional activity. *Carcinogenesis* 37, 656–668. doi: 10.1093/carcin/bgw048

Menazza, S., Sun, J., Appachi, S., Chambliss, K. L., Kim, S. H., Aponte, A., et al. (2017). Non-nuclear estrogen receptor alpha activation in endothelium reduces cardiac ischemia-reperfusion injury in mice. *J. Mol. Cell Cardiol.* 107, 41–51. doi: 10.1016/j.yjmcc.2017.04.004

Mendelsohn, M. E., and Karas, R. H. (2005). Molecular and cellular basis of cardiovascular gender differences. *Science* 308, 1583–1587. doi: 10.1126/science.1112062

Pagliaro, P., Mancardi, D., Rastaldo, R., Penna, C., Gattullo, D., Miranda, K. M., et al. (2003). Nitroxyl affords thiol-sensitive myocardial protective effects akin to early preconditioning. *Free Radic. Biol. Med.* 34, 33–43.

Pannella, M., Caliceti, C., Fortini, F., Aquila, G., Vieceli Dalla Sega, F., Pannuti, A., et al. (2016). Serum from advanced heart failure patients promotes angiogenic sprouting and affects the notch pathway in human endothelial cells. *J. Cell. Physiol.* 231, 2700–2710. doi: 10.1002/jcp.25373

Pasqua, T., Tota, B., Penna, C., Corti, A., Cerra, M. C., Loh, Y., et al. (2015). pGlu-serpinin protects the normotensive and hypertensive heart from ischemic injury. *J. Endocrinol.* 227, 167–178. doi: 10.1530/JOE-15-0199

Pei, H., Yu, Q., Xue, Q., Guo, Y., Sun, L., Hong, Z., et al. (2013). Notch1 cardioprotection in myocardial ischemia/reperfusion involves reduction of oxidative/nitrative stress. *Basic Res. Cardiol.* 108:373. doi: 10.1007/s00395-013-0373-x

Penna, C., Brancaccio, M., Tullio, F., Rubinetto, C., Perrelli, M. G., Angotti, C., et al. (2014). Overexpression of the muscle-specific protein, melusin, protects from cardiac ischemia/reperfusion injury. *Basic Res. Cardiol.* 109:418. doi: 10.1007/s00395-014-0418-9

Penna, C., Pasqua, T., Perrelli, M. G., Pagliaro, P., Cerra, M. C., and Angelone, T. (2012). Postconditioning with glucagon like peptide-2 reduces ischemia/reperfusion injury in isolated rat hearts: role of survival kinases and mitochondrial KATP channels. *Basic Res. Cardiol.* 107:272. doi: 10.1007/s00395-012-0272-6

Penna, C., Tullio, F., Femminò, S., Rocca, C., Angelone, T., Cerra, M. C., et al. (2017). Obestatin regulates cardiovascular function and promotes cardioprotection through the nitric oxide pathway. *J. Cell. Mol. Med.* 21, 3670–3678. doi: 10.1111/jcmm.13277

Penna, C., Tullio, F., Merlino, A., Moro, F., Raimondo, S., Rastaldo, R., et al. (2009). Postconditioning cardioprotection against infarct size and post-ischemic systolic dysfunction is influenced by gender. *Basic Res. Cardiol.* 104, 390–402. doi: 10.1007/s00395-008-0762-8

Penna, C., Tullio, F., Moro, F., Folino, A., Merlino, A., and Pagliaro, P. (2010). Effects of a protocol of ischemic postconditioning and/or captopril in hearts of normotensive and hypertensive rats. *Basic Res. Cardiol.* 105, 181–192. doi: 10.1007/s00395-009-0075-6

Penna, C., Tullio, F., Perrelli, M. G., Moro, F., Abbadessa, G., Piccione, F., et al. (2011). Ischemia/reperfusion injury is increased and cardioprotection by a postconditioning protocol is lost as cardiac hypertrophy develops in nandrolone treated rats. *Basic Res. Cardiol.* 106, 409–420. doi: 10.1007/s00395-010-0143-y

Perrelli, M. G., Tullio, F., Angotti, C., Cerra, M. C., Angelone, T., Tota, B., et al. (2013). Catestatin reduces myocardial ischaemia/reperfusion injury: involvement of PI3K/Akt, PKCs, mitochondrial KATP channels and ROS signalling. *Pflugers Arch.* 465, 1031–1040. doi: 10.1007/s00424-013-1217-0

Pupo, M., Maggiolini, M., and Musti, A. M. (2016). GPER mediates non-genomic effects of estrogen. *Methods Mol. Biol.* 1366, 471–488. doi: 10.1007/978-1-4939-3127-9_37

Pupo, M., Pisano, A., Abonante, S., Maggiolini, M., and Musti, A. M. (2014). GPER activates Notch signaling in breast cancer cells and cancer-associated fibroblasts (CAFs). *Int. J. Biochem. Cell Biol.* 46, 56–67. doi: 10.1016/j.biocel.2013.11.011

Rizzo, P., Bollini, S., Bertero, E., Ferrari, R., and Ameri, P. (2017). Beyond cardiomyocyte loss: role of notch in cardiac aging. *J. Cell. Physiol.* 233, 5670–5683. doi: 10.1002/jcp.26417

Rizzo, P., Mele, D., Caliceti, C., Pannella, M., Fortini, C., Clementz, A. G., et al. (2015). The role of notch in the cardiovascular system: potential adverse effects of investigational notch inhibitors. *Front. Oncol.* 4:384. doi: 10.3389/fonc.2014.00384

Rocca, C., Scavello, F., Granieri, M. C., Pasqua, T., Amodio, N., Imbrogno, S., et al. (2018). Phoenixin-14: detection and novel physiological implications in cardiac modulation and cardioprotection. *Cell. Mol. Life Sci.* 75, 743–756. doi: 10.1007/s00018-017-2661-3

Wang, M., Crisostomo, P., Wairiuko, G. M., and Meldrum, D. R. (2006). Estrogen receptor-alpha mediates acute myocardial protection in females. *Am. J. Physiol. Heart Circ. Physiol.* 290, H2204–H2209. doi: 10.1152/ajpheart.01219.2005

Wang, M., Wang, Y., Weil, B., Abarbanell, A., Herrmann, J., Tan, J., et al. (2009). Estrogen receptor beta mediates increased activation of PI3K/Akt signaling and improved myocardial function in female hearts following acute ischemia. *Am. J. Physiol. Regul. Integr. Comp. Physiol.* 296, R972–R978. doi: 10.1152/ajpregu.00045.2009

Yin, Y., Guan, Y., Duan, J., Wei, G., Zhu, Y., Quan, W., et al. (2013). Cardioprotective effect of Danshensu against myocardial ischemia/reperfusion injury and inhibits apoptosis of H9c2 cardiomyocytes via Akt and ERK1/2 phosphorylation. *Eur. J. Pharmacol.* 699, 219–226. doi: 10.1016/j.ejphar.2012.11.005

Zhou, X. L., Wan, L., Xu, Q. R., Zhao, Y., and Liu, J. C. (2013). Notch signaling activation contributes to cardioprotection provided by ischemic preconditioning and postconditioning. *J. Transl. Med.* 11:251. doi: 10.1186/1479-5876-11-251

Zimmerman, M. A., Budish, R. A., Kashyap, S., and Lindsey, S. H. (2016). GPER-novel membrane oestrogen receptor. *Clin. Sci.* 130, 1005–1016. doi: 10.1042/CS20160114

19

Chamazulene Attenuates ROS Levels in Bovine Aortic Endothelial Cells Exposed to High Glucose Concentrations and Hydrogen Peroxide

Giulia Querio[1], Susanna Antoniotti[1], Federica Foglietta[2], Cinzia M. Bertea[1], Roberto Canaparo[2], Maria P. Gallo[1] and Renzo Levi[1]*

[1] Department of Life Sciences and Systems Biology, University of Turin, Turin, Italy, [2] Department of Drug Science and Technology, University of Turin, Turin, Italy

Edited by:
Mariarosaria Santillo,
University of Naples Federico II, Italy

Reviewed by:
Chun-An Chen,
The Ohio State University,
United States
Vincenzo Lionetti,
Sant'Anna School of Advanced
Studies, Italy

***Correspondence:**
Maria P. Gallo
mariapia.gallo@unito.it

Endothelial cells surround the lumen of blood vessels and modulate many physiological processes, including vascular tone, blood fluidity, inflammation, immunity and neovascularization. Many pathological conditions, including hyperglycemia, may alter endothelial function through oxidative stress, leading to impaired nitric oxide bioavailability and to the onset of an inflammatory state. As widely shown in the last decade, dietary intervention could represent a good strategy to control endothelial dysfunction and atherosclerosis. In particular, extensive research in the field of antioxidant natural derivatives has been conducted. In this study, we evaluated the capability of Chamazulene (Cham), an azulene compound from chamomile essential oil, to attenuate ROS levels in bovine aortic endothelial cells (BAECs) stressed with either high glucose or H_2O_2. Cell viability at different concentrations of Cham was evaluated through the WST-1 assay, while ROS production acutely induced by High Glucose (HG, 4.5 g/L) treatment or H_2O_2 (0.5 mM) for 3 h, was quantified with 2′-7′-Dichlorofluorescein diacetate (DCFH-DA) probe using confocal microscopy and flow cytometry. Our results showed a reduction in ROS produced after simultaneous treatment with High Glucose or H_2O_2 and Cham, thus suggesting an *in vitro* antioxidant activity of the compound. On the whole, this study shows for the first time the potential role of Cham as a scavenging molecule, suggesting its possible use to prevent the rise of endothelial ROS levels and the consequent vascular damage.

Keywords: Chamazulene, oxidative stress, H_2O_2, glucose, bovine aortic endothelial cells, flow cytometry, confocal microscopy, ROS

INTRODUCTION

In recent years studies on free radicals, as reactive oxygen species (ROS) and reactive nitrogen species (RNS), and their role in mediating different functions in our organism are increasing. Free radicals, ROS and RNS normally produced in living cells, can increase due to external sources, such as X-rays, air pollutants or chemical compounds, or can be endogenously produced by essential enzymatic or non-enzymatic processes (Lobo et al., 2010). These molecules are involved in oxidation-reduction (redox) reactions. Indeed, free radicals are characterized by an unpaired electron that makes these molecules highly unstable and able to act both as oxidants or reductants. Such characteristics are fundamental in the regulation of different cellular functions, collectively indicated as "redox signaling" (Sies, 2015), and underline the role of these molecules both in physiological and pathological conditions. For example, ROS produced by phagocytic cells are fundamental in the first defense against infections (Finkel and Holbrook, 2000), but their uncontrolled rise with the consequent generation of a redox state, called the oxidative stress status, can be deleterious for cellular structures, like DNA, proteins and lipids, with the consequent modification of their function (Espinosa-Diez et al., 2015). Possible generation of systemic long term complications, such as chronic inflammation, endothelial dysfunction, atherosclerosis and cancer, can be related to this condition (Sies, 2015). To control the production of free radicals, ROS and RNS, animal cells use different systems generically called antioxidants, molecules able to donate an electron to free radicals, neutralizing them and confining cell damage. Antioxidants are classified in enzymatic and non-enzymatic molecules. Among enzymatic there are superoxide dismutase (SOD), catalase (CAT), glutathione peroxidase (GSH-Px), thioredoxins (TRX), peroxiredoxins (PRX), glutathione transferase (GST). Examples of non-enzymatic antioxidants are glutathione (GSH), ferritin, transferrin, uric acid, coenzyme Q (Birben et al., 2012). The importance of diet antioxidants that can modulate and sustain endogenous defenses is emerging: carotenoids, vitamin C, vitamin E, omega-3 fatty acids, β-glucans and polyphenols, present in food, can be used by the organisms to reinforce their antioxidant response (Kofuji et al., 2012; Pisoschi and Pop, 2015). Furthermore, in last years, the role of officinal plants as cellular endogenous defense enhancers or free radical *scavengers* emerged and the possible use of plant extracts, essential oils or isolated molecules of traditional relevance as antioxidants is nowadays strongly investigated (Agatonovic-Kustrin et al., 2015; Pisoschi and Pop, 2015). Among officinal plants, chamomile (*Matricaria chamomilla* L.) demonstrated several beneficial properties in cell cultures and in *in vivo* studies (McKay and Blumberg, 2006). In fact, chamomile infusions and extracts showed anti-inflammatory, anti-microbial, hypocholesterolemic and anti-genotoxic effects (Petronilho et al., 2012). Different studies showed that secondary metabolites, in particular terpenoids and flavonoids, isolated from chamomile, are able to neutralize the propagation of radical chains thank to their molecular structure, underlining the possibility to classify these molecules as natural antioxidants (Singh et al., 2010). Among bioactive compounds present in chamomile essential oil, Chamazulene (Cham), a sesquiterpene derived from matricine (Singh et al., 2010), has been proposed as a free radical scavenger. Results obtained with antioxidant assays, like that based on the 2,2′-azino-bis-3-ethylbenzthiazoline-6-sulphonic acid (ABTS) radical (Capuzzo et al., 2014; Agatonovic-Kustrin et al., 2015), suggested the possible antioxidant role of this molecule in a cell model of acute or chronic oxidative stress. Although available data in literature suggest Cham as a radical *scavenger*, there are no studies on its possible effect in a cell model of oxidative stress. In fact its chemical nature suggests its passage through the cell membrane and the possible interaction with radical species (**Figure 1**). Oxidative stress cell models can be determined in different ways depending on cell type and on their susceptibility to specific stressors that can cause pathophysiological conditions. For example, the diabetic state is characterized by endothelial dysfunction, induced by different stressors like high glucose concentrations (Zhou et al., 2015), which cause diminished production of nitric oxide, and, as a consequence, an imbalance in endothelium-derived relaxing and contracting factors, up-regulation of adhesion molecules, increased chemokine secretion, leukocyte adherence and cell permeability, low-density lipoprotein oxidation, platelet activation and vascular smooth muscle cell proliferation and migration (Hadi et al., 2005). The aim of this study was to evaluate the antioxidant properties of Cham on bovine aortic endothelial cells (BAECs) acutely treated with two different oxidative stressors already proposed in other studies (Zhou et al., 2015; Nadeev et al., 2016): High Glucose (HG, 4.5 g/L) concentrations or hydrogen peroxide (H_2O_2, 0.5 mM).

MATERIALS AND METHODS

Chemicals

Chamazulene purification from chamomile (*Matricaria chamomilla* L.) essential oil was performed according to Capuzzo et al. (2014). The compound used was solubilized in absolute ethanol (Sigma Aldrich Saint Louis, MO, USA) at the final concentration of 10 mg/ml. Unless otherwise specified, all reagents for cell culture and experiments were purchased from Sigma-Aldrich.

Cell Culture

Bovine aortic endothelial cells-1 (BAECs, ECACC, Salisbury, UK) were maintained in Dulbecco's modified eagle medium (DMEM) 1 g/L glucose supplemented with 10% FBS, 2 mM L-Glutamine and 50 μg/ml Gentamycin, incubated at 37°C in

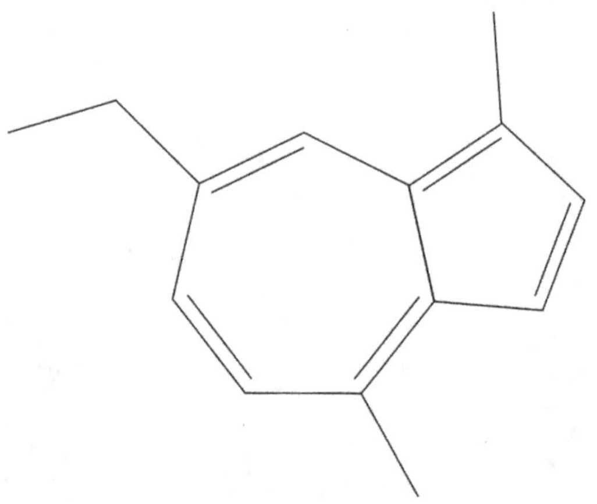

FIGURE 1 | Chemical structure of Chamazulene, C.A.S. n 529-05-5.

a humidified atmosphere containing 5% CO_2. High glucose (HG) treatment was performed using DMEM 4.5 g/L glucose supplemented with 10% FBS, 2 mM L-Glutamine and 50 µg/ml Gentamycin. H_2O_2 treatment was performed at the dilution of 0.5 mM in DMEM 1 g/L glucose. BAECs were used from passages 3 to 6.

Assessment of Cell Viability After Chamazulene Treatment

Cell proliferation reagent WST-1 (Roche Applied Science, Mannheim, Germany) based on the cleavage of a tetrazolium salt into a formazan product by living cell enzymes, in particular mitochondrial dehydrogenases, was used to assess cell viability. BAECs (1.6×10^3 cells/100 µl/well) were seeded into a 96-well plate in culture medium and incubated at 37°C for 24 h. Following incubation, cells were treated with increasing concentrations (10, 25, 100, 250 µg/ml) of Cham or its solvent, ethanol, at the same dilutions (1:1000; 1:400; 1:100; 1:40) for 3 h. WST-1 solution (1:10) was added 2 h before the end of the treatment. The absorbance at 450 nm was determined by a microplate reader (Microplate Reader, Bio-Rad, model 550). The effect of Cham on cell viability was calculated from the absorbance of soluble formazan dye generated by living cells and the results were expressed as percentage of cell viability compared to control, fixed at 100%.

Determination of the EC_{50} of Chamazulene

Half maximal effective concentration (EC_{50}) of Cham was obtained studying the effect of the compound at different concentrations (10, 25, 100, 250 µg/ml) for 3 h by means of the WST-1 Assay; from these data, the EC_{50} was calculated using the software CalcuSyn 2.11 (Biosoft, Cambridge, UK).

ROS Measurement With Confocal Microscopy

BAECs production of ROS was assessed with confocal microscopy using 2′-7′-Dichlorofluorescein diacetate probe (DCFH-DA, Sigma). BAECs were seeded (4.8×10^4 cells/ml) on uncoated glass bottom dishes of 35 mm diameter (MatTeck Corporation, Ashland, MA, USA) in DMEM 1 g/L glucose and incubated at 37°C for 24 h. Following incubation cells were treated with Cham 25 µg/ml, HG, H_2O_2 or simultaneously treated with Cham 25 µg/ml plus HG and Cham 25 µg/ml plus H_2O_2 for 3h; a control condition with ethanol 1:400, correspondent to that present in the 25 µg/ml Cham solution, was added to evaluate its effect alone on the cells. DCFH-DA solution (1 µl/ml) was added to each dish 30 min prior the end of the treatment, then cells were washed three times with PBS containing Ca^{2+} and Mg^{2+} to avoid cells loss. Fluorescence at 488 nm was determined with confocal microscopy (magnification 60x). Quantitative ROS production was calculated with the definition and measurement of Regions Of Interest (ROIs) using the software ImageJ (Rasband, W. S., ImageJ, U. S. National Institutes of Health, Bethesda, Maryland, USA, https://imagej.nih.gov/ij/, 1997-2017) and expressed as relative Medium Fluorescence Index (MFI) compared to control, fixed at 1.

ROS Measurement With Flow Cytometry

BAECs ROS production was assessed with flow cytometry (C6 Accuri, BD Bioscience) using DCFH-DA probe. BAECs were seeded into a 6-well plate (7×10^4 cells/well) in culture medium and incubated at 37°C for 24 h. Following incubation, cells were treated for 3 h with Cham 25 µg/ml, HG, H_2O_2 or simultaneously treated with Cham 25 µg/ml plus HG and Cham 25 µg/ml plus H_2O_2; a control condition with ethanol 1:400 was added to evaluate its role in mediating the effect of Chamazulene. DCFH-DA solution (1 µl/ml) was added to each well 30 min prior the determination of the fluorescence. A total of 10,000 events were considered and ROS levels were recorded at 5 min. Quantitative ROS production was calculated as relative Medium Fluorescence Index (MFI) compared to control, fixed at 1.

Statistical Analysis

All data were expressed as mean ± Standard Deviations of the mean. For differences between mean values Bonferroni's multiple comparisons test was performed. Differences with $P < 0.05$ were regarded as statistically significant.

RESULTS

BAECs Viability After Exposure to Different Concentrations of Chamazulene

To assess Cham toxicity BAECs were exposed to different concentrations of the compound (10, 25, 100, 250 µg/ml) for 3 h; its effects were evaluated by means of the WST-1 assay. None of the concentrations tested was toxic at 3 h; and, as shown in **Figure 2**, cells viability was not affected by ethanol at any of the concentrations used, corresponding to the amount of the solvent present in each Cham treatment.

These data were used to calculate the EC_{50} of Cham with the software CalcuSyn and, as confirmed in **Figure 2**, 25 µg/ml increased cells viability at 50% in 3 h and represented the EC_{50} dose of the compound in these experiments. This concentration was used in this preliminary evaluation of the antioxidant activity of Cham in cells.

Chamazulene and ROS Levels After HG Treatment

ROS production in BAECs after HG treatment was at first evaluated by confocal microscopy using the DCFH-DA probe (**Figures 3A,B**). Cells were treated for 3 h with HG, Cham 25 µg/ml or simultaneously with both. High Glucose treatment for 3 h induced augmented ROS levels that was balanced by the simultaneous addition of Cham. A control condition with ethanol 1:400, corresponding to the amount of solvent added to cells with the 25 µg/ml Cham treatment, had no effect on BAECs. Results of confocal microscopy experiments were confirmed by flow cytometry: high glucose treatment induced a significant

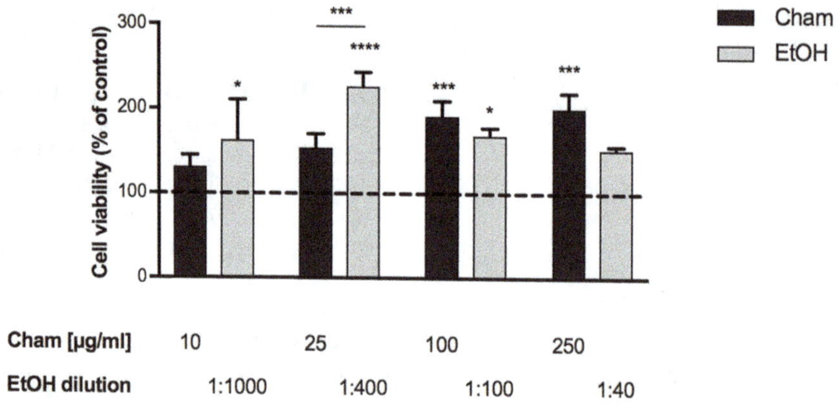

FIGURE 2 | Effect of Chamazulene on BAECs at 3 h of treatment, as assessed by the WST-1 Assay. None of the concentrations used was toxic for BAECs. Cell viability was not affected by ethanol (light gray bars) used at the same amount present in each Cham treatment. Data shown are mean ± SD of three independent experiments and are expressed as percentage toward control (Data are presented from the lowest to the highest concentration used. Cham: 131.08 ± 13.91; 153.81 ± 16.50; 191.56 ± 18.18; 200.36 ± 18.38. EtOH: 162.68 ± 48.13; 226.67 ± 16.97; 168.90 ± 9.02; 152.22 ± 3.94); $^*P < 0.05$, $^{***}P < 0.001$, $^{****}P < 0.0001$.

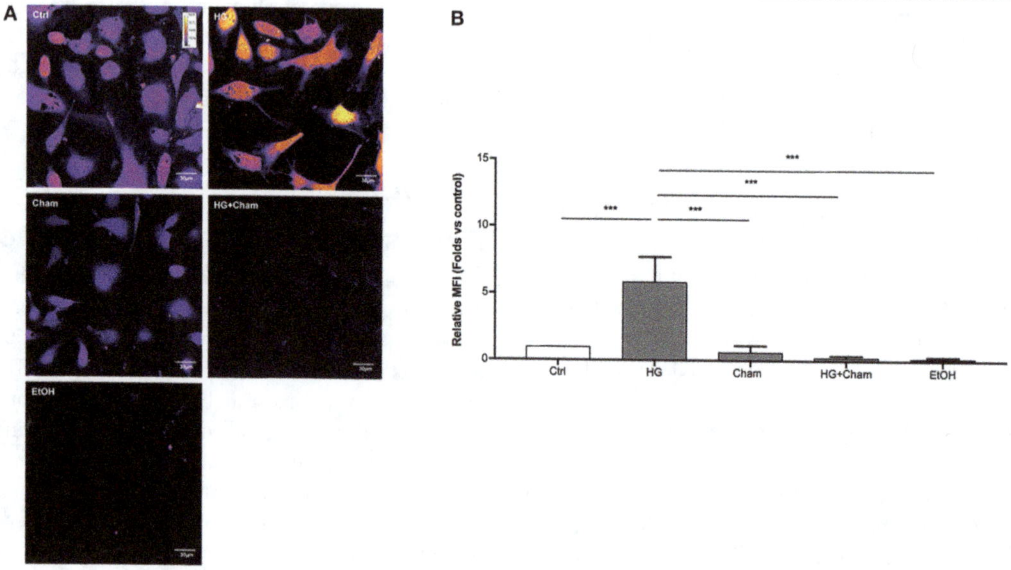

FIGURE 3 | Chamazulene and ROS levels in confocal microscopy after HG treatment. **(A)** Images obtained with confocal microscopy and DCFH-DA probe (magnification 60x). Fluorescence intensity is represented in pseudo color scale ("fire" in ImageJ software): HG treatment for 3 h induced augmented ROS levels as underlined by the changing color of cells compared to control and it was balanced by the simultaneous treatment with Cham. **(B)** Histograms illustrate the relative MFI toward control derived from images analysis and show augmented ROS levels when cells are treated with HG and their decrease in a simultaneous treatment with Cham. Cham effect is not affected by ethanol. Data shown are mean±SD of three independent experiments (HG: 5.89±1.84; Cham: 0.65±0.47; HG + Cham: 0.29 ± 0.10; EtOH: 0.22 ± 0.09); $^{***}P < 0.001$.

ROS increase in BAECs, as compared to cells maintained in low glucose medium; Cham added together with HG was able to attenuate the effect of HG while nor Cham nor EtOH alone did not have any effect on ROS production (**Figures 4A,B**).

Chamazulene and ROS Levels After H_2O_2 Treatment

ROS levels, due to H_2O_2 treatment for 3h, and their possible reduction induced by Cham, were quantified in a second set of experiments with confocal microscopy and flow cytometry using DCFH-DA probe. In confocal experiments, as shown in **Figures 5A,B**, BAECs stressed with H_2O_2 for 3 h revealed a higher production of ROS and this condition was reverted by simultaneous treatment with Cham 25 µg/ml. As shown, treatment with ethanol in which Cham was solubilized confirmed that ethanol had no effect on ROS production, not even Cham 25 µg/ml added alone to the culture medium had any effect on ROS levels.

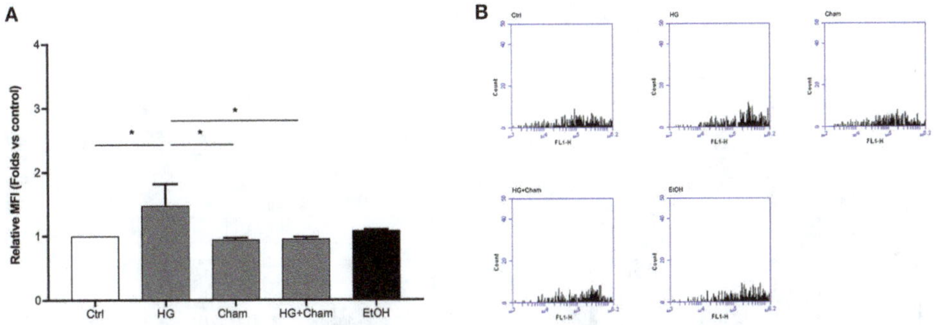

FIGURE 4 | Chamazulene and ROS levels in flow cytometry after HG treatment. **(A)** Histograms illustrate the relative MFI toward control derived from flow cytometry and show ROS levels when cells are treated with HG and their decrease in a simultaneous treatment with Cham and HG. Cham effect is not affected by ethanol. Data shown are mean ± SD of three independent experiments (HG: 1.47 ± 0.35; Cham: 0.94 ± 0.03; HG + Cham: 0.96 ± 0.02; EtOH: 1.08 ± 0.02); $^{*}P < 0.05$ **(B)** Representative graphs of flow cytometry in which is illustrated the variation in fluorescence in different treatments.

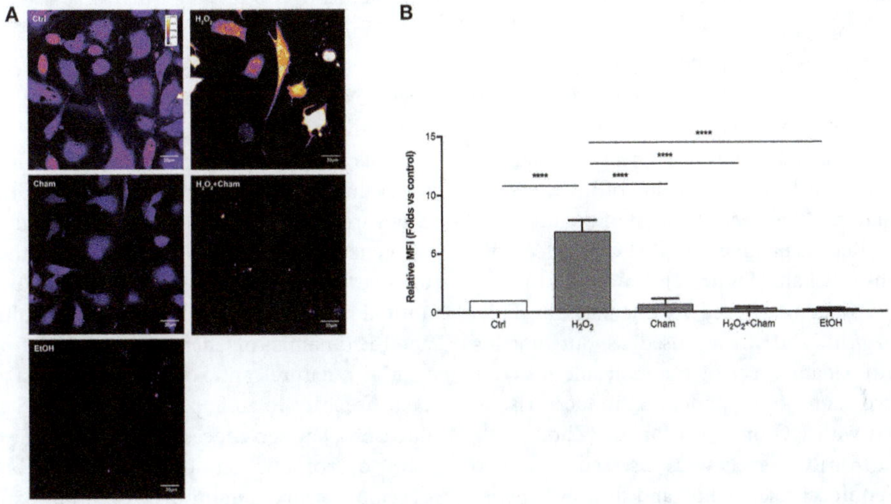

FIGURE 5 | Chamazulene and ROS levels in confocal microscopy after H_2O_2 treatment. **(A)** Images obtained with confocal microscopy and DCFH-DA probe (magnification 60x). Fluorescence intensity is represented in pseudo color scale ("fire" in ImageJ software): H_2O_2 treatment for 3h induce augmented ROS levels as underlined by the changing color of cells compared to control and it was balanced by the simultaneous treatment with Cham. **(B)** Histograms illustrate the relative MFI toward control derived from images analysis and show high ROS levels when cells are treated with H_2O_2 and their decrease in a simultaneous treatment with Cham and H_2O_2. Ethanol does not affect ROS level. Data shown are mean±SD of three independent experiments (H_2O_2: 6.86±1.00; Cham: 0.65±0.47; H_2O_2+Cham: 0.30±0.13; EtOH: 0.22±0.09); $^{****}P < 0.0001$.

These results were confirmed by flow cytometry experiments (**Figures 6A,B**).

DISCUSSION

Cells are continuously exposed to physical and chemical stressors. When endogenous and exogenous defenses are not sufficient to balance the production of free radicals, ROS and RNS, cells enter in an oxidative stress status which can be deleterious for the structure and function of important molecules like nucleic acids, proteins and lipids (Birben et al., 2012). Several pathological conditions can contribute to the definition of such status, characterized by the rise of reactive molecules; as an example, endothelial cells exposure to high concentrations of glucose, as it occurs in diabetic disease, can increase ROS production, enhancing endothelial dysfunction that characterizes this condition (Rahimi et al., 2005). In this scenario, the role of antioxidant molecules endogenously produced in cells or derived from exogenous sources, represents the first line of investigation in order to assess any increased cell defense against oxidative stress status and thus preventing further cell damage. Scavenger activity of exogenous antioxidants is usually tested primarily with chemical assays, like the ABTS assay (Floegel et al., 2011). Then, in order to classify a molecule as an antioxidant in complex systems such as living cells, it is important to evaluate how the molecule behaves in a cell model of oxidative stress status. A molecule recently studied for its capability to scavenge free radicals is Cham (Capuzzo et al., 2014), a sesquiterpene spontaneously derived from matricine and present in high concentrations in chamomile (*Matricaria chamomilla* L.) essential oil. Previous studies on Cham underline its antioxidant activity as the molecule is able to scavenge preformed free radicals

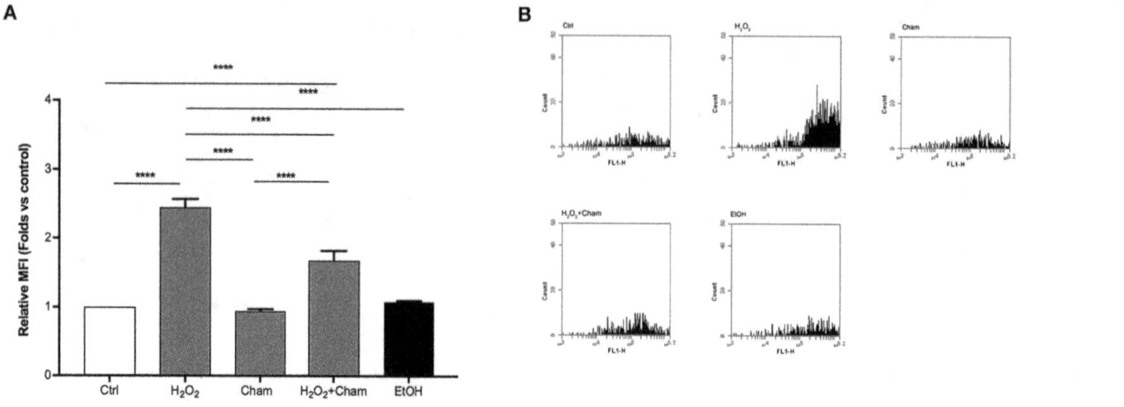

FIGURE 6 | Chamazulene and ROS levels in flow cytometry after H_2O_2 treatment. **(A)** Histograms illustrate the relative MFI toward control derived from flow cytometry and show high ROS levels when cells are treated with H_2O_2 and their decrease in a simultaneous treatment with Cham and H_2O_2. Cham effect is not affected by ethanol. Data shown are mean ± SD of three independent experiments (H_2O_2: 2.44 ± 0.13; Cham: 0.94 ± 0.03; H_2O_2+Cham: 1.68 ± 0.14; EtOH: 1.08 ± 0.02); $^{****}P < 0.0001$ **(B)** Representative graphs of flow cytometry in which is illustrated the variation in fluorescence in different treatments.

(Capuzzo et al., 2014; Formisano et al., 2015). Our aim, in this research paper, was to evaluate for the first time the role of Cham as an antioxidant in endothelial cells in two different models of oxidative stress. Since data showing the effect of Cham in cultured cells are still unavailable, our first line of investigation aimed to the determination of the concentration of the molecule by which treating cells. Results obtained on BAECs treated with different concentrations of Cham (**Figure 2**) showed no toxicity of the molecule. These data were used to calculate the EC_{50} of Cham at 3 h, 25 µg/ml, and it was used as our starting point to study any antioxidant effect of the molecule on cells. Cham was tested in two acute stress model that induced rise in ROS: cells were treated with HG or H_2O_2 for 3 h (Zhou et al., 2015; Nadeev et al., 2016). ROS levels were assessed using two different approaches: confocal microscopy and flow cytometry. Results obtained in confocal microscopy analysis showed a reduction in ROS levels when cells were simultaneously treated with HG or H_2O_2 and Cham (**Figures 3, 5**), and these data were confirmed by flow cytometry analysis (**Figures 4, 6**). These experiments underline the effect of Cham respect to different stimuli, high glucose and H_2O_2. High glucose was chosen to mimic the hyperglycemic state characteristic of diabetes. In this condition endothelial oxidative stress occurs thorough many pathways, including formation of peroxynitrite, reduced NO production, inactivation and/or reduction of expression of antioxidant enzymes, formation of AGEs (advanced glycation end products; Incalza et al., 2018). H_2O_2 represents a direct stronger insult that is able to induce covalent modifications of cysteine thiolate residues located in active and allosteric sites of specific proteins resulting in alterations on their activity and function. Moreover, high concentration of H_2O_2 evokes inflammatory responses leading to growth arrest and ultimately cell death (Sies, 2017).

Therefore, in these models ROS levels rise in different ways, but, in both conditions, Chamazulene was able to balance them. The novelty of this study can be pointed out, as done before, underlining that it has been the first work in which antioxidant activity of Cham has been tested on a cell model, even if, as previously said, results obtained were linked to short treatment times, reflecting only acute effects and not long term events such as gene expression. Furthermore, it could be interesting to evaluate how Cham acts in a cell model increasing the exposure time to different stressors and evaluating the effect on gene transcription. Another aspect that can be interesting to investigate, essential for the complete determination of its antioxidant activity, could be the determination of the kinetics and the dinamics of Chamazulene in *in vivo* studies.

Many natural antioxidants counteract oxidative stress, and their use leads to an improvement in ROS generation-associated diseases. New substances with antioxidant properties to balance ROS overproduction and favor NO bioavailability can be developed with the aim of preventing oxidative stress-induced vascular damage, and Cham could be included in the list of these molecules. Further studies on Cham and its potential application will reinforce the efficacy of natural beneficial nutritional components in delaying the onset of vascular dysfunction and maintaining or restoring vascular health.

AUTHOR CONTRIBUTIONS

CB, RC, MG, and RL conceived the study, assisted its design and revised the manuscript for important intellectual content. GQ, RL, FF, and SA carried out the experiments, statistical analysis, and interpreted the results with the other authors. GQ wrote the manuscript. All authors read, edited and approved the final manuscript.

ACKNOWLEDGMENTS

The authors thank Dr. Andrea Capuzzo for the technical support during isolation and analysis of Chamazulene from chamomile essential oil and Prof. Loredana Serpe for the support in cytofluorimetric analysis. This work was supported by the local founding of the University of Turin (GQ, MG and RL).

REFERENCES

Agatonovic-Kustrin, S., Ortakand, D. B., Morton, D. W., and Yusof, A. P. (2015). Rapid evaluation and comparison of natural products and antioxidant activity in calendula, feverfew, and German chamomile extracts. *J. Chromatogr. A* 1385, 103–110. doi: 10.1016/j.chroma.2015.01.067

Birben, E., Sahiner, U. M., Sackesen, C., Erzurum, S., and Kalayci, O. (2012). Oxidative stress and antioxidant defense. *WAO J.* 5, 9–19. doi: 10.1097/WOX.0b013e3182439613

Capuzzo, A., Occhipinti, A., and Maffei, M. E. (2014). Antioxidant and radical scavenging activities of chamazulene. *Natural Product Res. Form. Nat. Product Lett.* 28, 2321–2323. doi: 10.1080/14786419.2014.931393

Espinosa-Diez, C., Miguel, V., Mennerich, D., Kietzmann, T., Sánchez-Pérez, P., Cadenas, S., et al. (2015). Antioxidant responses and cellular adjustments to oxidative stress. *Redox Biol.* 6, 183–197. doi: 10.1016/j.redox.2015.07.008

Finkel, T., and Holbrook, N. J. (2000). Oxidants, oxidation stress and the biology of ageing. *Nature* 408, 239–247. doi: 10.1038/35041687

Floegel, A., Kim, D., Chung, S., Koo, S. I., and Chun, O. K. (2011). Comparison of ABTS/DPPH assays to measure antioxidant capacity in popular antioxidant-rich US foods. *J. Food Composit. Anal.* 24, 1043–1048. doi: 10.1016/j.jfca.2011.01.008

Formisano, C., Delfine, S., Oliviero, F., Tenore, G. C., Rigano, D., and Senatore, F. (2015). Correlation among environmental factors, chemical composition and antioxidative properties of essential oil and extracts of chamomile (*Matricaria recutita L.*) collected in Molise (South-central Italy). *Ind. Crops Prod.* 63, 256–263. doi: 10.1016/j.indcrop.2014.09.042

Hadi, H. A. R., Carr, C. S., and Al Suwaidi, J. (2005). Endothelial dysfunction: cardiovascular risk factors, therapy, and outcome. *Vasc. Health Risk Manag.* 1, 183–198.

Incalza, M. A., D'Oria, R., Natalicchio, A., Perrini, S., and Laviola, L. (2018). Oxidative stress and reactive oxygen species in endothelial dysfunction associated with cardiovascular and metabolic diseases. *Vascul. Pharmacol.* 100, 1–19. doi: 10.1016/j.vph.2017.05.005

Kofuji, K., Aoki, A., Tsubaki, K., Konishi, M., Isobe, T., and Murata, Y. (2012). Antioxidant activity of β-Glucan. *ISRN Pharm.* 2012:125864. doi: 10.5402/2012/125864

Lobo, V., Patil, A., Phatak, A., and Chandra, N. (2010). Free radicals, antioxidants and functional foods: impact on human health. *Pharmacogn. Rev.* 4, 118–126. doi: 10.4103/0973-7847.70902

McKay, D. L., and Blumberg, J. B. A. (2006). Review of the Bioactivity and Potential Health Benefits of Chamomile Tea (*Matricaria recutita* L.) *Phytother. Res.* 20, 519–530. doi: 10.1002/ptr.1900

Nadeev, A. D., Kudryavtsev, I. V., Serebriakova, M. K., Avdonin, P. V., Zinchenko, V. P., and GonCharov, N. V. (2016). Dual proapoptotic and pronecrotic effect of hydrogen peroxide on human umbilical vein endothelial cells. *Cell Tisue Biol.* 10, 145–151. doi: 10.1134/S1990519X16020097

Petronilho, S., Maraschin, M., Coimbra, M. A., and Rocha, S. M. (2012). *In vitro* and *in vivo* studies of natural products: a challenge for their valuation. The case study of chamomile *(Matricaria recutita* L.) *Indust. Crops Prod.* 40, 1–12. doi: 10.1016/j.indcrop.2012.02.041

Pisoschi, A. M., and Pop, A. (2015). The role of antioxidants in the chemistry of oxidative stress: a review. *Eur. J. Med. Chem.* 97, 55–74. doi: 10.1016/j.ejmech.2015.04.040

Rahimi, R., Nikfar, S., Larijani, B., and Abdollahi, M. (2005). A review on the role of antioxidants in the management of diabetes and its complications. *Biomed. Pharmacother.* 59, 365–373. doi: 10.1016/j.biopha.2005.07.002

Sies, H. (2015). Oxidative stress: a concept in redox biology and medicine. *Redox Biol.* 4, 180–183. doi: 10.1016/j.redox.2015.01.002

Sies, H. (2017). Hydrogen peroxide as a central redox signaling molecule in physiological oxidative stress: oxidative eustress. *Redox Biol.* 11, 613–619. doi: 10.1016/j.redox.2016.12.035

Singh, O., Khanam, Z., Misra, N., and Srivastava, M. K. (2010). Chamomile *(Matricaria chamomilla L.)*: an overview. *Pharmacogn. Rev.* 5, 82–95. doi: 10.4103/0973-7847.79103

Zhou, D.-Y., Su, Y., Gao, P., Yang, Q.-H., Wang, Z., and Xu, Q. (2015). Resveratrol ameliorates high glucose-induced oxidative stress injury in human umbilical endothelial cells by activating AMPK. *Life Sci.* 136, 94–99. doi: 10.1016/j.lfs.2015.07.008

20

Metabolomic Approach to Redox and Nitrosative Reactions in Cardiovascular Diseases

Martino Deidda†, Antonio Noto†, Pier P. Bassareo, Christian Cadeddu Dessalvi and Giuseppe Mercuro*

Department of Medical Sciences and Public Health, University of Cagliari, Sardinia, Italy

Edited by:
Pasquale Pagliaro,
Università degli Studi di Torino, Italy

Reviewed by:
Nina Kaludercic,
Università degli Studi di Padova, Italy
Felicia Carotenuto,
Università degli Studi di Roma Tor Vergata, Italy

****Correspondence:***
Martino Deidda
martino.deidda@unica.it;
martino.deidda@tiscali.it

† These authors have contributed equally to this work.

Metabolomics, also referred to as metabonomics, is one of the most recent innovative technologies in medicine. It offers a direct functional read-out of phenotypes by the detection, identification, and quantification of a large number of metabolites within a biological sample such as urine and blood. Metabolites (<1500 Da) represent the output of cellular metabolism, accounting for expression and activity of genes, transcripts, and proteins, and offering unique insights into small molecule regulation, which may uncover new biochemical patterns. Metabolomics research has considerable potential for translating the metabolic fingerprint into personalized therapeutic strategies. Within the field of interest, cardiovascular disease (CVD) is one of the most developed areas. However, CVD remains the leading cause of death worldwide with a marked increase in mortality rates over the past six decades. In this scenario, recent findings indicate the important role of redox and nitrosative (RN) reactions in CVD development and progression. RN reactions are generally involved in the homeostatic modulation of a wide number of cellular and organ functions. Conversely, the imbalance of these reactions may lead to a condition of allostasis that in turn can cause CVD. The aim of this review is to highlight how the use of metabolomics may be useful for the study of RN reactions related to CVD, providing a tool to understand the mechanisms underlying reactions that could lead to impaired ROS or RNS formation.

Keywords: metabolomics, cardiovascular diseases, nitric oxide, reactive oxygen species, redox and nitrosative reactions

INTRODUCTION

Cardiovascular diseases (CVDs) represent the leading cause of mortality in developed countries. Several risk factors are associated with CVDs. These are multifactorial diseases and involve a complex interplay between fixed (genotype, age, gender, and reproductive status) and modifiable (diet, smoking, exercise, and ethanol consumption) causative factors (Mozaffarian et al., 2015).

In both health and diseased states, redox and nitrosative (RN) reactions, as well as signaling, are involved in the modulation of a wide number of cellular and organ functions, such as the regulation of vascular tone by endothelial and smooth muscle cells, or the excitation-contraction coupling in cardiomyocytes (Fearon and Faux, 2009; He and Zuo, 2015).

Numerous review papers have provided overviews concerning the use of metabolomics approaches for the study of cardiac diseases, (Mercuro et al., 2011; Deidda et al., 2015a; Kordalewska and Markuszewski, 2015; Ussher et al., 2016) but none have specifically emphasized the complex area of oxidative stress. In this paper, we will review the various approaches that have employed metabolomics in order to investigate RN reactions and signaling.

METABOLOMICS

Metabolomics is one of the most recent innovative technologies that aims to understand the metabolic processes within cells, tissues, organs, and organisms (Griffin et al., 2011). It is focused on the quantitative analysis of large numbers of metabolites. The latter represent the end products of genes, transcripts, and protein functions, and provide an instantaneous snapshot of biological status. While progress in genomics and proteomics analysis has allowed understanding of altered genes and proteins under a variety of perturbations, including disease conditions, metabolomics offers an alternative approach to help understand altered metabolic pathways and discover new gene functions (Griffin et al., 2011). The strong interest in metabolomics is based on the fact that even subtle changes in genes, abundance of transcripts, or levels of protein can substantially change the quantity and dynamics of metabolites. Therefore, analysis of metabolites represents a sensitive measure of biological status in health or disease (Klupczyńska et al., 2015). Altered metabolic fingerprints, which are unique to every individual, offer novel opportunities to better understand systems biology, detect or identify potential risks for various diseases, and ultimately help achieve the goal of "personalized medicine." (Cheng et al., 2017) In this regard, a sizable number of findings have been tested for translational applications focusing on disease diagnostics ranging from early detection (Deidda et al., 2015b), to therapy prediction and prognosis,(Ussher et al., 2016) monitoring treatment and recurrence detection, as well as the important area of therapeutic target discovery (Griffin et al., 2011; Deidda et al., 2015a; Ussher et al., 2016). Moreover, current advances in analytical techniques ensure quantitation of biomarkers from even small amounts of biological samples using non-invasive or minimally invasive approaches, and facilitate high-throughput analysis required for real-time applications in clinical settings.

In this review, we focus on the application of metabolomics to the investigation of redox reactions and NO pathways, highlighting, through the presented studies, how metabolomic analysis may be applied in this research setting.

CARDIO-METABOLOMICS AND OXIDATIVE STRESS

Among the metabolites that can be measured by metabolomics there are some that can be used to understand the mechanisms underlying reactions leading to impaired reactive oxygen species (ROS). ROS are the result of aerobic metabolism, they include the superoxide anion (O_2^-), hydrogen peroxide (H_2O_2), and hydroxyl radicals (•OH), all of which have intrinsic chemical reactive properties involving distinctive biological targets such as lipids, proteins, and DNA. Usually, ROS are correlated with oxidative stress conditions, the damaging process that involves lipids, proteins, and DNA, which suggests that ROS are the cause of several pathologies. However, it was recently demonstrated (Schieber and Chandel, 2014) that ROS also operate as signaling molecules for regulating biological processes. On the other hand, when organisms generate ROS at a greater rate than they can be balanced by the regulating systems, there is a condition of oxidative stress (Schieber and Chandel, 2014). Moreover, as previously mentioned, ROS are generated during aerobic metabolism and in particular in the trycarboxylic acid (TCA) cycle, which is known to be heavily involved in the production of metabolic intermediates and generation of reducing potential. The purpose of TCA and oxidative phosphorylation is to completely oxidize molecules of acetyl-CoA and store the chemical energy in the synthesis of molecules of ATP from ADP and phosphate. ATP is used for a variety of anabolic (energy requiring) activities of the cell. These high rate reactions can, however, also produce ROS. Another main source of ROS formation is the metabolism of purines via the xanthine oxidase pathway. In fact, ATP is rapidly depleted in hypoxia-anoxia conditions, resulting in formation of ADP, AMP, adenosine, inosine and hypoxanthine. The enzyme xanthine oxidase produces ROS as hypoxanthine is being further metabolized to uric acid in the final steps of purine degradation.

The organism compensates for ROS production with antioxidant enzymes (superoxide dismutase, catalase, and glutathione peroxidase) and intracellular molecules such as glutathione that exist in reduced (GSH) and oxidized (GSSG) forms (Lu, 2009). In addition, there are circulating antioxidants such as uric acid, ascorbate, α-tocopherol, thiols, and bilirubin.

Early pioneering studies have reported an association between cardiac diseases and the presence of abnormal metabolites related to the presence of ROS in bodily fluids (Dhalla et al., 2000). Today, current knowledge points to the important role of metabolites derived from the production of ROS and cardiac disease (**Table 1**), because these metabolites can modulate phenotypes, influencing host metabolic pathways and the immune system and determining an individual susceptibility to disease. A milestone paper was published in 2014 from Murphy's group, which has identified how novel metabolic pathways become activated to fuel mitochondrial ROS production during ischemia-reperfusion (IR) injury (Chouchani et al., 2014). IR injury occurs when the blood supply to an organ is interrupted and then restored, and triggers many disorders, such as heart attack and stroke. To this aim, authors have used a male mouse model. Mice were allocated into four groups and exposed to 5, 30, and 30 min ischemia along with 5 min reperfusion and 30 min sham. Subsequently, LC-MS metabolomics analysis was performed on heart tissues. The resulting analysis showed that accumulation of succinate, via fumarate production and reversal of succinate dehydrogenase, is a universal metabolic signature of ischemia *in vivo*. In addition, during reperfusion, succinate dehydrogenase rapidly re-oxidized succinate in the respiratory chain thus driving mitochondrial ROS formation through RET at complex I. In conclusion, these data demonstrate that preventing succinate accumulation during ischemia is protective against IR injury *in vivo*, suggesting novel therapeutic targets for IR injury in various pathologies.

TABLE 1 | Presented studies on metabolomics and ROS.

Reference	Species	Technique	Setting	Biofluid/ Tissue	Discriminate Metabolites/ Metabolism
Li et al., 2015	LDLR−/− mice C57BL/J6 mice	NMR, GC-FID/MS	Atherosclerosis	Plasma, urine Liver, Kidney and myocardial Tissue	Significant drop in PUFA-to-MUFA (and PUFA-to-UFA) ratios in both the plasma and liver of WD-fed mice
Chouchani et al., 2014	C57BL/6J mice	LC-MS	Ischemia-reperfusion injury	Heart	Significant increase in succinate
Lu et al., 2017	Human	QTOF/MS	Coronary Heart Disease	Plasma	glycerophospholipid metabolism including phosphatidylcholine, lysophosphatidylcholine (lysoPC), phospha- tidylethanolamine, lysophosphatidylethanolamine (lysoPE), phos-phatidylserine, lysophosphatidylserine, phosphatidylino- sitol, and lysophosphatidic acids. Among them, lysoPC (20:0), lysoPC (20:1), lysoPC (20:2), lysoPC (20:5), lysoPC (22:5), lysoPE (18:3), and glycerophosphocholine
Wang et al., 2017	Sprague-Dawley rats	UPLC-TOF/MS	Pulmonary Arterial Hypertension	Right Ventricular Tissue	Significant increase in oxidized glutathione, xanthine and uric acid and a reduction in α-tocopherol nicotinate
Varvarousis et al., 2017	Landrace/large-white pigs	NMR, LC-MS/MS	Asphyxial cardiac arrest	Plasma	Significant increase in succinate

NMR, ^1H Nuclear magnetic resonance spectroscopy; GC-FID/MS, gas chromatography with flame ionization detection – mass spectrometry; LC-MS, liquid chromatography – mass spectrometry; QTOF/MS, quadrupole time of flight mass spectrometry; UPLC-TOF/MS, ultra performance liquid chromatography – time of flight mass spectrometry; PUFA, poly-unsaturated fatty acids; MUFA, mono-unsaturated fatty acids; UFA, unsaturated fatty acids; WD, western diet; LysoPC, lysophosphatidylcholine.

In the same year, Li and co-workers studied the origin of CVD resulting from hyperlipidemia and atherosclerosis. To this aim, The authors have analyzed metabolomic changes by means of NMR and GC-FID/MS using a well-established mouse model. This animal model is a knock-out (KO) for the low-density lipoprotein (LDL) receptor gene and is considered the preeminent animal model for experimentally investigating the pathogenesis and progression of atherosclerosis because this model can mimic the progress of hyperlipidemia-induced aortic plaques (Ishibashi et al., 1993, 1994a,b). The animals were randomly divided into three groups [control diet (CD), Western diet (WD), and diet-switched (DS)]. The CD and WD groups were fed with normal chow diet and WD, respectively, for 12 weeks, whereas the DS group was fed with WD for 6 weeks, followed by CD for a further 6 weeks. Metabolomics analyses were performed using samples of plasma, heart, kidney, liver, and urine. Among the important pathways modified by the WD diet, they found changes in energy metabolism with disruptions to glucose homeostasis including decreases in plasma glucose, renal lactate, and urinary excretion of TCA intermediates. Because of the significant presence of intermediates such as succinate, fumarate, and allantoin and the significant decrease of polyunsaturated fatty acid, it was hypothesized that the metabolic profile was associated with a condition of oxidative stress (Li et al., 2015).

Regarding succinate and fumarate, the mechanism was previously mentioned in the text (Chouchani et al., 2014); concerning allantoin and polyunsaturated fatty acid, the former was indicated by Grootveld as a product of oxidative stress resulting from oxidation of uric acid. Authors hypothesized that measurement of changes in allantoin concentration may be a useful index of free-radical reactions (Grootveld and Halliwell, 1987), whearase the latter [a reduced (PUFA/MUFA) ratio concentration] has been suggested as indicator of oxidative stress and lipid peroxidation (Galli et al., 2001).

Lu et al. (2017) performed a comprehensive metabolomics study in patients with coronary heart disease (CHD). (Lu et al., 2017) CHD is the most common type of heart disease. It is the leading cause of death in the United States in both men and women. It accounts for 30% of deaths worldwide, including 40% in high-income countries and approximately 28% in developing nations (Dalen et al., 2014; Herrington et al., 2016). CHD refers to a group of diseases that include stable angina, unstable angina, myocardial infarction, and sudden cardiac death. In order to gain a more comprehensive understanding of the pathophysiology of CHD at the molecular level, The authors have included two different groups of diseases: the stable angina (SA) and the myocardial infarction (MI) groups, which were then compared with a healthy control group (HC). All the patients recruited in this study were diagnosed and classified based on symptoms and coronary angiography (Lu et al., 2017). A plasma sample was collected from each subject and immediately frozen. Subsequently, metabolomics analysis was performed using an ultra-high performance liquid chromatography – quadrupole time-of-flight mass spectrometry (UHPLC-QTOF/MS) platform. The resulting data matrix was investigated by univariate and multivariate statistical analysis and 18, 37, and 36 metabolites were identified and recognized as being differential metabolites that distinguish SA from HC, MI from SA, and MI from HC, respectively. Among the important pathways, glycerophospholipid (GPL) metabolism emerged as the most-significantly disturbed, in particular oxidized PL on the surface of low density lipoprotein (LDL) particles and their hydrolyzed fatty acids were closely associated with CHD, however, the underlying molecular mechanisms remain poorly defined. The authors concluded that MI patients were characterized by high oxidative stress and lipid peroxidation, which is a known contributing factor in CHD.

Another interesting study was published by Wang et al., 2017 in regarding the presence of oxidative stress in right heart failure (RV) using a rat animal model (Wang et al., 2017). RV is the main cause of mortality among patients with pulmonary arterial hypertension (PAH). Recently, an experimental animal model of PAH was developed by injecting an inhibitor of VEGF receptor tyrosine kinase and ovalbumin (OVA). 2 out of 10 of animals developing PAH were dying because of RV failure within 8 weeks (Mizuno et al., 2012). Based on this experimental animal model, authors induced PAH by administering OVA and Sugen5416 to male rats and at day 50 animals were sacrificed and lung and heart tissues were collected for histological, proteomic, and metabolomics investigations. For metabolomics analysis, the collected RV tissue underwent metabolites extraction using methanol/acetonitrile followed by centrifugation. The samples were successively injected into a UHPLC-QTOF/MS system. The resulting data matrix was explored by means of partial least square-discriminant analysis (PLS-DA), which indicated the existence of a different metabolic profile between PAH RV rodents and controls. Among the discriminant metabolites, PAH RV rats had a 3.8-fold increase in xanthine and a 4.9-fold increase in uric acid, whose increased levels are index of augmented xanthine oxidase activity that is common during hypoxia and ischemia and is a well-known marker of oxidative stress. In addition, metabolomics results revealed that PAH caused a 2.1-fold increase in oxidized glutathione and a 28.2-fold reduction in α-tocopherol nicotinate, which can be because of ROS production. The authors concluded by suggesting that this model may help understanding of oxidative stress in PAH-induced RV modifications.

The idea to identify a metabolic profile in an experimental model of asphyxial cardiac arrest (ACA) compared with a model of ventricular fibrillation cardiac arrest (VFCA) was recently published by Varvarousis et al. (2017). These authors focused their attention on the metabolic differences existing between ACA and VFCA, which have not been studied yet although they represent the two most common types of CA. To this purpose, they have used landrace/large-white female pigs in which ACA and VFCA were induced. The metabolic content was characterized at different time points: at CA, during cardiopulmonary resuscitation, and in the post-resuscitation period. Plasma samples were analyzed by high resolution ^{1}H-NMR spectroscopy and LC-MS/MS spectrometry in order to identify the metabolomic profiles characterizing the two pathological entities during the different phases of the experiment. Major alterations in plasma concentrations of metabolites involved the key energy production pathways. In particular, asphyxia and ventricular fibrillation differed significantly with regard to the metabolic disturbances during the peri-arrest period. Among the important metabolites the accumulation of plasma succinate was detected in the animals undergoing ACA and with worse outcome. Based on the mechanism identified by Chouchani et al., 2014, by which ROS are produced by the RET mechanism, authors concluded by suggesting a potential prognostic role for this metabolite as an indicator of ROS production and poorer outcomes.

CARDIO-METABOLOMICS AND NO PATHWAYS

Nitric oxide (NO) plays an important role in the development of CVD; it is a highly reactive, short-lived free radical, that exerts a wide range of biological functions, critical for the normal physiology of cardiovascular system. NO effects include cardiac contractility, regulation of vasodilation, fibrinolysis, and inhibition of several biological processes such as atherogenesis, platelet aggregation, leukocyte adhesion, and smooth muscle cell proliferation (Fearon and Faux, 2009).

In pathological states (i.e., oxidative stress) there is an impairment in NO production and its actions are consequently reduced. It is also rapidly catabolized to ONOO when it reacts with O_2^-.

Nitric oxide synthesis takes place through the NADPH and tetrahydrobiopterin-dependent oxidation of the amino acid L-arginine to L-citrulline (**Figure 1**), mediated by NO synthases (NOS), a family of three isoforms including two constitutive forms, neuronal NOS (nNOS) and endothelial NOS (eNOS), and an inducible isoform, iNOS. The intracellular availability of arginine is the rate-limiting step in NO production, while argininosuccinate lyase, the enzyme that produces arginine from citrulline, seems to be important both to synthesize intracellular arginine and to utilize extracellular arginine for NO synthesis (van Dyk et al., 2015).

Although NO cannot be directly measured by techniques used in metabolomics, NO-signaling in CVDs can be investigated as described in the studies presented below (**Table 2**).

Wang et al. (2009) evaluated the relationship between post-translational modification products of arginine methylation and CHD, concluding that "factors beyond direct NOS inhibition contribute to the clinical associations between methylarginines and CAD outcomes." (Wang et al., 2009) They performed a metabolomic study analyzing 1011 plasma samples from subjects undergoing elective diagnostic cardiac catheterization using stable isotope dilution HPLC-MS/MS in order to evaluate the association of specific metabolites with future major adverse cardiac events (MACE: myocardial infarction, stroke, and death). Patients were followed-up for 3 years. They evaluated plasma levels of asymmetrical dimethylarginine (ADMA, endogenous NOS inhibitor), symmetrical dimethylarginine (SDMA, which lacks NOS inhibitory activity), N-mono-methylarginine (MMA, a potent

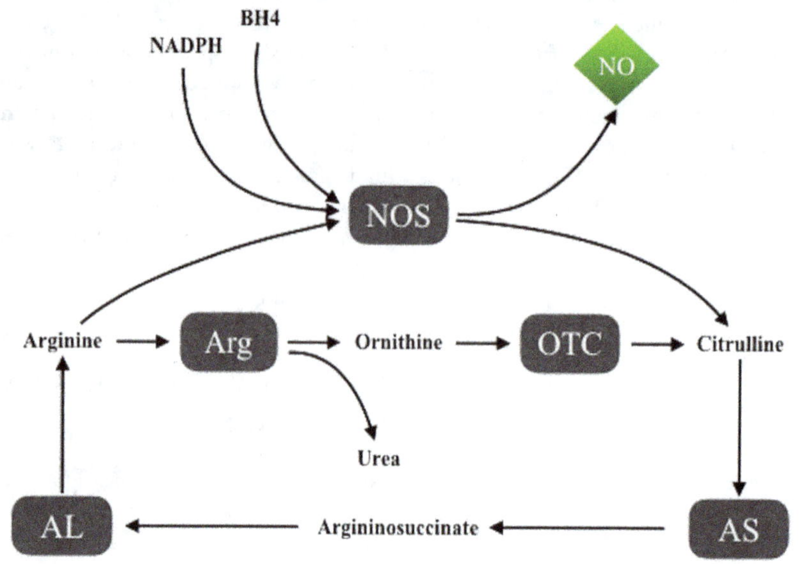

FIGURE 1 | NO synthesis through the NADPH and tetrahydrobiopterin-dependent oxidation of the amino acid L-arginine to L-citrulline by NO synthases. AL, argininosuccinate lyase; Arg, arginase; AS, argininosuccinate synthetase; BH4, tetrahydrobiopterin; NOS, NO synthases; OTC, ornithine transcarbamylase.

NOS inhibitor), methyl-lysine (Methyl-Lys, an unrelated methylated amino acid), arginine, and its major catabolites (citrulline and ornithine).

An augmented prevalence of obstructive CAD was observed in patients with higher levels of SDMA and lower abundance of MMA, whereas ADMA was not correlated. On the other hand, elevated levels of both SDMA and ADMA, as well as an integrated index of arginine methylation [ArgMI(ADMASDMA)/MMA] were shown to be independent predictors of MACE; of note, the latter result was predictive of MACE even after adjustments for global arginine bioavailability (Wang et al., 2009).

The authors suggested that ArgMI and the global arginine bioavailability ratio (GABR, an integrated index of arginine bioavailability), seems to be associated with different aspects of cardiovascular risk. In fact, ArgMI seems to have a superior prognostic utility when evaluated in the setting of secondary prevention, probably because of the association between later stages of atherosclerotic progression and pathways involving protein arginine methylation, proteolysis, and impairment in NO production. On the contrary, the capacity of GABR to enhance prognostic value in primary prevention could be related to a deeper link between the NO precursor arginine bioavailability and plaque initiation and development (Wang et al., 2009).

Various studies showed elevated levels of ADMA in both chronic (Usui et al., 1998) and acute heart failure (Mullens et al., 2003; Dückelmann et al., 2007; Tang et al., 2008). However, the mechanisms underlying this dysregulation in arginine metabolism in human heart failure are generally unknown.

In a study published in 2012 on Journal of American College of Cardiology (Shao et al., 2012), 68 patients affected by advanced decompensated heart failure and 57 subjects with stable chronic heart failure were enrolled. The authors measured ADMA plasma levels and the GABR (arginine/ornithine citrulline) using tandem mass spectrometry.

Results showed higher plasma ADMA levels and lower GABR in advanced decompensated heart failure subjects in comparison with values observed in chronic heart failure patients, and these features were associated with both higher systolic pulmonary artery and central venous pressures.

A relative deficiency of NO could result as a consequence of both reduced substrate (L- arginine) bioavailability and/or impaired production due to inhibition by ADMA and could contribute to disease progression, explaining, at least in part, a more favorable long-term outcome observed in advanced systolic heart failure subjects treated with drugs that release NO (Mullens et al., 2008, 2009).

On the other hand, The authors found increased myocardial levels of dimethylarginine dimethylaminohydrolase-1 in chronic heart failure patients with systolic pulmonary artery pressure (sPAP) >50 mmHg and diminished levels in those with sPAP <50 mmHg. Overall, the data of Shao et al. (2012) seem to suggest that impaired NO synthesis could lead to both an endothelial and myocardial dysfunction thus determining an increased in sPAP.

Trupp et al. (2012) performed a gas chromatography-time-of-flight mass-spectrometry-based metabolomic study to evaluate the effect of simvastatin treatment on intermediary metabolism. The authors enrolled 148 subjects who were profiled at basal time and after 6 weeks of treatment with 40 mg/day simvastatin, then randomly selected 100 patients among the LDL-C lowering treatment responders and 24 each from both the top and bottom 10% of the response distribution, thus identifying the "good" and "poor" responders, respectively. The drug exposure metabolic fingerprint of the whole group of responders included essential amino acids, lauric acid, and alpha-tocopherol. Simvastatin efficacy in lowering LDL correlated with

TABLE 2 | Presented studies on metabolomics and NO pathways.

Reference	Species	Technique	Setting	Biofluid/ Tissue	Discriminate Metabolites/ Metabolism
Wang et al., 2009	Human	HPLC-MS/MS	Coronary heart diseases	Plasma	Elevated levels of SDMA, ADMA and of the ArgMI index (ADMA+SDMA)/MMA)
Shao et al., 2012	Human	LC-MS/MS	Pulmonary Hypertension associated with Heart failure	Plasma	ADMA higher plasma levels and lower global arginine bioavailability ratio in acute vs. chronic heart failure. ↑ myocardial levels of dimethylarginine dimethylaminohydrolase-1 in HF patients with sPAP > 50 mmHg
Trupp et al., 2012	Human	GC-TOF/MS	Dyslipidemia	Plasma	Cystine, urea cycle intermediates, ornithine, citrulline and lysine. xanthine, 2-hydroxyvaleric acid, succinic acid, stearic acid, and fructose
Zhao et al., 2015	Human	UPLC/MS/MS GC-MS	Pulmonary Arterial Hypertension	Lung tissue	Sphingosine-1-phosphate metabolites Heme metabolites Arginine, creatine, ornithine, and urea
Lewis et al., 2016	Human C57Bl/6 mice	LC-MS	Pulmonary Arterial Hypertension	Plasma	Arginine, ornithine, citrulline, ADMA, SDMA. Indoleamine 2,3-dioxygenase (IDO)–dependent tryptophan metabolites, tricarboxylic acid intermediates, and purine metabolites.
Deidda et al., 2017	Human	NMR	Pulmonary Arterial Hypertension in systemic sclerosis	Plasma	Acetate, alanine, lactate, and lipoprotein. γ-aminobutyrate, arginine, betaine, choline, creatine, creatinine, glucose, glutamate, glutamine, glycine, histidine, phenylalanine, and tyrosine
Kirov et al., 2017	Human	GC-MS	Coronary artery diseases (CABG)	Arterial and Coronary sinus plasma	long-chain acylcarnitines, arginine, short-chain acylcarnitines and glycerophospholipids

HPLC-MS/MS, high performance liquid chromatography – tandem mass spectrometry; LC-MS/MS, liquid chromatography – tandem mass spectrometry; GC-TOF/MS, gas chromatography – time of flight mass spectrometry; UPLC-TOF/MS, ultra performance liquid chromatography – tandem mass spectrometry; GC-MS, gas chromatography – mass spectrometry; LC-MS, liquid chromatography – mass spectrometry; NMR, ^{1}H Nuclear magnetic resonance spectroscopy; SDMA, symmetrical dimethylarginine; ADMA, asymmetrical dimethylarginine; MMA, N-mono-methylarginine; ArgMI index, integrated index of arginine methylation; HF, heart failure; sPAP, systolic pulmonary artery pressure.

changes in concentration of cystine, an intermediate in the urea cycle, and the dibasic amino acids ornithine, citrulline and lysine. The latter share plasma membrane transporters with arginine, which is the rate-limiting substrate for NOS. Moreover, an orthogonal partial least square discriminant analysis (OPLS-DA) showed that xanthine, 2-hydroxyvaleric acid, succinic acid, stearic acid, and fructose were the metabolites whose basal pre-therapy levels were able to predict the good or the poor responses to simvastatin treatment (Trupp et al., 2012).

Notably, xanthine is the substrate of xanthine oxidase, whose enzymatic activity, producing H_2O_2, is implicated in ROS generation. Because ROS are able to uncouple NOS activity, a lower degree of xanthine and purine catabolism may lead to more intense NOS signaling. In line with these findings, hyperuricemia, which could result from increased purine degradation, is able to determine impaired NO production by inhibiting arginine transport at the level of NOS associated CAT-1 transporter (Trupp et al., 2012).

Pulmonary arterial hypertension is a vascular disease characterized by persistent pre-capillary pulmonary hypertension (PH), which can lead to premature death, often because of RV. In a study conducted on lung tissue of patients with PAH ($n = 8$) and controls ($n = 8$), Zhao et al. (2015) carried out a high-throughput liquid-and-gas-chromatography-mass spectrometry based metabolomic analysis, showing a genetic profile characterized by increases in both sphingosine-1-phosphate and heme metabolites, and a derangement of arginine/NO pathways, the latter represented by a decrease of arginine and an increase of creatine, ornithine, and urea (intermediates following arginine in the pathway) in PAH lung tissue compared to normal lung. The authors' findings showed that in PAH, expression of the gene Arginase-1 (*ARG1*) was significantly increased whereas that of NOS-1 (*NOS1*) was decreased and this phenomenon may be the result of feedback mechanisms due to disrupted arginine metabolism with excessive intracellular and extracellular NO levels. Furthermore, the latter, reacting with ROS, may lead to peroxynitrite production, thus exacerbating cellular damage (Zhao et al., 2015).

Lewis et al. (2016) conducted a metabolomic study to verify whether it might be possible to identify a metabolic profile of right ventricular-pulmonary vascular (RV-PV) dysfunction.

They enrolled 71 individuals who represented the discovery cohort and who underwent right heart catheterization (RHC) and radionuclide ventriculography at rest and during exercise. Subsequently, their plasma samples were analyzed using a GC-MS-based metabolomic technique. The authors analyzed plasma concentrations of 105 metabolites, validating the results in a second group that underwent invasive hemodynamic evaluations and in an independent cohort with or without PAH.

The authors identified a new association between RV-PV dysfunction and circulating indoleamine 2,3-dioxygenase (IDO)–dependent tryptophan metabolites (TMs), tricarboxylic acid intermediates, and purine metabolites; moreover, they confirmed previously described associations with arginine–NO metabolic pathway constituents. In fact, levels of arginine-NO metabolites (arginine, ornithine, citrulline, asymmetric dimethylarginine, and symmetric dimethylarginine) were related to RV-PV dysfunction indexes. The ratio of arginine to ornithine + citrulline, which previously emerged as an index of arginine bioavailability and a potential biomarker of specific forms of PH, was shown to be inversely related to pulmonary arterial pressure, pulmonary vascular resistance (PVR) and to changes in mean pulmonary arterial pressure relative to change in cardiac output; the latter seems to suggest that this ratio could indicate impaired NO-mediated vasodilation (Lewis et al., 2016).

In 2017, our group performed a metabolomics study on patients affected by systemic sclerosis (SSc) and who were free of pulmonary fibrosis (Deidda et al., 2017). All subjects underwent a RHC, during which a blood sample was collected at the level of the distal peripheral circulation of the pulmonary arteries. On the basis of values of PVR, we divided the population into 2 groups: A (PVR = 1.16 ± 0.23 WU) and B (PVR = 2.67 ± 0.67 WU; $p < 0.001$ vs. Group A). We applied an Orthogonal Signal Correction–PLS–DA to metabolomics data, obtaining clear clustering; SSc patients with PAH showed increases in acetate, alanine, lactate, and lipoprotein levels and decreases in γ-aminobutyrate, arginine, betaine, choline, creatine, creatinine, glucose, glutamate, glutamine, glycine, histidine, phenylalanine, and tyrosine levels.

Of relevance to this paper, and of particular interest, decreased levels of arginine, glutamine and glutamate were found in SSc patients with higher PVR and PAH (Group B).

In fact, arginine depletion has been correlated with pulmonary arterial vasoconstriction (Watts et al., 2012). Moreover, arginine deficiency can result in various important disease states, i.e., NO production preservation and reduction in superoxide anion generation.

On the other hand, glutamine and glutamate modulate NO production and the elastic response of the thoracic aortic wall (Schachter, 2007).

An interesting heart surgery metabolomic study was conducted in the setting of coronary artery bypass surgery, evaluating the differences between the off-pump and on-pump techniques. Twenty consecutive patients undergoing Coronary Artery Bypass Graft surgery (CABG) (10 operated off-pump and 10 on-pump) were enrolled in the study; blood samples obtained from paired arterial and coronary sinus were analyzed using a MS technique. Levels of thirteen metabolites were altered by the surgery; in detail, off-pump patients showed higher levels of long-chain acylcarnitines and lower levels of arginine, whereas those who underwent on-pump intervention had more short-chain acylcarnitines and less glycerophospholipids. Interestingly, the end-of-surgery concentration of plasma arginine, the NO precursor, showed an inverse correlation with amounts of post-operative vasopressor needed in the intensive care unit. In fact, arginine concentrations in off-pump patients were lower and required more vasopressor therapy, contrary to on-pump ones (Kirov et al., 2017).

Previous research (Czerny et al., 2000; Dybdahl et al., 2004; Tomic et al., 2005) has already found higher IL-10 levels at the end of surgery in on-pump patients than in off-pump. Because IL-10 is able to inhibit macrophage NOS2, it is plausible that IL-10 may inhibit iNOS in on-pump CABG, thus determining a reduction in NO production and, consequently, a decrease in arginine catabolism through iNOS. The consequence is higher arginine in plasma and less vascular dilatation requiring less vasopressin from noradrenaline.

Collectively, metabolomics can be used to indirectly investigate NO-pathways through the analysis of metabolites involved in NOS activity or modulation, such as arginine, ornithine, citrulline, glutamine and glutamate, ADMA and SDMA. Furthermore, other indices such as ArgMI and GABR could be useful in this kind of investigations.

CONCLUSION

The reported studies demonstrate the potential ability of metabolomics to investigate ROS and NO pathways and constitute a basis toward future and wider applications.

Metabolomic techniques have the limitation that they are not capable to directly identify ROS and NO; however, other molecules (see **Tables 1, 2**), involved in RN reactions, can be measured and analyzed, thus allowing an indirect investigation of these pathways.

The success of this approach depends on how metabolomic data are integrated and contextualized with clinical and instrumental data, as exemplified in the presented studies. Moreover, the knowledge of biochemical pathways related to identified metabolites and of their biological role, both in physiological and pathological states, is crucial for the correct interpretation of the findings resulting from the application of metabolomics to the investigation of ROS and NO metabolism and signaling.

Finally, the association with the other "omics" sciences can improve the capacity of metabolomics to be effectively applied to this particular setting of investigations.

AUTHOR CONTRIBUTIONS

MD and AN performed the bibliographic research. All authors evaluated retrieved papers and their reference lists to identify additional relevant articles. MD, AN, and PB wrote the manuscript. CC and GM supervised the manuscript.

REFERENCES

Cheng, S., Shah, S. H., Corwin, E. J., Fiehn, O., Fitzgerald, R. K., Gerszten, R. E., et al. (2017). Potential impact and study considerations of metabolomics in cardiovascular health and disease: a scientific statement from the American Heart Association. *Circ. Cardiovasc. Genet.* 10:e000032. doi: 10.1161/HCG.0000000000000032

Chouchani, E. T., Pell, V. R., Gaude, E., Aksentijević, D., Sundier, S. Y., Robb, E. L., et al. (2014). Ischaemic accumulation of succinate controls reperfusion injury through mitochondrial ROS. *Nature* 515, 431–435. doi: 10.1038/nature13909

Czerny, M., Baumer, H., Kilo, J., Lassnigg, A., Hamwi, A., Vukovich, T., et al. (2000). Inflammatory response and myocardial injury following coronary artery bypass grafting with or without cardiopulmonary bypass. *Eur. J. Cardiothorac. Surg.* 17, 737–742. doi: 10.1016/S1010-7940(00)00420-6

Dalen, J. E., Alpert, J. S., Goldberg, R. J., and Weinstein, R. S. (2014). The epidemic of the 20(th) century: coronary heart disease. *Am. J. Med.* 127, 807–812. doi: 10.1016/j.amjmed.2014.04.015

Deidda, M., Piras, C., Bassareo, P. P., Cadeddu Dessalvi, C., and Mercuro, G. (2015a). Metabolomics, a promising approach to translational research in cardiology. *IJC Metab. Endocr.* 9, 31–38. doi: 10.1016/j.ijcme.2015.10.001

Deidda, M., Piras, C., Dessalvi Cadeddu, C., Locci, E., Barberini, L., Torri, F., et al. (2015b). Metabolomic approach to profile functional and metabolic changes in heart failure. *J. Transl. Med.* 13:297. doi: 10.1186/s12967-015-0661-3

Deidda, M., Piras, C., Cadeddu Dessalvi, C., Locci, E., Barberini, L., Orofino, S., et al. (2017). Distinctive metabolomic fingerprint in scleroderma patients with pulmonary arterial hypertension. *Int. J. Cardiol.* 241, 401–406. doi: 10.1016/j.ijcard.2017.04.024

Dhalla, N. S., Temsah, R. M., and Netticadan, T. (2000). Role of oxidative stress in cardiovascular diseases. *J. Hypertens.* 18, 655–673. doi: 10.1097/00004872-200018060-00002

Dückelmann, C., Mittermayer, F., Haider, D. G., Altenberger, J., Eichinger, J., and Wolzt, M. (2007). Asymmetric dimethylarginine enhances cardiovascular risk prediction in patients with chronic heart failure. *Arterioscler. Thromb. Vasc. Biol.* 27, 2037–2042. doi: 10.1161/ATVBAHA.107.147595

Dybdahl, B., Wahba, A., Haaverstad, R., Kirkeby-Garstad, I., Kierulf, P., Espevik, T., et al. (2004). On-pump versus off-pump coronary artery bypass grafting: more heat-shock protein 70 is released after on-pump surgery. *Eur. J. Cardiothorac. Surg.* 25, 985–992. doi: 10.1016/j.ejcts.2004.03.002

Fearon, I. M., and Faux, S. P. (2009). Oxidative stress and cardiovascular disease: novel tools give (free) radical insight. *J. Mol. Cell Cardiol.* 47, 372–381. doi: 10.1016/j.yjmcc.2009.05.013

Galli, F., Varga, Z., Balla, J., Ferraro, B., Canestrari, F., Floridi, A., et al. (2001). Vitamin E, lipid profile, and peroxidation in hemodialysis patients. *Kidney Int.* 78(Suppl. 78), S148–S154. doi: 10.1046/j.1523-1755.2001.07846.x

Griffin, J. L., Atherton, H., Shockcor, J., and Atzori, L. (2011). Metabolomics as a tool for cardiac research. *Nat. Rev. Cardiol.* 8, 630–643. doi: 10.1038/nrcardio.2011.138

Grootveld, M., and Halliwell, B. (1987). Measurement of allantoin and uric acid in human body fluids. A potential index of free-radical reactions *in vivo*? *Biochem. J.* 243, 803–808.

He, F., and Zuo, L. (2015). Redox roles of reactive oxygen species in cardiovascular diseases. *Int. J. Mol. Sci.* 16, 27770–27780. doi: 10.3390/ijms161126059

Herrington, W., Lacey, B., Sherliker, P., Armitage, J., and Lewington, S. (2016). Epidemiology of atherosclerosis and the potential to reduce the global burden of atherothrombotic disease. *Circ. Res.* 118, 535–546. doi: 10.1161/CIRCRESAHA.115.307611

Ishibashi, S., Brown, M. S., Goldstein, J. L., Gerard, R. D., Hammer, R. E., and Herz, J. (1993). Hypercholesterolemia in low density lipoprotein receptor knockout mice and its reversal by adenovirus-mediated gene delivery. *J. Clin. Invest.* 92, 883–893. doi: 10.1172/JCI116663

Ishibashi, S., Goldstein, J. L., Brown, M. S., Herz, J., and Burns, D. K. (1994a). Massive xanthomatosis and atherosclerosis in cholesterol-fed low density lipoprotein receptor-negative mice. *J. Clin. Invest.* 93, 1885–1893.

Ishibashi, S., Herz, J., Maeda, N., Goldstein, J. L., and Brown, M. S. (1994b). The two-receptor model of lipoprotein clearance: tests of the hypothesis in "knockout" mice lacking the low density lipoprotein receptor, apolipoprotein E, or both proteins. *Proc. Natl. Acad. Sci. U.S.A.* 91, 4431–4435.

Kirov, H., Schwarzer, M., Neugebauer, S., Faerber, G., Diab, M., and Doenst, T. (2017). Metabolomic profiling in patients undergoing Off-Pump or On-Pump coronary artery bypass surgery. *BMC Cardiovasc. Disord.* 17:93. doi: 10.1186/s12872-017-0518-1

Klupczyńska, A., Dereziński, P., and Kokot, Z. J. (2015). Metabolomics in medical sciences–trends, challenges and perspectives. *Acta Pol. Pharm.* 72, 629–641. doi: 10.1016/j.jpba.2015.04.021

Kordalewska, M., and Markuszewski, M. J. (2015). Metabolomics in cardiovascular diseases. *J. Pharm. Biomed. Anal.* 113, 121–136. doi: 10.1016/j.jpba.2015.04.021

Lewis, G. D., Ngo, D., Hemnes, A. R., Farrell, L., Domos, C., Pappagianopoulos, P. P., et al. (2016). Metabolic profiling of right ventricular-pulmonary vascular function reveals circulating biomarkers of pulmonary hypertension. *J. Am. Coll. Cardiol.* 67, 174–189. doi: 10.1016/j.jacc.2015.10.072

Li, D., Zhang, L., Dong, F., Liu, Y., Li, N., Li, H., et al. (2015). Metabonomic changes associated with atherosclerosis progression for LDLR(−/−) mice. *J. Proteome Res.* 14, 2237–2254. doi: 10.1021/acs.jproteome.5b00032

Lu, J., Chen, B., Chen, T., Guo, S., Xue, X., Chen, Q., et al. (2017). Comprehensive metabolomics identified lipid peroxidation as a prominent feature in human plasma of patients with coronary heart diseases. *Redox Biol.* 12, 899–907. doi: 10.1016/j.redox.2017.04.032

Lu, S. C. (2009). Regulation of glutathione synthesis. *Mol. Aspects Med.* 30, 42–59. doi: 10.1016/j.mam.2008.05.005

Mercuro, G., Bassareo, P. P., Deidda, M., Cadeddu, C., Barberini, L., and Atzori, L. (2011). Metabolomics: a new era in cardiology? *J. Cardiovasc. Med. (Hagerstown).* 12, 800–805. doi: 10.2459/JCM.0b013e32834a658f

Mizuno, S., Farkas, L., Al Husseini, A., Farkas, D., Gomez-Arroyo, J., Kraskauskas, D., et al. (2012). Severe pulmonary arterial hypertension induced by SU5416 and ovalbumin immunization. *Am. J. Respir. Cell Mol. Biol.* 47, 679–687. doi: 10.1165/rcmb.2012-0077OC

Mozaffarian, D., Benjamin, E. J., Go, A. S., Arnett, D. K., Blaha, M. J., Cushman, M., et al. (2015). Heart disease and stroke statistics–2015 update: a report from the American Heart Association. *Circulation* 131, e29–e322. doi: 10.1161/CIR.0000000000000157

Mullens, W., Abrahams, Z., Francis, G. S., Skouri, H. N., Starling, R. C., Young, J. B., et al. (2008). Sodium nitroprusside for advanced low-output heart failure. *J. Am. Coll. Cardiol.* 52, 200–207. doi: 10.1016/j.jacc.2008.02.083

Mullens, W., Abrahams, Z., Francis, G. S., Sokos, G., Starling, R. C., Young, J. B., et al. (2003). High plasma level of asymmetric dimethylarginine in patients with acutely exacerbated congestive heart failure: role in reduction of plasma nitric oxide level. *Heart Vessels* 18, 177–182. doi: 10.1007/s00380-003-0715-y

Mullens, W., Abrahams, Z., Francis, G. S., Sokos, G., Starling, R. C., Young, J. B., et al. (2009). Usefulness of *Isosorbide Dinitrate* and *Hydralazine* as add-on therapy in patients discharged for advanced decompensated heart failure. *Am. J. Cardiol.* 103, 1113–1119. doi: 10.1016/j.amjcard.2008.12.028

Schachter, D. (2007). L-Glutamine in vitro regulates rat aortic glutamate content and modulates nitric oxide formation and contractility responses. *Am. J. Phys. Cell Phys.* 293, C142–C151. doi: 10.1152/ajpcell.00589.2006

Schieber, M., and Chandel, N. S. (2014). ROS function in redox signaling and oxidative stress. *Curr. Biol.* 24, R453–R462. doi: 10.1016/j.cub.2014.03.034

Shao, Z., Wang, Z., Shrestha, K., Thakur, A., Borowski, A. G., Sweet, W., et al. (2012). Pulmonary hypertension associated with advanced systolic heart failure: dysregulated arginine metabolism and importance of compensatory dimethylarginine dimethylaminohydrolase-1. *J. Am. Coll. Cardiol.* 59, 1150–1158. doi: 10.1016/j.jacc.2011.12.022

Tang, W. H., Tong, W., Shrestha, K., Wang, Z., Levison, B. S., Delfraino, B., et al. (2008). Differential effects of arginine methylation on diastolic dysfunction and disease progression in patients with chronic systolic heart failure. *Eur. Heart J.* 29, 2506–2513. doi: 10.1093/eurheartj/ehn360

Tomic, V., Russwurm, S., Möller, E., Claus, R. A., Blaess, M., Brunkhorst, F., et al. (2005). Transcriptomic and proteomic patterns of systemic inflammation in on-pump and off-pump coronary artery bypass grafting. *Circulation* 112, 2912–2920.

Trupp, M., Zhu, H., Wikoff, W. R., Baillie, R. A., Zeng, Z. B., Karp, P. D., et al. (2012). Metabolomics reveals amino acids contribute to variation in response to simvastatin treatment. *PLoS One* 7:e38386. doi: 10.1371/journal.pone.0038386

Ussher, J. R., Elmariah, S., Gerszten, R. E., and Dyck, J. R. (2016). The emerging role of metabolomics in the diagnosis and prognosis of cardiovascular disease. *J. Am. Coll. Cardiol.* 68, 2850–2870. doi: 10.1016/j.jacc.2016.09.972

Usui, M., Matsuoka, H., Miyazaki, H., Ueda, S., Okuda, S., and Imaizumi, T. (1998). Increased endogenous nitric oxide synthase inhibitor in patients with congestive heart failure. *Life Sci.* 62, 2425–2430. doi: 10.1016/S0024-3205(98)00225-2

van Dyk, M., Mangoni, A. A., McEvoy, M., Attia, J. R., Sorich, M. J., and Rowland, A. (2015). Targeted arginine metabolomics: A rapid, simple UPLC-QToF-MS(E) based approach for assessing the involvement of arginine metabolism in human disease. *Clin. Chim. Acta* 447, 59–65. doi: 10.1016/j.cca.2015.05.014

Varvarousis, D., Xanthos, T., Ferino, G., Noto, A., Iacovidou, N., Mura, M., et al. (2017). Metabolomics profiling reveals different patterns in an animal model of asphyxial and dysrhythmic cardiac arrest. *Sci. Rep.* 7:16575. doi: 10.1038/s41598-017-16857-6

Wang, X., Shults, N. V., and Suzuki, Y. J. (2017). Oxidative profiling of the failing right heart in rats with pulmonary hypertension. *PLoS One* 12:e0176887. doi: 10.1371/journal.pone.0176887

Wang, Z., Tang, W. H., Cho, L., Brennan, D. M., and Hazen, S. L. (2009). Targeted metabolomic evaluation of arginine methylation and cardiovascular risks: potential mechanisms beyond nitric oxide synthase inhibition. *Arterioscler. Thromb. Vasc. Biol.* 29, 1383–1391. doi: 10.1161/ATVBAHA.109.185645

Watts, J. A., Gellar, M. A., Fulkerson, M. B., Das, S. K., and Kline, J. A. (2012). Arginase depletes plasma l-arginine and decreases pulmonary vascular reserve during experimental pulmonary embolism. *Pulm. Pharmacol. Ther.* 25, 48–54. doi: 10.1016/j.pupt.2011.10.005

Zhao, Y. D., Chu, L., Lin, K., Granton, E., Yin, L., Peng, J., et al. (2015). A biochemical approach to understand the pathogenesis of advanced pulmonary arterial hypertension: metabolomic profiles of arginine, Sphingosine-1-Phosphate, and heme of human lung. *PLoS One* 10:e0134958. doi: 10.1371/journal.pone.0134958

21

Impaired Endothelial Function in Hereditary Angioedema During the Symptom-Free Period

Davide Firinu[1†], Pier P. Bassareo[2†], Angela M. Zedda[2], Maria P. Barca[1], Antonio Crisafulli[3], Giuseppe Mercuro[2] and Stefano Del Giacco[1]*

[1] Unit of Internal Medicine, Department of Medical Sciences and Public Health, Allergy and Clinical Immunology, University of Cagliari, Cagliari, Italy, [2] Unit of Cardiology and Angiology, Department of Medical Sciences and Public Health, University of Cagliari, Cagliari, Italy, [3] Sports Physiology Lab., Department of Medical Sciences and Public Health, University of Cagliari, Cagliari, Italy

Edited by:
Pasquale Pagliaro,
Università degli Studi di Torino, Italy

Reviewed by:
Massimo Piepoli,
Guglielmo da Saliceto Hospital, Italy
Fabio Mangiacapra,
Università Campus Bio-Medico, Italy

***Correspondence:**
Pier P. Bassareo
piercard@inwind.it

†These authors have contributed equally to this work.

Introduction: The presence of coronary endothelial dysfunction was previously shown in Hereditary Angioedema (HAE) patients. The aim of our study was to evaluate the effect of HAE on systemic endothelial function and whether there was a relationship among endothelial function, asymmetric dimethylarginine (ADMA) -which is a strong inhibitor of nitric oxide synthesis-, and disease severity scores.

Methods: Twenty-four HAE patients (18 females, aged 47.9 ± 2 years) without factors known to interfere with endothelial function were studied and compared with 24 healthy peers age- and gender-matched. Endothelial function was assessed by means of non-invasive finger plethysmography (reactive hyperaemia index: RHI) and ADMA levels by high-performance liquid chromatography. HAE severity scores have been calculated according to published literature.

Results: In HAE patients RHI was lower (2.03 ± 0.46 vs. 2.82 ± 0.34, $p < 0.0001$) and ADMA higher (0.636 ± 7 vs. 585 ± 5 micromol/L, $p < 0.01$) than in controls. A statistically significant inverse correlation was revealed between RHI and patients' ADMA levels ($r = -0.516$, $p = 0.009$) as well as between RHI and patients' chronological age ($r = -0.49$, $p = 0.015$). A statistically significant correlation between RHI and ADMA was confirmed even when excluding the possible influence of cholesterol ($r = -0.408$, $p = 0.048$). No other significant correlations were found with the examined laboratory and clinical parameters (chronological age, age at disease onset, disease duration, severity scores, and gender).

Conclusion: The dysfunction previously shown in HAE patients at the coronary arteries seems to involve the peripheral vessels as well, without a correlation with disease severity.

Keywords: hereditary angioedema, bradykinin, nitric oxide, asymmetric dimethylarginine, endothelium, atherosclerosis, flow mediated dilation

INTRODUCTION

Hereditary Angioedema (HAE) is a rare disease that is primarily caused by mutations in the *SERPING1* gene. This gene encodes for serine protease C1 inhibitor (C1-INH), with the HAE mutations resulting in quantitative (HAE type I, low C1-INH antigen levels) or functional deficiencies (HAE type II, normal C1-INH antigen levels); additionally, coagulation, fibrinolytic, complement and contact cascades are affected. This eventually leads to the overproduction of inflammatory molecules (Morgan, 2010; Longhurst and Cicardi, 2012; van Geffen et al., 2012), among which bradykinin (BK) plays a pivotal role (Nussberger et al., 1998; Cugno et al., 2003). BK is also involved in a subtype of HAE first recognized by Bork as HAE "type III" (Bork et al., 2000), and now named HAE with normal C1-INH function (Zuraw et al., 2012). A subgroup of patients bears mutations in the *F12* gene, and is defined as FXII-HAE (Firinu et al., 2015).

The main clinical HAE feature due to C1-INH deficiency and FXII-HAE is cutaneous or mucosal swelling, lasting between 1 and 5 days when untreated, and commonly involving the extremities, face, genitals, and gastrointestinal and respiratory tract (Zanichelli et al., 2015). Inflammatory BK may cause vasodilation and increased vascular leakage. The molecule binds to two distinct membrane receptors on endothelial cells: BK-receptor 1, inducible by proinflammatory cytokines, and BK-receptor 2, which is expressed constitutively and enhances vascular leakage (Kaplan et al., 2002).

In a study on coronary function in HAE patients, Demirtürk et al. showed the presence of early endothelial dysfunction, with development of atherosclerotic plaques (Demirtürk et al., 2012). A significant functional consequence of such endothelial damage is a reduction in the vasodilatory response to a range of pharmacological and physiological stimuli, such as reactive hyperemia. While endothelial function was previously assessed using only invasive techniques, non-invasive methods, such as the reactive hyperemia index (RHI), are currently available (Bassareo et al., 2010). Impaired endothelial function is correlated with future occurrence of adverse cardiovascular events and cardiac death (Celermajer et al., 1994).

Asymmetric dimethylarginine (ADMA) is a peptide in blood that is also a strong inhibitor of endothelial nitric oxide synthesis. High blood levels are associated with many pathological conditions related to atherosclerosis, including hypercholesterolemia, smoking, diabetes, hypertension, heart failure, chronic renal failure, erectile dysfunction, preeclampsia, and liver failure (Bassareo et al., 2014).

This study aimed to verify the presence of differences in RHI between HAE patients and healthy counterparts; to compare RHI in the two different subtypes of HAE included in the study; and to investigate the correlations between endothelial function in HAE patients and the laboratory and clinical parameters such as ADMA levels, lipid levels in blood, chronological age, age at disease onset, disease duration, severity scores, and sex.

MATERIALS AND METHODS

Study Subjects

The study included 24 C1-INH-HAE or FXII-HAE patients (18 women, 6 men), with mean age at the time of the study 47.9 ± 2 years, mean age at disease onset 20.0 ± 1 years, and mean disease duration 27.8 ± 2 years, that were followed at the outpatients' clinic of Allergy and Clinical Immunology, University of Cagliari, Italy. Patients were examined during remission state, which were asymptomatic for at least 15 days before sampling.

Exclusion criteria were presence of pathological or environmental conditions, such as diabetes and smoking, that are known to interfere with endothelial functions and administration of drugs that could influence endothelial function, apart from those strongly needed for prophylactic therapy against life-threatening HAE attacks (Celermajer et al., 1992; Vapaatalo and Mervaala, 2001).

The results in the HAE group were compared with those in a control group comprising healthy peers, matched for age and sex.

This study was approved by the ethics committee of the University of Cagliari (*Number NP/2013/3226, protocol 692/2013*) and was conducted in accordance with the Declaration of Helsinki. All participants gave their informed written consent.

Laboratory Tests for HAE Diagnosis

HAE was diagnosed by sequencing the *SERPING1* and *F12* genes (Firinu et al., 2013, 2015; Cicardi et al., 2014). Plasma levels of C1-INH antigen were measured using radial immunodiffusion (NOR Partigen C1-INH, Siemens Healthcare Diagnostics, Marburg, Germany); C4 antigen was measured using nephelometry. A chromogenic assay (Technochrom C1-Inhibitor, Technoclone, Vienna, Austria) was used to measure C1-INH activity. HAE severity scores were calculated according to published literature (Bygum et al., 2011; Gómez-Traseira et al., 2013).

Endothelial Function

Endothelial function was assessed using plethysmography-based probes placed on fingertips of the right hand (Endopath; Itamar Medical Ltd., Cesarea, Israel), a non-invasive, reliable, and reproducible method for quantifying RHI. The Endopath device allows measurement of changes in capillary diameter in the fingertips in response to an increase in shear stress (ischemia induced by occlusion of the brachial artery), which causes nitric oxide-dependent dilatation. The latter is reduced in a number of atherosclerosis-related pathological conditions (Bassareo et al., 2010). The strong reproducibility of this technique was demonstrated in a clinical study involving 19 centers in six European countries (Charakida et al., 2013). The clinical and predictive value of RHI measured at the fingertips is similar to that evaluated at the brachial artery (Zahedi et al., 2008).

This technique was approved by the American Food and Drug Administration as a diagnostic tool for use in the evaluation of endothelial function (Kuvin et al., 2003).

Blood Asymmetric Dimethylarginine Levels

One cm^3 of blood was collected from the antecubital vein using a heparin injector. Blood concentration of ADMA was assessed using high-performance liquid chromatography with highly-sensitive laser fluorescent detection (Bassareo et al., 2012). This laboratory technique allows us to separate and quantify ADMA from deproteinized human plasma using a specific reagent. The same polymeric cation-exchange column was used for all samples (HAE patients and controls). This method proved to be highly sensitive, selective, and reproducible for determining ADMA levels, not only when using a commercial assay, but also when using a home-made kit (Valtonen et al., 2005).

Statistics

Non-parametric Mann Whitney *U*-test for non-continuous variables and chi-square test for continuous variables were performed. Univariate analysis, Pearson correlation coefficients, and regression lines for relationships between the various parameters were used as well. Multivariate analysis was not applied, because of the small sample size. However, partial correlation analysis was applied, in order to separate the possible influence of a variable on another one, when these two are deeply correlated, such as ADMA and age. The minimum level of statistical significance was set at $p < 0.05$ (software SPSS version 22.0, SPSS Inc., Chicago, Illinois, USA).

RESULTS

The characteristics of HAE patients and controls are summarized in **Tables 1, 2.** Statistically significant differences were detected for RHI (2.03 ± 0.46 vs. 2.82 ± 0.34, $p <$ 0.0001) and ADMA (0.636 ± 7 vs. 585 ± 5 μmol/L, $p < 0.01$; see **Figures 1A,B**). When comparing RHI and ADMA in C1-INH-HAE and FXII-HAE subgroups, no statistically significant differences were found (2.02 ± 0.52 vs. 2.03 ± 0.38 and 0.640 ± 8 vs. 0.632 ± 6 μmol/L, both $p =$ ns).

A statistically significant correlation was found between RHI and ADMA ($r = -0.516$, $p =$ 0.009), as well as between RHI and chronological age ($r = -0.49$, $p = 0.015$). A statistically significant correlation was confirmed even when excluding the possible influence of cholesterol level on the relationship between RHI and ADMA ($r = -0.408$, $p = 0.048$). No significant correlations were detected between RHI and sex, severity scores, age at disease onset, and disease duration (all $p =$ ns).

TABLE 1 | Main clinical, laboratory data, and reactive hyperemia index results of patients affected by HAE studied with ENDOPAT.

Patient id	RHI	AI (%)	HR	Severity score*	Gender	Age	Age at onset	Disease duration	C4	C1-INH Ag	C1-INH Fn%
C1-INH-HAE 01	1,67	6	79	6	F	67	15	52	8	7,2	40
C1-INH-HAE 02	1,48	40	78	8	F	69	12	57	1	4,8	20
C1-INH-HAE 03	2,52	34	63	8	M	47	10	37	3	8	9
C1-INH-HAE 04	3,04	7	69	7	F	41	15	26	1	4,8	N.D.
C1-INH-HAE 05	2,47	2	68	7	F	54	10	44	3	7	33
C1-INH-HAE 06	2,41	−8	61	6	M	30	14	16	2	6	N.D.
C1-INH-HAE 07	2,56	5	64	4	F	31	19	12	N.D.	N.D.	N.D.
C1-INH-HAE 08	2,29	−9	82	4	F	29	18	11	N.D.	N.D.	N.D.
C1-INH-HAE 09	1,35	−4	71	0	M	40	N.A.	N.A.	5	6,5	N.D.
C1-INH-HAE 10	1,8	−16	97	0	M	44	N.A.	N.A.	6	8	N.D.
C1-INH-HAE 11	1,55	33	84	4	F	82	30	52	7	5,6	N.D.
C1-INH-HAE 12	1,74	32	66	6	M	47	11	36	5	6,4	15
C1-INH-HAE 13	1,49	18	86	7	F	52	12	40	2	5,6	22
C1-INH-HAE 14	1,97	33	70	6	F	48	15	33	1	7	27
Patient id	**RHI**	**AI (%)**	**HR**	**HAE-FXII score[§]**	**Gender**	**Age**	**Age at onset**	**Disease duration**	**C4**	**C1-INH Ag**	**C1-INH Fn%**
FXII-HAE 01	1,93	15	71	Asymptom	M	62	N.A.	N.A.	N.D.	N.D.	N.D.
FXII-HAE 02	1,6	−5	67	Severe	F	32	19	13	20	26,2	75
FXII-HAE 03	1,99	5	63	Moderate	F	38	14	24	19	22,2	N.D.
FXII-HAE 04	2,6	6	56	Moderate	F	31	23	8	14	17,4	85
FXII-HAE 05	1,93	−11	82	Mild	F	10	9	1	13	24	80
FXII-HAE 06	1,84	8	93	Severe	F	54	20	34	N.D.	N.D.	N.D.
FXII-HAE 07	2,1	9	60	Severe	F	43	33	10	13	28,1	80
FXII-HAE 08	2,01	29	64	Severe	F	58	21	37	16	26,8	N.D.
FXII-HAE 09	1,57	45	72	Mild	F	76	76	0	N.D.	N.D.	N.D.
FXII-HAE 10	2,77	70	69	Mild	F	66	24	42	N.D.	N.D.	N.D.

RHI, reactive hyperemia index; AI%, augmentation index; HR, heart rate.

**C1-INH-HAE score and [§]HAE-FXII severity score calculated according to reference 17 and 18.Normal ranges as follows:C1-INH Antigen (Ag) 21–39 mg/dl; C1-INH Function (Fn) 70–130%; Serum C4 antigen 10–40 mg/dl. N.D., Not determined for this study; N.A., Not applicable.*

TABLE 2 | Characteristics of patients, cardiovascular risk factors and specific HAE treatments of subjects enrolled in the study.

Patient id	HAE type	Attenuated androgens intake	HAE prophylaxis	HAE on demand treatment	Current or previous treatment for dyslipidemia	Hypertension, heart failure, diabetes, metabolic syndrome, kidney disease
C1-INH-HAE 01	C1-INH type I	No	None	Plasma derived C1-INH	No	No
C1-INH-HAE 02	C1-INH type I	No	Plasma derived C1-INH	Plasma derived C1-INH or icatibant	No	No
C1-INH-HAE 03	C1-INH type I	No	None	Plasma derived C1-INH	No	No
C1-INH-HAE 04	C1-INH type I	No	None	Plasma derived C1-INH or icatibant	No	No
C1-INH-HAE 05	C1-INH type I	No	None	Plasma derived C1-INH	No	No
C1-INH-HAE 06	C1-INH type I	No	None	Plasma derived C1-INH	No	No
C1-INH-HAE 07	C1-INH type I	No	None	Plasma derived C1-INH	No	No
C1-INH-HAE 08	C1-INH type I	No	None	Plasma derived C1-INH	No	No
C1-INH-HAE 09	C1-INH type I	No	None	Plasma derived C1-INH	No	No
C1-INH-HAE 10	C1-INH type I	No	None	Plasma derived C1-INH	No	No
C1-INH-HAE 11	C1-INH type I	No	None	Plasma derived C1-INH	No	No
C1-INH-HAE 12	C1-INH type I	No	None	Plasma derived C1-INH or icatibant	No	No
C1-INH-HAE 13	C1-INH type I	No	Plasma derived C1-INH	Plasma derived C1-INH	No	No
C1-INH-HAE 14	C1-INH type I	No	Plasma derived C1-INH	Plasma derived C1-INH or icatibant	No	No
FXII-HAE 01	FXII-HAE	No	None	Plasma derived C1-INH	No	No
FXII-HAE 02	FXII-HAE	No	Plasma derived C1-INH	Plasma derived C1-INH or icatibant	No	No
FXII-HAE 03	FXII-HAE	No	Plasma derived C1-INH	Plasma derived C1-INH or icatibant	No	No
FXII-HAE 04	FXII-HAE	No	None	Icatibant	No	No
FXII-HAE 05	FXII-HAE	No	None	Plasma derived C1-INH	No	No
FXII-HAE 06	FXII-HAE	No	None	Plasma derived C1-INH	No	No
FXII-HAE 07	FXII-HAE	No	None	Icatibant	No	No
FXII-HAE 08	FXII-HAE	No	None	Plasma derived C1-INH	No	No
FXII-HAE 09	FXII-HAE	No	None	Plasma derived C1-INH	No	No
FXII-HAE 10	FXII-HAE	No	None	Plasma derived C1-INH	No	No

DISCUSSION

Our findings revealed a significant decrease in endothelial function in HAE patients during the symptom-free period, when compared to a group of healthy peers. Furthermore, a strong correlation between RHI and ADMA was observed. While the pathological role in cardiovascular disease is somewhat unclear, ADMA is known to induce endothelial dysfunction, the earliest stage of atherosclerosis (Baum et al., 2016; Mangiacapra et al., 2016).

Our study was not designed to unravel the mechanisms behind the decrease in RHI and increase in ADMA, or their relationship. However, regarding a possible pathophysiological explanation, it might be hypothesized that both C1-INH-HAE and FXII-HAE subgroups had a shared endothelial dysfunction that was probably not caused by C1-INH deficiency or mutated coagulation FXII *per se*, but instead by bradykinin receptor-ADMA pathway activation. Although this metabolic pathway has not been adequately studied, ADMA levels increased after incubation with BK in a cellular model of human alveolar adenocarcinoma, while co-incubation with bradykinin B1 receptor inhibitor did not lead to a decrease in ADMA. This suggests that BK-dependent ADMA production may occur through bradykinin B2 receptor stimulation (Gamboa et al., 2015). Furthermore, previous studies showed that BK increases reactive oxygen species production through stimulation of NADPH oxidases; this in turn increases ADMA levels by increasing protein methylation while inhibiting ADMA degradation (Larsen et al., 2009; Luo et al., 2010). Another possible explanation for increased ADMA levels is the fact that BK may decrease dimethylarginine dimethylaminohydrolase activity, which is responsible for ADMA degradation (Gamboa et al., 2015). Again, C1-INH-HAE is able to dysregulate the activities of complement, coagulation, and contact systems (Kaplan and Joseph, 2014), and increased procoagulant and fibrinolytic activities were observed in HAE patients during

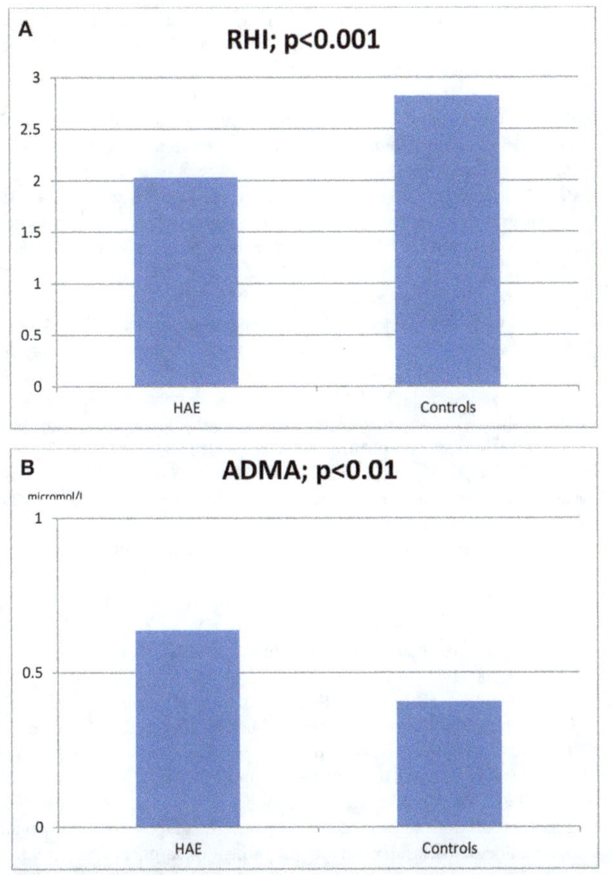

FIGURE 1 | Reactive hyperemia index (RHI, **A**) and asymmetric dimethylarginine blood levels (ADMA, **B**) in HAE patients and healthy controls.

attacks and remission phases (van Geffen et al., 2012; Reshef et al., 2015). The apparent thrombotic risk in patients with C1-INH-HAE, although not confirmed with clinical observations (Reshef et al., 2015), needs to be discussed in further studies, because of the endothelial dysfunction demonstrated in this work.

As none of the studied patients was taking attenuated androgens, our findings were not influenced by these drugs, which are known to impair lipid levels, thus leading to accelerated atherosclerosis (Széplaki et al., 2005). On the other hand, it was previously reported that in HAE subjects, most of the endothelial functions are normal in the inter-attack periods, as shown by normal blood levels of some markers of endothelial cell permeability (endothelin-1, von Willebrand factor) (Czúcz et al., 2012). However, increased endothelial nitric oxide synthase levels in attack-free periods were detected in C1-INH-HAE patients as well (Demirtürk et al., 2014; Costa et al., 2016).

More rapid development of coronary atherosclerosis in HAE patients was previously shown by altered coronary flow reserve measurement in the left anterior coronary artery. The latter is a non-invasive method useful for assessing coronary function, with results closely corresponding to invasive measurements (Caiati et al., 1999; Lethen et al., 2003). In a cohort of patients affected by C1-INH-HAE (most under long term prophylaxis with danazol), the coronary flow reserve was found to be decreased, even when the intima-media thickness in the carotid arteries was normal (Demirtürk et al., 2012). According to our findings, the early atherosclerosis detected with RHI was not related to disease severity scores or the duration of therapy (Demirtürk et al., 2012). Reduced coronary flow reserve is a sign of increased atherosclerosis, while reduced RHI is an early sign of atherosclerosis in peripheral vessels. The latter seems to occur more rapidly in HAE patients, in comparison with their healthy peers.

The present study has some limitations such as the small sample size. However, HAE is a rare disease, and groups of maximum 30 subjects were typically recruited in previous studies with similar design (Demirtürk et al., 2012; van Geffen et al., 2012; Wu et al., 2017). In addition, having studied HAE subjects only during inter-attack periods may have led to incomplete assessment of endothelial characteristics. Moreover, other factors potentially influencing endothelial response to ischemic stimuli, such as those that are usually administered for HAE attacks (plasma-derived C1-INH or icatibant), should be considered (Birjmohun et al., 2008). However, from an ethical point of view, it was obviously impossible to discontinue life-saving drugs in our patients.

In conclusion, this was the first study to report that the atherosclerotic process previously observed in coronary arteries also involves the peripheral vessels in HAE patients. Nitric oxide production impairment, through the still poorly-understood bradykinin receptor-ADMA pathway activation, was hypothesized to be involved (Rastaldo et al., 2007; Kim and Massett, 2016; Wang et al., 2016). This may indicate a much more extensive hardening of the arteries, involving the entire arterial tree. In practice, even though the main cause of death in HAE patients has been laryngeal involvement with subsequent asphyxia (25–30% of the patients in the first decades of life when untreated), the efficacy of the administered drugs has resulted in a decrease in mortality (0.35–0.5% in medically treated patients) (Varga and Farkas, 2008). In this respect, since atherosclerosis is a complex process that involves several mechanisms and is the leading cause of heart attacks, stroke, and peripheral vascular disease, regular cardiovascular follow-up is required in HAE patients (Penna et al., 2006; Yang et al., 2017).

AUTHOR CONTRIBUTIONS

DF and PB: interpretation of the data and manuscript writing. AZ and MB: aquisition of the data. AC, GM and SD: final approval of the manuscript to be published.

ACKNOWLEDGMENTS

The authors would thank the patients and their relatives who participated to this study and the Italian Association of HAE patients.

REFERENCES

Bassareo, P. P., Fanos, V., Puddu, M., Demuru, P., Cadeddu, F., Balzarini, M., et al. (2010). Reduced brachial flow-mediated vasodilation in young adult ex extremely low birth weight preterm: a condition predictive of increased cardiovascular risk? *J. Matern. Fetal Neonatal Med.* 23(Suppl. 3), 121–124. doi: 10.3109/14767058.2010.506811

Bassareo, P. P., Fanos, V., Puddu, M., Flore, G., and Mercuro, G. (2014). Advanced intrauterine growth restriction is associated with reduced excretion of asymmetric dimethylarginine. *Early Hum. Dev.* 90, 173–176. doi: 10.1016/j.earlhumdev.2014.01.010

Bassareo, P. P., Puddu, M., Flore, G., Deidda, M., Manconi, E., Melis, A., et al. (2012). Could ADMA levels in young adults born preterm predict an early endothelial dysfunction? *Int. J. Cardiol.* 159, 217–219. doi: 10.1016/j.ijcard.2011.02.069

Baum, C., Johannsen, S. S., Zeller, T., Atzler, D., Ojeda, F. M., Wild, P. S., et al. (2016). ADMA and arginine derivatives in relation to non-invasive vascular function in the general population. *Atherosclerosis* 244, 149–156. doi: 10.1016/j.atherosclerosis.2015.10.101

Birjmohun, R. S., Kees Hovingh, G., Stroes, E. S., Hofstra, J. J., Dallinga-Thie, G. M., Meijers, J. C., et al. (2008). Effects of short-term and long-term danazol treatment on lipoproteins, coagulation, and progression of atherosclerosis: two clinical trials in healthy volunteers and patients with hereditary angioedema. *Clin. Ther.* 30, 2314–2323. doi: 10.1016/j.clinthera.2008.12.021

Bork, K., Barnstedt, S. E., Koch, P., and Traupe, H. (2000). Hereditary angioedema with normal C1-inhibitor activity in women. *Lancet* 356, 213–217. doi: 10.1016/S0140-6736(00)02483-1

Bygum, A., Fagerberg, C. R., Ponard, D., Monnier, N., Lunardi, J., and Drouet, C. (2011). Mutational spectrum and phenotypes in Danish families with hereditary angioedema because of C1 inhibitor deficiency. *Allergy* 66, 76–84. doi: 10.1111/j.1398-9995.2010.02456.x

Caiati, C., Montaldo, C., Zedda, N., Bina, A., and Iliceto, S. (1999). New noninvasive method for coronary flow reserve assessment: contrast-enhanced transthoracic second harmonic echo Doppler. *Circulation* 99, 771–778. doi: 10.1161/01.CIR.99.6.771

Celermajer, D. S., Sorensen, K. E., Bull, C., Robinson, J., and Deanfield, J. E. (1994). Endothelium-dependent dilation in the systemic arteries of asymptomatic subjects relates to coronary risk factors and their interaction. *J. Am. Coll. Cardiol.* 24, 1468–1474. doi: 10.1016/0735-1097(94)90141-4

Celermajer, D. S., Sorensen, K. E., Gooch, V. M., Spiegelhalter, D. J., Miller, O. I., Sullivan, I. D., et al. (1992). Non-invasive detection of endothelial dysfunction in children and adults at risk of atherosclerosis. *Lancet* 340, 1111–1115. doi: 10.1016/0140-6736(92)93147-F

Charakida, M., de Groot, E., Loukogeorgakis, S. P., Khan, T., LUscher, T., Kastelein, J. J., et al. (2013). Variability and reproducibility of flow-mediated dilatation in a multicentre clinical study. *Eur Heart J.* 34, 3501–3507. doi: 10.1093/eurheartj/eht223

Cicardi, M., Aberer, W., Banerji, A., Bas, M., Bernstein, J. A., Bork, K., et al. (2014). Classification, diagnosis, and approach to treatment for angioedema: consensus report from the Hereditary Angioedema International Working Group. *Allergy* 69, 602–616. doi: 10.1111/all.12380

Costa, E. D., Rezende, B. A., Cortes, S. F., and Lemos, V. S. (2016). Neuronal nitric oxide synthase in vascular physiology and diseases. *Front. Physiol.* 7:206. doi: 10.3389/fphys.2016.00206

Cugno, M., Nussberger, J., Cicardi, M., and Agostoni, A. (2003). Bradykinin and the pathophysiology of angioedema. *Int. Immunopharmacol.* 3, 311–317. doi: 10.1016/S1567-5769(02)00162-5

Czúcz, J., Schaffer, G., Csuka, D., Walentin, S., Kunde, J., Prohaszka, Z., et al. (2012). Endothelial cell function in patients with hereditary angioedema: elevated soluble E-selectin level during inter-attack periods. *J. Clin. Immunol.* 32, 61–69. doi: 10.1007/s10875-011-9606-7

Demirtürk, M., Gelincik, A., Cinar, S., Kilercik, M., Onay-Ucar, E., Colakoglu, B., et al. (2014). Increased eNOS levels in hereditary angioedema. *Int. Immunopharmacol.* 20, 264–268. doi: 10.1016/j.intimp.2014.03.007

Demirtürk, M., Polat, N., Guz, G., Gurdal, A., Altun, I., Gelincik, A., et al. (2012). There is an increased risk of atherosclerosis in hereditary angioedema. *Int. Immunopharmacol.* 12, 212–216. doi: 10.1016/j.intimp.2011.11.013

Firinu, D., Bafunno, V., Vecchione, G., Barca, M. P., Manconi, P. E., Santacroce, R., et al. (2015). Characterization of patients with angioedema without wheals: the importance of F12 gene screening. *Clin. Immunol.* 157, 239–248. doi: 10.1016/j.clim.2015.02.013

Firinu, D., Colomba, P., Manconi, P. E., Barca, M. P., Fenu, L., Piseddu, G., et al. (2013). Identification of a novel and recurrent mutation in the SERPING1 gene in patients with hereditary angioedema. *Clin. Immunol.* 147, 129–132. doi: 10.1016/j.clim.2013.03.007

Gamboa, J. L., Pretorius, M., Sprinkel, K. C., Brown, N. J., and Ikizler, T. A. (2015). Angiotensin converting enzyme inhibition increases ADMA concentration in patients on maintenance hemodialysis–a randomized cross-over study. *BMC Nephrol.* 16:167. doi: 10.1186/s12882-015-0162-x

Gómez-Traseira, C., Lopez-Lera, A., Drouet, C., Lopez-Trascasa, M., Perez-Fernandez, E., Favier, B., et al. (2013). Hereditary angioedema caused by the p.Thr309Lys mutation in the F12 gene: a multifactorial disease. *J. Allergy Clin. Immunol.* 132, 986–989.e1. doi: 10.1016/j.jaci.2013.04.032

Kaplan, A. P., and Joseph, K. (2014). Pathogenic mechanisms of bradykinin mediated diseases: dysregulation of an innate inflammatory pathway. *Adv. Immunol.* 121, 41–89. doi: 10.1016/B978-0-12-800100-4.00002-7

Kaplan, A. P., Joseph, K., and Silverberg, M. (2002). Pathways for bradykinin formation and inflammatory disease. *J. Allergy Clin. Immunol.* 109, 195–209. doi: 10.1067/mai.2002.121316

Kim, S. K., and Massett, M. P. (2016). Genetic regulation of endothelial vasomotor function. *Front. Physiol.* 7:571. doi: 10.3389/fphys.2016.00571

Kuvin, J. T., Patel, A. R., Sliney, K. A., Pandian, N. G., Sheffy, J., Schnall, R. P., et al. (2003). Assessment of peripheral vascular endothelial function with finger arterial pulse wave amplitude. *Am. Heart J.* 146, 168–174. doi: 10.1016/S0002-8703(03)00094-2

Larsen, B. T., Bubolz, A. H., Mendoza, S. A., Pritchard, K. A. Jr., and Gutterman, D. D. (2009). Bradykinin-induced dilation of human coronary arterioles requires NADPH oxidase-derived reactive oxygen species. *Arterioscler Thromb Vasc Biol.* 29, 739–745. doi: 10.1161/ATVBAHA.108.169367

Lethen, H., Tries, H. P., Brechtken, J., Kersting, S., and Lambertz, H. (2003). Comparison of transthoracic Doppler echocardiography to intracoronary Doppler guidewire measurements for assessment of coronary flow reserve in the left anterior descending artery for detection of restenosis after coronary angioplasty. *Am. J. Cardiol.* 91, 412–417. doi: 10.1016/S0002-9149(02)03235-6

Longhurst, H., and Cicardi, M. (2012). Hereditary angio-oedema. *Lancet* 379, 474–481. doi: 10.1016/S0140-6736(11)60935-5

Luo, Z., Teerlink, T., Griendling, K., Aslam, S., Welch, W. J., and Wilcox, C. S. (2010). Angiotensin II. and NADPH oxidase increase ADMA in vascular smooth muscle cells. *Hypertension* 56, 498–504. doi: 10.1161/HYPERTENSIONAHA.110.152959

Mangiacapra, F., Conte, M., Demartini, C., Muller, O., Delrue, L., Dierickx, K., et al. (2016). Relationship of asymmetric dimethylarginine (ADMA) with extent and functional severity of coronary atherosclerosis. *Atherosclerosis* 220, 629–633. doi: 10.1016/j.ijcard.2016.06.254

Morgan, B. P. (2010). Hereditary angioedema–therapies old and new. *N. Engl. J. Med.* 363, 581–583. doi: 10.1056/NEJMe1006450

Nussberger, J., Cugno, M., Amstutz, C., Cicardi, M., Pellacani, A., and Agostoni, A. (1998). Plasma bradykinin in angio-oedema. *Lancet* 351, 1693–1697. doi: 10.1016/S0140-6736(97)09137-X

Penna, C., Rastaldo, R., Mancardi, D., Cappello, S., Pagliaro, P., Westerhof, N., et al. (2006). Effect of endothelins on the cardiovascular system. *J. Cardiovasc. Med.* 7, 645–652. doi: 10.2459/01.JCM.0000242996.19077.ba

Rastaldo, R., Pagliaro, P., Cappello, S., Penna, C., Mancardi, D., Westerhof, N., et al. (2007). Nitric oxide and cardiac function. *Life Sci.* 81, 779–793. doi: 10.1016/j.lfs.2007.07.019

Reshef, A., Zanichelli, A., Longhurst, H., Relan, A., and Hack, C. E. (2015). Elevated D-dimers in attacks of hereditary angioedema are not associated with increased thrombotic risk. *Allergy* 70, 506–513. doi: 10.1111/all.12587

Széplaki, G., Varga, L., Valentin, S., Kleiber, M., Karadi, I., Romics, L., et al. (2005). Adverse effects of danazol prophylaxis on the lipid profiles of patients with hereditary angioedema. *J. Allergy Clin. Immunol.* 115, 864–869. doi: 10.1016/j.jaci.2004.12.1130

Valtonen, P., Karppi, J., NyyssOnen, K., Valkonen, V. P., Halonen, T., and Punnonen, K. (2005). Comparison of HPLC method and commercial ELISA assay for asymmetric dimethylarginine (ADMA) determination in human serum. *J. Chromatogr. B Analyt. Technol. Biomed. Life Sci.* 828, 97–102. doi: 10.1016/j.jchromb.2005.09.023

van Geffen, M., Cugno, M., Lap, P., Loof, A., Cicardi, M., and van Heerde, W. (2012). Alterations of coagulation and fibrinolysis in patients with angioedema due to C1-inhibitor deficiency. *Clin. Exp. Immunol.* 167, 472–478. doi: 10.1111/j.1365-2249.2011.04541.x

Vapaatalo, H., and Mervaala, E. (2001). Clinically important factors influencing endothelial function. *Med. Sci. Monit.* 7, 1075–1085.

Varga, L., and Farkas, H. (2008). Treatment of type I and II hereditary angioedema with Rhucin, a recombinant human C1 inhibitor. *Expert Rev. Clin. Immunol.* 4, 653–651. doi: 10.1586/1744666X.4.6.653

Wang, H., Jiang, H., Liu, H., Zhang, X., Ran, G., He, H., et al. (2016). Modeling disease progression: angiotensin II indirectly inhibits nitric oxide production via ADMA accumulation in spontaneously Hipertensive Rats. *Front. Physiol.* 7:555. doi: 10.3389/fphys.2016.00555

Wu, M. A., Casella, F., Perego, F., Suffritti, C., Afifi Afifi, N., Tobaldini, E., et al. (2017). Hereditary angioedema: assessing the hypothesis for underlying autonomic dysfunction. *PLoS ONE* 12:e0187110. doi: 10.1371/journal.pone.0187110

Yang, X., Li, Y., Li, Y., Ren, X., Zhang, X., Hu, D., et al. (2017). Oxidative stress-mediated atherosclerosis: mechanisms and therapies. *Front. Physiol.* 8:600. doi: 10.3389/fphys.2017.00600

Zahedi, E., Jaafar, R., Ali, M. A., Mohamed, A. L., and Maskon, O. (2008). Finger photoplethysmogram pulse amplitude changes induced by flow-mediated dilation. *Physiol. Meas.* 29, 625–637. doi: 10.1088/0967-3334/29/5/008

Zanichelli, A., Arcoleo, F., Barca, M. P., Borrelli, P., Bova, M., Cancian, M., et al. (2015). A nationwide survey of hereditary angioedema due to C1 inhibitor deficiency in Italy. *Orphanet J. Rare Dis.* 10:11. doi: 10.1186/s13023-015-0233-x

Zuraw, B. L., Bork, K., Binkley, K. E., Banerji, A., Christiansen, S. C., Castaldo, A., et al. (2012). Hereditary angioedema with normal C1 inhibitor function: consensus of an international expert panel. *Allergy Asthma Proc.* 33(Suppl. 1), S145–S156. doi: 10.2500/aap.2012.33.3627

22

Hypoxia Tolerance in Teleosts: Implications of Cardiac Nitrosative Signals

Alfonsina Gattuso[†*], *Filippo Garofalo*[†], *Maria C. Cerra*[*] *and Sandra Imbrogno*

Department of Biology, Ecology and Earth Sciences, University of Calabria, Rende, Italy

Edited by:
Mariarosaria Santillo, University of Naples Federico II, Italy

Reviewed by:
Philip Aaronson, King's College London, United Kingdom
Giovanna Zoccoli, Università degli Studi di Bologna, Italy

***Correspondence:**
Alfonsina Gattuso
alfonsina.gattuso@unical.it
Maria C. Cerra
maria_carmela.cerra@unical.it

[†]*These authors have contributed equally to this work.*

Changes in environmental oxygen (O_2) are naturally occurring phenomena which ectotherms have to face on. Many species exhibit a striking capacity to survive and remain active for long periods under hypoxia, even tolerating anoxia. Some fundamental adaptations contribute to this capacity: metabolic suppression, tolerance of pH and ionic unbalance, avoidance and/or repair of free-radical-induced cell injury during reoxygenation. A remarkable feature of these species is their ability to preserve a normal cardiovascular performance during hypoxia/anoxia to match peripheral (tissue pO_2) requirements. In this review, we will refer to paradigms of hypoxia- and anoxia-tolerant teleost fish to illustrate cardiac physiological strategies that, by involving nitric oxide and its metabolites, play a critical role in the adaptive responses to O_2 limitation. The information here reported may contribute to clarify the molecular and cellular mechanisms underlying heart vulnerability vs. resistance in relation to O_2 availability.

Keywords: heart, hypoxia, nitric oxide, nitrite, teleosts

INTRODUCTION

Molecular oxygen (O_2) is essential for life. A limited O_2 supply leads to tissue hypoxia which often results in organ damage.

When compared to terrestrial animals, water-breathing organisms are more likely to be exposed to wider temporal and spatial variations of O_2 supply. This is largely due to the inherent properties of the water and to the rapid fluctuations in the pattern of O_2 production and consumption (Nikinmaa et al., 2011). Several animal species are adapted to tolerate regular and often severe hypoxia. This is the case of various fish, frog, and turtle species that tolerate anoxia, and some snakes and insects that can endure severe hypoxia (Hermes-Lima and Zenteno-Savín, 2002). Teleost fish exhibit a very large spectrum of O_2 sensitivity, moving from species showing an extraordinary ability to tolerate hypoxia and anoxia to species that dramatically suffer O_2 deprivation. Among teleost fish, examples of hypoxia/anoxia resistance are the members of the cyprinid genus Carassius, such as the goldfish (*Carassius auratus*), and the crucian carp (*Carassius carassius*), which exhibit a striking capacity to survive and remain active for long periods under low O_2, even tolerating anoxia (Bickler and Buck, 2007). This capacity is correlated with the ability to generate ethanol as anaerobic end-product, which is acid–base neutral, in contrast with the normal glycolytic end-product lactic acid. Among cyprinids, the zebrafish (*Danio rerio*) is characterized by a growth-dependent transition from hypoxia tolerance to sensitivity (Padilla and Roth, 2001). Its genome is fully sequenced and this is of benefit for studying the components of hypoxia-resistance pathways in fish.

Despite the different abilities of vertebrates to tolerate a limited O_2 availability in the environment or in internal tissues, many studies in mammalian and non-mammalian models (see Fago and Jensen, 2015, for references) suggest a common set of concerted physiological responses. They basically include depression of O_2 consumption rates, protection against oxidative damage, and, at least in air-breathing species, redistribution of blood flow into the circulation. All these responses require the activation of a complex network of intracellular cascades, such as those related to nitric oxide (NO) and its metabolites, nitrite and nitrate, that represent common signaling molecules able to control and coordinate the molecular circuits that sustain adaptive hypoxia-dependent physiological responses (Fago and Jensen, 2015).

The heart is a major target of hypoxia. As largely documented in mammals, O_2 deprivation is accompanied by changes in cardiac muscle metabolism, reactivation of fetal gene programs and hypertrophy responses, modifications of the extracellular matrix composition, mitochondrial biogenesis and arrangement, as well as of the expression of intracellular effectors [i.e., the NO pathway, hypoxamiRs, Hypoxia Inducible Factor (HIF), etc.] (Fago and Jensen, 2015). A large number of studies on mammals have recognized the critical role of NO and its metabolites, in particular nitrite and S-nitrosothiols (SNO; formed when Cys thiols react with NO^+), in the mechanisms which control the cardiac response to low O_2 availability. This role has been recently extended to non-mammalian vertebrates, including fish, in which a growing body of evidence has documented the cardioprotective role of NO and its related nitrosative signals, under hypoxic challenges.

In this review we will illustrate the cardiac role of the nitric oxide synthase (NOS)/NO/nitrite system with emphasis to hypoxia-activated cardio-protective effects of nitrite, a major source of NO under low O_2. We will mainly provide information on the cardiac nitrosative signaling of teleost species characterized by a high ability to tolerate hypoxia/anoxia. This feature makes them valuable models to whom deserve a renewed attention to explore the mechanisms that contribute to survive low O_2, also in a translational perspective for human cardioprotection. For the reader who is unfamiliar with the adaptive physiology of fish, we will outline their phenotypic plasticity in relation to anoxia and hypoxia, and to the different mechanisms that allow O_2 detection. In the subsequent adaptive response, the heart, as a major effector, is modulated to properly sustain organism requirements.

ENVIRONMENTAL STRESS RESPONSE IN VERTEBRATES

Many vertebrate species are able to face a wide range of environmental changes in abiotic parameters that include O_2 availability, temperature, pH, and salinity. A common universal strategy characterizes the homeostatic response to different environmental stresses. This strategy requires important modifications from molecular to organismal level. An example is the response to hypoxia/anoxia that, as in case of the thermal stress, is characterized by a decrement in bioenergetic demand/production whose consequences are energy conservation, osmotic balance, and substrate economy (Boutilier, 2001 and references therein). The universal nature of the stress response is confirmed by genomic and post-genomic studies showing that the phenotypic flexibility of many species in response to hypoxia (as well as to hypothermia) involves the same pattern of genes that influence ATP and protein turnover, energy conservation, and stress factors release (Hochachka and Somero, 2002).

Two physiological adaptations confer the ability to cope with environmental stresses: "capacity adaptations" (i.e., the condition in which organisms preserve normal levels of both activity and homeostasis, enabling them "to grow and reproduce under the harsh conditions") and "resistance adaptations" (i.e., the condition in which organisms enhance their resistance even losing homeostasis, enabling them "to avoid or survive the stress until conditions become favorable again") (Cossins and Bowler, 1987). The reaction to stressors varies between individual members of a given species and represents a combination of factors, i.e., the appraisal of the environmental change and the ability to cope (Broom and Johnson, 1993; Koolhaas et al., 1999). As stated by Wilson et al. (1994), phenotypes within one species have a differential fitness and this differentiation represents adaptive individual differences in resource use and response to risk.

The different responses to stress can be clustered in two different phenotypes within the same species: proactive and reactive (Wilson et al., 1994). Proactive animals are characterized by high sympathetic and locomotor activity, while reactive individuals show low mobility and sympathetic activity (Van Raaij et al., 1996). Proactive individuals are usually audacious and more aggressive with respect to their reactive counterparts; these different activity levels between the two phenotypes have been observed both in wild (Montiglio et al., 2010) and laboratory environments (Tran and Gerlai, 2013). As observed in the teleost rainbow trout (*Oncorhynchus mykiss*) exposed to hypoxia, the proactive phenotype corresponds to an escaping and "non-surviving fish," showing a strong avoidance behavior with a consequent high energy expenditure and instantaneous beginning of anaerobic metabolism. In contrast, the reactive fish remains quiet and survives thanks to the delaying activation of anaerobic mechanisms (Schjolden et al., 2005 and references therein).

Another trait of the adaptive response to low O_2 is its relationship with animal development and growth. In general, it can be assumed that adults are less hypoxia-tolerant than neonatal and embryonic vertebrates (Crowder et al., 1998). If exposure to hypoxia occurs during juvenile or adult life, the effect is reversible. In contrast, if the stress takes place during the development, its influence persists throughout the life (Padilla and Roth, 2001).

ANOXIA AND HYPOXIA TOLERANCE OF THE FISH HEART

Fish, as well as amphibians and reptiles, are characterized by an impressive ability to survive long period of partial and/or complete O_2 deprivation. Three major adaptations allow these animals to face anoxia: deep metabolic depression, tolerance of acidosis and osmotic stress, prevention and/or restoration of cell damage induced by the huge radical production during re-oxygenation (see for review Driedzic and Gesser, 1994; Bickler and Buck, 2007). Moreover, long-term survival to anoxic stress requires massive accumulations of glycogen in critical tissues, and an extreme metabolic depression in specific body districts, and this allows the extension of anoxia tolerance to the whole organism (Hochachka, 1986).

Fish show a very high variety of phenotypes characterized by different abilities to cope with O_2 fluctuations. At the basis of this plasticity is the expression of specific genes. Many investigations have recently attempted to identify these genes, and this resulted in the development of a database of Fish Hypoxia Responsive Genes (HRGFish) which currently covers 818 gene sequences and 35 genes (including HIF, myoglobin, and glucose transporters) from 38 fishes (Rashid et al., 2017).

The formidable adaptations shown by teleost fish to face low and very low O_2 availability is typically related to the anaerobic capacity of the animal. This is exemplified by an early study by Mathur (1967) on the Indian cyprinid *Rasbora daniconius* showing that, if placed in a hermetically sealed glass jar, this teleost survives for more than 100 days. This resistance to protracted anoxia is supported by a notable anaerobic potential and the ability to escape from acidosis caused by the anaerobic waste-product increase (e.g., lactate).

Because of their very high resistance to minimum rates of water O_2 saturation and a wide range of temperatures (from <4°C up to >38°C), Cyprinids, such as the common carp *Cyprinus carpio*, and its related specie, the crucian carp *C. carassius*, are largely recognized as major experimental models in which analyze morpho-functional adaptation to environmental or laboratory hypoxia. In these species, a significant metabolic down-regulation (down to 30%), which allows glycogen storing, is fundamental to surviving anoxia (Nilsson, 2001; Lutz and Nilsson, 2004).

Information on these fascinating models of hypoxia/anoxia resistance mainly comes from studies aimed to explore the mechanisms of defense of their hearts. Remarkable cardiac interspecific differences have emerged. In fact, while in the common carp, a critical decrease in heart function occurs during 24 h of severe hypoxia, the crucian carp conserves normal cardiac activity and autonomic cardiovascular control up to 5 days of anoxia at 8°C (Stecyk et al., 2004). This preserved cardiovascular function allows the crucian carp to effectively perfuse with blood both gills and liver. The appropriate perfusion mobilizes huge amount of glucose from the large hepatic glycogen store to all tissues, allowing, at the same time, lactate transport to the muscle where it is converted to ethanol (Nilsson, 2001). This, being less harmful than lactate, prevents acidosis. Additionally, the easily diffusible ethanol is quickly removed by the branchial epithelium thanks to the very effective blood perfusion. Accordingly, a preserved heart performance is the basis for improving anoxia resistance of the whole piscine organism thanks to the improved metabolic and functional cooperation among single organs (**Figure 1**). In this context, also the cooperation between different cardiac regions contributes to the response to low O_2. In the cardiac ventricle of the bluefin tuna (*Thunnus thynnus*), the subendocardial trabeculae (*spongiosa*), essentially perfused by venous blood, are capable to metabolize lactate more than the compact subepicardial myocardium, which is completely perfused by oxygenated blood through the coronary vessels coming from the gills (**Figure 2**); this allows the *spongiosa* to face a reduced O_2 availability (reviewed in Tota et al., 2011).

The role of fuel substrates, in relation to the response to low O_2 availability, has been also analyzed. Studies on the isolated and perfused eel heart show that glucose supply is essential for maintaining the cardiac performance during acute anoxic stress (see references in Imbrogno, 2013). In *Anguilla rostrata*, characterized by a marked anoxic endurance, if oxidative phosphorylation is blocked by perfusion with NaCN, endogenous glycogen stores are consumed regardless of the presence or absence of glucose in the medium (Bailey et al., 2000). Of note, down-regulation of oxidative phosphorylation is critical for heart endurance under protracted anoxia. As shown in the *Carassius* species, a strong metabolic depression is essential for the conservation of glycogen stores allowing fish to resist very long period of anoxia (Bickler and Buck, 2007; Vornanen and Haverinen, 2016).

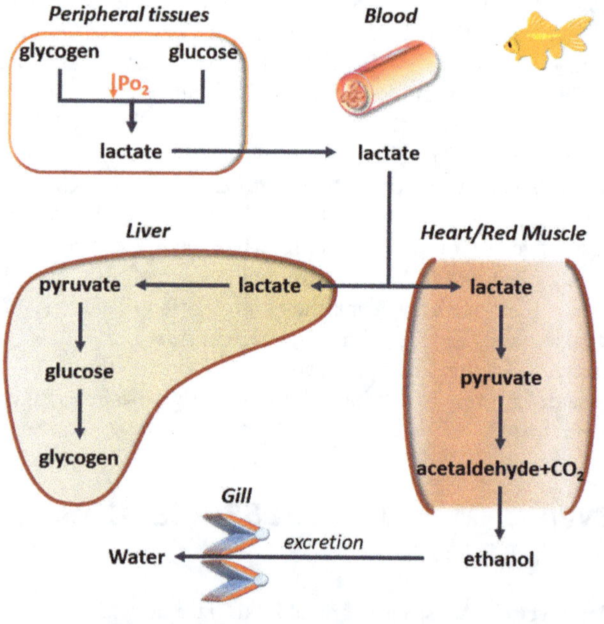

FIGURE 1 | A simplified scheme illustrating the metabolic cooperation among different tissues in hypoxia-tolerant Cyprinid in the presence of low O_2. Under these conditions, the muscle is able to activate the conversion of lactate (also produced by other organs) to ethanol. This is excreted by the gills, thus preventing lactate accumulation.

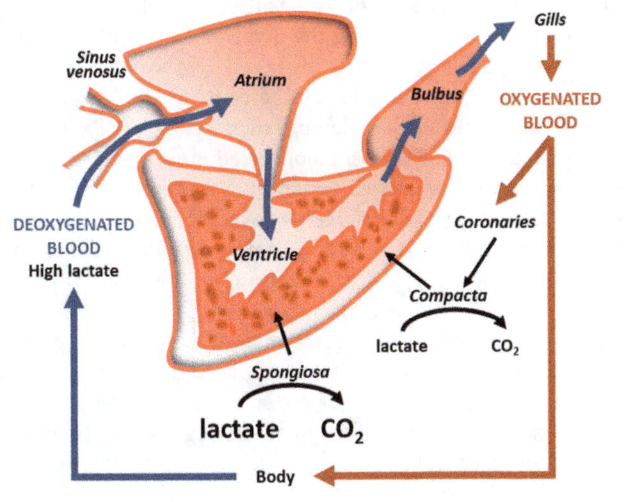

FIGURE 2 | Intracardiac cooperation in a coronarized teleost heart (e.g., tuna). With respect to the compact layer, supplied with coronary oxygenated blood, the spongy layer, supplied by venous blood, has a greater capability to oxidize lactate to CO_2 (modified from Tota et al., 2011 with permission).

During anoxia exposure, anoxia tolerant hearts show an *in vivo* cardiac ATP demand lower than their cardiac maximum glycolytic potential (i.e., the maximum ATP production solely from glycolysis) (Farrell and Stecyk, 2007). Two strategies, for achieving this have been proposed: a naturally low routine cardiac ATP demand that can be sustained by anaerobic glycolysis (as in the case of crucian carp, *C. carassius*), or a considerably down-regulation of cardiac ATP demand to a level that can be sustained by glycolytic ATP production (e.g., in *C. carpio*). In the case of the *C. carpio*, hypoxic bradycardia may represent a strategy to protect the heart since it allows the depression of cardiac power output and thus ATP requirement, reducing the need of oxygen for several hours (Farrell, 2007). In the case of *C. carassius*, during anoxia, anaerobic ATP production is sufficient to power the heart to pump, thus it is not necessary to activate bradycardia (Stecyk et al., 2004).

OXYGEN-SENSING AND HYPOXIA/ANOXIA RESPONSES

Detection of environmental, hematic, or tissue O_2 is a crucial task of the homeostatic response of vertebrates to hypoxia/anoxia. Complex and integrated systems and effectors are present in the different classes, phyla, and species, and even within the same species. A critical step is the activation of sensors which detect O_2 during the initial, acute phase of hypoxia. As a consequence, catecholamines are secreted and the cardiovascular activity is modulated so that vascular tissue perfusion is adjusted to balance O_2 supply and demand (Buckler, 2007; Milsom and Burleson, 2007). If the hypoxia persists, these mechanisms activate long-term responses that require the regulation of gene expression [i.e., the hypoxia inducible factor (HIF) transcription factor family] and this sustains and potentiates the initial response.

Detection of environmental and blood hypoxia relies on the activation of extremely specialized chemoreceptors. They are characterized by a very high sensitivity to small changes in PO_2 in either the external environment, or the internal micro environment, depending on their position. They are strategically located in regions exposed to O_2 fluctuations, as in the case of the neuroepithelial cells (NECs) of the gills, the neuroepithelial bodies of the airways, and the carotid bodies in the vasculature.

In fish, regardless their phyletic position, a major role in O_2-sensing is attributed to branchial NECs whose location and orientation is not uniform across species. They can be distributed either across the gill arches, or outside the gills in the oro-branchial cavity (see Milsom, 2012 for references; Gilmour and Perry, 2007; Milsom and Burleson, 2007). In addition, NECs may be oriented externally or internally or both, and this provides the animals with a selective ability to detect PO_2 variations in water, and blood, or in both environments (reviewed by Milsom, 2012). It is generally assumed that hypoxia-tolerant species responds primarily to arterial hypoxaemia, while less tolerant fish respond more immediately to aquatic hypoxia (Sundin et al., 2000).

Externally-oriented chemoreceptors represent a primitive O_2 sensing mechanism that disappeared early in vertebrate evolution, since they are absent in the obligate air-breathing South American lungfish, *Lepidosiren paradoxa* (Sanchez et al., 2001). In this fish, only blood hypoxia, but not water hypoxia, induces a rapid ventilator response, suggesting a prevalent role of internal rather than of branchial receptors.

Branchial NECs are differently sensitive to low PO_2 and this correlates with the degree of hypoxia tolerance/intolerance of the various species. For example, in the hypoxia tolerant goldfish, isolated NECs do not respond to low PO_2 until severe hypoxic or even anoxic levels. An increased ventilation is observed only if goldfish are exposed at water PO_2 that are lower (25 mmHg: Tzaneva et al., 2011) than those (110 mmHg) eliciting the ventilatory response in the hypoxia sensitive zebrafish (Vulesevic et al., 2006). This may be advantageous during prolonged environmental anoxia to avoid continuous stimulation of stimulation of chemoreceptors without the possibility of increasing O_2 uptake.

An interesting aspect of fish O_2-sensitivity is the relationship with development. As observed in zebrafish, animals may change from hypoxia/anoxia tolerance to hypoxia sensitivity during growth. The zebrafish embryo is initially anoxia-tolerant but becomes hypoxia-sensitive between 2 and 3 days post-fertilization (dpf), when it begins to show hyperventilation under hypoxia (Padilla and Roth, 2001; Mendelsohn et al., 2008). This suggests that the chemoreflex induced by hypoxia appears before gill NECs are fully functional, and is presumably mediated by extrabranchial chemoreceptors (Jonz et al., 2015).

THREE HYPOTHESES FOR OXYGEN-SENSING AND DOWNSTREAM RESPONSES

Studies in mammals have proposed three hypotheses for O_2 sensing: a "membrane hypothesis," a "mitochondrial/metabolic hypothesis," and a more recent recent "gasotransmitter hypothesis" (reviewed by Prabhakar and Peers, 2014; Dzal et al., 2015; López-Barneo et al., 2016). Once activated, all these mechanisms converge on K^+ currents of chemoreceptors cells with consequent neurotransmitter release and activation of the physiological modulation of ventilation and perfusion to maintain homeostasis.

Membrane Hypothesis

In mammals, chemoreceptor-dependent O_2 sensing relies on the modulation of plasmalemmal K^+ channels. Different types of K^+ channels are involved, including background K^+ (K_B) channels (Buckler, 1999), large conductance Ca^{2+}-activated K^+ currents (K_{Ca}) (Peers, 1990; Wyatt and Peers, 1995), TASK-like background K^+ channels (Buckler, 2007), and kv3 and kv4 channels (Sanchez et al., 2002; Pérez-García et al., 2004). Modulation of these channels regulates membrane permeability and cell excitability, according to a common scheme for chemotransduction. Inhibition of the resting K^+ current allows membrane depolarization, opening of voltage-dependent Ca^{2+} channels, neurotransmitter secretion and excitation of afferent neurons to cardio-respiratory centers (Nurse, 2005).

Available data suggest that also in fish, hypoxic chemotransduction involves O_2-sensitive K^+ currents, as supported by evidence in gill NECs of zebrafish (Jonz et al., 2004; Qin et al., 2010) and channel catfish (*Ictalurus punctatus*) (Burleson et al., 2006). While in zebrafish, the cell current appears to be mediated by background K^+ (K_B) channels (Jonz et al., 2004; Qin et al., 2010), similar to TASK-like background K^+ channels of the mammalian carotid body (Buckler, 2007), in catfish the hypoxic response seems to be mediated by O_2-sensitive voltage-dependent outward K^+ (K_v) current (Burleson et al., 2006).

Variations in membrane Ca^{2+} fluxes and intracellular Ca^{2+} concentrations, with consequent stimulation of neurotransmitter release, are presumably also involved in fish O_2 chemoreception (Jonz, 2014). However, while in both zebrafish and catfish, gill NECs express a small number of Ca^{2+}-activated K^+ channels (K_{Ca}) (Jonz et al., 2004; Burleson et al., 2006; Qin et al., 2010), the goldfish gill NECs express predominantly K_{Ca} channels, with a minor contribution of K_B and Kv (Zachar and Jonz, 2012) and L-type Ca^{2+} channels (Zachar et al., 2017). These data suggest a species-specific expression of ion channels that, modulated as a consequence of PO_2 changes, participate to O_2 sensing.

Mitochondrial/Metabolic Hypothesis

Under hypoxia, the mitochondrial ATP generation is reduced and this affects many intracellular effectors, and thus a large spectrum of cell functions. Two major cellular events are proposed downstream the hypoxia-dependent ATP decrease. One is the inhibition of K^+ TASK-like background channels. This may result in membrane depolarization and initiation of the electric activity and of voltage-dependent Ca^{2+} entry (Varas et al., 2007). The second is the increased cytosolic AMP/ATP ratio followed by the activation of AMP-activated protein kinase (AMPK). This, by inhibiting O_2 sensitive K^+ channels (K_B and K_{Ca}) leads to chemoreceptors depolarization (Evans et al., 2005, 2009; Wyatt and Evans, 2007; Wyatt et al., 2007). In fish, no data are available concerning the involvement of mitochondria in O_2 sensing. Only few data suggest a role for AMPK in the downstream response to anoxia of tolerant species. As observed in heart and brain of the tolerant crucian carp, AMPK induces metabolic depression and ethanol secretion only under anoxia, but not under hypoxia (Stensløkken et al., 2008), consistent with a quiescent kinase until complete anoxia is achieved (Pamenter, 2014). This may be an advantage for hypoxia-tolerant species since may allow to increase the depth and/or duration of hypoxia they can tolerate before the activation of AMPK-mediated metabolic adjustments becomes a necessity. In this way, protein synthesis, and other AMPK downregulated anabolic pathways, continue to function under hypoxia along with the ability to preferentially shunt blood flow to at-risk organs (e.g., brain and heart) (Pamenter, 2014).

Gasotransmitters Hypothesis

NO, Carbon Monoxide (CO), and Hydrogen sulfide (H_2S), are mediators of O_2 sensing in chemoreceptors. As shown in the mammalian carotid body, under normoxia, NO and CO are inhibitory, while H_2S is excitatory. Regardless the type of response, their effects occur via ion channels modulation: NO causes glomus cell hyperpolarization by inhibiting Ca^{2+} channels and activating K^+ channels; CO also activates these latter channels, preventing cell depolarization, while H_2S inhibit them (for review see Prabhakar and Peers, 2014). Under hypoxia, both NO and CO production decrease, as their enzymatic activity requires molecular O_2, leading to a reduced inhibition of L-type Ca^{2+} channels and to the closure of K^+ channels. In contrast, H_2S generation increases under hypoxia. This condition is associated with the inhibition of maxiK and TASK-like channels (see Prabhakar and Peers, 2014). All the above effects result in membrane potential depolarization, neurotransmitter release, and afferent neurons activation.

In fish, few data suggest a role for NO and CO in O_2 chemoreception and in the control of breathing, while more robust information indicates that H_2S is directly involved in O_2 sensing and in the hypoxic response (Olson et al., 2008).

A NO-dependent O_2-sensing mechanism has been proposed based on the identification of nNOS in neuroepithelial cells of adult and larvae of the zebrafish (Porteus et al., 2015). According to Perry and Tzaneva (2016), like in mammalian glomus cells (Summers et al., 1999), NO may inhibit ion channels involved in neurosecretion. This is supported by the NO-dependent regulation of intracellular Ca^{2+} observed in the melanophore of the Indian snakehead *Channa punctatus* (Biswas et al., 2011) and in the growth hormone release of goldfish (Chang et al., 2014). Apart from its putative involvement in O_2 chemoreception, in teleosts, as well as in mammals, NO may play a role in the hypoxia-elicited response via a modulation of the ventilatory performance. This is supported by evidence in zebrafish that NO produced by nNOS expressed in branchial NECs, modulates the response to hypoxic stimuli by inhibiting and stimulating ventilation in adult and larvae, respectively (Porteus et al., 2015). As hereafter discussed, NO and its metabolites play a crucial role in the responses to O_2 limitation, representing signaling molecules able to control and coordinate the molecular circuits that sustain adaptive hypoxia-dependent physiological responses.

In fish, as in mammals, O_2 sensing involves the HO-dependent generation of CO. As observed in the goldfish, HO-1 (the hypoxia inducible isoform) is present in branchial NECs and its inhibitory effect on ventilation in goldfish acclimated to 7°C may reflect the HO-1-mediated production of CO within NECs (Tzaneva and Perry, 2014). The involvement of CO in the control of the ventilatory response has been also proposed by data in zebrafish, in which HO-1 expression in both larvae (skin NECs) and adult (gill NECs), is indicative of an endogenous CO production (Tzaneva and Perry, 2016). Once produced in branchial peripheral chemoreceptors, CO may affect the piscine ventilatory response via a modulation of intracellular Ca^{2+} and neurotransmitter release (Tzaneva and Perry, 2014), as in mammalian glomus cells (Overholt and Prabhakar, 1997; Prabhakar, 1999). This view is supported by the presence of both L-type Ca^{2+} and K_{Ca} channels in gill NECs of the goldfish which respond to hypoxia by increasing intracellular Ca^{2+} and synaptic vesicle activity (Zachar et al., 2017).

Several evidence in mammals indicate that H_2S acts as an O_2 sensor (Olson, 2011) and a mediator of hypoxic signaling (Peng et al., 2010). H_2S generation, by constitutive cystathionine γ-lyase (CSE), cystathionine β-synthase (CBS), and 3-mercaptopyruvate sulfurtransferase (3-MST)/cysteine aminotransferase (CAT) (Kimura, 2011), is linked to O_2 availability. In fact, it is present at low levels under normoxia, because of its oxidation by the mitochondrial electron transport chain enzymes, but increases under hypoxia, when the activity of the mitochondrial electron transport chain is reduced (Olson, 2011). In the carotid body, the mechanism involves a reduced activity of HO-2 which in turn increases CSE activity and thus H_2S production; however, the role of CSE and H_2S in the hypoxia sensing is not universally accepted. Recently, Wang et al. (2017) reported that in glomus cells from $CSE^{-/-}$ mice, hypoxia-dependent effects on TASK-like channels, intracellular calcium, and ventilation were not modified. Even if the study does not provide a role for CSE in acute hypoxia sensing, this cannot be excluded (Wang et al., 2017), also considering that CSE inhibition affects the hypoxia response in chronic pathological states (Yuan et al., 2016).

H_2S plays a role in O_2 sensing also in fish. The first evidence was obtained in rainbow trout and zebrafish where, under hypoxia, the gas initiates the cardiorespiratory response by promoting membrane depolarization of chemoreceptive NECs (Olson et al., 2008; Porteus et al., 2014). This is also supported by the identification of CBS and CSE in the gills of rainbow trout and zebrafish whose inhibition, or gene knockdown (in zebrafish larvae), abolishes or attenuates the hyperventilatory response to hypoxia (Porteus et al., 2014). In addition, under normoxia, Na_2S (H_2S donor) induces membrane depolarization of trout branchial NECs (Olson et al., 2008), and increases intracellular Ca^{2+} in zebrafish (Porteus et al., 2014). Also for this gasotransmitter, the mechanism appears similar to that described in mammals.

CARDIAC NITROSATIVE SIGNALS

Generation of NO and its Metabolites

In almost all animal tissues, NO is generated by the family of NOS isoenzymes [i.e., the constitutive endothelial (eNOS) and neuronal (nNOS), and the inducible (iNOS), isoforms], which convert L-arginine into L-citrulline and NO, in the presence of O_2 and NADPH as essential cofactors. This reaction, because of the obligatory requirement for molecular O_2, is vulnerable to hypoxia (Moncada and Higgs, 1993; Bryan, 2006; Lundberg et al., 2008).

NOS enzymes are the products of different genes, and show different localization, regulation, catalytic properties and inhibitor sensitivity (Pautz et al., 2010; Imbrogno et al., 2011). The constitutive NOSs produce, in the steady-state, nanomolar concentrations of NO. In contrast iNOS, if induced by immunologic and inflammatory stimuli, generates micromolar cytotoxic amounts of the gas (Vallance et al., 2000).

NO exerts its physiological effects by reversible binding and/or reacting with hemes, thiols or amines, forming iron-nitrosyl (FeNO), S-nitroso (SNO) and N-nitroso (NNO) compounds (Hill et al., 2010). NO has a very short half-life. It is rapidly metabolized to nitrite in reaction with O_2 (Lundberg et al., 2008), and is inactivated by oxidation to nitrate in reaction with oxygenated hemoglobin (Hb) and myoglobin (Mb). NO can also react with O_2, yielding peroxynitrite ($ONOO^-$) (Ronson et al., 1999), and this depletes the bioactivity of the gas (Guzik et al., 2002). $ONOO^-$ itself is not only a signaling molecule, but also a highly reactive species (Pacher et al., 2007), being able to form additional types of reactive nitrogen species, including nitrogen dioxide (NO_2) and dinitrogen trioxide (N_2O_3). All reactive nitrogen species are responsible for protein post-translational modifications because of either ability to induce either S-nitrosation [the formation of a covalent bond between an NO^+ equivalent and a nucleophilic center (amine or thiol)], or S-nitrosylation [the addition of NO without changing the formal charge of the substrate (metal center or radical species)] (Heinrich et al., 2013). Often, S-nitrosation and S-nitrosylation are used interchangeably to refer to the same substrate modification, i.e., the process leading to S-nitrosothiols (SNO) formation within proteins (for specific chemical terminology, see Heinrich et al., 2013). Likely, an uncontrolled nitrosation/nitrosylation of cysteine residues may induce nitrosative stress, with important effects on proteins activity, stability, conformation and/or ability to interact with other molecules (Foster et al., 2009).

In the presence of a reduced O_2 availability, when the conversion of L-arginine in L-citrulline and NO is compromised, nitrite can be reduced back to NO, providing an alternative pathway for gas generation (Gladwin et al., 2005; Lundberg et al., 2009; van Faassen et al., 2009). This NO regeneration occurs through acidic disproportionation (Zweier et al., 1999) and enzymatic reduction via xanthine oxidoreductase (Millar et al., 1998), mitochondrial enzymes (Kozlov et al., 1999; Castello et al., 2006), or deoxygenated Hb (Cosby et al., 2003; Nagababu et al., 2003), Mb (Shiva et al., 2007a) and neuroglobin (Petersen et al., 2008). Under anoxia, also eNOS is capable of reducing nitrite to NO (Gautier et al., 2006). Thus, in the presence of low O_2, NO production is gradually taken over by nitrite reduction, nitrite functioning as a pool of NO availability (Lundberg et al., 2008; van Faassen et al., 2009; Angelone et al., 2012).

Also nitrate contributes to NO homeostasis since it can be slowly reduced to nitrite by the ubiquitous enzyme xanthine oxidoreductase (Jansson et al., 2008). The nitrate-nitrite-NO pathway may be considered complementary to the classical L-arginine-NOS pathway. All these pathways partly work in parallel, but when O_2 availability is reduced and NOS activity is decreased, nitrite reduction to NO becomes more pronounced. Thus, according to the general concept of the NO cycle in mammals, first proposed by Reutov (Reutov, 2002), NO_2^- and NO_3^- ions are formed as a result of non-enzymatic/enzymatic NO oxidation: L-Arg => NO =>NO_2^-/NO_3^-; the reduction of NO_2^- ions to NO: NO_2^- + e- => NO takes place through the nitrite reductase reaction (reviewed in Tota et al., 2010). The NOS and nitrite-reductase component of the NO cycle are schematically reported in **Figure 3**.

The Cardiac NO Signaling in the Response to Hypoxia

Mammals

In mammals, the cardiac physiological role of NO in relation to O_2 availability is well established. A hypoxia-dependent increase of NO helps mammalian myocardial cells to limit cardiac injury caused by low O_2 supply. For example NO, by down-regulating O_2 consumption rate, both competitively and uncompetitively inhibits O_2 binding to mitochondrial cytochrome c oxidase (Mason et al., 2006; Erusalimsky and Moncada, 2007; Cooper et al., 2008). NO inhibition of cellular respiration mainly occurs at low O_2 tensions; thus, particularly under hypoxia, NO may protect cellular functions by extending O_2 availability (Hagen et al., 2003; Misfeldt et al., 2009). In oxygenated heart muscle from guinea pig, NO has been found to increase metabolic efficiency, determined by the coupling between myocardial O_2 consumption and cardiac performance and the coupling between myocardial O_2 consumption and ATP synthesis (Shen et al., 2001).

Of note, in the presence of ischemia, the NO-dependent suppression of the electron-transport chain, by reducing mitochondrial energy production, limits the cardiac damages induced by ischemia/reperfusion (IR) (Shiva et al., 2007b).

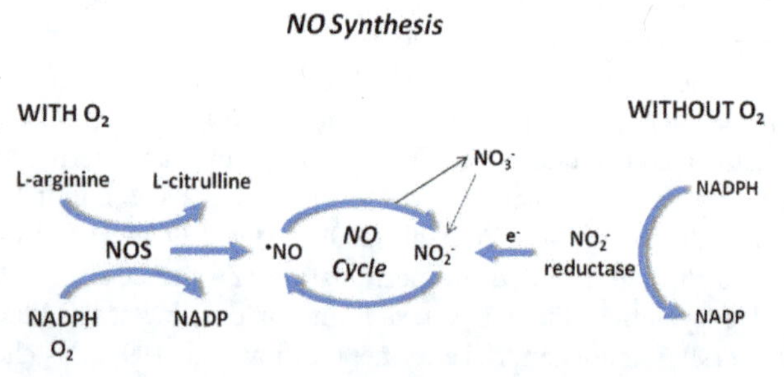

FIGURE 3 | NO synthesis in the presence **(Left)** and absence **(Right)** of O_2. Note NOS and nitrite reductase components involved in the NO formation.

Fish

In fish, the role of NO as a major organizer of complex cardiac transduction signals has been widely assessed, and to date many data are available about its wide cardiac repertoire of actions (see for example Garofalo et al., 2009a, 2012; Imbrogno et al., 2010, 2013, 2017, 2018; Filice et al., 2017; Imbrogno and Cerra, 2017). Very recent studies extended the large variety of NO functions in fish to the mechanisms which allow to maintain the cardiovascular status and control the response to low O_2. It is well established in fish that, if NOS activity is compromised by limited O_2, an increased NOS expression or, alternatively, a nitrite reduction to NO, stabilize NO levels, and this contributes to protect the hypoxic myocardium (Hansen and Jensen, 2010; Sandvik et al., 2012; Imbrogno et al., 2014). A similar NOS enhanced expression can be also observed in the vasculature of the trout in response to hypoxia (McNeill and Perry, 2006).

Experimental evidences indicating the NO involvement in cardiac homeostasis of teleosts fish under hypoxic/anoxic conditions mainly derive from studies on the goldfish *C. auratus*, a champion of hypoxia tolerance. In the goldfish heart, NO inhibits mitochondrial respiration without affecting contractility (Pedersen et al., 2010). This increases myocardial efficiency (i.e., the force generated per O_2 consumed), thus importantly contributing to maintain fish myocardial function in the presence of hypoxia or anoxia (Stecyk et al., 2004). In line with these observations, Imbrogno et al. (2014) showed that, during acute hypoxia, the goldfish heart enhances its basal performance, as well as the sensitivity to heterometric (i.e., Frank-Starling) regulation. This has been considered an important mechanism for maintaining functional and metabolic interactions between organs and tissues, required for the hypoxia tolerance of the organism. Interestingly, in the goldfish, exposure to hypoxia is accompanied by an increased myocardial NOS expression, pointing to NO generation as a crucial step for adjusting the cardiac function of the goldfish during hypoxic challenges (Imbrogno et al., 2014).

It has been also reported that the hypoxia-induced increase in NO production in goldfish heart could activate sarcolemmal K_{ATP} channels, a response that may enhance tolerance of hypoxia in this species (Cameron et al., 2003). This mechanism represents a point of convergence with the mammalian preconditioning protection of ischemic myocardium in which the opening of ATP-sensitive K^+ channels is a crucial event (Noma, 1983).

Of note, in the hypoxic goldfish heart, the increased NOS expression is accompanied by an enhanced expression of HIF-1α. Such hypoxia-dependent cross-talk between NOS and HIF-1α represents an evolutionary conserved trait of the vertebrate response to low O_2. In fact, in the mammalian heart, under hypoxic stress (i.e., during ischemia), HIF-1α activates a number of critical genes (Hochachka and Lutz, 2001; Liu and Simon, 2004; Semenza, 2007), including NOS (Jugdutt, 2002), and this contributes to cell survival. At the same time, high NO concentrations (>1 μM) stabilize HIF-1α (Mateo et al., 2003), thus increasing the dimeric form of the protein that, via binding to HIF responsive elements (HREs), promotes NOS expression (Mateo et al., 2003). Interestingly, in hypoxia-resistant fish, as in the case of the crucian carp, HIF-1α stabilization occurs even under normoxic conditions, suggesting a high basal expression of hypoxic-regulated genes, including NOS (Sollid et al., 2006).

As illustrated above, under hypoxic conditions, a significant source of NO is represented by nitrite. Compared to terrestrial animals, fish are exposed to an additional direct uptake of exogenous nitrite from the environmental water across the respiratory surfaces (Jensen, 2009). This external nitrite supply is an important source for the internal NO generation during severe hypoxia. An example is the crucian carp that, when exposed to deep hypoxia, takes up ambient nitrite across the gills and directs it to tissues, including the heart (Hansen et al., 2016).

In hypoxia-tolerant fish, such as the goldfish and the crucian carp, basal plasma nitrite levels are around 0.75–1.75 μM. These values are higher than those observed not only in mammals, but also in fish that are hypoxia intolerant (e.g., flounder, eelpout, oyster toadfish, brown trout) (about 0.2 μM) (Jensen, 2009; Hansen and Jensen, 2010; Sandvik et al., 2012). The reason for these high nitrite plasma levels in hypoxia-tolerant species is unclear. Presumably, this depends on the high overall NOS activity/expression under normoxia (Kleinbongard et al., 2003). Of note, fish living in nitrite-contaminated environments, have significantly high plasma nitrite, concentrations reaching the millimolar range (Bath and Eddy, 1980). At high concentrations, nitrite is toxic and can influence ion, respiratory and circulatory homeostasis (Jensen, 2009). As shown in the zebrafish, exposure to high nitrite is accompanied by very high levels of HbNO, a biomarker of NO generation from nitrate (Jensen, 2007). The consequent high nitrite-derived NO could perturb physiological processes, and may induce tissues nitrosative stress, resulting in high levels of S-nitrosylated proteins and cell damage (Jensen, 2009). For these reasons, fish need to balance the advantages of a rich ambient pool of nitrite for internal NO production with the potentially dangerous effects of nitrite-polluted habitats (Jensen and Hansen, 2011). At the same time, the possibility to maintain internal nitrite levels is particularly important for securing a source for NO production during hypoxia and anoxia, where NOS enzymes are unable to produce NO. At this purpose, the goldfish and the crucian carp possess an intrinsic ability to increase intracellular nitrite concentration and nitrosylated compounds during deep hypoxia and anoxia in tissues with high myoglobin and mitochondria content, such as the heart (Sandvik et al., 2012; Jensen et al., 2014; Hansen et al., 2016). This occurs at the expenses of extracellular nitrite. The extracellular-intracellular transfer of nitrite is facilitated by nitrite binding to intracellular proteins that, by keeping low the cytosolic concentration of free nitrite, allows inward diffusion (Hansen and Jensen, 2010). As shown in the crucian carp, anoxia increases tissue nitrite in the heart, but not in the white muscle. This is indicative of a role for Mb nitrite reductase activity, which is present at high levels in the heart and in the red musculature (Jensen et al., 2014).

Although no clear evidence is available, in fish, mitochondria may play a role in elevating intracellular nitrite during hypoxia and anoxia. Indeed, the cytoprotective effects of nitrite under low O_2 are largely directed at the mitochondria (Walters et al., 2012; de Lima Portella et al., 2015). In mammalian mitochondria, nitrite S-nitrosates complex I, attenuating ROS generation during early reperfusion (Dezfulian et al., 2009; Chouchani et al., 2013), and nitrosylates complex IV, which inhibits O_2 consumption rates (Hendgen-Cotta et al., 2008). Unlike mammals, in hypoxia-tolerant ectotherms, as presumably in all ectotherms, reoxygenation does not affect mitochondria, which maintain their capacity to produce energy. For example, reoxygenation does not result in mitochondria Ca^{2+} overload and/or in reversing ATP-synthase into an ATPase (Galli and Richards, 2014 for references). At the same time, mitochondrial proton leak is kept low (Galli and Richards, 2014 for references). With respect to hypoxia-intolerant, in hypoxia-tolerant species, mitochondria respiration appears more resistant to hypoxic stresses. For example, among elasmobranchs, cardiac mitochondria from the hypoxia-tolerant epaulet shark (*Hemiscyllium ocellatum*) produce less reactive oxidative species than the hypoxia sensitive shovelnose ray (*Aptychotrema rostrata*) (Hickey et al., 2012). For this purpose, the dynamic organization of respiratory chain complexes and ATP synthase (Cogliati et al., 2016) results crucial for mitochondrial respiration under hypoxia.

Unique natural animal models to analyse the role of NO, nitrite and Mb in the response to hypoxia are Antarctic teleosts. Some of them are example of disaptation, being naturally deprived of Hb, and/or of cardiac Mb, as in the case of the icefish *Chionodraco hamatus* (Hb^-/Mb^+), *Chenocephalus aceratus* (Hb^-/Mb^-), and their red-blooded counterparts *Trematomus bernacchii* (Hb^+/Mb^+) (Garofalo et al., 2009b). This condition makes these teleosts well suited for comparatively studying evolutionary and mechanistic aspects of the NO-nitrite system in relation to cardiac homeostasis and adaptation, including the response to varying O_2 levels (see for references Garofalo et al., 2009b). This aspect is crucial in the stably ice Antarctic waters, which are highly oxygenated but, at the same time, exposed to changes in O_2 content. At the moment, no data are available in Antarctic teleost on the putative role of the NO/nitrite equilibrium in relation to the response to low O_2. In the heart of *C. hamatus* and *T. bernacchii*, under normoxia, nitrite influences cardiac performance by inducing a concentration-dependent increase of contractility (Garofalo et al., 2015). In the Antarctic Hb- and Mb-less (Hb^-/Mb^-) icefish *C. aceratus*, intracardiac NOS expression is lower than in its Mb^+ counterpart, the Hb^-/Mb^+ *C. hamatus* (Amelio et al., 2006). Compared to the Mb expressing *C. hamatus*, in *C. aceratus* the heart is more sensitive to NOS stimulation by L-arginine (Cerra et al., 2009). Since the nitrite reductase activity of cardiac Mb is absent and NOS is poorly expressed, other mechanisms have been proposed to contribute to local NO production. For example, in the absence of the Mb-mediated scavenging effect, NO half-life is increased; the consequent larger availability of free NO may compensate for the reduced NOS expression. Contrarily, in *C. hamatus*, cardiac Mb may contribute to local NO generation and this maintains the nitrergic homeostasis. Interestingly, in *C. hamatus*, very low concentrations of exogenous nitrite (0.1 μmol/l) increase cardiac contractility, an effect similar to that elicited by NO (Cerra et al., 2009). At the same time, as in mammals (Vanin et al., 2007), the largely expressed NOS equipment might represent a rich source of NO from nitrite. Of note, in Hb^{-}/Mb^{-} icefish, the high NO levels occurring in the absence of both respiratory proteins correlate with major cardiovascular and subcellular compensations, including mitochondrial enlargement within myocardiocytes (Urschel and O'Brien, 2008). This contributes to myocardial oxidative equilibrium and hence to heart protection under hypoxia.

CONCLUSIONS

This review emphasizes the amazing flexibility of teleost fish in relation to their peculiar ability to cope with low O_2. Teleosts possess complex equipments for sensing O_2 that activate intricate downstream molecular signal-transduction networks crucial to balance tissue O_2 supply and demand. Although much still remains to be investigated, the available information indicate the critical role played by NO and its metabolites in the physiological strategies that in teleost allow cardiac adaptive responses to O_2 limitation, also contributing to better understand the extraordinary morphofunctional plasticity and adaptation that determined their evolutionary success.

AUTHOR CONTRIBUTIONS

AG and FG participated in drafting, writing, and editing the manuscript. MCC and SI participated in writing and editing the manuscript. All Authors approved it for publication.

FUNDING

This work was supported by the MIUR of Italy (ex 60%) and the Dottorato di Ricerca in Scienze della Vita.

REFERENCES

Amelio, D., Garofalo, F., Pellegrino, D., Giordano, F., Tota, B., and Cerra, M. C. (2006). Cardiac expression and distribution of nitric oxide synthases in the ventricle of the cold-adapted Antarctic teleosts, the hemoglobinless *Chionodraco hamatus* and the red-blooded *Trematomus bernacchii*. *Nitric Oxide* 15, 190–198. doi: 10.1016/j.niox.2005.12.007

Angelone, T., Gattuso, A., Imbrogno, S., Mazza, R., and Tota, B. (2012). Nitrite is a positive modulator of the Frank-Starling response in the vertebrate heart. *Am. J. Physiol.* 302, R1271–R1281. doi: 10.1152/ajpregu.00616.2011

Bailey, J. R., Rodnick, K. J., MacDougall, R., Clowe, S., and Driedzic, W. R. (2000). Anoxic performance of the American eel (*Anguilla rostrata* L.) heart requires extracellular glucose. *J. Exp. Zool.* 286, 699–706. doi: 10.1002/(SICI)1097-010X(20000601)286:7<699::AID-JEZ4>3.0.CO;2-G

Bath, R. N., and Eddy, F. B. (1980). Transport of nitrite across fish gills, J. *Exp. Zool.* 214, 119–121. doi: 10.1002/jez.1402140115

Bickler, P. E., and Buck, L. T. (2007). Hypoxia tolerance in reptiles, amphibians, and fishes: life with variable oxygen availability. *Annu. Rev. Physiol.* 69, 5.1–5.26. doi: 10.1146/annurev.physiol.69.031905.162529

Biswas, S. P., Palande, N. V., and Jadhao, A. G. (2011). Nitric oxide inhibited the melanophore aggregation induced by extracellular calcium concentration in snakehead fish, *Channa punctatus*. *Fish Physiol. Biochem.* 37, 919–927. doi: 10.1007/s10695-011-9489-9

Boutilier, R. G. (2001). Mechanisms of cell survival in hypoxia and hypothermia. *J. Exp. Biol.* 204(Pt 18), 3171–3181.

Broom, D. M., and Johnson, K. G. (1993). *Stress and Animal Welfare*. London: Chapman and Hall.

Bryan, N. S. (2006). Nitrite in nitric oxide biology: cause or consequence? A systems-based review. *Free Radic. Biol. Med.* 41, 691–701. doi: 10.1016/j.freeradbiomed.2006.05.019

Buckler, K. J. (1999). Background leak K^{+}-currents and oxygen sensing in carotid body type 1 cells. *Respir. Physiol.* 115, 179–187. doi: 10.1016/S0034-5687(99)00015-8

Buckler, K. J. (2007). TASK-like potassium channels and oxygen sensing in the carotid body. *Respir. Physiol. Neurobiol.* 157, 55–64. doi: 10.1016/j.resp.2007.02.013

Burleson, M. L., Mercer, S. E., and Wilk-Blaszczak, M. A. (2006). Isolation and characterization of putative O_2 chemoreceptor cells from the gills of channel catfish (*Ictalurus punctatus*). *Brain Res.* 1092, 100–107. doi: 10.1016/j.brainres.2006.03.085

Cameron, J. S., Hoffmann, K. E., Zia, C., Hemmett, H. M., Kronsteiner, A., and Lee, C. M. (2003). A role for nitric oxide in hypoxia-induced activation of cardiac KATP channels in goldfish (*Carassius auratus*). *J. Exp. Biol.* 206, 4057–4065. doi: 10.1242/jeb.00655

Castello, P. R., David, P. S., McClure, T., Crook, Z., and Poyton, R. O. (2006). Mitochondrial cytochrome oxidase produces nitric oxide under hypoxic conditions: implications for oxygen sensing and hypoxic signaling in eukaryotes. *Cell Metab.* 3, 277–287. doi: 10.1016/j.cmet.2006.02.011

Cerra, M. C., Angelone, T., Parisella, M. L., Pellegrino, D., and Tota, B. (2009). Nitrite modulates contractility of teleost (*Anguilla anguilla* and *Chionodraco hamatus*, i.e. the Antarctic hemoglobinless icefish) and frog (Rana esculenta) hearts. *Biochim. Biophys. Acta* 1787, 849–855. doi: 10.1016/j.bbabio.2009.03.008

Chang, J. P., Sawisky, G. R., Davis, P. J., Pemberton, J. G., Rieger, A. M., and Barreda, D. R. (2014). Relationship between nitric oxide- and calcium-dependent signal transduction pathways in growth hormone release from dispersed goldfish pituitary cells. *Gen. Comp. Endocrinol.* 206, 118–129. doi: 10.1016/j.ygcen.2014.07.006

Chouchani, E. T., Methner, C., Nadtochiy, S. M., Logan, A., Pell, V. R., Ding, S., et al. (2013). Cardioprotection by S-nitrosation of a cysteine switch on mitochondrial complex I. *Nat. Med.* 19, 753–759. doi: 10.1038/nm.3212

Cogliati, S., Enriquez, J. A., and Scorrano, L. (2016). Mitochondrial Cristae: where beauty meets functionality. *Trends Biochem. Sci.* 41, 261–273. doi: 10.1016/j.tibs.2016.01.001

Cooper, C. E., Mason, M. G., and Nicholls, P. (2008). A dynamic model of nitric oxide inhibition of mitochondrial cytochrome c oxidase. *Biochim. Biophys. Acta* 1777, 867–876. doi: 10.1016/j.bbabio.2008.03.021

Cosby, K., Partovi, K. S., Crawford, J. H., Patel, R. P., Reiter, C. D., Martyr, S., et al. (2003). Nitrite reduction to nitric oxide by deoxyhemoglobin vasodilates the human circulation. *Nat. Med.* 9, 1498–1505. doi: 10.1038/nm954

Cossins, A. R., and Bowler, K. (1987). *Temperature Biology of Animals*. London: Chapman and Hall.

Crowder, W. C., Nie, M., and Ultsch, G. R. (1998). Oxygen uptake in bullfrog tadpoles (Rana catesbeiana). *J. Exp. Zool.* 280, 121–134. doi: 10.1002/(SICI)1097-010X(19980201)280:2<121::AID-JEZ3>3.0.CO;2-Q

de Lima Portella, R., Bickta, J., and Shiva, S. (2015). Nitrite confers preconditioning and cytoprotection after Ischemia/reperfusion injury through the modulation of mitochondrial function. *Antioxid. Redox Signal.* 23, 307–327. doi: 10.1089/ars.2015.6260

Dezfulian, C., Shiva, S., Alekseyenko, A., Pendyal, A., Beiser, D. G., Munasinghe, J., et al. (2009). Nitrite therapy after cardiac arrest reduces reactive oxygen species generation, improves cardiac and neurological function, and enhances survival via reversible inhibition of mitochondrial complex I. *Circulation* 120, 897–905. doi: 10.1161/CIRCULATIONAHA.109.853267

Driedzic, W. R., and Gesser, H. (1994). Energy metabolism and contractility in ectothermic vertebrate hearts: hypoxia, acidosis, and low temperature. *Physiol. Rev.* 74, 221–258. doi: 10.1152/physrev.1994.74.1.221

Dzal, Y. A., Jenkin, S. E., Lague, S. L., Reichert, M. N., York, J. M., and Pamenter, M. E. (2015). Oxygen in demand: How oxygen has shaped vertebrate physiology. *Comp. Biochem. Physiol. A Mol. Integr. Physiol.* 186, 4–26. doi: 10.1016/j.cbpa.2014.10.029

Erusalimsky, J. D., and Moncada, S. (2007). Nitric oxide and mitochondrial signaling: from physiology to pathophysiology. *Arterioscler. Thromb. Vasc. Biol.* 27, 2524–2531. doi: 10.1161/ATVBAHA.107.151167

Evans, A. M., Hardie, D. G., Peers, C., Wyatt, C. N., Viollet, B., Kumar, P., et al. (2009). Ion channel regulation by AMPK: the route of hypoxia-response coupling in thecarotid body and pulmonary artery. *Ann. N. Y. Acad. Sci.* 1177, 89–100. doi: 10.1111/j.1749-6632.2009.05041.x

Evans, A. M., Mustard, K. J., Wyatt, C. N., Peers, C., Dipp, M., Kumar, P., et al. (2005). Does AMP-activated protein kinase couple inhibition of mitochondrial oxidative phosphorylation by hypoxia to calcium signaling in O_2-sensing cells? *J. Biol. Chem.* 280, 41504–41511. doi: 10.1074/jbc.M5100 40200

Fago, A., and Jensen, F. B. (2015). Hypoxia tolerance, nitric oxide, and nitrite: lessons from extreme animals. *Physiology (Bethesda).* 30, 116–126. doi: 10.1152/physiol.00051.2014

Farrell, A. P. (2007). Tribute to P. L. Lutz: a message from the heart – why hypoxic bradycardia in fishes? *J. Exp. Biol.* 210, 1715–1725. doi: 10.1242/jeb.02781

Farrell, A. P., and Stecyk, J. A. (2007). The heart as a working model to explore themes and strategies for anoxic survival in ectothermic vertebrates. *Comp. Biochem. Physiol. A* 147, 300–312. doi: 10.1016/j.cbpa.2007.01.021

Filice, M., Amelio, D., Garofalo, F., David, S., Fucarino, A., Jensen, F. B., et al. (2017). Angiotensin II dependent cardiac remodeling in the eel *Anguilla anguilla* involves the NOS/NO system. *Nitric Oxide* 65, 50–59. doi: 10.1016/j.niox.2017.02.007

Foster, M. W., Hess, D. T., and Stamler, J. S. (2009). Protein S-nitrosylation in health and disease: a current perspective. *Trends Mol. Med.* 15, 391–404. doi: 10.1016/j.molmed.2009.06.007

Galli, G. L., and Richards, J. G. (2014). Mitochondria from anoxia-tolerant animals reveal common strategies to survive without oxygen. *J. Comp. Physiol. B.* 184, 285–302. doi: 10.1007/s00360-014-0806-3

Garofalo, F., Amelio, D., Gattuso, A., Cerra, M. C., and Pellegrino, D. (2015). Cardiac contractility in Antarctic teleost is modulated by nitrite through xanthine oxidase and cytochrome p-450 nitrite reductase. *Nitric Oxide* 49, 1–7. doi: 10.1016/j.niox.2015.05.002

Garofalo, F., Imbrogno, S., Tota, B., and Amelio, D. (2012). Morpho-functional characterization of the goldfish (*Carassius auratus* L.) heart. *Comp. Biochem. Physiol.* 163, 215–222. doi: 10.1016/j.cbpa.2012.05.206

Garofalo, F., Parisella, M. L., Amelio, D., Tota, B., and Imbrogno, S. (2009a). Phospholamban S-nitrosylation modulates starling response in fish heart. *Proc. R. Soc. B: Biol. Sci.* 276, 4043–4052. doi: 10.1098/rspb.200 9.1189

Garofalo, F., Pellegrino, D., Amelio, D., and Tota, B. (2009b). The Antarctic hemoglobinless icefish, fifty five years later: a unique cardiocirculatory interplay of disaptation and phenotypic plasticity. *Comp. Biochem. Physiol. A Mol. Integr. Physiol.* 154, 10–28. doi: 10.1016/j.cbpa.2009.04.621

Gautier, C., van Faassen, E., Mikula, I., Martasek, P., and Slama-Schwok, A. (2006). Endothelial nitric oxide synthase reduces nitrite anions to NO under anoxia, Biochem. *Biophys. Res. Commun.* 341, 816–821. doi: 10.1016/j.bbrc.2006.01.031

Gilmour, K. M., and Perry, S. F. (2007). "Branchial chemoreceptor regulation of cardiorespiratory function," in *Fish Physiology v25 Sensory Systems Neuroscience*, eds T. J. Hara and B. Zielinski (San Diego, CA: Academic Press), 97–151.

Gladwin, M. T., Schechter, A. N., Kim-Shapiro, D. B., Patel, R. P., Hogg, N., Shiva, S., et al. (2005). The emerging biology of the nitrite anion. *Nat. Chem. Biol.* 1, 308–314. doi: 10.1038/nchembio1105-308

Guzik, T. J., West, N. E., Pillai, R., Taggart, D. P., and Channon, K. M. (2002). Nitric oxide modulates superoxide release and peroxynitrite formation in human blood vessels. *Hypertension* 39, 1088–1094. doi: 10.1161/01.HYP.0000018041.48432.B5

Hagen, T., Taylor, C. T., Lam, F., and Moncada, S. (2003). Redistribution of intracellular oxygen in hypoxia by nitric oxide: effect on HIF1alpha. *Science* 302, 1975–1978. doi: 10.1126/science.1088805

Hansen, M. N., Gerber, L., and Jensen, F. B. (2016). Nitric oxide availability in deeply hypoxic crucian carp: acute and chronic changes and utilization of ambient nitrite reservoirs. *Am. J. Physiol. Regul. Integr. Comp. Physiol.* 310, R532–R540. doi: 10.1152/ajpregu.00515.2015

Hansen, M. N., and Jensen, F. B. (2010). Nitric oxide metabolites in goldfish under normoxic and hypoxic conditions. *J. Exp. Biol.* 213, 3593–3602. doi: 10.1242/jeb.048140

Heinrich, T. A., da Silva, R. S., Miranda, K. M., Switzer, C. H., Wink, D. A., and Fukuto, J. M. (2013). Biological nitric oxide signalling: chemistry and terminology. *Br. J. Pharmacol.* 169, 1417–1429. doi: 10.1111/bph.12217

Hendgen-Cotta, U. B., Merx, M. W., Shiva, S., Schmitz, J., Becher, S., Klare, J. P., et al. (2008). Nitrite reductase activity of myoglobin regulates respiration and cellular viability in myocardial ischemia-reperfusion injury. *Proc. Natl. Acad. Sci. U.S.A.* 105, 10256–10261. doi: 10.1073/pnas.0801 336105

Hermes-Lima, M., and Zenteno-Savín, T. (2002). Animal response to drastic changes in oxygen availability and physiological oxidative stress. *Comp. Biochem. Physiol. C Toxicol. Pharmacol.* 133, 537–556.

Hickey, A. J., Renshaw, G. M., Speers-Roesch, B., Richards, J. G., Wang, Y., Farrell, A. P., et al. (2012). A radical approach to beating hypoxia: depressed free radical release from heart fibres of the hypoxia-tolerant epaulette shark (*Hemiscyllum ocellatum*). *J. Comp. Physiol. B* 182, 91–100. doi: 10.1007/s00360-011-0 599-6

Hill, B. G., Dranka, B. P., Bailey, S. M., Lancaster, J. R. Jr., and Darley-Usmar, V. M. (2010). What part of NO don't you understand? Some answers to the cardinal questions in nitric oxide biology. *J. Biol. Chem.* 285, 19699–19704. doi: 10.1074/jbc.R110.101618

Hochachka, P. W. (1986). Defense strategies against hypoxia and hypothermia. *Science* 231, 234–241. doi: 10.1126/science.2417316

Hochachka, P. W., and Lutz, P. L. (2001). Mechanism, origin, and evolution of anoxia tolerance in animals. *Comp. Biochem. Physiol. B Biochem. Mol. Biol.* 130, 435–459. doi: 10.1016/S1096-4959(01)00408-0

Hochachka, P. W., and Somero, G. N. (2002). *Biochemical Adaptation: Mechanism and Process in Physiological Evolution.* New York, NY: Oxford University Press.

Imbrogno, S. (2013). The eel heart: multilevel insights into functional organ plasticity. *J. Exp. Biol.* 216, 3575–3586. doi: 10.1242/jeb.089292

Imbrogno, S., Capria, C., Tota, B., and Jensen, F. B. (2014). Nitric oxide improves the hemodynamic performance of the hypoxic goldfish (*Carassius auratus*) heart. *Nitric Oxide* 42, 24–31. doi: 10.1016/j.niox.2014.08.012

Imbrogno, S., and Cerra, M. C. (2017). "Hormonal and autacoid control of cardiac function," in *Fish Physiology: The Cardiovascular System: Design, Control and Function, 1st Edn.*, Vol. 36, eds A. K. Gamperl, A. P. Farrell, and C. J. Brauner (Oxford: Academic Press), 265–315.

Imbrogno, S., Filice, M., Cerra, M. C., and Gattuso, A. (2018). NO, CO, and H_2S: what about gasotransmitters in fish and amphibian hearts? *Acta Physiologica (Oxf).* doi: 10.1111/apha.13035. [Epub ahead of print].

Imbrogno, S., Garofalo, F., Amelio, D., Capria, C., and Cerra, M. C. (2013). Humoral control of cardiac remodeling in fish: role of Angiotensin, II. *Gen. Comp. Endocrinol.* 194, 189–197. doi: 10.1016/j.ygcen.2013.09.009

Imbrogno, S., Garofalo, F., Cerra, M. C., Mahata, S. K., and Tota, B. (2010). The catecholamine release-inhibitory peptide catestatin (chromogranin A344-363) modulates myocardial function in fish. *J. Exp. Biol.* 213, 3636–3643. doi: 10.1242/jeb.045567

Imbrogno, S., Mazza, R., Pugliese, C., Filice, M., Angelone, T., Loh, Y. P., et al. (2017). The Chromogranin A-derived sympathomimetic serpinin depresses myocardial performance in teleost and amphibian hearts. *Gen. Comp. Endocrinol.* 240, 1–9. doi: 10.1016/j.ygcen.2016.09.004

Imbrogno, S., Tota, B., and Gattuso, A. (2011). The evolutionary functions of cardiac NOS/NO in vertebrates tracked by fish and amphibian paradigms. *Nitric Oxide* 25, 1–10. doi: 10.1016/j.niox.2011.05.001

Jansson, E. A., Huang, L., Malkey, R., Govoni, M., Nihlén, C., Olsson, A., et al. (2008). A mammalian functional nitrate reductase that regulates nitrite and nitric oxide homeostasis. *Nat. Chem. Biol.* 4, 411–417. doi: 10.1038/nchembio.92

Jensen, F. B. (2007). Nitric oxide formation from nitrite in zebrafish *J. Exp. Biol.* 210, 3387–3394. doi: 10.1242/jeb.008748

Jensen, F. B. (2009). The role of nitrite in nitric oxide homeostasis: a comparative perspective. *Biochim. Biophys. Acta* 1787, 841–848. doi: 10.1016/j.bbabio.2009.02.010

Jensen, F. B., and Hansen, M. N. (2011). Differential uptake and metabolism of nitrite in normoxic and hypoxic goldfish. *Aquat. Toxicol.* 101, 318–325. doi: 10.1016/j.aquatox.2010.11.007

Jensen, F. B., Hansen, M. N., Montesanti, G., and Wang, T. (2014). Nitric oxide metabolites during anoxia and reoxygenation in the anoxia-tolerant vertebrate *Trachemys scripta*. *J. Exp. Biol.* 217, 423–431. doi: 10.1242/jeb.093179

Jonz, M. G. (2014). "Oxygen sensing," in *The Physiology of Fishes 4th Edn.*, eds D. H. Evans, J. B. Claiborne, and S. Currie (Boca Raton, FL: CRC Press), 149–174.

Jonz, M. G., Fearon, I. M., and Nurse, C. A. (2004). Neuroepithelial oxygen chemoreceptors of the zebrafish gill. *J. Physiol.* 560, 737–752. doi: 10.1113/jphysiol.2004.069294

Jonz, M. G., Zachar, P. C., Da Fonte, D. F., and Mierzwa, A. S. (2015). Peripheral chemoreceptors in fish: a brief history and a look ahead. *Comp. Biochem. Physiol. A Mol. Integr. Physiol.* 186, 27–38. doi: 10.1016/j.cbpa.2014.09.002

Jugdutt, B. I. (2002). Nitric oxide and cardioprotection during ischemia-reperfusion. *Heart Fail. Rev.* 7, 391–405.

Kimura, H. (2011). Hydrogen sulfide: its production, release and functions. *Amino Acids*, 41, 113–121. doi: 10.1007/s00726-010-0510-x

Kleinbongard, P., Dejam, A., Lauer, T., Rassaf, T., Schindler, A., Picker, O., et al. (2003). Plasma nitrite reflects constitutive nitric oxide synthase activity in mammals. *Free Radic. Biol. Med.* 35, 790–796. doi: 10.1016/S0891-5849(03)00406-4

Koolhaas, J. M., Korte, S. M., De Boer, S. F., Van Der Vegt, B. J., Van Reenen, C. G., Hopster, H., et al. (1999). Coping styles in animals: current status in behavior and stress-physiology. *Neurosci. Biobehav. Rev.* 23, 925–935. doi: 10.1016/S0149-7634(99)00026-3

Kozlov, A. V., Staniek, K., and Nohl, H. (1999). Nitrite reductase activity is a novel function of mammalian mitochondria. *FEBS Lett.* 454, 127–130. doi: 10.1016/S0014-5793(99)00788-7

Liu, L., and Simon, M. C. (2004). Regulation of transcription and translation by hypoxia. *Cancer Biol. Ther.* 3, 492–497. doi: 10.4161/cbt.3.6.1010

López-Barneo, J., González-Rodríguez, P., Gao, L., Fernández-Agüera, M. C., Pardal, R., and Ortega-Sáenz, P. (2016). Oxygen sensing by the carotid body: mechanisms and role in adaptation to hypoxia. *Am. J. Physiol. Cell. Physiol.* 310, C629–C642. doi: 10.1152/ajpcell.00265.2015

Lundberg, J. O., Gladwin, M. T., Ahluwalia, A., Benjamin, N., Bryan, N. S., Butler, A., et al. (2009). Nitrate and nitrite in biology, nutrition and therapeutics. *Nat. Chem. Biol.* 5, 865–869. doi: 10.1038/nchembio.260

Lundberg, J. O., Weitzberg, E., and Gladwin, M. T. (2008). The nitrate-nitrite-nitric oxide pathway in physiology and therapeutics. *Nat. Rev. Drug Discov.* 7, 156–167. doi: 10.1038/nrd2466

Lutz, P. L., and Nilsson, G. E. (2004). Vertebrate brains at the pilot light. *Respir. Physiol. Neurobiol.* 141, 285–296. doi: 10.1016/j.resp.2004.03.013

Mason, M. G., Nicholls, P., Wilson, M. T., and Cooper, C. E. (2006). Nitric oxide inhibition of respiration involves both competitive (heme) and noncompetitive (copper) binding to cytochrome c oxidase. *Proc. Natl. Acad. Sci. U.S.A.* 103, 708–713. doi: 10.1073/pnas.0506562103

Mateo, J., García-Lecea, M., Cadenas, S., Hernández, C., and Moncada, S. (2003). Regulation of hypoxia-inducible factor-1alpha by nitric oxide through mitochondria-dependent and -independent pathways. *Biochem. J.* 376, 537–544. doi: 10.1042/bj20031155

Mathur, G. B. (1967). Anaerobic respiration in a cyprinoid fish *Rasbora daniconius* (Ham). *Nature* 214, 318–319. doi: 10.1038/214318b0

McNeill, B., and Perry, S. F. (2006). The interactive effects of hypoxia and nitric oxide on catecholamine secretion in rainbow trout (*Oncorhynchus mykiss*). *J. Exp. Biol.* 209, 4214–4223. doi: 10.1242/jeb.02519

Mendelsohn, B. A., Kassebaum, B. L., and Gitlin, J. D. (2008). The zebrafish embryo as a dynamic model of anoxia tolerance. *Dev. Dyn.* 237, 1780–1788. doi: 10.1002/dvdy.21581

Millar, T. M., Stevens, C. R., Benjamin, N., Eisenthal, R., Harrison, R., and Blake, D. R. (1998). Xanthine oxidoreductase catalyses the reduction of nitrates and nitrite to nitric oxide under hypoxic conditions. *FEBS Lett.* 427, 225–228. doi: 10.1016/S0014-5793(98)00430-X

Milsom, W. K. (2012). New insights into gill chemoreception: receptor distribution and roles in water and air breathing fish. *Respir. Physiol. Neurobiol.* 184, 326–339. doi: 10.1016/j.resp.2012.07.013

Milsom, W. K., and Burleson, M. L. (2007). Peripheral arterial chemoreceptors and the evolution of the carotid body. *Respir. Physiol. Neurobiol.* 157, 4–11. doi: 10.1016/j.resp.2007.02.007

Misfeldt, M., Fago, A., and Gesser, H. (2009). Nitric oxide increases myocardial efficiency in the hypoxia-tolerant turtle *Trachemys scripta*. *J. Exp. Biol.* 212, 954–960. doi: 10.1242/jeb.025171

Moncada, S., and Higgs, A. (1993). The L-arginine-nitric oxide pathway. *N. Engl. J. Med.* 329, 2002–2012. doi: 10.1056/NEJM199312303292706

Montiglio, P. O., Garant, D., Thomas, D., and Re'ale, D. (2010). Individual variation in temporal activity patterns in open-field tests. *Anim. Behav.* 80, 905–912. doi: 10.1016/j.anbehav.2010.08.014

Nagababu, E., Ramasamy, S., Abernethy, D. R., and Rifkind, J. M. (2003). Active nitric oxide produced in the red cell under hypoxic conditions by deoxyhemoglobin-mediated nitrite reduction, J. *Biol. Chem.* 278, 46349–46356. doi: 10.1074/jbc.M307572200

Nikinmaa, M., Gassmann, M., and Bogdanova, A. (2011). "Oxygen sensing: the role of reactive oxygen species," in *Oxidative Stress in Aquatic Ecosystems*, eds D. Abele, J. P. Vàzquez- Medina, and T. Zenteno-Savin (Chichester: John Wiley & Sons Ltd), 165–177.

Nilsson, G. E. (2001). Surviving anoxia with the brain turned on. *News Physiol. Sci.* 16, 218–221. doi: 10.1152/physiologyonline.2001.16.5.217

Noma, A. (1983). ATP-regulated K+ channels in cardiac muscle. *Nature* 305, 147–158. doi: 10.1038/305147a0

Nurse, C. A. (2005). Neurotransmission and neuromodulation in the chemosensory carotid body. *Auton. Neurosci.* 120, 1–9. doi: 10.1016/j.autneu.2005.04.008

Olson, K. R. (2011). Hydrogen sulfide is an oxygen sensor in the carotid body. *Respir. Physiol. Neurobiol.* 179, 103–110. doi: 10.1016/j.resp.2011.09.010

Olson, K. R., Healy, M. J., Qin, Z., Skovgaard, N., Vulesevic, B., Duff, D. W., et al. (2008). Hydrogen sulfide as an oxygen sensor in trout gill chemoreceptors. *Am. J. Physiol. Regul. Integr. Comp. Physiol.* 295, R669–R680. doi: 10.1152/ajpregu.00807.2007

Overholt, J. L., and Prabhakar, N. R. (1997). Ca^{2+} current in rabbit carotid body glomus cells is conducted by multiple types of high-voltage-activated Ca^{2+} channels. *J. Neurophysiol.* 78, 2467–2474. doi: 10.1152/jn.1997.78.5.2467

Pacher, P., Beckman, J. S., and Liaudet, L. (2007). Nitric oxide and peroxynitrite in health and disease. *Physiol. Rev.* 87, 315–424. doi: 10.1152/physrev.00029.2006

Padilla, P. A., and Roth, M. B. (2001). Oxygen deprivation causes suspended animation in the zebrafish embryo. *Proc. Natl. Acad. Sci. U.S.A.* 98, 7331–7335. doi: 10.1073/pnas.131213198

Pamenter, M. E. (2014). Mitochondria: a multimodal hub of hypoxia tolerance. *Can. J. Zool.* 92, 569–589. doi: 10.1139/cjz-2013-0247

Pautz, A., Art, J., Hahn, S., Nowag, S., Voss, C., and Kleinert, H. (2010). Regulation of the expression of inducible nitric oxide synthase. *Nitric Oxide* 23, 75–93. doi: 10.1016/j.niox.2010.04.007

Pedersen, C. L., Faggiano, S., Helbo, S., Gesser, H., and Fago, A. (2010). Roles of nitric oxide, nitrite and myoglobin on myocardial efficiency in trout (*Oncorhynchus mykiss*) and goldfish (*Carassius auratus*): implications for hypoxia tolerance. *J. Exp. Biol.* 213, 2755–2762. doi: 10.1242/jeb.041624

Peers, C. (1990). Hypoxic suppression of K^+ currents in type I carotid body cells: selective effect on the Ca^{2+}-activated K^+ current. *Neurosci. Lett.* 2, 253–256. doi: 10.1016/0304-3940(90)90846-2

Peng, Y. J., Nanduri, J., Raghuraman, G., Souvannakitti, D., Gadalla, M. M., Kumar, G. K., et al. (2010). H_2S mediates O_2 sensing in the carotid body. *Proc. Natl. Acad. Sci. U.S.A.* 107, 10719–10724. doi: 10.1073/pnas.1005866107

Pérez-García, M. T., Colinas, O., Miguel-Velado, E., Moreno-Domínguez, A., and López-López, J. R. (2004). Characterization of the Kv channels of mouse carotid body chemoreceptor cells and their role in oxygen sensing. *J. Physiol.* 557, 457–471. doi: 10.1113/jphysiol.2004.062281

Perry, S. F., and Tzaneva, V. (2016). The sensing of respiratory gases in fish: Mechanisms and signalling pathways. *Respir. Physiol. Neurobiol.* 224, 71–79. doi: 10.1016/j.resp.2015.06.007

Petersen, M. G., Dewilde, S., and Fago, A. (2008). Reactions of ferrous neuroglobin and cytoglobin with nitrite under anaerobic conditions *J. Inorg. Biochem.* 102, 1777–1782. doi: 10.1016/j.jinorgbio.2008.05.008

Porteus, C. S., Abdallah, S. J., Pollack, J., Kumai, Y., Kwong, R. W., Yew, H. M., et al. (2014). The role of hydrogen sulphide in the control of breathing in hypoxic zebrafish (*Danio rerio*). *J. Physiol.* 592, 3075–3088. doi: 10.1113/jphysiol.2014.271098

Porteus, C. S., Pollack, J., Tzaneva, V., Kwong, R. W., Kumai, Y., Abdallah, S. J., et al. (2015). A role for nitric oxide in the control of breathing in zebrafish (*Danio rerio*). *J. Exp. Biol.* 218, 3746–3753. doi: 10.1242/jeb.127795

Prabhakar, N. R. (1999). NO and CO as second messengers in oxygen sensing in the carotid body. *Respir. Physiol.* 115, 161–168. doi: 10.1016/S0034-5687(99)00019-5

Prabhakar, N. R., and Peers, C. (2014). Gasotransmitter regulation of ion channels: a key step in O_2 sensing by the carotid body. *Physiology (Bethesda)* 29, 49–57. doi: 10.1152/physiol.00034.2013

Qin, Z., Lewis, J. E., and Perry, S. F. (2010). Zebrafish (*Danio rerio*) gill neuroepithelial cells are sensitive chemoreceptors for environmental CO_2. *J. Physiol.* 588, 861–872. doi: 10.1113/jphysiol.2009.184739

Rashid, I., Nagpure, N. S., Srivastava, P., Kumar, R., Pathak, A. K., Singh, M., et al. (2017). HRGFish: a database of hypoxia responsive genes in fishes. *Sci. Rep.* 7:42346. doi: 10.1038/srep42346

Reutov, V. P. (2002). Nitric oxide cycle in mammals and the cyclicity principle. *Biochemistry (Mosc)* 67, 293–311. doi: 10.1023/A:1014832416073

Ronson, R. S., Nakamura, M., and Vinten-Johansen, J. (1999). The cardiovascular effects and implications of peroxynitrite. *Cardiovasc. Res.* 44, 47–59. doi: 10.1016/S0008-6363(99)00184-4

Sanchez, A., Soncini, R., Wang, T., Koldkjaer, P., Taylor, E. W., and Glass, M. L. (2001). The differential cardio-respiratory responses to ambient hypoxia and systemic hypoxaemia in the South American lungfish, *Lepidosiren paradoxa. Comp. Biochem. Physiol. Part A Mol. Integr. Physiol.* 130, 677–687. doi: 10.1016/S1095-6433(01)00395-6

Sanchez, D., López-López, J. R., Pérez-García, M. T., Sanz-Alfayate, G., Obeso, A., Ganfornina, M. D., et al. (2002). Molecular identification of Kvalpha subunits that contribute to the oxygen-sensitive K^+ current of chemoreceptor cells of the rabbit carotid body. *J. Physiol.* 542, 369–382. doi: 10.1113/jphysiol.2002.018382

Sandvik, G. K., Nilsson, G. E., and Jensen, F. B. (2012). Dramatic increase of nitrite levels in hearts of anoxia-exposed crucian carp supporting a role in cardioprotection. *Am. J. Physiol. Regul. Integr. Comp. Physiol.* 302, R468–R477. doi: 10.1152/ajpregu.00538.2011

Schjolden, J., Stoskhus, A., and Winberg, S. (2005). Does individual variation in stress responses and agonistic behavior reflect divergent stress coping strategies in juvenile rainbow trout? *Physiol. Biochem. Zool.* 78, 715–723. doi: 10.1086/432153

Semenza, G. L. (2007). Hypoxia-inducible factor 1 (HIF-1) pathway. *Sci STKE.* 407:cm8.

Shen, W., Tian, R., Saupe, W. K., Spindler, M., and Ingwall, S. J. (2001). Endogenous nitric oxide enhances coupling between O_2 consumption and ATP synthesis in guinea pig hearts. *Am. J. Physiol. Heart Circ. Physiol.* 281, 838–846. doi: 10.1152/ajpheart.2001.281.2.H838

Shiva, S., Huang, Z., Grubina, R., Sun, J., and Ringwood, L. A., MacArthur, et al. (2007a). Deoxymyoglobin is a nitrite reductase that generates nitric oxide and regulates mitochondrial respiration. *Circ. Res.* 100, 654–661. doi: 10.1161/01.RES.0000260171.52224.6b

Shiva, S., Sack, M. N., Greer, J. J., Duranski, M., Ringwood, L. A., Burwell, L., et al. (2007b). Nitrite augments tolerance to ischemia/reperfusion injury via the modulation of mitochondrial electron transfer. *J. Exp. Med.* 204, 2089–2102. doi: 10.1084/jem.20070198

Sloan Wilson D., Clark, A. B., Coleman, K., and Dearstyne, T. (1994). Shyness and boldness in humans and other animals. *Trends Ecol. Evol.* 9, 442–446. doi: 10.1016/0169-5347(94)90134-1

Sollid, J., Rissanen, E., Tranberg, H. K., Thorstensen, T., Vuori, K. A., Nikinmaa, M., et al. (2006). HIF-1alpha and iNOS levels in crucian carp gills during hypoxia-induced transformation. *J. Comp. Physiol. B.* 176, 359–369. doi: 10.1007/s00360-005-0059-2

Stecyk, J. A., Stenløcken, K. O., Farrell, A. P., and Nilsson, G. E. (2004). Maintained cardiac pumping in anoxic crucian carp. *Science* 306:77. doi: 10.1126/science.1100763

Stensløkken, K. O., Ellefsen, S., Stecyk, J. A., Dahl, M. B., Nilsson, G. E., and Vaage, J. (2008). Differential regulation of AMP-activated kinase and AKT kinase in response to oxygen availability in crucian carp (*Carassius carassius*). *Am. J. Physiol. Regul. Integr. Comp. Physiol.* 295, R1803–R1814. doi: 10.1152/ajpregu.90590.2008

Summers, B. A., Overholt, J. L., and Prabhakar, N. R. (1999). Nitric oxide inhibits L-type Ca2+ current in glomus cells of the rabbit carotid body via a cGMP-independent mechanism. *J. Neurophysiol.* 81, 1449–1457. doi: 10.1152/jn.1999.81.4.1449

Sundin, L., Reid, S. G., Rantin, F. T., and Milsom, W. K. (2000). Branchial receptors and cardiorespiratory reflexes in a neotropical fish, the tambaqui (*Colossoma macropomum*). *J. Exp. Biol.* 203(Pt 7), 1225–1239.

Tota, B., Angelone, T., Mancardi, D., and Cerra, M. C. (2011). Hypoxia and anoxia tolerance of vertebrate hearts: an evolutionary perspective. *Antioxid. Redox Signal.* 14, 851–862. doi: 10.1089/ars.2010.3310

Tota, B., Quintieri, A. M., and Angelone, T. (2010). The emerging role of nitrite as an endogenous modulator and therapeutic agent of cardiovascular function. *Curr. Med. Chem.* 17, 1915–1925. doi: 10.2174/092986710791163948

Tran, S., and Gerlai, R. (2013). Individual differences in activity levels in zebrafish (*Danio rerio*). *Behav. Brain Res.* 257, 224–229. doi: 10.1016/j.bbr.2013.09.040

Tzaneva, V., Bailey, S., and Perry, S. F. (2011). The interactive effects of hypoxemia, hyperoxia, and temperature on the gill morphology of goldfish (*Carassius auratus*). *Am. J. Physiol. Regul. Integr. Comp. Physiol.* 300, R1344–R1351. doi: 10.1152/ajpregu.00530.2010

Tzaneva, V., and Perry, S. F. (2014). Heme oxygenase-1 (HO-1) mediated respiratory responses to hypoxia in the goldfish, *Carassius auratus. Respir. Physiol. Neurobiol.* 199, 1–8. doi: 10.1016/j.resp.2014.04.006

Tzaneva, V., and Perry, S. F. (2016). Role of endogenous carbon monoxide in the control of breathing in zebrafish (*Danio rerio*). *Am. J. Physiol. Regul. Integr. Comp. Physiol.* 311, R1262–R1270. doi: 10.1152/ajpregu.00094.2016

Urschel, M. R., and O'Brien, K. M. (2008). High mitochondrial densities in the hearts of Antarctic icefishes are maintained by an increase in mitochondrial size rather than mitochondrial biogenesis. *J. Exp. Biol.* 211, 2638–2646. doi: 10.1242/jeb.018598

Vallance, P., Rees, D., and Moncada, S. (2000). "Therapeutic potential of NOS inhibitors in septic shock," in *Handbook of Experimental Pharmacology*, Vol. 143, ed B. Mayer (Berlin: Springer-Verlag), 385–397.

van Faassen, E. E., Bahrami, S., Feelisch, M., Hogg, N., Kelm, M., Kim-Shapiro, D. B., et al. (2009). Nitrite as regulator of hypoxic signaling in mammalian physiology. *Med. Res. Rev.* 29, 683–741. doi: 10.1002/med.20151

Vanin, A. F., Bevers, L. M., Slama-Schwok, A., and van Faassen, E. E. (2007). Nitric oxide synthase reduces nitrite to NO under anoxia. *Cell. Mol. Life Sci.* 64, 96–103. doi: 10.1007/s00018-006-6374-2

Van Raaij, M., Van den Thillart, G., Vianen, G. J., Pit, D. S., Balm, P. H., and Steffens, A. B. (1996). Substrate mobilization and hormonal changes in rainbow trout (Oncorhynchus mykiss, L.) and common carp (Cyprinus carpio, L.) during deep hypoxia and subsequent recovery. *J. Comp. Physiol.* 166, 443–452. doi: 10.1007/BF02337889

Varas, R., Wyatt, C. N., and Buckler, K. J. (2007). Modulation of TASK-like background potassium channels in rat arterial chemoreceptor cells by intracellular ATP and other nucleotides. *J. Physiol.* 583, 521–536. doi: 10.1113/jphysiol.2007.135657

Vornanen, M., and Haverinen, J. (2016). Glycogen dynamics of crucian carp (*Carassius carassius*) in prolonged anoxia. *J. Comp. Physiol. B.* 186, 999–1007. doi: 10.1007/s00360-016-1007-z

Vulesevic, B., McNeill, B., and Perry, S. F. (2006). Chemoreceptor plasticity and respiratory acclimation in the zebrafish *Danio rerio. J. Exp. Biol.* 209(Pt 7), 1261–1273. doi: 10.1242/jeb.02058

Walters, A. M., Porter, G. A., and Brookes, P. S. (2012). Mitochondria as a drug target in Ischemic heart disease and cardiomyopathy. *Circ. Res.* 111, 1222–1236. doi: 10.1161/CIRCRESAHA.112.265660

Wang, J., Hogan, J. O., Wang, R., White, C., and Kim, D. (2017). Role of cystathionine-γ-lyase in hypoxia-induced changes in TASK activity, intracellular [Ca2+] and ventilation in mice. Respir. Physiol. *Neurobiol.* 246, 98–106. doi: 10.1016/j.resp.2017.08.009

Wyatt, C. N., and Evans, A. M. (2007). AMP-activated protein kinase and chemotransduction in the carotid body. *Respir. Physiol. Neurobiol.* 157, 22–29. doi: 10.1016/j.resp.2007.01.021

Wyatt, C. N., Mustard, K. J., Pearson, S. A., Dallas, M. L., Atkinson, L., Kumar, P., et al. (2007). AMP-activated protein kinase mediates carotid body excitation by hypoxia. *J. Biol. Chem.* 282, 8092–8098. doi: 10.1074/jbc.M608742200

Wyatt, C. N., and Peers, C. (1995). Ca^{2+-}activated K^+ channels in isolated type I cells of the neonatal rat carotid body. *J. Physiol.* 483, 559–565. doi: 10.1113/jphysiol.1995.sp020606

Yuan, G., Peng, Y. J., Khan, S. A., Nanduri, J., Singh, A., Vasavda, C., et al. (2016). H_2S production by reactive oxygen species in the carotid body triggers hypertension in a rodent model of sleep apnea. *Sci. Signal.* 9:ra80. doi: 10.1126/scisignal.aaf3204

Zachar, P. C., and Jonz, M. G. (2012). Oxygen sensitivity of gill neuroepithelial cells in the anoxia-tolerant goldfish. *Adv. Exp. Med. Biol.* 758, 167–172. doi: 10.1007/978-94-007-4584-1_23

Zachar, P. C., Pan, W., and Jonz, M. G. (2017). Characterization of ion channels and O_2 sensitivity in gill neuroepithelial cells of the anoxia-tolerant goldfish (*Carassius auratus*). *J. Neurophysiol.* 118, 3014–3023. doi: 10.1152/jn.00237.2017

Zweier, J. L., Samouilov, A., and Kuppusamy, P. (1999). Non-enzymatic nitric oxide synthesis in biological systems. *Biochim. Biophys. Acta* 1411, 250–262. doi: 10.1016/S0005-2728(99)00018-3

23

Cardiovascular Benefits of Dietary Melatonin: A Myth or a Reality?

*Zukiswa Jiki, Sandrine Lecour and Frederic Nduhirabandi**

Cardioprotection Group, Hatter Institute for Cardiovascular Research in Africa, Department of Medicine, Faculty of Health Sciences, University of Cape Town, Cape Town, South Africa

Edited by:
Pasquale Pagliaro,
Università degli Studi di Torino, Italy

Reviewed by:
Vincenzo Lionetti,
Scuola Sant'Anna di Studi Avanzati, Italy
Antonio Colantuoni,
University of Naples Federico II, Italy

****Correspondence:***
Frederic Nduhirabandi
frederic.nduhirabandi@uct.ac.za

The role of the diet as well as the impact of the dietary habits on human health and disease is well established. Apart from its sleep regulatory effect, the indoleamine melatonin is a well-established antioxidant molecule with multiple health benefits. Convincing evidence supports the presence of melatonin in plants and foods with the intake of such foods affecting circulating melatonin levels in humans. While numerous actions of both endogenous melatonin and melatonin supplementation are well described, little is known about the influence of the dietary melatonin intake on human health. In the present review, evidence for the cardiovascular health benefits of melatonin supplementation and dietary melatonin is discussed. Current knowledge on the biological significance as well as the underlying physiological mechanism of action of the dietary melatonin is also summarized. Whether dietary melatonin constitutes an alternative preventive treatment for cardiovascular disease is addressed.

Keywords: antioxidant, cardiovascular diseases, hypertension, melatonin, myocardial infarction

INTRODUCTION

The role of the diet as well as the impact of the dietary habits on human health and disease has been described since the antiquity (Skiadas and Lascaratos, 2001). In ancient Greece, excess food intake was considered as unhealthy and a cause of illness, whereas a moderate diet made of cereals, legumes, fruits, milk, honey and fish with a modest consumption of meat, confectionery and wine, as currently found in the common Mediterranean diet, was recommended as healthy (Skiadas and Lascaratos, 2001). Today, the health benefits of the Mediterranean diet are well established (Estruch et al., 2013; Afshin et al., 2014). Accordingly, supplementation of the Mediterranean diet with extra-virgin olive oil or nuts is associated with a reduction in the risk of major cardiovascular events among high-risk persons (Estruch et al., 2013). The health-promoting properties of the Mediterranean diet are attributed to its various food ingredients including, amongst others, flavonoids (Kruger et al., 2014) and, more recently, melatonin (Lecour and Lamont, 2011), therefore supporting the current growing interest in the dietary sources and bioactivities of melatonin (Peuhkuri et al., 2012; Johns et al., 2013; Sae-Teaw et al., 2013; Tan et al., 2014; Iriti and Varoni, 2015; Meng et al., 2017b).

Melatonin or N-acetyl-5-methoxytryptamine is a highly conserved indoleamine molecule found in all microorganisms (Hardeland and Fuhrberg, 1996), plants and animals (Reiter et al., 2001; Tan et al., 2012). Originally identified in the bovine pineal gland (Lerner et al., 1958), melatonin is also produced by a wide range of tissues including the retina, thymus, spleen, heart, muscle, liver, stomach, pancreas, intestine, placenta, testis, ovaries, bone marrow, skin and hair follicle, cerebral cortex, and striatum (Stefulj et al., 2001; Venegas et al., 2012; Acuna-Castroviejo et al., 2014). The content of melatonin in these tissues varies and decreases with age to a similar extent as its pineal production (Sanchez-Hidalgo et al., 2009; Scholtens et al., 2016). After biosynthesis, pineal melatonin is immediately released into the circulatory system and reaches all biological fluids including cerebrospinal fluid, bile, saliva, synovial fluid, semen, ovarian follicular fluid, amniotic fluid, breast milk and tears (Illnerova et al., 1993; Acuna-Castroviejo et al., 2014; Carracedo et al., 2017). In physiological conditions, the extra-pineal melatonin does not seem to significantly contribute to the circulating levels of melatonin (Acuna-Castroviejo et al., 2014).

Historically, the isolation and identification of melatonin in the bovine pineal gland in 1958 (Lerner et al., 1958) was motivated by the potential dermatological effects of the pineal gland extracts reported early in 1917 with the hypothesis that melatonin could play a major role in the skin lightening (McCord and Allen, 1917). Unfortunately, the skin lightening properties could not be further demonstrated (Lerner et al., 1958; McElhinney et al., 1994) and the project was then abandoned. In the early 1990s, the research conducted on melatonin received popular attention with the media to the point that its multiple actions including its potential anti-ageing activities were at some extent described as "a miracle" or "a mystery" due to a lack of scientific evidence (Reppert and Weaver, 1995). Also, the role of melatonin in the physiological regulation of seasonal and circadian rhythms (Arendt, 1998), its antioxidant properties (Tan et al., 1993) and the presence of its specific receptors (Hattori et al., 1995) were progressively established in various experimental models. Since then, numerous studies have demonstrated additional properties of melatonin (for review, see Acuna-Castroviejo et al., 2014; Reiter et al., 2016; Favero et al., 2017), making the wide range of actions of melatonin a reality and not a myth. It is now well established that endogenous melatonin induces multiple physiological responses in humans including, amongst others, synchronizing the circadian rhythms of the body, regulation of the sleep-wakefulness cycle, antioxidant capacity, modulation of the immune system and the cardiovascular system (Hardeland et al., 2011; Reiter et al., 2016).

The health benefits of melatonin as a nutritional supplement are widely accepted [EFSA Panel on Dietetic Products,Nutrition and Allergies (NDA), 2011]. Currently, melatonin is only prescribed for the regulation of sleeping patterns such as in the jet lag (Herxheimer and Petrie, 2002) and adult sleep disorders (Auld et al., 2017). However, growing evidence supports the multi-organ effects of melatonin (Opie and Lecour, 2016) with a therapeutic potential in cardiovascular pathologies (Sun et al., 2016; Pandi-Perumal et al., 2017), neurodegenerative diseases (Trotti and Karroum, 2016), reproductive diseases (Reiter et al., 2009), bone diseases (osteopenia, osteoporosis, and periodontal disease) (Maria and Witt-Enderby, 2014), various cancers (Reiter et al., 2017), skin diseases (Fischer et al., 2013) and metabolic disorders (Nduhirabandi et al., 2012; Navarro-Alarcon et al., 2014). Interestingly, melatonin is present in edible plants, meats, fruits, beverage and other food stuffs (Dubbels et al., 1995; Hattori et al., 1995; Hardeland and Pandi-Perumal, 2005; Stürtz et al., 2011; Tan et al., 2014; Herrera et al., 2018). Although the levels of melatonin in foods are much lower than those of melatonin given as a nutritional supplement, consumption of foods rich in melatonin significantly increases circulating melatonin levels in the range of the physiological concentrations (Maldonado et al., 2009; Johns et al., 2013; Sae-Teaw et al., 2013). However, little is known about the influence of the dietary melatonin intake on human health. In this review, evidence for cardiovascular health benefits of endogenous melatonin and melatonin supplementation as a pharmacological agent or from the diet is discussed.

EVIDENCE FOR CARDIOVASCULAR BENEFITS OF ENDOGENOUS MELATONIN AND MELATONIN SUPPLEMENTATION

A strong inverse relationship exists between endogenous melatonin levels and cardiovascular disease (Dominguez-Rodriguez et al., 2010). Epidemiological studies report that both nocturnal melatonin synthesis and circulating levels are reduced in patients with coronary heart disease (Brugger et al., 1995; Altun et al., 2002; Dominguez-Rodriguez et al., 2002), hypertension (Kozirog et al., 2011; Dominguez-Rodriguez et al., 2014), heart failure (Girotti et al., 2003; Dzida et al., 2013; Kimak et al., 2014; Dominguez-Rodriguez et al., 2016) and cardiovascular risk conditions such as diabetes (McMullan et al., 2013) and obesity (Mantele et al., 2012). Incidence for adverse cardiac events, including myocardial infarction (Dominguez-Rodriguez et al., 2002), sudden cardiac death (Muller et al., 1987) and cardiac arrhythmias (Siegel et al., 1992) increases in the early morning, when circulating melatonin levels are considerably lower (Altun et al., 2002). Similarly, low melatonin secretion levels are associated with a greater risk of incidence for myocardial infarction in women with increased body mass index (McMullan et al., 2017), supporting the crucial role of endogenous melatonin in cardiovascular pathologies.

Solid evidence supports the beneficial effects of melatonin supplementation in various cardiovascular pathologies (for review, see Paulis and Simko, 2007; Reiter et al., 2010; Sun et al., 2016). Since the cardiovascular benefits of melatonin have recently been reviewed elsewhere (Sun et al., 2016), only the evidence for the benefits of melatonin supplementation in hypertension, pulmonary hypertension and ischemic heart disease is summarized below.

Melatonin and Hypertension and Other Vascular Pathologies

Endogenous and exogenous melatonin play an important role in hypertension and other vascular pathologies (Grossman et al., 2006; Paulis and Simko, 2007; Mozdzan et al., 2014; Simko et al., 2016). In animal studies, continuous light exposure or pinealectomy with a subsequent melatonin deficiency (Brown et al., 1991; Iigo et al., 1995) results in an increase in blood pressure (BP), a condition which is reversed by melatonin supplementation (Simko

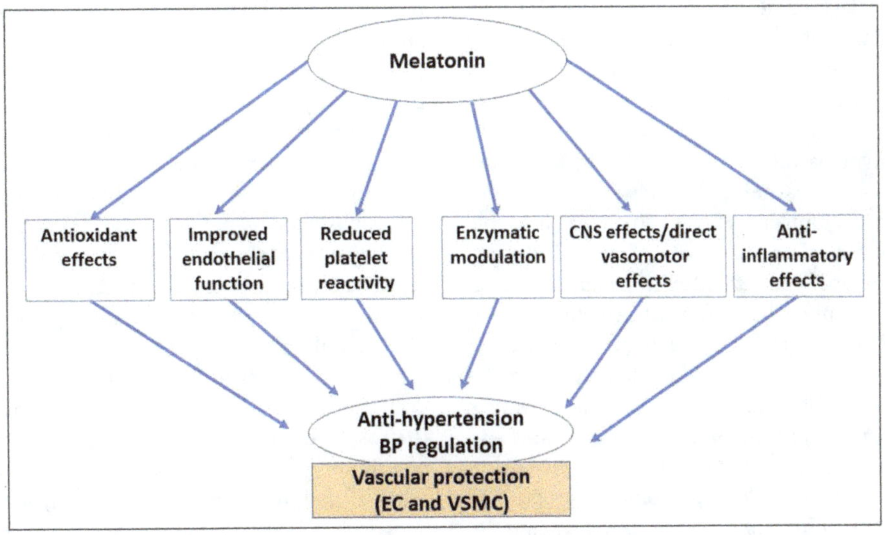

FIGURE 1 | Benefits of melatonin in hypertension and vascular pathologies. Melatonin positively affects vascular function (endothelial and smooth vascular muscle cells) via its direct and indirect regulatory effects associated with its strong antioxidant, anti-inflammatory, anti-lipidemic and vasomotor properties (vasodilation), all contributing to BP regulation (anti-hypertensive effects). These effects are also associated with enzymatic modulation, improved endothelial function and a reduced platelet reactivity. BP, blood pressure; CNS, central nervous system; EC, endothelial cells; CSMC, vascular smooth muscle cells.

et al., 2014b). A similar finding is also reported in spontaneous hypertensive (Tain et al., 2010) and metabolic syndrome (Kantar et al., 2015) rats supplemented with melatonin, thereby confirming its therapeutic potential in hypertension.

In human studies, night time melatonin administration (2–5 mg/day for 3–4 weeks) reduces BP values of hypertensive men (Scheer et al., 2004; Grossman et al., 2006) or women (Cagnacci et al., 2005) as well as normotensive women (Cagnacci et al., 2005). In patients with metabolic syndrome, melatonin supplementation (5 mg/day, 2 h before bedtime) for 2 months reduces the systolic and diastolic BP, low-density lipoprotein cholesterol (LDL-C), thiobarbituric acid reactive substrates (TBARS, a marker of oxidative stress) and increases antioxidant defense (catalase activity) (Kozirog et al., 2011). These beneficial effects are also observed in patients with essential hypertension receiving medical treatment where melatonin (3 mg or 5 mg for 4 weeks) restores the normal circadian rhythm of BP (Mozdzan et al., 2014). However, in patients with postural tachycardia syndrome (characterized by an excessive increase in heart rate with upright posture accompanied by palpitations), melatonin does not affect systolic BP despite a modest decrease in standing tachycardia (Green et al., 2014).

Figure 1 summarizes the mechanisms of actions of melatonin in hypertension and vascular pathologies. These mechanisms involve the indirect regulation of blood pressure via the central nervous system and the modulation of catecholamine secretion, the direct antioxidative and anti-inflammatory activities, the relaxation of the smooth muscle in blood vessels via α1-adrenergic receptors, nitric oxide production and calcium signaling, and the improvement of insulin signaling in insulin resistance states (Paulis and Simko, 2007; Paulis et al., 2010; Kantar et al., 2015; Agabiti-Rosei et al., 2017). In high-fat-fed rabbits, melatonin ameliorates vascular endothelial dysfunction and inflammation (Hu et al., 2013), the major contributing factors of the initiation and progression of atherosclerosis. Melatonin also improves endothelial vascular function and oxidative stress in type 2 diabetic rats (Salmanoglu et al., 2016) and insulin-resistant mice (Sartori et al., 2009). In a senescence-accelerated prone mice (SAMP8, a model of age-related vascular dysfunction), a 10-month melatonin treatment increases the expression of adiponectin and adiponectin receptor 1 in the visceral adipose tissue, the markers of vasoprotection (upregulation of eNOS and sirtuin 1 (SIRT1) and downregulation of endothelin-1 and iNOS) and inhibits aorta hypertrophy (by reducing oxidative stress and inflammation) while restoring the anticontractile effect of the perivascular adipose tissue (Agabiti-Rosei et al., 2017).

As a potential therapy in vascular disease, melatonin improves vascular function by decreasing the expression of platelets, endothelial cells adhesion molecule-1 (CD31), intercellular adhesion molecule-1 (ICAM-1), vascular cell adhesion molecule-1 (VCAM-1) and endothelin-1 (ET-1) while it increases endothelial nitric oxide synthase (eNOS), nuclear erythroid 2-related factor 2 (Nrf2), NAD(P)H quinone oxidoreductase 1 (NQO-1), catalytic glutamate cysteine ligase (GCLC) and heme oxygenase-1 (HO-1) in a rat model of a smoke-induced vascular injury (Wang et al., 2016). Similarly, in a population smoking more than 10 cigarettes per day for at least 1 year, supplementation of melatonin (3 mg/day for 2 weeks) reduces the concentration of fibrinogen and free fatty acids, the expression of ICAM-1, VCAM-1 and ET-1, and increases the expressions of Nrf2 and HO-1 (Wang et al., 2016).

Melatonin and Pulmonary Hypertension

Hypoxia-induced inflammation and excessive proliferation of pulmonary artery smooth muscle cells (PASMCs) play an important role in the pathological process of pulmonary hypertension and subsequent heart failure (Jin et al., 2014). Melatonin improves hypoxia-induced pulmonary hypertension by suppressing the hypoxia-induced high expression of proliferating cell nuclear antigen (PCNA), hypoxia-inducible factor-1α (HIF-1α), and nuclear factor-κB (NF-κB) (Jin et al., 2014). These effects are associated with inhibition of proliferation of PASMCs, the levels of phosphorylation of protein kinase B (PKB/Akt) and extracellular signal-regulated kinases1/2 (ERK1/2) caused by hypoxia (Jin et al., 2014), supporting the preventive activities of melatonin via its anti-inflammatory and anti-proliferative mechanisms. Similar findings are also reported in a new born sheep model of pulmonary hypertension (Torres et al., 2015). In this model, melatonin improves the vasodilator function of small pulmonary arteries, enhancing the endothelial-and muscular-dependent pathways associated with enhanced nitric oxide-dependent and independent vasodilator components and increased bioavailability of nitric oxide in lung tissue (Torres et al., 2015).

Melatonin and Cardiac Diseases

Melatonin induces multiple actions in various cardiac pathologies (Reiter et al., 2010; Lochner et al., 2013; Yang et al., 2014; Sun et al., 2016; Favero et al., 2017). In this paper, only relevant evidence in myocardial infarction, myocardial ischemia/reperfusion (I/R) injury and heart failure is included (**Tables 1, 2**).

Melatonin supplementation protects the heart in several experimental models of myocardial infarction and myocardial I/R injuries (Lochner et al., 2013; Yang et al., 2014). Tan and co-workers were first to demonstrate the beneficial effects of melatonin in isolated rat hearts subjected to cardiac I/R-induced arrhythmias: infusion of melatonin (during the period of ischemia and reperfusion or reperfusion only) reduces premature ventricular contraction and ventricular fibrillation due to occlusion and reopening of the anterior descending coronary artery (Tan et al., 1998). This finding is also reported in other animal models of cardiac arrhythmias (Lagneux et al., 2000; Sahna et al., 2002; Diez et al., 2013), confirming the therapeutic potential for melatonin in reducing the incidence of sudden cardiac death (Sahna et al., 2002). Additional studies show that short-and long-term melatonin supplementation is cardioprotective in various *in vivo* and *ex vivo* myocardial models of I/R injury (Lagneux et al., 2000; Lochner et al., 2006; Lamont et al., 2011; Nduhirabandi et al., 2011, 2014, 2016; Maarman et al., 2015; Zhai et al., 2017a,b). In these studies, administration of melatonin before or after ischemia preserves the microstructure of the cardiomyocyte and reduced myocardial I/R injury as indicated by a reduction in myocardial infarct size (for review, see Lochner et al., 2013).

The mechanisms of cardioprotection induced with melatonin against myocardial infarction or I/R injury are complex and not well understood. As presented in the **Figure 2**, melatonin may directly and indirectly affect cardiac pathologies via multiple mechanisms including amongst others, antihypertensive, antilipidemic, antiadrenergic, and immunomodulatory activities. It also reduces oxidative stress, apoptosis, necrosis, mitochondrial permeability transition pore opening, lipid peroxidation and inflammation (for more details, see Yang et al., 2014). Recent findings in the mechanisms of melatonin-induced cardioprotection suggest the involvement of the intracellular survival signaling pathways including, mainly, the activation of the survivor activating factor enhancement (SAFE), the reperfusion injury salvage kinase risk (RISK), Notch1 and sirtuins (SIRT1 and SIRT 3) signaling pathways (Lochner et al., 2013; Nduhirabandi et al., 2014, 2016; Yu et al., 2017b; Zhai et al., 2017a) as well as the crucial role of the mitochondria in cell death and survival (necrosis, apoptosis, autophagy, mitophagy) (Petrosillo et al., 2009; Pei et al., 2016; Hu et al., 2017). The description of these cardioprotective mechanisms is beyond the focus of the present paper (for details, see Lochner et al., 2013; Yang et al., 2014; Sun et al., 2016).

Melatonin supplementation is also beneficial for the treatment of pathological cardiac remodeling and heart failure (Chua et al., 2016; Hu et al., 2017; Zhai et al., 2017b). For example, in a mouse model of myocardial infarction, melatonin significantly reduces adverse left ventricle remodeling and post-myocardial infarction remodeling and dysfunction by increasing autophagy, reducing apoptosis, and reversing mitochondrial dysfunction (Hu et al., 2017). As underlying mechanisms, these effects are associated with a significant activation of adenosine monophosphate-activated protein kinase (AMPK) and an inhibition of macrophage-stimulating 1 (MST) phosphorylation while increasing the expression of SIRT1 and SIRT3, peroxisome proliferator-activated receptor gamma (PPARγ) co-activator 1-protein (PGC-1α), the translocase of the outer membrane 70 (Tom 70), a receptor for translocases in the outer mitochondrial membrane complex (Hu et al., 2017; Pei et al., 2017; Yu et al., 2017b). Furthermore, in a murine model of pathological cardiac hypertrophy induced by transverse aortic constriction (TAC), melatonin supplementation for 4–8 weeks reverses the pathological hypertrophy via the reduction of the pulmonary congestion (Zhai et al., 2017b). These effects are associated with an upregulation of the level of α-myosin heavy chain expression, a downregulation of the levels of β-myosin heavy chain and atrial natriuretic peptide expression, an inhibition of oxidative stress (as expressed by the levels of malondialdehyde (MDA) and superoxide dismutase (SOD) activity), and the activation of PGC-1β as well as the reduction of the cardiac fibrosis (Zhai et al., 2017b). Similar protective effects of melatonin with its antifibrotic properties are also reported in a rat model of cardiorenal syndrome (Chua et al., 2016) and in other animal models of heart failure such as myocardial damage induced by chronic intermittent hypoxia (Yeung et al., 2015), isoproterenol (Patel et al., 2010) or epinephrine (Vazan and Ravingerova, 2015), chemotherapy drugs (Liu et al., 2002), sepsis-induced myocardial injury (An et al., 2016), and diabetic cardiomyopathy (Zhang et al., 2017).

In view of the above benefits in animal studies, melatonin supplementation is highly regarded as an effective therapy in cardiac diseases (Yang et al., 2014; Opie and Lecour, 2016;

TABLE 1 | The effect of melatonin supplementation on cardiac diseases: animal studies.

Animal model		Genre and strain	Age or weight	Sample size	Melatonin administration		Effect	References
					Dose	Mode and duration		
Arrhythmias	Myocardial I/R Arrhythmias in normal rats (*in vitro*)	Male Sprague-Dawley rats	280–320 g	$n = 10$/group	1, 10, 50 μM	In the perfusate either during entire experiment or 2 min before reperfusion	Cardioprotection	Tan et al., 1998
	Myocardial I/R Arrhythmias normal rats (*ex vivo*)	Male Wistar rats	280–350 g	$n = 6$/group	1 or 10 mg/kg	I.P. at 10 min before ischemia	Cardioprotection	Lagneux et al., 2000
	Myocardial I/R Arrhythmias in pinealectomized rats (*in vivo*)	Male Wistar rats	150–200 g	$n = 16$/group	0.4 / 4 mg/kg	I.V. at 10 min before ischemia or just prior to reperfusion	Cardioprotection No effect in non-pinealectomized rats	Sahna et al., 2002
	Myocardial I/R Arrhythmias in spontaneously hypertensive and fructose-induced metabolic syndrome rats (*ex vivo*)	Male Wistar Kyoto (WKY) rats	12 wk	$n = 12$/group	50 μM	In the perfusate at reperfusion (15 min regional ischemia)	Cardioprotection	Diez et al., 2013
Myocardial I/R injury	Myocardial I/R in normal rabbits (*in vivo*)	Male New Zealand white rabbits	2.2–3.2 kg	$n = 8$/group	10 mg/kg/day	I.V. at 10 min before ischemia and 15 min before reperfusion	No effect	Dave et al., 1998
	Myocardial I/R injury in normal rats (*ex vivo*)	Male Wistar rats	250–300 g	$n = 6$/group	50 μM	In the perfusate for 15 min before ischemia and during 2h of reperfusion	Cardioprotection	Petrosillo et al., 2009
	Myocardial I/R injury in diet induced obesity rats (*ex vivo*)	Male Wistar rats	4 wk 180–220 g	$n = 6$/group	4 mg/kg/day	Oral for 6 or 3 wk	Cardioprotection	Nduhirabandi et al., 2014
	Myocardial I/R injury in normal rats and mice (*in vivo* and *ex vivo*)	Male Wistar rats and C57BL6 mice	240–300 g (Rats) 12–16 wk (Mice)	$n > 5$/group	75 ng/L	Oral for 2 wk before I/R injury	Cardioprotection	Lamont et al., 2015
	Myocardial I/R injury in normal mice (*ex vivo*)	Male C57BL mice	12–16 wk	$n = 6$/group	75 ng/L	In the perfusate before ischemia	Cardioprotection	Nduhirabandi et al., 2016
	Myocardial I/R injury in normal rats (*ex vivo*)	Male Wistar rats	240–300 g	$n = 36$ (5–7/group)	75 ng/L	In the perfusate before ischemia	Cardioprotection	Nduhirabandi et al., 2016
	Myocardial I/R injury in a closed-chest porcine model in normal pigs (*in vivo*)	Female Danish Landrace pigs	Not given	$n = 20$	5 mg/kg (0.4 mg/mL)	IV infusion at 5 min before reperfusion for 30 min and intracoronary infusion at 1 min to reperfusion for 2 min	No effect	Ekelof et al., 2016
	Myocardial I/R injury in hyper- glycaemic rats (*in vivo*)	Male Sprague-Dawley rats	200–220 g	$n = 6$/group	10 mg/kg/day	I.V. at 5 min before and during ischemia and 4 h reperfusion	Cardioprotection	Yu et al., 2017a
	Myocardial I/R injury in diabetic rats (*in vivo*)	Male Sprague-Dawley rats	8 wk 180–220 g	$n = 6$/group	10 mg/kg/day	Oral for 5 days and I.P at 10 min before reperfusion	Cardioprotection	Yu et al., 2017b
	Myocardial I/R injury in normal fed mice (*in vivo*)	Male C57BL/6 mice	8 wk 20–22 g	$n = 8$ group	20 mg/kg/day	I.P at 10 min before reperfusion.	Cardioprotection	Zhai et al., 2017a

(Continued)

TABLE 1 | Continued

Animal model		Genre and strain	Age or weight	Sample size	Melatonin administration		Effect	References
					Dose	Mode and duration		
Heart failure	Myocardial infarction-induced heart failure in normal rats (*in vivo*)	Male Wistar albino rats	200–250 g	$n = 6$/group	10 mg/kg/day	I.P for 4 wk	Cardioprotection	Sehirli et al., 2013
	Post-infarction cardiac remodeling and dysfunction in normal mice (*in vivo*)	Male C57BL Mice	8–12 wk	$n = 6$/group	20 mg/kg/day	Oral for 1 wk before MI	Cardioprotection	Hu et al., 2017
	Isoproterenol-induced myocardial infarction in normal rats (*in vivo*)	Male Sprague-Dawley rats	10 wk 175–225 g	$n = 6$/group	10 mg/kg/day	I.P. for 1 wk	Cardioprotection	Patel et al., 2010
	Isoproterenol-induced heart failure in normal rats (*in vivo*)	Male Wistar rats	12 wk	$n = 12$/group	10 mg/kg/day	Oral for 2 or 4 wk	Cardioprotection But no effect on LV or RV hypertrophy	Simko et al., 2014a
	Pathological cardiac hypertrophy induced by transverse aortic constriction in normal mice (*in vivo*)	Male C57BL/6 mice	20–25g 8–10 wk	$n = 85$ ($n =$ 10–40/group)	20 mg/kg/day	Oral for 4 or 8 wk	Cardioprotection	Zhai et al., 2017b
Pulmonary hypertension	Chronic hypoxia-induced RV hypertrophy and pulmonary hypertension (*in vivo*)	Male Sprague–Dawley rats	200–250g	$n = 7$/group	15 mg/kg/day	I.P. morning /wk prior to hypoxic and 4 wk hypoxia	Cardioprotection	Jin et al., 2014
	Monocrotaline-induced pulmonary hypertensive rats (*ex vivo* heart perfusion)	Male Long Evans rats	150–175g	$n = 6$/group	75 ng/L 6 mg/kg/day	Oral for 2 or 4 wk	Cardioprotection	Maarman et al., 2015
Hypertensive heart disease	Continuous light-induced hypertensive rats (6 wk) (*in vivo*)	Male Wistar rats	12 wk	$n = 10$/group	10 mg/kg/day	Oral for 6 wk	Cardioprotection But no effect on LV hypertrophy	Simko et al., 2014b

I/R, ischemia reperfusion; MI, myocardial infarction; LV, left ventricular; RV, right ventricular; IV, intravenous injection; IP, intraperitoneal injection; wk, week.

TABLE 2 | The effect of melatonin supplementation on cardiac diseases: human studies.

Type of the study	Sample size (*n*)	Age of patients (years)	Male/female ratio	Melatonin administration (dose, delivery mode and duration)	Effect	References
A randomized triple-blinded, placebo-controlled study including patients undergoing coronary artery bypass grafting (CABG) surgery	58	58.1 ± 9.8 (42–75)	14/1	10 mg tablet once daily for 4 wk before surgery	Cardioprotection	Haghjooy-Javanmard et al., 2013
A prospective, randomized, double-blinded, placebo-controlled clinical trial including patients undergoing surgery for abdominal aortic aneurisms (AAA)	50	67 (45–80)	23/3	50 mg infusion over a 2-h period intra-operative, and oral 10 mg for the first 3 nights after surgery	Cardioprotection	Gogenur et al., 2014
A double blinded placebo-control study including patients undergoing coronary artery bypass grafting (CABG) surgery	45	52.3 (45–65) and 53.9 (45–64)	13/2 (10 mg) and 11/4 (20 mg)	10 and 20 mg, capsules once daily for 5 days before surgery	Cardioprotection	Dwaich et al., 2016
A prospective, multicenter, randomized, double-blind, placebo-controlled study for the Melatonin adjunct in the acute myocardial infarction treated with angioplasty (MARIA) trial	125	57.3 ± 10	50/13	IV: 51.7 μmol for 60 min starting immediately before percutaneous coronary intervention and IC bolus of 8.6 μmol through-PCI guiding catheter within the first 60 seconds of reperfusion	No effect	Dominguez-Rodriguez et al., 2017b
A *post-hoc* analysis of the randomized, double-blinded, placebo-controlled study for the Melatonin adjunct in the acute myocardial infarction treated with angioplasty (patients with ST-elevation myocardial infarction) (MARIA) trial	125 1st, 2nd,3rd tertiles: 41, 43, 41	1st: 54 ± 10 2nd: 58 ± 10 3rd: 60 ± 11	1st: 18/3 2nd: 20/6 3rd: 18/5	IV 51.7 μmol for 60 min starting immediately before percutaneous coronary intervention and IC bolus of 8.6 μmol through PCI-guiding catheter within the first 60 seconds of reperfusion	Cardioprotection in the 1st tertile (early after symptom onset) No effect in 2nd and 3rd tertiles	Dominguez-Rodriguez et al., 2017a
A randomized, double-blinded, placebo-controlled trial for intracoronary and systemic melatonin to patients with ST-elevation myocardial infarction (IMPACT) trial	48	61.7 (56.2–66.9)	20/3	50 mg; IC and IV infusion starting immediately after PCI with a flow rate fixed at 80 ml/h for 6 h	No effect	Ekeloef et al., 2017

PCI, percutaneous coronary intervention; IV, intravenous; IC, Intracoronary; wk, week.

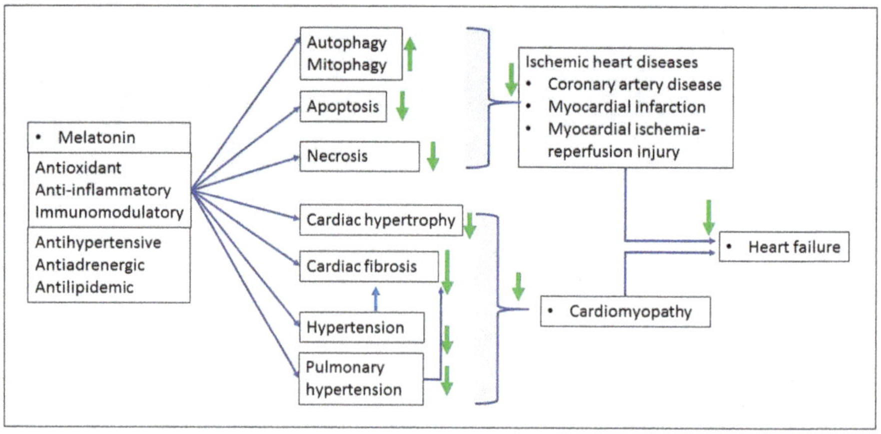

FIGURE 2 | Benefits of melatonin in cardiac pathologies. Melatonin, via its antioxidant, anti-inflammatory and immunomodulatory properties protects against ischemic heart disease as well as subsequent ischemic heart failure characterized by myocardial cell death (necrosis, apoptosis, autophagy) and cardiac dysfunction. Hypertension and pulmonary hypertension induce both cardiac fibrosis and pathological hypertrophy (cardiomyopathy) and subsequent heart failure. Melatonin reverses these effects as indicated with green arrows (↓: increase, ↑: reduce).

Sun et al., 2016). Unfortunately, very few clinical trials have investigated the effects of exogenous melatonin in cardiac diseases (Dominguez-Rodriguez et al., 2007; Gogenur et al., 2014; Ekelof et al., 2016) (**Table 2**). In patients undergoing surgery for abdominal aortic aneurisms, an infusion of 50 mg melatonin over a 2 h period followed by oral administration of 10 mg melatonin for the first three nights after surgery, protects the heart against reperfusion injury by reducing cardiac morbidity as well as the occurrence of myocardial ischemia after abdominal aortic aneurism repair (Gogenur et al., 2014). In patients undergoing coronary artery bypass grafting surgery, melatonin supplementation (10 or 20 mg capsule once a day) increases significantly the ejection fraction and the outcomes together with a remarkable decrease in pro-inflammatory and apoptotic markers, supporting its promising benefits in myocardial I/R injury (Dwaich et al., 2016).

The therapeutic potential of melatonin in cardiac diseases has recently received controversial comments with the publication of the study of melatonin as an adjunct in patients with acute myocardial infarction undergoing primary angioplasty (MARIA trial) (Dominguez-Rodriguez et al., 2007, 2017a,b; Hausenloy et al., 2017). Despite the acceptable safety and tolerability, the MARIA trial reports a lack of cardioprotection in patients treated with formulation of melatonin in polyethylene glycol solution (51.7 μmoles given 60 min before intervention and a bolus of 8.6 μmoles 60 min after intervention) (Dominguez-Rodriguez et al., 2017b). A lack of beneficial effects of melatonin is also reported in other clinical study (Ekeloef et al., 2017). Interestingly, preclinical testing showed that melatonin fails to protect the heart in a closed-chest porcine model of acute myocardial infarction (Halladin et al., 2014; Ekelof et al., 2016) and in a rabbit model of myocardial I/R injury (Dave et al., 1998). It is possible that the intracoronary and intravenous administrations, as opposed to the preferred oral administration, may contribute to the neutral outcomes as suggested by other studies (Dwaich et al., 2016). In addition, ischemic duration and other methodological issues (for review, see Heusch, 2017) may also play a role in the outcomes of above clinical trials, suggesting a re-evaluation of the therapeutic effects of melatonin in a well-planed study.

In the light of the very low physiological concentrations of melatonin, it remains unknown whether consumption of melatonin-rich foods, which increases circulating melatonin concentration into physiological range, may be more effective for cardioprotection.

OVERVIEW OF CARDIOVASCULAR BENEFITS OF MELATONIN-RICH FOOD

The presence of melatonin in edible plants and other types of food is well established (Tan et al., 2012, 2014). Melatonin-rich foods include various food components from both animal and plant origins such as chicken, lamb, pork, cow milk, strawberries, tomatoes, olives, grapes, wines, cereals and cherries (for review, see Iriti et al., 2010; Tan et al., 2014) (see **Table 3**). Interestingly, melatonin concentrations are significantly higher in plants than in animals (Byeon et al., 2014). This is most likely due to differences between the biosynthetic pathways of melatonin in plants and animals (see **Figure 3**). Plants synthesize tryptophan themselves via the shikimic acid pathway, which increases their melatonin synthetic capacity (Byeon et al., 2014). Animals produce melatonin from tryptophan (essential amino acid from the food) (Byeon et al., 2014). For more details on the biosynthesis of melatonin as well as the dietary source of melatonin, see reviews (Park et al., 2013; Byeon et al., 2014; Tan et al., 2016).

It is likely that the consumption of melatonin-rich food influences endogenous melatonin production (for review, see Peuhkuri et al., 2012). For example, in chickens, circulating melatonin levels increase more than 3.5-folds 1.5 h after the intake of chick food composed of corn, milo, beans, and rice (3 ng/g melatonin) (Hattori et al., 1995). A similar observation is

TABLE 3 | Some examples of melatonin content in different plants and foods.

Plant or food	Melatonin content	References
Tomato	3–114 ng/g	Stürtz et al., 2011
Walnuts	3–4 ng/g	Reiter et al., 2005
Cereals (rice, barley)	300–1,000 pg/g	Hattori et al., 1995
Strawberry	1–11 ng/g	Iriti et al., 2010
Olive oil	53–119 pg/ml	de la Puerta et al., 2007
Wine	50–230 pg/ml	Murch et al., 2010
Beer	52–170 pg/ml	Maldonado et al., 2009
Cow's milk (unprocessed)	3–25 pg/ml	Májovský et al., 2017
Night-time milk	10–40 ng/ml	Tan et al., 2014
Whole yellow corn	0.28–1.3 ng/g	Tan et al., 2014
Whole chicken meat and skin	0.23–2.3 ng/g	Tan et al., 2014
Chicken heart and liver blend	1.0–1.2 ng/g	Tan et al., 2014

reported in other studies after the consumption of melatonin-rich foods such as walnuts, olive oil, wine, fruits and legumes as well as germinated kidney beans (Peuhkuri et al., 2012; Johns et al., 2013; Sae-Teaw et al., 2013; Tan et al., 2014; Aguilera et al., 2016). However, it remains unclear whether the acute variation of circulating melatonin levels induced by the consumption of melatonin-rich foods correlates with their influence on the cardiovascular system (Bazzano et al., 2001; Al Abdrabalnabi et al., 2017; Aune et al., 2017; Micha et al., 2017). The evidence for cardiovascular benefits of some melatonin containing foods including, walnuts, tropical fruits and grape products are reviewed below.

Walnuts Consumption

Long and short-term observational and intervention studies show that regular consumption of walnuts reduces the risk of CVDs (Kris-Etherton, 2014; Al Abdrabalnabi et al., 2017). In an elderly population, a daily consumption of walnuts improves blood lipids and BP after a one-year trial (Al Abdrabalnabi et al., 2017). In rats fed walnuts an increase in the blood concentration of melatonin and antioxidant capacity is observed (Reiter et al., 2005) However, the correlation between the variation of melatonin levels and the cardiovascular benefits of walnuts remains to be established.

Tropical Fruits Consumption

Fruits consumption is associated with reduced CVDs (Aune et al., 2017; Micha et al., 2017). Melatonin is present in tropical fruits, namely banana, pineapple, orange, papaya, mango (Johns et al., 2013). Apart from papaya and mango, the consumption of these fruits increases the circulating melatonin as measured by 6-sulphatoxymelatonin in healthy volunteers (Johns et al., 2013). Interestingly, the rise in serum melatonin levels is positively associated with the antioxidant capacity but not the melatonin content in fruits (Johns et al., 2013; Sae-Teaw et al., 2013). However, it remains unknown whether increasing circulating melatonin levels with fruits consumption is beneficial for patients with reduced levels of endogenous melatonin or CVDs and other illnesses involving oxidative damage.

Grapes and Wine Consumption

Chronic and moderate consumption of red wine is associated with a reduced risk of CVDs and other diseases such as diabetes and neurological diseases (Opie and Lecour, 2007). Melatonin is present in grapes and wines; and consumption of grape products may affect endogenous melatonin levels (Iriti, 2009; Murch et al., 2010; Meng et al., 2017a). In young, middle-aged and elderly individuals, intake of 200 mL of grape juice twice a day significantly increases urinary 6-sulfatoxymelatonin and total antioxidant capacity (Gonzalez-Flores et al., 2012). However, whether grape juice-induced elevated circulating melatonin is associated with improved disease conditions is still unknown.

Interestingly, despite the presence of melatonin in grape, melatonin found in wine is mainly synthesized by yeast during alcoholic fermentation (Rodriguez-Naranjo et al., 2011). The concentrations of melatonin in human serum significantly increase after drinking alcoholic beer (Maldonado et al., 2009). Conversely, other studies report a decrease in endogenous melatonin production following alcohol consumption (Peuhkuri et al., 2012) thereby making the influence of alcohol found in wine on melatonin levels inconsistent. Nevertheless, as described below, melatonin present in red wine significantly induces cardioprotective effects (Lamont et al., 2015).

ROLE OF DIETARY MELATONIN IN CVDs

Dietary melatonin refers commonly to melatonin content that is present in diet or melatonin-rich food (Iriti and Varoni, 2015; Meng et al., 2017b). Very few studies have investigated the role of dietary melatonin in CVD. These are limited to the exploration of the cardioprotective effect of melatonin in red wine against myocardial I/R injury (Lamont et al., 2011, 2012, 2015; Nduhirabandi et al., 2016) and pulmonary hypertension (Maarman et al., 2015).

Dietary Melatonin and Myocardial I/R Injury

Using both *in vivo* and *in vitro* models of myocardial I/R, studies from our laboratory demonstrate that the presence of melatonin in red wine may contributes to the protective effect of red wine against lethal I/R damage (Lamont et al., 2011, 2015). This is supported by the findings that: (1) lowering the alcohol content of red wine does not alter its cardioprotective properties (Lamont et al., 2012); and (2) melatonin, given acutely and directly to the isolated heart at the concentration found in wine (75 ng/L) protects the isolated mouse and rat hearts against I/R injury by reducing myocardial infarct size and improving functional recovery (Lamont et al., 2011). (3) The cardioprotective effect of the consumption chronic and moderate red wine against I/R damage is partially abolished in the presence of prazosin, an inhibitor of melatonin receptor type 3 (M3) (Lamont et al., 2015). Further findings from our laboratory show that drinking water supplemented daily with a moderate amount of red wine or melatonin given at the concentration found in the red wine (75 pg/mL) for 14 days protects the rat and mouse hearts subjected

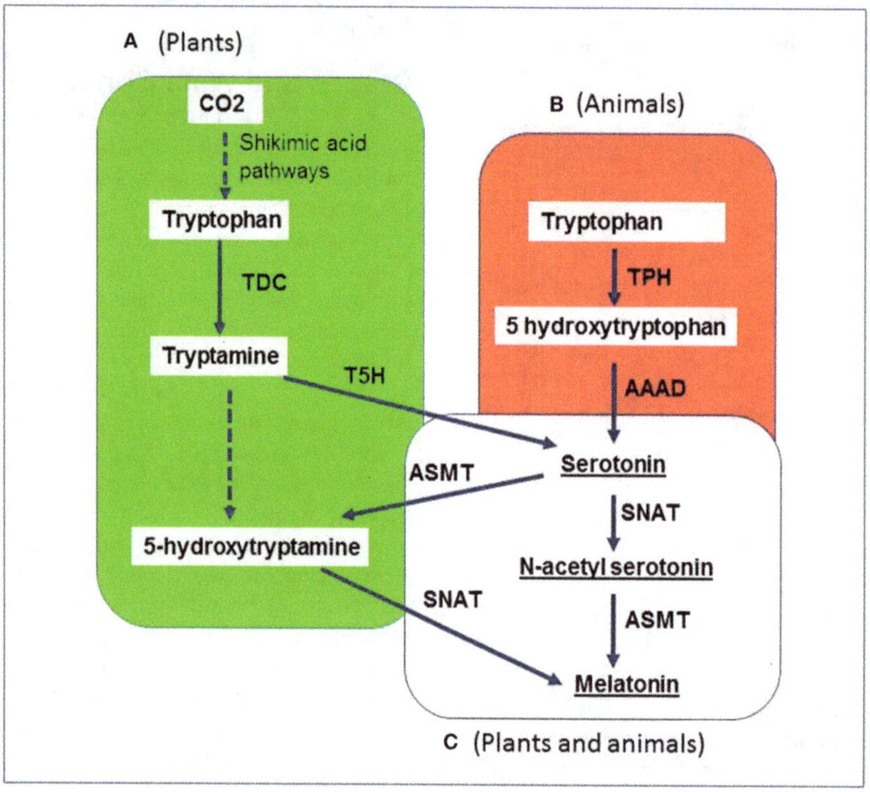

FIGURE 3 | Simplified representation of the biosynthetic pathways of melatonin in plants and animals. Tryptophan is the common precursor of melatonin in all species. **(A)** In plants (green), melatonin is synthesized under two pathways: (1) tryptophan-tryptamine-serotonin-N-acetyl serotonin-melatonin pathway (under normal growth conditions); (2) tryptophan-tryptamine-serotonin-5-methoxytryptamine-melatonin pathway (upon senescence, when plants produce large amounts of serotonin); **(B)** In animals (red); tryptophan is converted in serotonin via hydroxytryptophan; **(C)** In both plants and animals (white), melatonin production from serotonin is the same two-step process and includes the conversion of serotonin to N-acetylserotonin by the rate-limiting enzyme AA-NAT (arylalkylamine N-acetyltransferase) also called as serotonin N-acetyltransferase followed by the conversion of N-acetylserotonin to melatonin by acetylserotonin O-methyltransferase. CO2, carbon dioxide; TPH, tryptophan hydroxylase; AAAD, aromatic amino acid decarboxylase; SNAT, serotonin N-acetyltransferase; ASMT, N-acetylserotonin O-methyltransferase; TDC, tryptophan decarboxylase; T5H, tryptamine 5-hydroxylase.

to *in vivo* or *ex vivo* I/R by reducing their infarct size (Lamont et al., 2015).

The mechanism of cardioprotection induced with dietary melatonin is complex and still under investigation. As indicated above, melatonin exhibits its physiological functions through its antioxidant, anti-inflammatory, immune-modulatory and vasomotor activities (Pandi-Perumal et al., 2006). Acute (Lamont et al., 2011; Nduhirabandi et al., 2016) and chronic (Lamont et al., 2015) physiological concentrations of melatonin at the concentration found in red wine protect the heart against I/R injury via its membrane receptors related cell survival signaling (Lamont et al., 2015; Nduhirabandi et al., 2016). This is associated with an increased level of activation of myocardial signal transducer and activator of transcription 3 (STAT3) prior to ischemic insult by 79% (Lamont et al., 2011). The importance of STAT3 activation is that it is associated with the activation of SAFE pathway, a well-known powerful cardioprotective signaling pathway (Lamont et al., 2015; Nduhirabandi et al., 2016). Interestingly, luzindole, a specific inhibitor of membrane melatonin receptors 1 and 2 (MT1 and MT 2) (2.3 mg/kg/day, intraperitoneally) does not affect wine treatment, while prazosin, an inhibitor of M3 receptor (2.5 mg/kg/day, intraperitoneally) abolishes wine-induced cardioprotection, therefore suggesting the crucial role of both melatonin and M3 receptor in the cardioprotective effect of red wine (Lamont et al., 2015).

However, how moderate red wine consumption or dietary melatonin affects the SAFE pathway is still unclear. Our recent data suggest that melatonin confers cardioprotection via toll-like receptor 4 (TLR4) which, in turn, activates tumor necrosis factor-α (TNFα)/STAT3 pathway (Nduhirabandi et al., 2016). In view of the pro-inflammatory effects of TLR4 stimulation (Yang et al., 2000), this finding is surprising considering the well-known anti-inflammatory activities of melatonin with its TLR4 suppressing activities (Hu et al., 2013; Mauriz et al., 2013); but it is consistent with the current view of melatonin as an immune system buffer acting as a stimulant under basal or immunosuppressive conditions or as an anti-inflammatory compound in the presence of exacerbated immune responses (for review, see Carrillo-Vico et al., 2013).

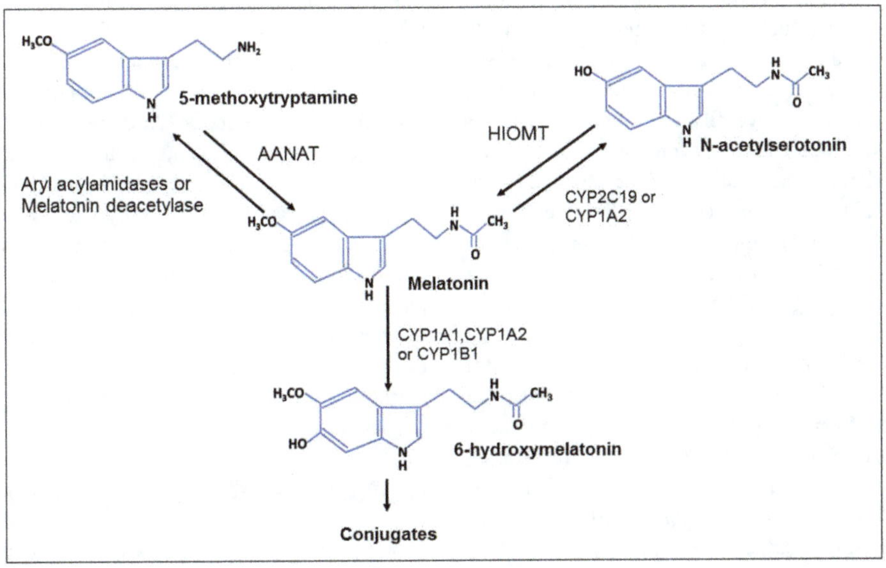

FIGURE 4 | Metabolism of melatonin: enzymatic pathways. Melatonin given orally is principally metabolized in the liver by cytochrome P-450 isoforms (CYP1A1, CYP1A2, and CYP1B1) in 6-hydroxylation to yield 6-hydroxymelatonin which is thereafter conjugated with sulfates to 6-sulfatoxymelatonin and eliminated in urine. Melatonin may also be transformed by deacetylation or by CYP2C19 and CYP1A2 mediated O-demethylation in 5-methoxytryptamine or N-acetylserotonin, respectively. N-acetylserotonin and 5-methoxytryptamine can be converted in melatonin by hydroxyindole-O-methyltransferase (HIOMT) and arylalkylamine N-acetyltransferase (AANAT).

Dietary Melatonin and Pulmonary Hypertension

Pulmonary hypertension is associated with an increased oxidative stress and leads to right ventricle (RV) hypertrophy and cardiac fibrosis with the hallmarks of the heart failure (Maarman et al., 2015). A single subcutaneous injection of monocrotaline (80 mg/kg) induces pulmonary hypertension with RV hypertrophy and dysfunction, increase in interstitial fibrosis and plasma oxidative stress (Maarman et al., 2015). In this model, a chronic dietary melatonin treatment (75 ng/L) reduces RV hypertrophy, improves RV function, reduces plasma oxidative stress and reduces cardiac interstitial fibrosis, therefore supporting the beneficial effects of curative and preventive treatments of dietary melatonin in pulmonary hypertension (Maarman et al., 2015). These effects of melatonin are associated with a reduction in oxidative stress and an increase in enzymatic and non-enzymatic antioxidant capacity (Maarman et al., 2015; Torres et al., 2015).

CURRENT CHALLENGES, LIMITATIONS AND NEW PERSPECTIVES FOR THE USE OF MELATONIN IN CVDs

The dietary supplementation of melatonin appears as an effective option to compensate the physiological decline in the production of pineal gland melatonin with ageing; however, the role of dietary melatonin in health and disease is still not well established (Kennaway, 2017; Meng et al., 2017b). The strong limitation for the studies of dietary melatonin is the lack of standardized methods to determine melatonin concentration in foods with adequate sample treatment to obtain accurate results, thus making some of its proposed benefits hard to swallow (Kennaway, 2017). In addition, most of the studies on dietary melatonin measure melatonin content in food, but very few evaluate the bioavailability of melatonin after melatonin-rich food consumption. It is well established that the bioavailability of melatonin after oral and intravenous melatonin administration in human is very low (approximately 15%) with a maximal half-life of 10–60 min (Harpsoe et al., 2015). Although other factors (such as age, disease conditions, specific drugs, cigarette smoking and caffeine intake) may also influence the bioavailability of melatonin which is mostly metabolized by the enzymatic catabolism in the liver (Ma et al., 2005). As shown in the **Figure 4**, melatonin is principally metabolized in the liver by cytochrome P-450 isoforms (CYP1A1, CYP1A2, and CYP1B1) in 6-hydroxylation to yield 6-hydroxymelatonin which is thereafter conjugated with sulfates to 6-sulfatoxymelatonin and eliminated in urine (Ma et al., 2005; Pandi-Perumal et al., 2006). Melatonin may also be transformed to a less extend by CYP2C19 and CYP1A2 mediated O-demethylation in N-acetylserotonin (N-acetyl-5-hydroxytryptamine) or by deacetylation to 5-methoxytryptamine which can be reconverted to melatonin (Ma et al., 2005).

Furthermore, how melatonin-rich food contributes to the overall endogenous melatonin production is complex and still unclear. Besides the melatonin content in the food, food intake may also influence endogenous melatonin concentration, suggesting that the overall beneficial effect could be a result of a combined action of more components found in these food stuffs. Indeed, an increase in blood melatonin levels may be a result of other components found in food that may stimulate endogenous melatonin production such as in the case of ingestion of tryptophan (Huether et al., 1992; Bravo et al., 2013) or serotonin (Esteban et al., 2004). These possible effects make more challenging the delimitation of the contribution of the dietary melatonin to the overall cardiovascular benefits of melatonin-rich foods. Moreover, to avoid bias due to drug interaction, the drugs that are metabolized by cytochrome P-450 such as fluvoxamine, caffeine, and oral contraceptives need to be considered (Harpsoe et al., 2015). Since these drugs compete with melatonin for the same enzyme, they may increase the plasma levels of melatonin after exogenous melatonin administration (Harpsoe et al., 2015).

Due to the very low bioavailability of melatonin after oral or intravenous administration, new developments to optimize the intake of melatonin as supplement or food consider various alternative administrative routes, namely: intranasal, transdermal, subcutaneous, and oral transmucosal (such as sublingual and trans buccal) administration or other forms of preparations (spray, elastic liposomes, gels, pastes) (for review, see Zetner et al., 2016). These alternative routes are very important because they: (1) bypass the liver metabolism, (2) are painless, and (3) provide possible sustained release with a subsequent increase in the bioavailability of melatonin (Zetner et al., 2016).

Although melatonin supplementation is safe in patients with myocardial infarction (Dominguez-Rodriguez et al., 2017b) and nocturnal hypertension (Grossman et al., 2011; Simko et al., 2016), melatonin is contra-indicated for patients with high normal BP to avoid the danger of the diurnal arterial hypertension (Rechcinski et al., 2010). In addition, in children with age of 1-year, increased serum melatonin levels may be associated with severe heart failure (Wu et al., 2017), raising the alarming issue of a high dose of melatonin supplementation in children at this age. While this association is surprising in view of low circulating melatonin levels in adult patients with heart failure, it may be explained by either compensatory mechanisms (of heart failure) or potential detrimental effects of high dose of melatonin in infants (Wu et al., 2017).

Thus far, there is no evidence for the dose-dependent effect of melatonin in the context of cardiovascular diseases. Current data show that both high and low doses of short-term melatonin treatment confer cardiovascular protection in experimental animal models. According to recent clinical trials, although the overall melatonin treatment is safe, it may cause mild adverse effects from transient sedation, daytime sleepiness, mild headache to worsening of dyspnea, and combining melatonin with any drug associated with these effects is contra-indicated (for review, see Andersen et al., 2016). However, further investigation is needed to determine the optimal dose of melatonin and the effects of long-term of melatonin supplementation in humans.

Recent data from clinical studies using melatonin in cardiac diseases show more inconsistencies regarding its cardioprotective effects (Andersen et al., 2016; Dominguez-Rodriguez et al., 2017b; Ekeloef et al., 2017). Apart from dosage issues and mode of administration, previous failures could be partially explained by the use of young and healthy animals with eventual lack of various cardiovascular risk factors, comorbidities and comedications which are characteristics of patients suffering an acute myocardial infarction or undergoing cardiovascular surgery (Heusch, 2017). Considering the current disappointment, further well-planned preclinical and clinical studies are needed to better delineate the cardiovascular benefits of melatonin.

CONCLUSION

In summary, preclinical studies clearly suggest the cardiovascular health benefit of both endogenous and supplementary melatonin. Melatonin is an important safe molecule with a wide range of physiological functions in animals and humans with a strong therapeutic potential in CVDs. Despite the current difficulties to translate the basic research findings into a clinical setting, cardiovascular protective action of melatonin supplementation is promising but a better understanding of this action is needed. Most importantly, consumption of melatonin-rich foods such as grape juice, wine, cereals, tropical fruits and walnuts increases circulating melatonin levels and antioxidant capacity. Preclinical studies suggest that melatonin, given at dietary levels, confers cardioprotection. However, a better understanding of the mechanisms involved in this effect are required before it can be considered as an adjuvant for effective preventive and curative therapy in CVDs.

AUTHOR CONTRIBUTIONS

ZJ: wrote the first draft of the manuscript; SL: conception, critical comments on the different drafts of the manuscript (content review); FN: conception, literature choice, figures and tables, revised the final draft manuscript.

ACKNOWLEDGMENTS

This work was supported by the South African National Research Foundation (NRF), the University of Cape Town and the Wine Industry Network for Expertise and Technology (Winetech) (SL). FN received a National Research Foundation (NRF) Postdoctoral Research Fellowship and European Research Council (ERC)/NRF partnership award.

REFERENCES

Acuna-Castroviejo, D., Escames, G., Venegas, C., Diaz-Casado, M. E., Lima-Cabello, E., Lopez, L. C., et al. (2014). Extrapineal melatonin: sources, regulation, and potential functions. *Cell Mol. Life Sci.* 71, 2997–3025. doi: 10.1007/s00018-014-1579-2

Afshin, A., Micha, R., Khatibzadeh, S., and Mozaffarian, D. (2014). Consumption of nuts and legumes and risk of incident ischemic heart disease, stroke, and diabetes: a systematic review and meta-analysis. *Am. J. Clin. Nutr.* 100, 278–288. doi: 10.3945/ajcn.113.076901

Agabiti-Rosei, C., Favero, G., De Ciuceis, C., Rossini, C., Porteri, E., Rodella, L. F., et al. (2017). Effect of long-term treatment with melatonin on vascular markers of oxidative stress/inflammation and on the anticontractile activity of perivascular fat in aging mice. *Hypertens. Res.* 40, 41–50. doi: 10.1038/hr.2016.103

Aguilera, Y., Rebollo-Hernanz, M., Herrera, T., Cayuelas, L. T., Rodríguez-Rodríguez, P., de Pablo, Á. L., et al. (2016). Intake of bean sprouts influences melatonin and antioxidant capacity biomarker levels in rats. *Food Funct.* 7, 1438–1445. doi: 10.1039/C5FO01538C

Al Abdrabalnabi, A., Bitok, E., Rajaram, S., Rizzo, N., and Sabaté, J. (2017). A year-long trial to examine the effects of a daily dose of walnuts on cardiometabolic risk markers in an elderly population. *FASEB J.* 31:447.1.

Altun, A., Yaprak, M., Aktoz, M., Vardar, A., Betul, U. A., and Ozbay, G. (2002). Impaired nocturnal synthesis of melatonin in patients with cardiac syndrome X. *Neurosci. Lett.* 327, 143–145. doi: 10.1016/S0304-3940(02)00368-3

An, R., Zhao, L., Xi, C., Li, H., Shen, G., Liu, H., et al. (2016). Melatonin attenuates sepsis-induced cardiac dysfunction via a PI3K/Akt-dependent mechanism. *Basic Res. Cardiol.* 111:8-015-0526-1. doi: 10.1007/s00395-015-0526-1

Andersen, L. P., Gogenur, I., Rosenberg, J., and Reiter, R. J. (2016). The safety of melatonin in humans. *Clin. Drug Investig.* 36, 169–175. doi: 10.1007/s40261-015-0368-5

Arendt, J. (1998). Melatonin and the pineal gland: influence on mammalian seasonal and circadian physiology. *Rev. Reprod.* 3, 13–22. doi: 10.1530/ror.0.0030013

Auld, F., Maschauer, E. L., Morrison, I., Skene, D. J., and Riha, R. L. (2017). Evidence for the efficacy of melatonin in the treatment of primary adult sleep disorders. *Sleep Med. Rev.* 34, 10–22. doi: 10.1016/j.smrv.2016.06.005

Aune, D., Giovannucci, E., Boffetta, P., Fadnes, L. T., Keum, N., Norat, T., et al. (2017). Fruit and vegetable intake and the risk of cardiovascular disease, total cancer and all-cause mortality-a systematic review and dose-response meta-analysis of prospective studies. *Int. J. Epidemiol.* 46, 1029–1056. doi: 10.1093/ije/dyw319

Bazzano, L. A., He, J., Ogden, L. G., Loria, C., Vupputuri, S., Myers, L., et al. (2001). Legume consumption and risk of coronary heart disease in US men and women: NHANES I Epidemiologic Follow-up Study. *Arch. Intern. Med.* 161, 2573–2578. doi: 10.1001/archinte.161.21.2573

Bravo, R., Matito, S., Cubero, J., Paredes, S., Franco, L., Rivero, M., et al. (2013). Tryptophan-enriched cereal intake improves nocturnal sleep, melatonin, serotonin, and total antioxidant capacity levels and mood in elderly humans. *Age (Dordr).* 35, 1277–1285. doi: 10.1007/s11357-012-9419-5

Brown, G. M., Bar-Or, A., Grossi, D., Kashur, S., Johannson, E., and Yie, S. M. (1991). Urinary 6-sulphatoxymelatonin, an index of pineal function in the rat. *J. Pineal Res.* 10, 141–147. doi: 10.1111/j.1600-079X.1991.tb00831.x

Brugger, P., Marktl, W., and Herold, M. (1995). Impaired nocturnal secretion of melatonin in coronary heart disease. *Lancet* 345:1408.

Byeon, Y., Lee, H. Y., Lee, K., Park, S., and Back, K. (2014). Cellular localization and kinetics of the rice melatonin biosynthetic enzymes SNAT and ASMT. *J. Pineal Res.* 56, 107–114. doi: 10.1111/jpi.12103

Cagnacci, A., Cannoletta, M., Renzi, A., Baldassari, F., Arangino, S., and Volpe, A. (2005). Prolonged melatonin administration decreases nocturnal blood pressure in women. *Am. J. Hypertens.* 18, 1614–1618. doi: 10.1016/j.amjhyper.2005.05.008

Carracedo, G., Carpena, C., Concepción, P., Díaz, V., García-García, M., Jemni, N., et al. (2017). Presence of melatonin in human tears. *J. Optom.* 10, 3–4. doi: 10.1016/j.optom.2016.03.002

Carrillo-Vico, A., Lardone, P. J., Alvarez-Sanchez, N., Rodriguez-Rodriguez, A., and Guerrero, J. M. (2013). Melatonin: buffering the immune system. *Int. J. Mol. Sci.* 14, 8638–8683. doi: 10.3390/ijms14048638

Chua, S., Lee, F. Y., Chiang, H. J., Chen, K. H., Lu, H. I., Chen, Y. T., et al. (2016). The cardioprotective effect of melatonin and exendin-4 treatment in a rat model of cardiorenal syndrome. *J. Pineal Res.* 61, 438–456. doi: 10.1111/jpi.12357

Dave, R. H., Hale, S. L., and Kloner, R. A. (1998). The effect of melatonin on hemodynamics, blood flow, and myocardial infarct size in a rabbit model of ischemia-reperfusion. *J. Cardiovasc. Pharmacol. Ther.* 3, 153–160. doi: 10.1177/107424849800300208

de la Puerta, C., Carrascosa-Salmoral, M. P., García-Luna, P. P., Lardone, P. J., Herrera, J. L., Fernández-Montesinos, R., et al. (2007). Melatonin is a phytochemical in olive oil. *Food Chem.* 104, 609–612. doi: 10.1016/j.foodchem.2006.12.010

Diez, E. R., Renna, N. F., Prado, N. J., Lembo, C., Ponce Zumino, A. Z., Vazquez-Prieto, M., et al. (2013). Melatonin, given at the time of reperfusion, prevents ventricular arrhythmias in isolated hearts from fructose-fed rats and spontaneously hypertensive rats. *J. Pineal Res.* 55, 166–173. doi: 10.1111/jpi.12059

Dominguez-Rodriguez, A., Abreu-Gonzalez, P., de la Torre-Hernandez, J. M., Consuegra-Sanchez, L., Piccolo, R., Gonzalez-Gonzalez, J., et al. (2017a). Usefulness of early treatment with melatonin to reduce infarct size in patients with ST-segment elevation myocardial infarction receiving percutaneous coronary intervention (from the melatonin adjunct in the acute myocardial infarction treated with angioplasty trial). *Am. J. Cardiol.* 120, 522–526. doi: 10.1016/j.amjcard.2017.05.018

Dominguez-Rodriguez, A., Abreu-Gonzalez, P., de la Torre-Hernandez, J. M., Gonzalez-Gonzalez, J., Garcia-Camarero, T., Consuegra-Sanchez, L., et al. (2017b). Effect of intravenous and intracoronary melatonin as an adjunct to primary percutaneous coronary intervention for acute ST-elevation myocardial infarction: results of the Melatonin Adjunct in the acute myocaRdial Infarction treated with Angioplasty trial. *J. Pineal Res.* 62:e12374. doi: 10.1111/jpi.12374

Dominguez-Rodriguez, A., Abreu-Gonzalez, P., Garcia, M. J., Sanchez, J., Marrero, F., and de Armas-Trujillo, D. (2002). Decreased nocturnal melatonin levels during acute myocardial infarction. *J. Pineal Res.* 33, 248–252. doi: 10.1034/j.1600-079X.2002.02938.x

Dominguez-Rodriguez, A., Abreu-Gonzalez, P., Garcia-Gonzalez, M. J., Kaski, J. C., Reiter, R. J., and Jimenez-Sosa, A. (2007). A unicenter, randomized, double-blind, parallel-group, placebo-controlled study of Melatonin as an Adjunct in patients with acute myocaRdial Infarction undergoing primary Angioplasty The Melatonin Adjunct in the acute myocaRdial Infarction treated with Angioplasty (MARIA) trial: study design and rationale. *Contemp. Clin. Trials* 28, 532–539. doi: 10.1016/j.cct.2006.10.007

Dominguez-Rodriguez, A., Abreu-Gonzalez, P., Piccolo, R., Galasso, G., and Reiter, R. J. (2016). Melatonin is associated with reverse remodeling after cardiac resynchronization therapy in patients with heart failure and ventricular dyssynchrony. *Int. J. Cardiol.* 221, 359–363. doi: 10.1016/j.ijcard.2016.07.056

Dominguez-Rodriguez, A., Abreu-Gonzalez, P., and Reiter, R. J. (2014). The potential usefulness of serum melatonin level to predict heart failure in patients with hypertensive cardiomyopathy. *Int. J. Cardiol.* 174, 415–417. doi: 10.1016/j.ijcard.2014.04.044

Dominguez-Rodriguez, A., Abreu-Gonzalez, P., Sanchez-Sanchez, J. J., Kaski, J. C., and Reiter, R. J. (2010). Melatonin and circadian biology in human cardiovascular disease. *J. Pineal Res.* 49, 14–22. doi: 10.1111/j.1600-079X.2010.00773.x

Dubbels, R., Reiter, R. J., Klenke, E., Goebel, A., Schnakenberg, E., Ehlers, C., et al. (1995). Melatonin in edible plants identified by radioimmunoassay and by high performance liquid chromatography-mass spectrometry. *J. Pineal Res.* 18, 28–31. doi: 10.1111/j.1600-079X.1995.tb00136.x

Dwaich, K. H., Al-Amran, F. G., Al-Sheibani, B. I., and Al-Aubaidy, H. A. (2016). Melatonin effects on myocardial ischemia–reperfusion injury: impact on the outcome in patients undergoing coronary artery bypass grafting surgery. *Int. J. Cardiol.* 221, 977–986. doi: 10.1016/j.ijcard.2016.07.108

Dzida, G., Prystupa, A., Lachowska-Kotowska, P., Kadas, T., Kamienski, P., Kimak, E., et al. (2013). Alteration in diurnal and nocturnal melatonin serum level in patients with chronic heart failure. *Ann. Agric. Environ. Med.* 20, 745–748.

EFSA (European Food Safety Authority), Panel on Dietetic Products, Nutrition and Allergies (NDA) (2011). Scientific Opinion on the substantiation of a health claim related to melatonin and reduction of sleep onset latency (ID 1698, 1780, 4080) pursuant to Article 13(1) of Regulation (EC) No 1924/2006. *EFSA J.* 9:2241. doi: 10.2903/j.efsa.2011.2241

Ekeloef, S., Halladin, N., Fonnes, S., Jensen, S. E., Zaremba, T., Rosenberg, J., et al. (2017). Effect of intracoronary and intravenous melatonin on myocardial salvage index in patients with ST-elevation myocardial infarction: a randomized placebo controlled trial. *J. Cardiovasc. Transl. Res.* 10, 470–479. doi: 10.1007/s12265-017-9768-7

Ekelof, S. V., Halladin, N. L., Jensen, S. E., Zaremba, T., Aaroe, J., Kjaergaard, B., et al. (2016). Effects of intracoronary melatonin on ischemia-reperfusion injury in ST-elevation myocardial infarction. *Heart Vessels* 31, 88–95. doi: 10.1007/s00380-014-0589-1

Esteban, S., Nicolaus, C., Garmundi, A., Rial, R. V., Rodriguez, A. B., Ortega, E., et al. (2004). Effect of orally administered L-tryptophan on serotonin, melatonin, and the innate immune response in the rat. *Mol. Cell. Biochem.* 267, 39–46. doi: 10.1023/B:MCBI.0000049363.97713.74

Estruch, R., Ros, E., Salas-Salvado, J., Covas, M. I., Corella, D., and Aros, F. (2013). Primary prevention of cardiovascular disease with a Mediterranean diet. *N. Engl. J. Med.* 368, 1279–1290. doi: 10.1056/NEJMoa1200303

Favero, G., Franceschetti, L., Buffoli, B., Moghadasian, M. H., Reiter, R. J., Rodella, L. F., et al. (2017). Melatonin: protection against age-related cardiac pathology. *Ageing Res. Rev.* 35, 336–349. doi: 10.1016/j.arr.2016.11.007

Fischer, T. W., Kleszczynski, K., Hardkop, L. H., Kruse, N., and Zillikens, D. (2013). Melatonin enhances antioxidative enzyme gene expression (CAT, GPx, SOD), prevents their UVR-induced depletion, and protects against the formation of DNA damage (8-hydroxy-2′-deoxyguanosine) in *ex vivo* human skin. *J. Pineal Res.* 54, 303–312. doi: 10.1111/jpi.12018

Girotti, L., Lago, M., Ianovsky, O., Elizari, M. V., Dini, A., Perez Lloret, S., et al. (2003). Low urinary 6-sulfatoxymelatonin levels in patients with severe congestive heart failure. *Endocrine* 22, 245–248. doi: 10.1385/ENDO:22:3:245

Gogenur, I., Kucukakin, B., Panduro Jensen, L., Reiter, R. J., and Rosenberg, J. (2014). Melatonin reduces cardiac morbidity and markers of myocardial ischemia after elective abdominal aortic aneurism repair: a randomized, placebo-controlled, clinical trial. *J. Pineal Res.* 57, 10–15. doi: 10.1111/jpi.12138

Gonzalez-Flores, D., Gamero, E., Garrido, M., Ramirez, R., Moreno, D., Delgado, J., et al. (2012). Urinary 6-sulfatoxymelatonin and total antioxidant capacity increase after the intake of a grape juice cv. Tempranillo stabilized with HHP. *Food Funct.* 3, 34–39. doi: 10.1039/C1FO10146C

Green, E. A., Black, B. K., Biaggioni, I., Paranjape, S. Y., Bagai, K., Shibao, C., et al. (2014). Melatonin reduces tachycardia in postural tachycardia syndrome: a randomized, crossover trial. *Cardiovasc. Ther.* 32, 105–112. doi: 10.1111/1755-5922.12067

Grossman, E., Laudon, M., Yalcin, R., Zengil, H., Peleg, E., Sharabi, Y., et al. (2006). Melatonin reduces night blood pressure in patients with nocturnal hypertension. *Am. J. Med.* 119, 898–902. doi: 10.1016/j.amjmed.2006.02.002

Grossman, E., Laudon, M., and Zisapel, N. (2011). Effect of melatonin on nocturnal blood pressure: meta-analysis of randomized controlled trials. *Vasc. Health. Risk Manag.* 7, 577–584. doi: 10.2147/VHRM.S24603

Haghjooy-Javanmard, S., Ziaei, A., Ziaei, S., Ziaei, E., and Mirmohammad-Sadeghi, M. (2013). The effect of preoperative melatonin on nuclear erythroid 2-related factor 2 activation in patients undergoing coronary artery bypass grafting surgery. *Oxid Med. Cell. Longev* 2013:676829. doi: 10.1155/2013/676829

Halladin, N. L., Ekelof, S., Jensen, S. E., Aaroe, J., Kjaergaard, B., Heegaard, P. M., et al. (2014). Melatonin does not affect oxidative/inflammatory biomarkers in a closed-chest porcine model of acute myocardial infarction. *In Vivo* 28, 483–488.

Hardeland, R., and Fuhrberg, B. (1996). Ubiquitous melatonin–presence and effects in unicells, plants and animals. *Trends Comp. Biochem. Physiol.* 2, 25–45.

Hardeland, R., Cardinali, D. P., Srinivasan, V., Spence, D. W., Brown, G. M., and Pandi-Perumal, S. R. (2011). Melatonin–a pleiotropic, orchestrating regulator molecule. *Prog. Neurobiol.* 93, 350–384. doi: 10.1016/j.pneurobio.2010.12.004

Hardeland, R., and Pandi-Perumal, S. R. (2005). Melatonin, a potent agent in antioxidative defense: actions as a natural food constituent, gastrointestinal factor, drug and prodrug. *Nutr. Metab. (Lond)* 2:22. doi: 10.1186/1743-7075-2-22

Harpsoe, N. G., Andersen, L. P., Gogenur, I., and Rosenberg, J. (2015). Clinical pharmacokinetics of melatonin: a systematic review. *Eur. J. Clin. Pharmacol.* 71, 901–909. doi: 10.1007/s00228-015-1873-4

Hattori, A., Migitaka, H., Iigo, M., Itoh, M., Yamamoto, K., Ohtani-Kaneko, R., et al. (1995). Identification of melatonin in plants and its effects on plasma melatonin levels and binding to melatonin receptors in vertebrates. *Biochem. Mol. Biol. Int.* 35, 627–634.

Hausenloy, D. J., Garcia-Dorado, D., Erik Botker, H., Davidson, S. M., Downey, J., Engel, F. B., et al. (2017). Melatonin as a cardioprotective therapy following ST-segment elevation myocardial infarction: is it really promising? Reply. *Cardiovasc. Res.* 113, 1418–1419. doi: 10.1093/cvr/cvx137

Herrera, T., Aguilera, Y., Rebollo-Hernanz, M., Bravo, E., Benítez, V., Martínez-Sáez, N., et al. (2018). Teas and herbal infusions as sources of melatonin and other bioactive non-nutrient components. *Food Sci. Technol.* 89, 65–73. doi: 10.1016/j.lwt.2017.10.031

Herxheimer, A., and Petrie, K. J. (2002). Melatonin for the prevention and treatment of jet lag. *Cochrane Database Syst. Rev.* 2:CD001520. doi: 10.1002/14651858.CD001520

Heusch, G. (2017). Critical issues for the translation of cardioprotection. *Circ. Res.* 120, 1477–1486. doi: 10.1161/CIRCRESAHA.117.310820

Hu, J., Zhang, L., Yang, Y., Guo, Y., Fan, Y., Zhang, M., et al. (2017). Melatonin alleviates postinfarction cardiac remodeling and dysfunction by inhibiting Mst1. *J. Pineal Res.* 62:e12368. doi: 10.1111/jpi.12368

Hu, Z. P., Fang, X. L., Fang, N., Wang, X. B., Qian, H. Y., Cao, Z., et al. (2013). Melatonin ameliorates vascular endothelial dysfunction, inflammation, and atherosclerosis by suppressing the TLR4/NF-kappaB system in high-fat-fed rabbits. *J. Pineal Res.* 55, 388–398. doi: 10.1111/jpi.12085

Huether, G., Poeggeler, B., Reimer, A., and George, A. (1992). Effect of tryptophan administration on circulating melatonin levels in chicks and rats: evidence for stimulation of melatonin synthesis and release in the gastrointestinal tract. *Life Sci.* 51, 945–953. doi: 10.1016/0024-3205(92)90402-B

Iigo, M., Furukawa, K., Hattori, A., Hara, M., Ohtani-Kaneko, R., Suzuki, T., et al. (1995). Effects of pinealectomy and constant light exposure on day-night changes of melatonin binding sites in the goldfish brain. *Neurosci. Lett.* 197, 61–64. doi: 10.1016/0304-3940(95)11903-A

Illnerova, H., Buresova, M., and Presl, J. (1993). Melatonin rhythm in human milk. *J. Clin. Endocrinol. Metab.* 77, 838–841.

Iriti, M. (2009). Melatonin in grape, not just a myth, maybe a panacea. *J. Pineal Res.* 46, 353–353. doi: 10.1111/j.1600-079X.2008.00616.x

Iriti, M., and Varoni, E. M. (2015). Melatonin in Mediterranean diet, a new perspective. *J. Sci. Food Agric.* 95, 2355–2359. doi: 10.1002/jsfa.7051

Iriti, M., Varoni, E. M., and Vitalini, S. (2010). Melatonin in traditional Mediterranean diets. *J. Pineal Res.* 49, 101–105. doi: 10.1111/j.1600-079X.2010.00777.x

Jin, H., Wang, Y., Zhou, L., Liu, L., Zhang, P., Deng, W., et al. (2014). Melatonin attenuates hypoxic pulmonary hypertension by inhibiting the inflammation and the proliferation of pulmonary arterial smooth muscle cells. *J. Pineal Res.* 57, 442–450. doi: 10.1111/jpi.12184

Johns, N. P., Johns, J., Porasuphatana, S., Plaimee, P., and Sae-Teaw, M. (2013). Dietary intake of melatonin from tropical fruit altered urinary excretion of 6-sulfatoxymelatonin in healthy volunteers. *J. Agric. Food Chem.* 61, 913–919. doi: 10.1021/jf300359a

Kantar, S., Turkozkan, N., Bircan, F. S., and Pasaoglu, O. T. (2015). Beneficial effects of melatonin on serum nitric oxide, homocysteine, and ADMA levels in fructose-fed rats. *Pharm. Biol.* 53, 1035–1041. doi: 10.3109/13880209.2014.957782

Kennaway, D. J. (2017). Are the proposed benefits of melatonin-rich foods too hard to swallow? *Crit. Rev. Food Sci. Nutr.* 57, 958–962. doi: 10.1080/10408398.2014.962686

Kimak, E., Dzida, G., Duma, D., Prystupa, A., Halabis, M., Kimak, A., et al. (2014). Association between concentration of melatonin, and lipoproteins, LPO, hsCRP, NTproBNP in chronic heart failure patients. *Curr. Issues Pharm. Med. Sci.* 27, 159–164. doi: 10.1515/cipms-2015-0007

Kozirog, M., Poliwczak, A. R., Duchnowicz, P., Koter-Michalak, M., Sikora, J., and Broncel, M. (2011). Melatonin treatment improves blood pressure, lipid profile, and parameters of oxidative stress in patients with metabolic syndrome. *J. Pineal Res.* 50, 261–266. doi: 10.1111/j.1600-079X.2010.00835.x

Kris-Etherton, P. M. (2014). Walnuts decrease risk of cardiovascular disease: a summary of efficacy and biologic mechanisms. *J. Nutr.* 144, 547S–554S. doi: 10.3945/jn.113.182907

Kruger, M. J., Davies, N., Myburgh, K. H., and Lecour, S. (2014). Proanthocyanidins, anthocyanins and cardiovascular diseases. *Food. Res. Int.* 59, 41–52. doi: 10.1016/j.foodres.2014.01.046

Lagneux, C., Joyeux, M., Demenge, P., Ribuot, C., and Godin-Ribuot, D. (2000). Protective effects of melatonin against ischemia-reperfusion injury in the isolated rat heart. *Life Sci.* 66, 503–509. doi: 10.1016/S0024-3205(99)00620-7

Lamont, K., Blackhurst, D., Albertyn, Z., Marais, D., and Lecour, S. (2012). Lowering the alcohol content of red wine does not alter its cardioprotective properties. *S. Afr. Med. J.* 102, 565–567. doi: 10.7196/SAMJ.5733

Lamont, K., Nduhirabandi, F., Adam, T., Thomas, D. P., Opie, L. H., and Lecour, S. (2015). Role of melatonin, melatonin receptors and STAT3 in the cardioprotective effect of chronic and moderate consumption of red wine. *Biochem. Biophys. Res. Commun.* 465, 719–724. doi: 10.1016/j.bbrc.2015.08.064

Lamont, K. T., Somers, S., Lacerda, L., Opie, L. H., and Lecour, S. (2011). Is red wine a SAFE sip away from cardioprotection? Mechanisms involved in resveratrol- and melatonin-induced cardioprotection. *J. Pineal Res.* 50, 374–380. doi: 10.1111/j.1600-079X.2010.00853.x

Lecour, S., and Lamont, K. T. (2011). Natural polyphenols and cardioprotection. *Mini Rev. Med. Chem.* 11, 1191–1199. doi: 10.2174/13895575111091191

Lerner, A. B., Case, J. D., Takahashi, Y., Lee, T. H., and Mori, W. (1958). Isolation of melatonin, the pineal gland factor that lightens melanocyteS1. *J. Am. Chem. Soc.* 80, 2587–2587. doi: 10.1021/ja01543a060

Liu, X., Chen, Z., Chua, C. C., Ma, Y. S., Youngberg, G. A., Hamdy, R., et al. (2002). Melatonin as an effective protector against doxorubicin-induced cardiotoxicity. *Am. J. Physiol. Heart Circ. Physiol.* 283, H254–H263. doi: 10.1152/ajpheart.01023.2001

Lochner, A., Genade, S., Davids, A., Ytrehus, K., and Moolman, J. A. (2006). Short- and long-term effects of melatonin on myocardial post-ischemic recovery. *J. Pineal Res.* 40, 56–63. doi: 10.1111/j.1600-079X.2005.00280.x

Lochner, A., Huisamen, B., and Nduhirabandi, F. (2013). Cardioprotective effect of melatonin against ischaemia/reperfusion damage. *Front. Biosci. (Elite Ed)* 5, 305–315. doi: 10.2741/E617

Ma, X., Idle, J. R., Krausz, K. W., and Gonzalez, F. J. (2005). Metabolism of melatonin by human cytochromes p450. *Drug Metab. Dispos.* 33, 489–494. doi: 10.1124/dmd.104.002410

Maarman, G., Blackhurst, D., Thienemann, F., Blauwet, L., Butrous, G., Davies, N., et al. (2015). Melatonin as a preventive and curative therapy against pulmonary hypertension. *J. Pineal Res.* 59, 343–353. doi: 10.1111/jpi.12263

Májovský, M., Řezáčová, L., Sumová, A., Pospíšilová, L., Netuka, D., Bradáč, O., et al. (2017). Melatonin and cortisol secretion profile in patients with pineal cyst before and after pineal cyst resection. *J. Clin. Neurosci.* 39, 155–163. doi: 10.1016/j.jocn.2017.01.022

Maldonado, M. D., Moreno, H., and Calvo, J. R. (2009). Melatonin present in beer contributes to increase the levels of melatonin and antioxidant capacity of the human serum. *Clin. Nutr.* 28, 188–191. doi: 10.1016/j.clnu.2009.02.001

Mantele, S., Otway, D. T., Middleton, B., Bretschneider, S., Wright, J., Robertson, M. D., et al. (2012). Daily rhythms of plasma melatonin, but not plasma leptin or leptin mRNA, vary between lean, obese and type 2 diabetic men. *PLoS ONE* 7:e37123. doi: 10.1371/journal.pone.0037123

Maria, S., and Witt-Enderby, P. A. (2014). Melatonin effects on bone: potential use for the prevention and treatment for osteopenia, osteoporosis, and periodontal disease and for use in bone-grafting procedures. *J. Pineal Res.* 56, 115–125. doi: 10.1111/jpi.12116

Mauriz, J. L., Collado, P. S., Veneroso, C., Reiter, R. J., and Gonzalez-Gallego, J. (2013). A review of the molecular aspects of melatonin's anti-inflammatory actions: recent insights and new perspectives. *J. Pineal Res.* 54, 1–14. doi: 10.1111/j.1600-079X.2012.01014.x

McCord, C. P., and Allen, F. P. (1917). Evidences associating pineal gland function with alterations in pigmentation. *J. Exp. Zool.* 23, 207–224. doi: 10.1002/jez.1400230108

McElhinney, D. B., Hoffman, S. J., Robinson, W. A., and Ferguson, J. (1994). Effect of melatonin on human skin color. *J. Invest. Dermatol.* 102, 258–259. doi: 10.1111/1523-1747.ep12371773

McMullan, C. J., Rimm, E. B., Schernhammer, E. S., and Forman, J. P. (2017). A nested case-control study of the association between melatonin secretion and incident myocardial infarction. *Heart* 103, 694–701. doi: 10.1136/heartjnl-2016-310098

McMullan, C. J., Schernhammer, E. S., Rimm, E. B., Hu, F. B., and Forman, J. P. (2013). Melatonin secretion and the incidence of type 2 diabetes. *JAMA* 309, 1388–1396. doi: 10.1001/jama.2013.2710

Meng, J., Shi, T., Song, S., Zhang, Z., and Fang, Y. (2017a). Melatonin in grapes and grape-related foodstuffs: a review. *Food Chem.* 231, 185–191. doi: 10.1016/j.foodchem.2017.03.137

Meng, X., Li, Y., Li, S., Zhou, Y., Gan, R. Y., Xu, D. P., et al. (2017b). Dietary sources and bioactivities of melatonin. *Nutrients* 9:367. doi: 10.3390/nu9040367

Micha, R., Penalvo, J. L., Cudhea, F., Imamura, F., Rehm, C. D., and Mozaffarian, D. (2017). Association between dietary factors and mortality from heart disease, stroke, and type 2 diabetes in the United States. *JAMA* 317, 912–924. doi: 10.1001/jama.2017.0947

Mozdzan, M., Mozdzan, M., Chalubinski, M., Wojdan, K., and Broncel, M. (2014). The effect of melatonin on circadian blood pressure in patients with type 2 diabetes and essential hypertension. *Arch. Med. Sci.* 10, 669–675. doi: 10.5114/aoms.2014.44858

Muller, J. E., Ludmer, P. L., Willich, S. N., Tofler, G. H., Aylmer, G., Klangos, I., et al. (1987). Circadian variation in the frequency of sudden cardiac death. *Circulation* 75, 131–138. doi: 10.1161/01.CIR.75.1.131

Murch, S. J., Hall, B. A., Le, C. H., and Saxena, P. K. (2010). Changes in the levels of indoleamine phytochemicals during véraison and ripening of wine grapes. *J. Pineal Res.* 49, 95–100. doi: 10.1111/j.1600-079X.2010.00774.x

Navarro-Alarcon, M., Ruiz-Ojeda, F. J., Blanca-Herrera, R. M., Serrano, M. M., Acuna-Castroviejo, D., Fernandez-Vazquez, G., et al. (2014). Melatonin and metabolic regulation: a review. *Food Funct.* 5, 2806–2832. doi: 10.1039/C4FO00317A

Nduhirabandi, F., Du Toit, E. F., Blackhurst, D., Marais, D., and Lochner, A. (2011). Chronic melatonin consumption prevents obesity-related metabolic abnormalities and protects the heart against myocardial ischemia and reperfusion injury in a prediabetic model of diet-induced obesity. *J. Pineal Res.* 50, 171–182. doi: 10.1111/j.1600-079X.2010.00826.x

Nduhirabandi, F., du Toit, E. F., and Lochner, A. (2012). Melatonin and the metabolic syndrome: a tool for effective therapy in obesity-associated abnormalities? *Acta Physiol. (Oxf)* 205, 209–223. doi: 10.1111/j.1748-1716.2012.02410.x

Nduhirabandi, F., Huisamen, B., Strijdom, H., Blackhurst, D., and Lochner, A. (2014). Short-term melatonin consumption protects the heart of obese rats independent of body weight change and visceral adiposity. *J. Pineal Res.* 57, 317–332. doi: 10.1111/jpi.12171

Nduhirabandi, F., Lamont, K., Albertyn, Z., Opie, L. H., and Lecour, S. (2016). Role of toll-like receptor 4 in melatonin-induced cardioprotection. *J. Pineal Res.* 60, 39–47. doi: 10.1111/jpi.12286

Opie, L. H., and Lecour, S. (2016). Melatonin has multiorgan effects. *Eur. Heart J. Cardiovasc. Pharmacother.* 2, 258–265. doi: 10.1093/ehjcvp/pvv037

Opie, L. H., and Lecour, S. (2007). The red wine hypothesis: from concepts to protective signalling molecules. *Eur. Heart J.* 28, 1683–1693. doi: 10.1093/eurheartj/ehm149

Pandi-Perumal, S., BaHammam, A. S., Ojike, N. I., Akinseye, O. A., Kendzerska, T., Buttoo, K., et al. (2017). Melatonin and human cardiovascular disease. *J. Cardiovasc. Pharmacol. Ther.* 22, 122–132. doi: 10.1177/1074248416660622

Pandi-Perumal, S. R., Srinivasan, V., Maestroni, G. J., Cardinali, D. P., Poeggeler, B., and Hardeland, R. (2006). Melatonin: nature's most versatile biological signal? *FEBS J.* 273, 2813–2838. doi: 10.1111/j.1742-4658.2006.05322.x

Park, S., Byeon, Y., and Back, K. (2013). Transcriptional suppression of tryptamine 5-hydroxylase, a terminal serotonin biosynthetic gene, induces melatonin biosynthesis in rice (*Oryza sativa* L.). *J. Pineal Res.* 55, 131–137. doi: 10.1111/jpi.12053

Patel, V., Upaganlawar, A., Zalawadia, R., and Balaraman, R. (2010). Cardioprotective effect of melatonin against isoproterenol induced myocardial infarction in rats: a biochemical, electrocardiographic and histoarchitectural evaluation. *Eur. J. Pharmacol.* 644, 160–168. doi: 10.1016/j.ejphar.2010.06.065

Paulis, L., Pechanova, O., Zicha, J., Barta, A., Gardlik, R., Celec, P., et al. (2010). Melatonin interactions with blood pressure and vascular function during L-NAME-induced hypertension. *J. Pineal Res.* 48, 102–108. doi: 10.1111/j.1600-079X.2009.00732.x

Paulis, L., and Simko, F. (2007). Blood pressure modulation and cardiovascular protection by melatonin: potential mechanisms behind. *Physiol. Res.* 56, 671–684.

Pei, H., Du, J., Song, X., He, L., Zhang, Y., Li, X., et al. (2016). Melatonin prevents adverse myocardial infarction remodeling via Notch1/Mfn2 pathway. *Free Radic. Biol. Med.* 97:e1237. 408–417. doi: 10.1016/j.freeradbiomed.2016.06.015

Pei, H. F., Hou, J. N., Wei, F. P., Xue, Q., Zhang, F., Peng, C. F., et al. (2017). Melatonin attenuates postmyocardial infarction injury via increasing Tom70 expression. *J. Pineal Res.* 62:e12371. doi: 10.1111/jpi.12371

Petrosillo, G., Colantuono, G., Moro, N., Ruggiero, F. M., Tiravanti, E., Di Venosa, N., et al. (2009). Melatonin protects against heart ischemia-reperfusion injury by inhibiting mitochondrial permeability transition pore opening. *Am. J. Physiol. Heart Circ. Physiol.* 297, H1487–H1493. doi: 10.1152/ajpheart.00163.2009

Peuhkuri, K., Sihvola, N., and Korpela, R. (2012). Dietary factors and fluctuating levels of melatonin. *Food Nutr. Res.* 56:17252. doi: 10.3402/fnr.v56i0.17252

Rechcinski, T., Trzos, E., Wierzbowska-Drabik, K., Krzeminska-Pakula, M., and Kurpesa, M. (2010). Melatonin for nondippers with coronary artery disease: assessment of blood pressure profile and heart rate variability. *Hypertens. Res.* 33, 56–61. doi: 10.1038/hr.2009.174

Reiter, R. J., Manchester, L. C., and Tan, D. X. (2005). Melatonin in walnuts: influence on levels of melatonin and total antioxidant capacity of blood. *Nutrition* 21, 920–924. doi: 10.1016/j.nut.2005.02.005

Reiter, R. J., Mayo, J. C., Tan, D. X., Sainz, R. M., Alatorre-Jimenez, M., and Qin, L. (2016). Melatonin as an antioxidant: under promises but over delivers. *J. Pineal Res.* 61, 253–278. doi: 10.1111/jpi.12360

Reiter, R. J., Rosales-Corral, S. A., Tan, D. X., Acuna-Castroviejo, D., Qin, L., Yang, S. F., et al. (2017). Melatonin, a full service anti-cancer agent: inhibition of initiation, progression and metastasis. *Int. J. Mol. Sci.* 18:843. doi: 10.3390/ijms18040843

Reiter, R. J., Tan, D. X., Burkhardt, S., and Manchester, L. C. (2001). Melatonin in plants. *Nutr. Rev.* 59, 286–290. doi: 10.1111/j.1753-4887.2001.tb07018.x

Reiter, R. J., Tan, D. X., Manchester, L. C., Paredes, S. D., Mayo, J. C., and Sainz, R. M. (2009). Melatonin and reproduction revisited. *Biol. Reprod.* 81, 445–456. doi: 10.1095/biolreprod.108.075655

Reiter, R. J., Tan, D. X., Paredes, S. D., and Fuentes-Broto, L. (2010). Beneficial effects of melatonin in cardiovascular disease. *Ann. Med.* 42, 276–285. doi: 10.3109/07853890903485748

Reppert, S. M., and Weaver, D. R. (1995). Melatonin madness. *Cell* 83, 1059–1062. doi: 10.1016/0092-8674(95)90131-0

Rodriguez-Naranjo, M. I., Gil-Izquierdo, A., Troncoso, A. M., Cantos-Villar, E., and Garcia-Parrilla, M. C. (2011). Melatonin is synthesised by yeast during alcoholic fermentation in wines. *Food Chem.* 126, 1608–1613. doi: 10.1016/j.foodchem.2010.12.038

Sae-Teaw, M., Johns, J., Johns, N. P., and Subongkot, S. (2013). Serum melatonin levels and antioxidant capacities after consumption of pineapple, orange, or banana by healthy male volunteers. *J. Pineal Res.* 55, 58–64. doi: 10.1111/jpi.12025

Sahna, E., Olmez, E., and Acet, A. (2002). Effects of physiological and pharmacological concentrations of melatonin on ischemia-reperfusion arrhythmias in rats: can the incidence of sudden cardiac death be reduced? *J. Pineal Res.* 32, 194–198. doi: 10.1034/j.1600-079x.2002.1o853.x

Salmanoglu, D. S., Gurpinar, T., Vural, K., Ekerbicer, N., Dariverenli, E., and Var, A. (2016). Melatonin and L-carnitin improves endothelial disfunction and oxidative stress in Type 2 diabetic rats. *Redox Biol.* 8, 199–204. doi: 10.1016/j.redox.2015.11.007

Sanchez-Hidalgo, M., Guerrero Montavez, J. M., Carrascosa-Salmoral Mdel, P., Naranjo Gutierrez Mdel, C., Lardone, P. J., and de la Lastra Romero, C. A. (2009). Decreased MT1 and MT2 melatonin receptor expression in extrapineal tissues of the rat during physiological aging. *J. Pineal Res.* 46, 29–35. doi: 10.1111/j.1600-079X.2008.00604.x

Sartori, C., Dessen, P., Mathieu, C., Monney, A., Bloch, J., Nicod, P., et al. (2009). Melatonin improves glucose homeostasis and endothelial vascular function in high-fat diet-fed insulin-resistant mice. *Endocrinology* 150, 5311–5317. doi: 10.1210/en.2009-0425

Scheer, F. A., Van Montfrans, G. A., van Someren, E. J., Mairuhu, G., and Buijs, R. M. (2004). Daily nighttime melatonin reduces blood pressure in male patients with essential hypertension. *Hypertension* 43, 192–197. doi: 10.1161/01.HYP.0000113293.15186.3b

Scholtens, R. M., van Munster, B. C., van Kempen, M. F., and de Rooij, S. E. (2016). Physiological melatonin levels in healthy older people: a systematic review. *J. Psychosom. Res.* 86, 20–27. doi: 10.1016/j.jpsychores.2016.05.005

Sehirli, A. O., Koyun, D., Tetik, S., Ozsavci, D., Yiginer, O., Cetinel, S., et al. (2013). Melatonin protects against ischemic heart failure in rats. *J. Pineal Res.* 55, 138–148. doi: 10.1111/jpi.12054

Siegel, D., Black, D. M., Seeley, D. G., and Hulley, S. B. (1992). Circadian variation in ventricular arrhythmias in hypertensive men. *Am. J. Cardiol.* 69, 344–347. doi: 10.1016/0002-9149(92)90231-M

Simko, F., Baka, T., Paulis, L., and Reiter, R. J. (2016). Elevated heart rate and nondipping heart rate as potential targets for melatonin: a review. *J. Pineal Res.* 61, 127–137. doi: 10.1111/jpi.12348

Simko, F., Bednarova, K. R., Krajcirovicova, K., Hrenak, J., Celec, P., Kamodyova, N., et al. (2014a). Melatonin reduces cardiac remodeling and improves survival in rats with isoproterenol-induced heart failure. *J. Pineal Res.* 57, 177–184. doi: 10.1111/jpi.12154

Simko, F., Pechanova, O., Repova Bednarova, K., Krajcirovicova, K., Celec, P., Kamodyova, N., et al. (2014b). Hypertension and cardiovascular remodelling in rats exposed to continuous light: protection by ACE-inhibition and melatonin. *Mediators Inflamm.* 2014:703175. doi: 10.1155/2014/703175

Skiadas, P. K., and Lascaratos, J. G. (2001). Dietetics in ancient Greek philosophy: plato's concepts of healthy diet. *Eur. J. Clin. Nutr.* 55, 532–537. doi: 10.1038/sj.ejcn.1601179

Stefulj, J., Hortner, M., Ghosh, M., Schauenstein, K., Rinner, I., Wolfler, A., et al. (2001). Gene expression of the key enzymes of melatonin synthesis in extrapineal tissues of the rat. *J. Pineal Res.* 30, 243–247. doi: 10.1034/j.1600-079X.2001.300408.x

Stürtz, M., Cerezo, A. B., Cantos-Villar, E., and Garcia-Parrilla, M. C. (2011). Determination of the melatonin content of different varieties of tomatoes (Lycopersicon esculentum) and strawberries (*Fragaria ananassa*). *Food Chem.* 127, 1329–1334. doi: 10.1016/j.foodchem.2011.01.093

Sun, H., Gusdon, A. M., and Qu, S. (2016). Effects of melatonin on cardiovascular diseases: progress in the past year. *Curr. Opin. Lipidol.* 27, 408–413. doi: 10.1097/MOL.0000000000000314

Tain, Y. L., Huang, L. T., Lin, I. C., Lau, Y. T., and Lin, C. Y. (2010). Melatonin prevents hypertension and increased asymmetric dimethylarginine in young spontaneous hypertensive rats. *J. Pineal Res.* 49, 390–398. doi: 10.1111/j.1600-079X.2010.00806.x

Tan, D. X., Chen, L. D., Poeggeler, B., Manchester, L. C., and Reiter, R. J. (1993). Melatonin: a potent, endogenous hydroxyl radical scavenger. *Endocr. J.* 1, 57–60.

Tan, D., Manchester, L. C., Reiter, R. J., Qi, W., Kim, S. J., and El-Sokkary, G. H. (1998). Ischemia/reperfusion-induced arrhythmias in the isolated rat heart: prevention by melatonin. *J. Pineal Res.* 25, 184–191. doi: 10.1111/j.1600-079X.1998.tb00558.x

Tan, D. X., Hardeland, R., Back, K., Manchester, L. C., Alatorre-Jimenez, M. A., and Reiter, R. J. (2016). On the significance of an alternate pathway of melatonin synthesis via 5-methoxytryptamine: comparisons across species. *J. Pineal Res.* 61, 27–40. doi: 10.1111/jpi.12336

Tan, D. X., Hardeland, R., Manchester, L. C., Korkmaz, A., Ma, S., Rosales-Corral, S., et al. (2012). Functional roles of melatonin in plants, and perspectives in nutritional and agricultural science. *J. Exp. Bot.* 63, 577–597. doi: 10.1093/jxb/err256

Tan, D. X., Zanghi, B. M., Manchester, L. C., and Reiter, R. J. (2014). Melatonin identified in meats and other food stuffs: potentially nutritional impact. *J. Pineal Res.* 57, 213–218. doi: 10.1111/jpi.12152

Torres, F., Gonzalez-Candia, A., Montt, C., Ebensperger, G., Chubretovic, M., Seron-Ferre, M., et al. (2015). Melatonin reduces oxidative stress and improves vascular function in pulmonary hypertensive newborn sheep. *J. Pineal Res.* 58, 362–373. doi: 10.1111/jpi.12222

Trotti, L. M., and Karroum, E. G. (2016). Melatonin for sleep disorders in patients with neurodegenerative diseases. *Curr. Neurol. Neurosci. Rep.* 16:63. doi: 10.1007/s11910-016-0664-3

Vazan, R., and Ravingerova, T. (2015). Protective effect of melatonin against myocardial injury induced by epinephrine. *J. Physiol. Biochem.* 71, 43–49. doi: 10.1007/s13105-014-0377-5

Venegas, C., Garcia, J. A., Escames, G., Ortiz, F., Lopez, A., Doerrier, C., et al. (2012). Extrapineal melatonin: analysis of its subcellular distribution and daily fluctuations. *J. Pineal Res.* 52, 217–227. doi: 10.1111/j.1600-079X.2011.00931.x

Wang, Z., Ni, L., Wang, J., Lu, C., Ren, M., Han, W., et al. (2016). The protective effect of melatonin on smoke-induced vascular injury in rats and humans: a randomized controlled trial. *J. Pineal Res.* 60, 217–227. doi: 10.1111/jpi.12305

Wu, Y., Si, F., Luo, L., and Yi, Q. (2017). Serum levels of melatonin may contribute to the pathogenesis of heart failure in children with median age of 1 year. *J. Pediatr.* doi: 10.1016/j.jped.2017.06.023. [Epub ahead of print].

Yang, H., Young, D. W., Gusovsky, F., and Chow, J. C. (2000). Cellular events mediated by lipopolysaccharide-stimulated toll-like receptor 4. MD-2 is required for activation of mitogen-activated protein kinases and Elk-1. *J. Biol. Chem.* 275, 20861–20866. doi: 10.1074/jbc.M002896200

Yang, Y., Sun, Y., Yi, W., Li, Y., Fan, C., Xin, Z., et al. (2014). A review of melatonin as a suitable antioxidant against myocardial ischemia-reperfusion injury and clinical heart diseases. *J. Pineal Res.* 57, 357–366. doi: 10.1111/jpi.12175

Yeung, H. M., Hung, M. W., Lau, C. F., and Fung, M. L. (2015). Cardioprotective effects of melatonin against myocardial injuries induced by chronic intermittent hypoxia in rats. *J. Pineal Res.* 58, 12–25. doi: 10.1111/jpi.12190

Yu, L., Fan, C., Li, Z., Zhang, J., Xue, X., Xu, Y., et al. (2017a). Melatonin rescues cardiac thioredoxin system during ischemia-reperfusion injury in acute hyperglycemic state by restoring Notch1/Hes1/Akt signaling in a membrane receptor-dependent manner. *J. Pineal Res.* 62:e12375. doi: 10.1111/jpi.12375

Yu, L., Gong, B., Duan, W., Fan, C., Zhang, J., Li, Z., et al. (2017b). Melatonin ameliorates myocardial ischemia/reperfusion injury in type 1 diabetic rats by preserving mitochondrial function: role of AMPK-PGC-1alpha-SIRT3 signaling. *Sci. Rep.* 7:41337. doi: 10.1038/srep41337

Zetner, D., Andersen, L. P., and Rosenberg, J. (2016). Pharmacokinetics of alternative administration routes of melatonin: a systematic review. *Drug Res. (Stuttg)* 66, 169–173. doi: 10.1055/s-0035-1565083

Zhai, M., Li, B., Duan, W., Jing, L., Zhang, B., Zhang, M., et al. (2017a). Melatonin ameliorates myocardial ischemia reperfusion injury through SIRT3-dependent regulation of oxidative stress and apoptosis. *J. Pineal Res.* 63:e12419. doi: 10.1111/jpi.12419

Zhai, M., Liu, Z., Zhang, B., Jing, L., Li, B., Li, K., et al. (2017b). Melatonin protects against the pathological cardiac hypertrophy induced by transverse aortic constriction through activating PGC-1beta: *in vivo* and *in vitro* studies. *J. Pineal Res.* 63:3. doi: 10.1111/jpi.12433

Zhang, M., Lin, J., Wang, S., Cheng, Z., Hu, J., Wang, T., et al. (2017). Melatonin protects against diabetic cardiomyopathy through Mst1/Sirt3 signaling. *J. Pineal Res.* 63:e12418. doi: 10.1111/jpi.12418

Permissions

All chapters in this book were first published in RNSCSFPRD, by Frontiers; hereby published with permission under the Creative Commons Attribution License or equivalent. Every chapter published in this book has been scrutinized by our experts. Their significance has been extensively debated. The topics covered herein carry significant findings which will fuel the growth of the discipline. They may even be implemented as practical applications or may be referred to as a beginning point for another development.

The contributors of this book come from diverse backgrounds, making this book a truly international effort. This book will bring forth new frontiers with its revolutionizing research information and detailed analysis of the nascent developments around the world.

We would like to thank all the contributing authors for lending their expertise to make the book truly unique. They have played a crucial role in the development of this book. Without their invaluable contributions this book wouldn't have been possible. They have made vital efforts to compile up to date information on the varied aspects of this subject to make this book a valuable addition to the collection of many professionals and students.

This book was conceptualized with the vision of imparting up-to-date information and advanced data in this field. To ensure the same, a matchless editorial board was set up. Every individual on the board went through rigorous rounds of assessment to prove their worth. After which they invested a large part of their time researching and compiling the most relevant data for our readers.

The editorial board has been involved in producing this book since its inception. They have spent rigorous hours researching and exploring the diverse topics which have resulted in the successful publishing of this book. They have passed on their knowledge of decades through this book. To expedite this challenging task, the publisher supported the team at every step. A small team of assistant editors was also appointed to further simplify the editing procedure and attain best results for the readers.

Apart from the editorial board, the designing team has also invested a significant amount of their time in understanding the subject and creating the most relevant covers. They scrutinized every image to scout for the most suitable representation of the subject and create an appropriate cover for the book.

The publishing team has been an ardent support to the editorial, designing and production team. Their endless efforts to recruit the best for this project, has resulted in the accomplishment of this book. They are a veteran in the field of academics and their pool of knowledge is as vast as their experience in printing. Their expertise and guidance has proved useful at every step. Their uncompromising quality standards have made this book an exceptional effort. Their encouragement from time to time has been an inspiration for everyone.

The publisher and the editorial board hope that this book will prove to be a valuable piece of knowledge for researchers, students, practitioners and scholars across the globe.

List of Contributors

Ioanna Andreadou, Panagiotis Efentakis and Panagiota-Efstathia Nikolaou
Laboratory of Pharmacology, Faculty of Pharmacy, School of Health Sciences, National and Kapodistrian University of Athens, Athens, Greece

Evangelos Balafas and Nikolaos Kostomitsopoulos
Academy of Athens Biomedical Research Foundation, Centre of Clinical Experimental Surgery andTranslational Research, Athens, Greece

Gabriele Togliatto and Maria F. Brizzi
Department of Medical Sciences, University of Turin, Turin, Italy

Constantinos H. Davos, Aimilia Varela and Constantinos A. Dimitriou
Cardiovascular Research Laboratory, Biomedical Research Foundation, Academy of Athens, Athens, Greece

Eirini Maratou
Hellenic National Center for Research, Prevention and Treatment of Diabetes Mellitus and Its Complications, Athens, Greece

Vaia Lambadiari and George Dimitriadis
Department of Internal Medicine, Research Institute and Diabetes Center, National and Kapodistrian University of Athens, "Attikon"University Hospital, Athens, Greece

Ignatios Ikonomidis and Efstathios K. Iliodromitis
University Department of Cardiology, Medical School, National and Kapodistrian University of Athens, Athens, Greece

Isabella Russo, Cristina Barale and Stefano Geuna
Department of Clinical and Biological Sciences, AOU San Luigi, University of Turin, Turin, Italy
Saveria Femminò, Francesca Tullio, Pasquale Pagliaro and Claudia Penna
Department of Clinical and Biological Sciences, AOU San Luigi, University of Turin, Turin, Italy
Istituto Nazionale Ricerche Cardiovascolari (INRC), Bologna, Italy

Franco Cavalot
Internal Medicine and Metabolic Disease Unit, AOU San Luigi, University of Turin, Turin, Italy
Ospedale San Luigi Gonzaga, Orbassano, Italy

Kerstin Boengler, Klaus-Dieter Schlüter and Rainer Schulz
Physiologisches Institut, Justus-Liebig-Universität, Giessen, Germany

Judit Pipis
Pharmahungary Group, Szeged, Hungary
Péter Bencsik, János Palóczi, Krisztina Kiss, Márton Pipicz
Pharmahungary Group Szeged, Hungary
Cardiovascular Research Group, Department of Biochemistry, University of Szeged, Szeged, Hungary

Péter Ferdinandy
Pharmahungary Group, Szeged, Hungary
Cardiovascular Research Group, Department of Biochemistry, University of Szeged, Szeged, Hungary
Department of Pharmacology and Pharmacotherapy, Semmelweis University, Budapest, Hungary

Gabriele G. Schiattarella, Nicola Boccella, Roberta Paolillo, Stefania D'Apice, Giuseppe Giugliano, Giovanni Esposito and Cinzia Perrino
Department of Advanced Biomedical Sciences, University of Naples Federico II, Naples, Italy

Laura Rinaldi, Domenica Borzacchiello and Antonio Feliciello
Department of Molecular Medicine and Medical Biotechnologies, University of Naples Federico II, Naples, Italy

Valentina Trimarco
Department of Neuroscience, Reproductive Science and Odontostomatology, University of Naples Federico II, Naples, Italy

Anna Franzone
Department of Advanced Biomedical Sciences, University of Naples Federico II, Naples, Italy
Department of Cardiology, Inselspital, Universitätsspital Bern, Bern, Switzerland

Alessandra Gentile and Assunta Lombardi
Department of Biology, University of Naples Federico II, Naples, Italy

Fabio Cattaneo
Department of Advanced Biomedical Sciences, University of Naples Federico II, Naples, Italy
Department of Biology, University of Naples Federico II, Naples, Italy

Pasquale Pagliaro, Saveria Femminò, Jasmin Popara and Claudia Penna
Department of Clinical and Biological Sciences, University of Turin, Turin, Italy

Carlo G. Tocchetti, Paolo Parrella, Flora Pirozzi, Antonio Pecoraro and Valentina Mercurio
Department of Translational Medical Sciences, University of Naples Federico II, Naples, Italy

Gilda Varricchi
Department of Translational Medical Sciences, University of Naples Federico II, Naples, Italy
Department of Translational Medical Sciences, Center for Basic and Clinical Immunology Research, University of Naples Federico II, Naples, Italy

Pietro Ameri, Paolo Spallarossa
Clinic of Cardiovascular Diseases, IRCCS San Martino IST, Genova, Italy

Christian Cadeddu, Giuseppe Mercuro
Department of Medical Sciences and Public Health,University of Cagliari, Cagliari, Italy

Alessandra Ghigo
Department of Molecular Biotechnology and Health Sciences, Molecular Biotechnology Center, University of Turin, Turin, Italy

Rosalinda Madonna
Institute of Cardiology, Center of Excellence on Aging, Università degli Studi"G. d'Annunzio" Chieti - Pescara, Chieti, Italy
Department of Internal Medicine, Texas Heart Institute and Center for Cardiovascular Biology and Atherosclerosis Research, University of Texas Health Science Center, Houston, TX,United States

Giancarlo Marone
Section of Hygiene, Department of Public Health, University of Naples Federico II, Naples, Italy
Monaldi Hospital Pharmacy, Naples, Italy

Ines Monte
Department of General Surgery and Medical-Surgery Specialities, University of Catania,Catania, Italy

Giuseppina Novo
U.O.C. Magnetic Resonance Imaging, Fondazione Toscana G. Monasterio C.N.R., Pisa, Italy

Concetta Zito
Division of Clinical and Experimental Cardiology, Department of Medicine and Pharmacology, Policlinico "G. Martino" University of Messina, Messina, Italy

Giorgio Aquila
Department of Medical Sciences, University of Ferrara, Ferrara, Italy

Claudia Penna, Saveria Femminò and Pasquale Pagliaro
Department of Clinical and Biological Sciences, University of Torino, Torino, Italy

Matteo Sorge and Mara Brancaccio
Department of Molecular Biotechnologyand Health Sciences, University of Torino, Torino, Italy

Vieceli Dalla Sega and Francesca Fortini
Department of Medical Sciences, University of Ferrara, Ferrara, Italy
Maria Cecilia Hospital, GVM Care & Research, E.S.Health Science Foundation, Cotignola, Italy
Department of Morphology, Surgery and Experimental Medicine, University of Ferrara, Ferrara, Italy

Giorgio Aquila
Department of Medical Sciences, University of Ferrara, Ferrara, Italy
Maria Cecilia Hospital, GVM Care & Research, E.S.Health Science Foundation, Cotignola, Italy

Rita Pavasini,Simone Biscaglia, Davide Bernucci, Annamaria Del Franco and Elisabetta Tonet
Cardiovascular Institute, Azienda Ospedaliero-Universitaria di Ferrara, Cona, Italy

Paola Rizzo
Department of Morphology, Surgery and Experimental Medicine, University of Ferrara, Ferrara, Italy
Laboratory for Technologies of Advanced Therapies, University of Ferrara, Ferrara, Italy

Roberto Ferrari
Maria Cecilia Hospital, GVM Care & Research, E.S.Health Science Foundation, Cotignola, Italy
Department of Morphology, Surgery and Experimental Medicine, University of Ferrara, Ferrara, Italy
Cardiovascular Institute, Azienda Ospedaliero-Universitaria di Ferrara, Cona, Italy

Gianluca Campo
Department of Morphology, Surgery and Experimental Medicine, University of Ferrara, Ferrara, Italy
Cardiovascular Institute, Azienda Ospedaliero-Universitaria di Ferrara, Cona, Italy

Roberto Paternò
Dipartimento di Medicina Clinica e Chirurgia, Università degli Studi di Napoli Federico II, Naples, Italy

Jean-Marc Chillon
Mécanismes Physiopathologiques et Conséquences des Calcifications Cardiovasculaires (EA 7517), Faculty of Pharmacy, University of Picardie Jules Verne, Amiens, France
Direction de la Recherche Clinique et de l'Innovation, CHU Amiens Picardie, Amiens, France

Kelvin J. A. Davies
Leonard Davis School of Gerontology of the Ethel Percy Andrus Gerontology Center, University of Southern California, LosAngeles, CA, United States
Molecular and Computational Biology Program, Department of Biological Sciences, Dornsife College of Letters, Arts, and Sciences, University of Southern California, Los Angeles, CA, United States
Department of Biochemistry and Molecular Medicine, USC Keck School of Medicine, University of Southern California, Los Angeles, CA, United States

Gábor Koncsos and Gábor J. Brenner
Cardiometabolic Research Group, Department of Pharmacology and Pharmacotherapy, Semmelweis University, Budapest, Hungary

Tamás Baranyai and Pál Pacher
Laboratory of Cardiovascular Physiology and Tissue Injury, National Institute on Alcohol Abuse and Alcoholism,National Institutes of Health, Bethesda, MD, United States

Zoltán V. Varga
Cardiometabolic Research Group, Department of Pharmacology and Pharmacotherapy, Semmelweis University, Budapest, Hungary
Laboratory of Cardiovascular Physiology and Tissue Injury, National Institute on Alcohol Abuse and Alcoholism, National Institutes of Health, Bethesda, MD, United States

Márton Pipicz, Júlia A. Baán and Tamás Csont
Department of Biochemistry, Faculty of Medicine, University of Szeged, Szeged, Hungary

Przemyslaw Leszek
Department of Heart Failure and Transplantology, Cardinal Stefan Wyszyn´ ski Institute of Cardiology, Warszawa, Poland

Mariusz Kuśmierczyk
Department of Cardiac Surgery and Transplantology, Cardinal Stefan Wyszyn´ ski Institute of Cardiology, Warszawa, Poland

Fátima Sánchez-Cabo
Bioinformatics Unit, Centro Nacional de Investigaciones Cardioavsculares Carlos III, Madrid, Spain

Pablo García-Pavía
Heart Failure and Inherited Cardiac Diseases Unit, Department of Cardiology, Hospital Universitario Puerta de Hierro Majadahonda, Madrid, Spain

Zoltán Giricz
Cardiometabolic Research Group, Department of Pharmacology and Pharmacotherapy, Semmelweis University, Budapest, Hungary
Pharmahungary Group, Szeged, Hungary

Luca Mendler
Department of Biochemistry, Faculty of Medicine, University of Szeged, Szeged, Hungary
Faculty of Medicine, Institute of Biochemistry II, Goethe University, Frankfurt, Germany

Enrique Lara-Pezzi
Centro de Investigaciones Cardiovasculares Carlos III, Madrid, Spain

Péter Ferdinandy
Cardiometabolic Research Group, Department of Pharmacology and Pharmacotherapy, Semmelweis University, Budapest, Hungary
Department of Biochemistry, Faculty of Medicine, University of Szeged, Szeged, Hungary
Pharmahungary Group, Szeged, Hungary

Gennaro Riccio
Department of Pharmacy, Federico II University, Naples, Italy

Salvatore Antonucci, Fabio Di Lisa and Carlo G.
Department of Biomedical Sciences and CNR Institute of Neuroscience, University of Padova, Padova, Italy

Carmela Coppola, Giovanna Piscopo and Carlo Maurea Nicola Maurea
Division of Cardiology, National Cancer Institute, G. Pascale Foundation, Naples, Italy

Chiara D'Avino and Claudia De Lorenzo
Department of Molecular Medicine and Medical Biotechnology, Federico II University, Naples, Italy
CEINGE Biotecnologie Avanzate, Naples, Italy

Danilo Fiore and Gerolama Condorelli
Department of Molecular Medicine and Medical Biotechnology, Federico II University, Naples, Italy

Michele Russo and Tocchetti
Department of Translational Medical Sciences, Federico II University, Naples, Italy

Domenica Rea and Claudio Arra
Department of Animal Experimental Research, National Cancer Institute, G. Pascale Foundation, Naples, Italy

Antonietta Messina, Vincenzo Monda and Marcellino Monde
Department of Experimental Medicine, Section of Human Physiology and Unit of Dietetics and Sports Medicine, Università degli Studi della Campania "Luigi Vanvitelli," Naples, Italy

Francesco Sessa, Anna Valenzano,Monica Salerno, Giuseppe Cibelli and Giovanni Messina
Department of Clinical and Experimental Medicine, University of Foggia, Foggia, Italy

Ilaria Bitetti, Francesco Precenzano, Roberta I. Ferrentino and Marco Carotenuto
Clinic of Child and Adolescent Neuropsychiatry, Department of Mental Health, Physical and Preventive Medicine, Università degli Studi della Campania "Luigi Vanvitelli," Naples, Italy

Rosa Marotta, Francesco Lavano and Serena M. Lavano,
Department of Health Sciences, University"Magna Graecia," Catanzaro, Italy

Margherita Salerno, Agata Maltese, Michele Roccella, Lucia Parisi
Child Neuropsychiatry, Department of Psychology and Pedagogical Sciences, University of Palermo, Palermo, Italy

Gabriele Tripi
Childhood Psychiatric Service for Neuro developmentals Disorders, Chinon, France

Beatrice Gallai
Department of Surgical and Biomedical Sciences, University of Perugia, Perugia, Italy

Nydegger, Ludwig von Segesser, Piergiorgio Tozzi and Giuseppina Milano
Laboratory of Cardiovascular Research, Department of Surgery and Anesthesiology, University Hospital of Lausanne, Lausanne, Switzerland

Carla Martinelli and Michele Samaja
Department of Health Science, University of Milan, Milan, Italy

Fabiano Di Marco and Gaetano Bulfamante
Department of Health Science, University of Milan, Milan, Italy
ASST Santi Paolo e Carlo, Milan, Italy

Daniela Sorriento, Nicola De Luca and Bruno Trimarco
Dipartimento di Scienze Biomediche Avanzate, Università Federico II, Napoli, Italy

Guido Iaccarino
Dipartimento di Medicina, Chirurgia e Odontoiatria, Università degli Studi di Salerno, Baronissi, Italy

Teresa Mastantuono, Martina Di Maro, Martina Chiurazzi, Laura Battiloro, Espedita Muscariello, Gilda Nasti, Antonio Colantuoni and Dominga Lapi
Department of Clinical Medicine and Surgery, "Federico II" University Medical School, Naples, Italy

Noemy Starita
Molecular Biology and Viral Oncology Unit, Istituto Nazionale Tumori IRCCS - "Fond. G. Pascale", Naples, Italy

Massimo Venturelli, Stefano Tamburin and Federico Schena
Department of Neurosciences, Biomedicine and Movement Sciences, University of Verona, Verona, Italy

Anna Pedrinolla
Department of Medicine, University of Verona, Verona, Italy

Ilaria Boscolo Galazzo
Department of Computer Science, University of Verona, Verona, Italy

Cristina Fonte and Nicola Smania
Department of Neurosciences, Biomedicine and Movement Sciences, University of Verona, Verona, Italy
Neuromotor and Cognitive Rehabilitation Research Centre, University of Verona, Verona, Italy

Ettore Muti
Mons. Mazzali Foundation, Mantua, Italy

Lucia Crispoltoni, Annamaria Stabile, Alessandra Pistilli and Mario Rende
Department of Surgical and Biomedical Sciences, Section of Human Anatomy, School of Medicine, University of Perugia, Perugia, Italy

Francesca B. Pizzini
Neuroradiology, Department of Diagnostics and Pathology, Verona University Hospital, Verona, Italy

Carmine Rocc and Teresa Pasqua
Laboratory of Molecular and Cellular Cardiac Physiology, Department of Biology, Ecology and E.S., University of Calabria, Rende, Italy

Saveria Femminò
Department of Biological and Clinical Sciences, University of Turin, Turin, Italy

Ernestina M. De Francesco, Damiano C. Rigiracciolo and Marcello Maggiolini
Department of Pharmacy, Health and Nutritional Sciences, University of Calabria, Rende, Italy

Francesca Fortini
Department of Medical Sciences, University of Ferrara, Ferrara, Italy
Maria Cecilia Hospital, GVM Care & Research, E.S. Health Science Foundation, Cotignola, Italy

Maria C. Cerra and Tommaso Angelone
Laboratory of Molecular and Cellular Cardiac Physiology, Department of Biology, Ecology and E.S., University of Calabria, Rende, Italy
National Institute for Cardiovascular Research, Bologna, Italy

Pasquale Pagliaro and Claudia Penna
Department of Biological and Clinical Sciences, University of Turin, Turin, Italy
National Institute for Cardiovascular Research, Bologna, Italy

Paola Rizzo
Department of Morphology, Surgery and Experimental Medicine, University of Ferrara, Ferrara, Italy
Laboratory for Technologies of Advanced Therapies, University of Ferrara,Ferrara, Italy

Giulia Querio, Susanna Antoniotti, Cinzia M. Bertea, Maria P. Gallo and Renzo Levi
Department of Life Sciences and Systems Biology, University of Turin, Turin, Italy

Roberto Canaparo and Federica Foglietta
Department of Drug Science and Technology, University of Turin, Turin, Italy

Martino Deidda, Antonio Noto, Pier P. Bassareo, Christian Cadeddu Dessalvi and Giuseppe Mercuro
Department of Medical Sciences and Public Health, University of Cagliari, Sardinia, Italy

Davide Firinu, Maria P. Barca and Stefano Del Giacco
Unit of Internal Medicine, Department of Medical Sciences and Public Health, Allergy and Clinical Immunology, University of Cagliari, Cagliari, Italy

Giuseppe Mercuro and Pier P. Bassareo, Angela M. Zedda
Unit of Cardiology and Angiology, Department of Medical Sciences and Public Health, University of Cagliari, Cagliari, Italy

Antonio Crisafulli
Sports Physiology Lab., Department of Medical Sciences and Public Health, University of Cagliari, Cagliari, Italy

Zukiswa Jiki, Sandrine Lecour and Frederic Nduhirbbandi
Cardioprotection Group, Hatter Institute for Cardiovascular Research in Africa, Department of Medicine, Faculty of Health Sciences, University of Cape Town, Cape Town

Index

O

P

R

S

T

V

www.ingramcontent.com/pod-product-compliance
Lightning Source LLC
LaVergne TN
LVHW080926210926
848485LV00004B/737